ANTE BILIĆ D.M.D.
41000 ZAGREB — NAZOROVA 2
Telefon: (041) 437-012
YUGOSLAVIA

VIRULENCE MECHANISMS OF BACTERIAL PATHOGENS

VIRULENCE MECHANISMS OF BACTERIAL PATHOGENS

JAMES A. ROTH
Editor

Department of Veterinary Microbiology and Preventive Medicine
College of Veterinary Medicine
Iowa State University
Ames, Iowa

American Society for Microbiology
Washington, D.C.

Library of Congress Cataloging-in-Publication Data

Virulence mechanisms of bacterial pathogens / James A. Roth, editor.
    p. cm.
  Based on a conference held at the Iowa State University, Ames, Iowa, June 1987.
  Includes index.
    1. Virulence (Microbiology)—Congresses.   2. Bacteria, Pathogenic—Congresses.
I. Roth, James A.
    [DNLM: 1. Bacteria—pathogenicity—congresses. 2. Virulence—congresses.
QW 730 V821 1987]
QR175.V57 1988
616'.014—dc19

ISBN 0-914826-99-9

Cover: Microcolony of *Bordetella avium* among the cilia of a tracheal epithelial cell
  from a young turkey. (Provided by L. H. Arp.)

CONTENTS

V. STRATEGIES TO OVERCOME BACTERIAL
VIRULENCE MECHANISMS

VI. PAST, PRESENT, AND FUTURE STUDIES

ORGANIZING COMMITTEE

JAMES A. ROTH (Chair)

Department of Veterinary Microbiology, Iowa State University, Ames, IA 50011

LAWRENCE H. ARP

Department of Veterinary Pathology, College of Veterinary Medicine, Iowa State University, Ames, IA 50011

LYNETTE B. CORBEIL

University of California-San Diego Medical Center, San Diego, CA 92103

CHARLES J. CZUPRYNSKI

Department of Pathobiological Sciences, School of Veterinary Medicine, University of Wisconsin, Madison, WI 53706

THEODORE T. KRAMER

Department of Veterinary Microbiology, Iowa State University, Ames, IA 50011

HARLEY W. MOON

Department of Bacteriology, National Animal Disease Center, U.S. Department of Agriculture, Agricultural Research Service, Ames, IA 50010

ROBERT NERVIG

U.S. Department of Agriculture, National Veterinary Services Laboratory, Ames, IA 50010

CHARLES PILET

Animal and Comparative Immunology Institute, Ecole Veterinaire d'Alfort, 94704 Maisons-Alfort, France

RICHARD F. ROSS

Veterinary Medical Research Institute, Iowa State University, Ames, IA 50011

PATRICIA E. SHEWEN

Department of Veterinary Microbiology and Immunology, University of Guelph, Guelph, Ontario, Canada N1G 2W1

LEN R. STEPHENS

Regional Veterinary Laboratory, Bairnsdale, Victoria 3875, Australia

WILLIAM P. SWITZER

College of Veterinary Medicine, Iowa State University, Ames, IA 50011

ALEX WINTER

Veterinary Microbiology, New York State College of Veterinary Medicine, Cornell University, Ithaca, NY 14853

AUTHORS

LAWRENCE H. ARP
  Department of Veterinary Pathology, College of Veterinary Medicine, Iowa State University, Ames, IA 50011

H. CHART
  Division of Enteric Pathogens, Public Health Laboratory Service, Central Public Health Laboratory, London NW9 5EQ, England

FRANK M. COLLINS
  Trudeau Institute, Inc., Saranac Lake, NY 12983

LYNETTE B. CORBEIL
  Department of Pathology, University of California-San Diego Medical Center, San Diego, CA 92103

ROY CURTISS III
  Department of Biology, Washington University, St. Louis, MO 63130

CHARLES J. CZUPRYNSKI
  Department of Pathobiological Sciences, School of Veterinary Medicine, University of Wisconsin, Madison, WI 53706

CLAUDIO DENZLINGER
  Biochemisches Institut, Universität Freiburg, D-7800 Freiburg, Federal Republic of Germany

DAVID L. EMERY
  Commonwealth Scientific and Industrial Research Organisation, Division of Animal Health, Animal Health Research Laboratory, Parkville 3052, Victoria, Australia

SAMUEL B. FORMAL
  Department of Enteric Infections, Walter Reed Army Institute of Research, Washington, DC 20307-5100

JOHN H. FREER
  Department of Microbiology, University of Glasgow, Glasgow G11 6NU, Scotland

ROLF FRETER
  Department of Microbiology and Immunology, The University of Michigan, Ann Arbor, MI 48109

JORGE E. GALÁN
  Department of Biology, Washington University, St. Louis, MO 63130

CLAUDIA R. GENTRY-WEEKS
  Department of Biology, Washington University, St. Louis, MO 63130

JOCHEN R. GOLECKI
  Institut Biologie II, Mikrobiologie, Universität Freiburg, D-7800 Freiburg, Federal Republic of Germany

MAYER B. GOREN
  Department of Molecular and Cellular Biology, National Jewish Center for Immunology and Respiratory Medicine, Denver, CO 80206

E. GRIFFITHS
  National Institute for Biological Standards and Control, Potters Bar, Hertfordshire EN6 3QG, England
PAUL A. GULIG
  Department of Biology, Washington University, St. Louis, MO 63130
CARLTON L. GYLES
  Department of Microbiology, Ontario Veterinary College, University of Guelph, Guelph, Ontario, Canada N1G 2W1
THOMAS LARRY HALE
  Department of Enteric Infections, Walter Reed Army Institute of Research, Washington, DC 20307-5100
DIETRICH K. HAMMER
  Max-Planck-Institut für Immunbiologie, D-7800 Freiburg, Federal Republic of Germany
KELTON P. HEPPER
  Marion Laboratories, Inc., Kansas City, MO 64134
RICHARD E. ISAACSON
  Department of Immunology and Infectious Diseases, Central Research Division, Pfizer, Incorporated, Groton, CT 06340
SANDRA M. KELLY
  Department of Biology, Washington University, St. Louis, MO 63130
DIETRICH KEPPLER
  Biochemisches Institut, Universität Freiburg, D-7800 Freiburg, Federal Republic of Germany
NATAN MOR
  Department of Molecular and Cellular Biology, National Jewish Center for Immunology and Respiratory Medicine, Denver, CO 80206
DONALD C. ROBERTSON
  Department of Microbiology, University of Kansas, Lawrence, KS 66045
JAMES A. ROTH
  Department of Veterinary Microbiology and Preventive Medicine, Iowa State University, Ames, IA 50011
J. M. RUTTER
  Agricultural and Food Research Council, Institute for Animal Disease Research, Compton Laboratory, Compton, Berkshire RG16 0NN, England
BARBARA SAILER-KRAMER
  Max-Planck-Institut für Immunbiologie, D-7800 Freiburg, Federal Republic of Germany
PETER H. SCHEUBER
  Max-Planck-Institut für Immunbiologie, D-7800 Freiburg, Federal Republic of Germany
K. L. SCHNORR
  Department of Veterinary Microbiology and Parasitology, School of Veterinary Medicine, Louisiana State University, Baton Rouge, LA 70803
PATRICIA E. SHEWEN
  Department of Veterinary Microbiology and Immunology, University of Guelph, Guelph, Ontario, Canada N1G 2W1

H. SMITH
  Department of Microbiology, University of Birmingham, Birmingham B15 2TT, United Kingdom

P. STEVENSON
  National Institute for Biological Standards and Control, Potters Bar, Hertfordshire EN6 3QG, England

J. STORZ
  Department of Veterinary Microbiology and Parasitology, School of Veterinary Medicine, Louisiana State University, Baton Rouge, LA 70803

PETER W. TAYLOR
  CIBA-GEIGY Pharmaceuticals, Horsham, West Sussex RH12 4AB, United Kingdom

W. J. TODD
  Department of Veterinary Microbiology and Parasitology, School of Veterinary Medicine, Louisiana State University, Baton Rouge, LA 70803

PHILLIP R. WIDDERS
  Department of Veterinary Microbiology and Pathology, Washington State University, Pullman, WA 99164-7040

DIETMAR WILKER
  Chirurgische Klinik Innenstadt der Universität München, D-8000 Munich, Federal Republic of Germany

JOHN B. WOOLCOCK
  Department of Veterinary Pathology and Public Health, University of Queensland, St. Lucia, Queensland 4067, Australia

PREFACE

Generation of new ideas and refinement or extension of established concepts are the essence of advances in knowledge. The former occurs infrequently, requires broad vision, and has the potential to open up new vistas for examination. The role of bacterial toxins in disease, recognized in the late 19th century, is an example of such a novel idea. The critical role of bacterial adherence to mucosal surfaces is a more recent example of a new concept in pathogenesis which has had a significant impact on our understanding of disease processes due to bacteria. Another broadly based mechanism of disease is the possession by pathogens of systems which enable them to compete with animal hosts for scarce substrates such as iron. Also, host factors, particularly cell-mediated immunity and immunity at mucosal surfaces, have increasingly been recognized to be critical in the outcome of bacterial disease.

Once formulated, new principles in bacterial pathogenesis tend to generate an aura of excitement and an intense search for answers to new questions. Scientists are driven to establish how widely applicable the concept is, to determine variations on the theme that undoubtedly exist in nature, to purify and characterize the bacterial components involved, to identify the host factors implicated, to understand the genetic regulation of both bacterial and host factors, and to fill in missing details. Pursuit of these questions often leads to discoveries which, by themselves or taken with other information, form the basis of new concepts.

Traditionally, the study of bacterial virulence mechanisms has been dominated by individuals trained as bacteriologists or immunologists and with a medical or veterinary background. In recent years there has been a dramatic shift in the investigation of bacterial virulence. We now want to understand things at the molecular level and have the capacity to do this. It is no longer good enough merely to identify the gross and microscopic lesions in tissues. We need to know the biochemical lesion and to identify the specific host reactions that are impaired. Furthermore, we have come to realize that the powerful new tools of molecular genetics can be of immense assistance as we try to understand how bacteria cause disease. Transposon mutagenesis, recombinant DNA technology, gene cloning and sequencing, understanding the substrate and temperature conditions which regulate genes involved in virulence, and synthesizing DNA of interest and peptides of value are now common methods and approaches in the quest for understanding disease processes. The possibility of a new generation of vaccines and pharmaceutical agents has spurred on research on pathogenesis: if we understand how the bacterium causes disease and how the host responds to infection, our chances of selecting the best strategies for prevention and therapy are enhanced.

Given the new emphasis, it is not surprising that the field of pathogenesis in general and of virulence mechanisms in particular has been invaded by basic scientists, especially molecular biologists, and has been enriched by their presence. This development represents a challenge for the rest of us to bring the sophistication and precision of the basic scientists to bear on our own studies and to work with these colleagues, because our combined skills can provide new insights.

Despite the unquestionable value of research at the molecular level, we need to ensure that deficits in information in areas beyond the interaction of host and pathogen at the molecular level are not ignored. To understand pathogenesis, we need to be fully informed about the habitat of the bacterium and the circumstances under which infection occurs. The biological context must not be lost amidst the glamor of the new technologies.

If we look continually at the same object under the same conditions, we lose the prospect of seeing anything new: our vision is framed by our limited experience and by our notion of what we expect to see. This book provides a unique opportunity for recognizing new perspectives on virulence mechanisms in bacterial diseases. Mechanisms of bacterial virulence do not respect the boundaries erected between humans and other animal species, and this volume brings together outstanding researchers who have looked at bacterial virulence from different vantage points and the experiences of a variety of disciplines: medicine, veterinary medicine, genetics, biochemistry, immunology, and microbiology. Although there are opportunities for examination of details, the big picture is still the overall theme: there can be no consideration of bacterial virulence without reference to the interaction of pathogen and host.

CARLTON L. GYLES
University of Guelph
Guelph, Ontario, Canada

ACKNOWLEDGMENTS

This volume resulted from the International Symposium on Virulence Mechanisms of Veterinary Bacterial Pathogens held in Ames, Iowa, 2 to 5 June 1987. The symposium was sponsored by the following organizations:

American Association of Veterinary Immunologists
World Association of Veterinary Immunologists, Microbiologists, and Specialists in Infectious Diseases
National Animal Disease Center (United States)
National Veterinary Services Laboratory (United States)
College of Veterinary Medicine, Iowa State University

The Organizing Committee thanks the following for their generous financial support of the symposium:

Supporters

Faculty Development Committee of the Iowa State University Biotechnology Council, Ames
National Animal Disease Center, Ames, Iowa
CIBA-GEIGY Limited, Basel, Switzerland
Norden Laboratories, Inc., Lincoln, Nebraska
Pfizer Central Research, Animal Health Research, Terre Haute, Indiana
Rhone Merieux, Lyon, France

Contributors

Bayer, Bayerwerk, Federal Republic of Germany
Beecham Laboratories, White Hall, Illinois
Boehringer Ingelheim Animal Health, Inc., St. Joseph, Missouri
Connaught Laboratories, Inc., Swiftwater, Pennsylvania
Diamond Scientific, Des Moines, Iowa
Eli Lilly and Company, Indianapolis, Indiana
Fort Dodge Laboratories, Fort Dodge, Iowa
Hoechst-Roussel Agri-Vet Company, Somerville, New Jersey
Intervet America Inc., Millsboro, Delaware
Mobay Corporation, Animal Health Division, Shawnee Mission, Kansas
Salsbury Laboratories, Inc., Charles City, Iowa
The Upjohn Company, Kalamazoo, Michigan

Section I: Mechanisms of Bacterial Adherence, Colonization, and Invasion

Bacterial Infection of Mucosal Surfaces: an Overview of Cellular and Molecular Mechanisms

LAWRENCE H. ARP

Department of Veterinary Pathology
College of Veterinary Medicine
Iowa State University
Ames, Iowa 50011

INTRODUCTION

Bacterial colonization of a mucosal surface requires that bacteria (i) establish close proximity to the mucosa, (ii) avoid being swept away, (iii) acquire essential nutrients for growth, (iv) replicate at a rate sufficient to maintain or expand their population, and (v) resist local host defenses. Mechanisms by which bacteria maintain close proximity to a mucosal surface can be loosely categorized as association, adhesion, and invasion according to the degree of intimacy between bacterial and mucosal surfaces. Association, the least intimate form of surface interaction, implies weak, reversible attachment or localization of bacteria along a surface (Fig. 1). Adhesion, a more intimate form of attachment than association, describes relatively stable, irreversible attachment mediated by specialized complementary molecules of the bacterial and mucosal surfaces. The most intimate form of bacterial-mucosal interaction is invasion, wherein pathogenic bacteria penetrate the mucosal barrier to establish themselves within epithelial cells or adjacent stromal

tissue. The purpose of this chapter is to review many of the cellular and molecular mechanisms of bacterial association, adhesion, and invasion within the context of mucosal colonization. Because many mechanisms are common to animal and human disease, an attempt is made to integrate some of the medical and veterinary literature that has contributed to our current understanding of bacterial infections of mucosal surfaces. The overview of bacterial colonization is followed by a discussion of virulence mechanisms of selected bacterial pathogens of the respiratory tract, ocular tissues, and skin.

COLONIZATION

Studies of bacterial adhesion and colonization were originated by marine and soil microbiologists in the 1930s and 1940s (86, 87). Early microbiologists used glass slides submerged in water or soil to collect and study adherent bacterial colonies (86). In 1940 Heukelekian and Heller found that nutrients, having a tendency to adsorb to and concentrate on

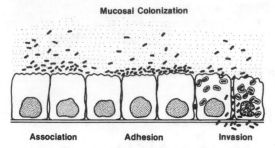

Mucosal Colonization

Association   Adhesion   Invasion

FIGURE 1. Types of bacterial-mucosal interaction involved in bacterial infection of mucosal surfaces.

surfaces, provided a fertile habitat for colonial growth of bacteria capable of attaching to the surface (87).

Although bacterial attachment to erythrocytes was reported by Guyot in 1908 (80), there were few systematic studies of bacterial attachment and colonization of mucosal surfaces in animals until the early 1970s. Pioneering studies of diarrheas (108, 155, 191), dental caries (73, 74), and gonorrhea (130, 201) caused by bacteria sparked widespread recognition of bacterial attachment as a critically important initial event in bacterial infection of mucosal surfaces (168). In the past decade, powerful new techniques in molecular biology have contributed to an information explosion concerning mechanisms of infection. Investigations of bacterial colonization have progressed from descriptions of diseases and their corresponding lesions to characterization of bacterial virulence mechanisms at the molecular and genetic level. Progress in understanding mechanisms of bacterial diarrheas in livestock species has provided an important background for continuing research of diarrheal disease and urinary tract infections of human patients (111, 169). In contrast, our understanding of bacterial infections of other mucosal surfaces of animals has generally lagged far behind comparable research in humans.

Colonization is the formation of a stable population of bacteria in a suitable habitat. Colonization requires sufficient multiplication of the localized bacterial population to replace bacteria lost to senescence, dispersion, and local bactericidal mechanisms. The fundamental mechanisms of bacterial colonization are similar regardless of whether the surface being colonized represents living tissues of plants and animals, rocks in a stream, heat exchanger pipes, hulls of ships, or culture plates (126). As stated by Costerton et al. (37), "the basic bacterial strategy is, clearly, to live within protected adherent microcolonies in nutritionally favorable environments and to dispatch mobile swarmer cells to reconnoiter neighboring niches and to establish new adherent microcolonies in the most favorable of them." Only a very limited number of bacterial species have the capacity to colonize mucosal surfaces, and of these even fewer establish a parasitic relationship with the host. Actually, one of the most important antibacterial defense mechanisms of mucosal surfaces is competition by indigenous microorganisms for receptors, space, and substrates (69, 172).

The fate of bacteria on mucosal surfaces is determined by the capacity of the bacteria to exploit the available habitat and by the adequacy of host antimicrobial mechanisms. The gene pool of the bacterial chromosome and plasmids determines the surface molecules available for interaction with host tissues, the enzyme systems available for substrate utilization, and the bacterial products released. Potential bacterial pathogens are exposed to constant selective pressure of nonspecific and immune-mediated host defenses, competition with indigenous organisms, and antimicrobial products (antibiotics and bacteriocins) of exogenous and endogenous origin.

As a critically important first step in mucosal infection, bacteria must establish and maintain their position in close proximity with the mucosal surface. The tracheal and small-intestinal mucosal linings are examples of surfaces subjected to substantial physical shear forces that sweep away all particles and bacteria lacking specific adhesive mechanisms. Bacteria colonizing the ciliated respiratory tract, oral cavity, small intestine, urethra, and cornea usually have specific adhesive surface molecules that bind with host cell receptors to initiate relatively irreversible attachment leading to colonization

(Fig. 2). In contrast, the large intestine, ruminant forestomachs, vagina, uterus, and skin represent epithelial surfaces which lack highly efficient physical clearing mechanisms. Therefore, bacterial pathogens colonizing these tissues may rely less on specific adhesion and more on the weak, reversible interaction termed association (Fig. 1). Such bacteria may maintain association with the mucosal surface by binding to mucus or by chemotaxis.

Although mechanisms of colonization are emphasized below, it must be remembered that bacterial virulence usually requires multiple factors. For example, production of both enterotoxin and colonizing factors is required for pathogenicity of enterotoxigenic strains of *Escherichia coli*. Loss of a single gene product may prevent an otherwise virulent organism from colonizing its usual mucosal habitat. However, many bacterial pathogens have multiple fail-safe mechanisms to help ensure at least some level of colonization. Some strains of enterotoxigenic *E. coli*, *Pseudomonas aeruginosa*, and *Bordetella pertussis* produce several different surface-adhesive molecules which bind the bacteria to the host epithelium. The loss of one colonization factor may only reduce adhesive efficiency. Since many virulence factors are en-

coded by plasmid DNA, these bacteria have a grand repertoire of potential virulence factors available to ensure successful colonization. Our challenge is to characterize molecular mechanisms of colonization, devise strategies to disrupt colonization by pathogens, and yet cause minimal perturbation of the indigenous microflora and host tissue.

ASSOCIATION

Association is a nonspecific term for the localization of bacteria on a surface; it does not specify the mechanisms involved (133). The term is used in this chapter to describe the loose, reversible attachment or localization of bacteria in close proximity with a mucosal surface. Association may precede specific adhesion or invasion (Fig. 1). Bacteria may maintain their position along a mucosal surface by associating with mucus or exudates, by establishing small numbers of noncovalent bonds between the bacterial and mucosal surfaces, or by chemotaxis.

Chemotaxis is a significant virulence mechanism of bacterial pathogens of mucosal surfaces. Studies with *Vibrio cholerae* and *Sal-*

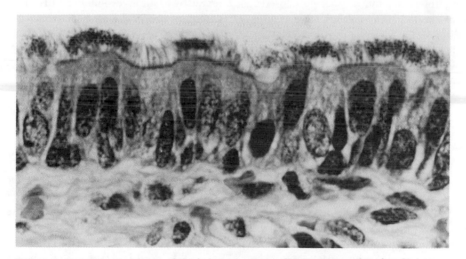

FIGURE 2. Bacterial colonization of the bronchial mucosa. Dense colonies of *B. bronchiseptica* are intimately attached to the cilia of bronchial epithelial cells in a young dog with kennel cough. The disease shares several similarities with whooping cough of humans.

monella typhimurium have shown that bacterial association with the intestinal mucosa is influenced by chemotactic stimuli (1, 68, 70). To be relevant in vivo, the chemotactic mechanism requires that the bacteria express flagella and the necessary array of taxin receptors. Chemotaxis enables bacteria to exploit mucosal regions of optimal substrate availability and also to penetrate the mucous blanket to enhance contact with receptors on the epithelial surface (67).

Motility may enhance the association of bacteria with mucosal surfaces by mechanisms other than chemotaxis. Dispatching of motile swarmer cells from established bacterial microcolonies (37) allows colonization of mucosal surfaces to progress in the opposite direction to physical clearance mechanisms. Despite a mucociliary clearance rate of 30 cm/min in tracheas of normal turkeys (63), motile *Bordetella avium* sp. nov. (109) bacteria progressively spread from the upper to the lower trachea within a few days (9). Lee et al. have recently demonstrated that there is significant antigenic cross-reactivity between flagellar proteins of gastrointestinal *Campylobacter* spp. that are pathogenic for humans and of gram-negative spiral bacteria that colonize the intestinal mucosa of rodents (120). It may be that bacteria colonizing intestinal mucus share a conserved portion of the flagellin molecule that is functionally important for colonization of the mucous layer (120). Additionally, flagella of *V. cholerae* may function as adhesins (13).

ADHESION

The term adhesion is used to describe the relatively stable, irreversible attachment of bacteria to a surface (107). Specific adhesion requires the interaction of specialized complementary molecules in a ligand-receptor fashion between surfaces of bacteria and substratum. This interaction typically occurs between bacterial surface proteins and carbohydrate-containing molecules of the eucaryotic cell membrane or glycocalyx (117). The term adherence

is often used synonymously with adhesion (16); however, some authors argue that adhesion is the preferable term for such bacterial attachment phenomena (133). The process whereby bacterial cells become collected in intimate contact, as in the formation of microcolonies, is aggregation (133). An adhesin is any bacterial structure or molecule that mediates adhesion, and adhesins which agglutinate erythrocytes are also hemagglutinins (96). Hemagglutinins behave as multivalent molecules which attach to and cause agglutination of erythrocytes. Receptors are components of the mucosal surface which bind in a complementary fashion with the active site of the corresponding adhesin during specific bacterial adhesion. When purified adhesins are shown to have hemagglutinating activity, it is likely that cell membranes of the host target cell and erythrocyte share a similar or identical receptor molecule.

Physicochemistry of Adhesion

Electrostatic charge and hydrophobicity are general characteristics of cell surfaces that profoundly affect adhesion. Glycoproteins, anchored by regions of hydrophobic amino acids, and glycolipids, anchored in the cell membrane by their hydrophobic tails, represent a variety of charged molecules which contribute to the cell glycocalyx (23, 35, 149). As the outermost layer of the bacterial surface, the glycocalyx is important in formation of microcolonies, resistance to host defenses, acquisition of nutrients, and concentration and conservation of bacterial enzymes. The glycocalyx of an epithelial cell is closely associated with the mucous layer and contributes to the negative surface charge of the cell (213). Being composed mainly of hydrated polysaccharide components of membrane glycoconjugates, the glycocalyx also provides many complex surface molecules that function in chemotaxis and adhesion (35).

Early studies of bacterial adhesion indicated that irreversible attachment was preceded by a weak, reversible phase (association) (134,

218). The initial, reversible phase of attachment may be the result of the combined effects of van der Waals forces, hydrogen bonds, and ionic and hydrophobic interactions (105). In contrast, specific irreversible adhesion probably requires more numerous noncovalent bonds concentrated between complementary macromolecules of the adjacent surfaces.

A possible physicochemical explanation for net adhesive interaction between two negatively charged surfaces is provided by the Derjaguin-Landau and Verwey-Overbeek (DLVO) theory (105, 107, 211). This theory of the physical interaction between colloid particles states that as two rigid bodies of like charge approach each other, they are affected by both attractive and repulsive forces, which vary independently with the distance between the bodies. Over relatively large distances (>10 nm) there is a net force of attraction, and the bodies are held in a state of weak, reversible association. At intermediate distances (1 to 10 nm), the concentration of ion clouds on the apposing surfaces causes a net repulsive force. Finally, if the intermediate zone of repulsion can be bridged, then there is a strong net attractive force at distances of <1 nm, and the bodies can establish strong, relatively irreversible adhesive interaction (Fig. 3). This stable, irreversible attachment is consistent with observations of specific bacterial adhesive mechanisms, but how do bacteria bridge the intermediate zone of repulsion?

A possible explanation is to consider what really constitutes the functional surfaces of bacteria and eucaryotic cells. Epithelial cell surfaces normally consist of microvilli, cilia, or folds covered by a complex layer of glycocalyx and mucus. Bacterial surfaces are commonly surrounded by complex polymers or filamentous appendages which project several micrometers into the surrounding milieu. Surface structures with small radii of curvature produce much less repulsive force than does the whole cell. Both attractive and repulsive forces are decreased by a reduction in the radii of curvature of the interacting surfaces. However, as radii of curvature become smaller, the decrease in repulsive forces is greater than the corresponding decrease in attractive forces, resulting in a net increase in attractive forces. Therefore, bacterial surface appendages and molecules of

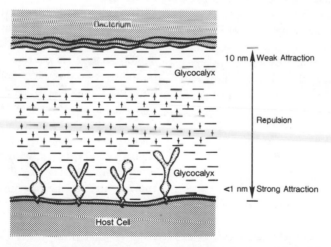

FIGURE 3. Reversible association of the negatively charged bacterial surface with the negatively charged epithelial cell surface at a distance of ca. 10 nm. The cells are weakly attached by noncovalent bonds, but more intimate attachment is prevented by the energy maximum generated by electrostatic forces at distances of 1 to 10 nm. Both bacterial and epithelial cells contain a glycocalyx of anionic polysaccharides, which contributes to the negative surface charge.

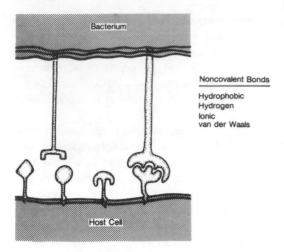

FIGURE 4. Irreversible adhesion of bacterium and epithelial cell surfaces mediated by specific adhesin-receptor interaction. Because the bacterial adhesins have small radii of curvature, they can bridge the zone of maximum repulsion to establish numerous noncovalent bonds with a specific receptor molecule of the epithelial surface. A mismatch between bacterial adhesins and epithelial cell receptors does not contribute to the adhesive process.

the bacterial glycocalyx having very small radii of curvature may be able to extend through the intermediate repulsive zone and establish stable ligand-receptor interactions (Fig. 4) (107, 211). Additionally, cations such as Ca^{2+}, Mn^{2+}, and Fe^{3+} may act as ionic bridges between negatively charged surface molecules (106, 160, 211). A more complete discussion of the physicochemistry of bacterial adhesion is provided in several excellent reviews (105, 107, 132, 177, 211).

Methods Used To Study Bacterial Adhesion

Attachment of bacteria to erythrocytes, leading to hemagglutination (HA), was first reported by Guyot in 1908 (80). Since that time, other investigators have used HA as an efficient in vitro indicator of bacterial adhesive activity (24, 48, 174). The capacity of bacteria to agglutinate erythrocytes of different animal species has facilitated characterization of adhesins and classification of bacterial strains (27, 58, 59). A major advance in the understanding

of bacterial adhesin-host cell receptor interaction occurred with the observation by Old that D-mannose inhibits the HA activity of *E. coli* (150). Inhibition of HA by D-mannose provided evidence that the monosaccharide may be a significant component of the eucaryotic cell receptor for type 1 fimbrial adhesins. The failure of D-mannose to block HA activity of other *E. coli* fimbrial adhesins (K88, K99, CFA/I, and CFA/II) led to the classification of bacterial hemagglutinins as either mannose sensitive or mannose resistant (non-mannose sensitive) (48). Although HA activity has contributed to the characterization of bacterial surface molecules, we must remember that not all adhesins cause HA and not all hemagglutinins have a recognized role in pathogenicity.

Mechanisms of bacterial adhesion have been studied extensively in vitro by using isolated host cells such as leukocytes, erythrocytes, and epithelial cells of the oral (31), intestinal (97), respiratory (104, 165, 206), and urogenital (20, 199) tracts. Some investigators have used the brush borders extracted from the luminal surface of intestinal epithelium for adhesion assays (106, 185). Adhesion was then quantitated by using light microscopy to count the number of bacteria associated with a given number of isolated cells. Alternatively, radiolabeled or living bacteria are mixed with isolated cells, and adherent bacteria are quantitated by scintillation or colony counting after nonadherent bacteria have been removed by filtration or centrifugation.

The surfaces of bacteria and eucaryotic cells grown in vivo are likely to differ significantly from those of cells grown in vitro. Isolated epithelial cells may have an altered glycocalyx and contain little of the mucous blanket found on mucosal surfaces. As stated by Costerton et al., "it is most unlikely that the surface of a derived tissue culture cell shows any more than a superficial resemblance to the cells of living tissues of an animal" (35). Mucosal epithelial cells in living animals are initially exposed to bacteria only on the apical cell membrane, whereas in vitro models may include adhesion to basolateral cell surfaces that would never be exposed to bacteria in the actual disease. Since apical and basolateral membranes have distinctly different receptor profiles, results of in vitro adhesion models must be interpreted with consideration for what is possible in living animals (69).

The expression of bacterial adhesins is markedly affected by culture conditions (95, 107, 151), and even when they are expressed, adhesins may be functionally blocked by excessive capsular material (175). Therefore, adhesins relevant to mucosal colonization and infection may or may not be the same adhesins produced by the bacteria grown in culture. Many bacteria are capable of expressing several different adhesins, depending upon culture conditions. Interpretation of adhesive events from in vitro models, therefore, must always be made with the benefit of supportive in vivo studies (69).

In contrast to the experimental limitations of bacterial disease research with human volunteers, animal disease researchers are free to choose between in vivo and in vitro models of bacterial colonization. Isolated intestinal loops in calves, pigs, and laboratory animals have been extensively used to characterize colonization and pathogenic mechanisms of intestinal pathogens. Isolated tracheal segments have been used to characterize adhesion and colonization by *B. avium* in young turkeys (8). Germfree animals are particularly valuable for the study of intestinal pathogens, but exclusion of the influence of indigenous flora makes interpretation of adhesion and colonization events difficult.

Bacterial Adhesins

Irreversible attachment of bacteria to mucosal surfaces is usually mediated by a variety of complex polymers on the bacterial surface. Adhesins described thus far in the literature are composed of protein (107), polysaccharides (74, 129), lipoteichoic acid (16), or conjugates of these. The majority of adhesins which have been characterized at the molecular and genetic level are surface proteins of gram-negative bacteria (107, 117). These proteinaceous adhesins have

the capacity for specific receptor interactions comparable to those of antibody molecules. Proteinaceous bacterial adhesins can be divided into those with fimbrial morphology and those lacking definite size and shape.

Fimbrial Adhesins

Fimbriae (48) and pili (24, 25) are morphologic terms used synonymously to denote nonflagellar, filamentous appendages that radiate from the bacterial surface. Therefore, adhesins with fimbrial morphology are fimbrial adhesins. Pili may function as mediators of adhesion or as appendages involved in transfer of genes between bacteria. To avoid confusion of these common terms, Jones and Isaacson (107) have suggested that the term fimbriae (fimbriated) be reserved for filamentous appendages involved in bacterial adhesion and colonization and that the term pili (piliated) be reserved for filamentous appendages involved directly in gene transfer.

The filamentous structure of most fimbriae is readily apparent on electron microscopy of negatively stained bacterial suspensions (107). Fimbriae are arranged in polar (64) or peritrichous fashion on the bacterial cell and vary in number from a few to several hundred. They are 2 to 7 nm in diameter and may extend up to 4 μm from the bacterial surface. Unlike flagella, which are thicker and smoothly curved, fimbriae are either straight, or kinked and flexible. The larger-diameter (ca. 7-nm) rigid fimbriae, typified by type 1 and 987P fimbriae of *E. coli*, have a central channel, whereas smaller-diameter (ca. 2 to 4 nm) flexible fimbriae do not (107). Type 1 fimbriae and possibly others grow longer by the addition of subunits at the base (128).

Most fimbrial adhesins can be isolated by subjecting the fimbriated bacteria to shearing in a high-speed mixer, removing bacterial cells by centrifugation, and precipitating the fimbriae from the supernatant (25, 46, 93, 99, 125, 178). Biochemically, fimbriae are polymers consisting of protein subunits (fimbrin or pilin) having a molecular mass of 15 to 26 ki-

TABLE 1
Characteristics of selected fimbrial adhesins

Adhesin[a]	Organism	Tissue tropism	Host	Putative receptor[b]
Type 1 (F1)	*Enterobacteriaceae*	Numerous cell types, mucus	Many	D-Mannosides
K88 (F4)	*E. coli*	Small intestine	Pigs	D-Galactoside
K99 (F5)	*E. coli*	Ileum	Calves, lambs, pigs	GM$_2$ ganglioside? D-Galactoside?
987P (F6)	*E. coli*	Ileum	Pigs	Glycoprotein, D-galactose, GalNac, L-fucose
F41	*E. coli*	Small intestine	Calves	GalNac, GlcNac, mucin
CFA/I (F2)	*E. coli*	Small intestine	Humans	GM$_2$ ganglioside
CFA/II (F3) CS1 CS2 CS3	*E. coli*	Small intestine	Humans	?
Type 4	*N. gonorrhoeae*	Urogenital tract	Humans	?
Type 4	*M. bovis*	Cornea Conjunctiva	Cattle	?
Type 4	*Bacteroides nodosus*	Epidermis of hoof	Sheep	?
Fimbriae	*Corynebacterium renale*	Urinary bladder Vulva	Cattle	?

[a] F1 to F6, Serologic classification of fimbrial adhesins proposed by Ørskov and Ørskov (153); types 1 and 4 classification proposed by Ottow (157).
[b] GalNac, *N*-Acetylgalactosamine; GlcNac, *N*-acetylglucosamine. ?, Unknown or uncertain.
[c] MS, Mannose sensitive; NMS, non-mannose sensitive.
[d] M. Lindahl and T. Wadström, Abstr. VIII Int. Symp. Glycoconjugates 1985, p. 366.

lodaltons (kDa) (107). In addition to protein, small amounts of phosphate, carbohydrate, and phospholipid are sometimes associated with the subunits.

The fimbrial adhesins of *E. coli* and many other bacterial species have been reviewed elsewhere (71, 96, 107, 111, 171). Therefore, only some of the molecular and genetic characteristics of fimbrial adhesins from selected bacterial pathogens of humans and animals are presented here (Table 1).

Nonfimbrial Proteinaceous Adhesins

A variety of bacterial species produce surface protein adhesins that lack definitive morphology. These tend to be outer membrane proteins or secreted proteins that remain loosely associated with the bacterial surface. *B. pertussis* produces two secreted proteins involved in adhesion to cilia of the respiratory epithelium (39). Despite the descriptive name of filamentous hemagglutinin for one of these proteins, it now appears that the protein does not have

TABLE 1
(continued)

Diam (nm)	Mol mass of subunits (kDa)	HA[c]	Plasmid encoded	References
7	14–22	MS	−	25, 48, 60, 62, 107
2.1	ca. 27.5	NMS	+	71, 108, 140, 155 107, 111
2.0	18.2	NMS	+	45, 93, 141, 154 61, 95, 192
7	20.0		−	43, 98, 99, 140
3.2	29.5	?	−	46, 142, 143, 145; Lindahl and Wadstrom[d]
ca. 3	15.0	NMS	+	57, 58, 61, 71, 110, 111
		NMS	+	56, 58, 71, 112
6–7	16.3			125, 193
6–7	15.3			146, 193
ca. 2	14.8			125, 193
ca. 6	17.5	NMS	?	162, 184, 201, 213
ca. 6	17–19	NMS	−	6, 75, 124, 190 123
ca. 6	16.5–19		−	3, 4, 54, 137
2.5–3	19.0		−	90, 115, 182, 214 85, 114

fimbrial morphology (11, 12). The other protein, pertussis toxin, has both toxic and adhesive roles in the production of pertussis (whooping cough) (205). These adhesins of *B. pertussis* are unique in that they bind to both cilia and the bacterial surface to form adherence bridges (203, 205). Additionally, Tuomanen has shown that other pathogenic bacteria, pretreated with these adhesins, acquire the specific ability to bind to cilia in vitro and in vivo (203). Adhesion of *Neisseria gonorrhoeae* to epithelial cells is mediated not only by fimbriae, but also by a group of closely related outer membrane proteins (protein II) (200). Protein II expression is responsible for opaque colony phenotype and increased aggregation of gonococci (21). *Staphylococcus aureus*, an important cause of posttraumatic skin and wound infection, produces a surface protein with specific affinity for fibronectin (55). Although *Streptococcus pyogenes* also binds specifically to fibronectin (195), the adhesin appears to be lipoteichoic acid rather than a surface protein (38).

Adhesins Composed of Carbohydrates or Lipids

Marine biologists originally observed that bacteria required some time to become firmly attached to solid surfaces (218). It was suggested that the bacteria secrete a mucilaginous slime which both mediates firm adhesion and provides for colony formation. The importance of the bacterial glycocalyx in colonization of living tissues has been emphasized by Costerton and Irvin (34). The anionic polysaccharide matrix of the glycocalyx enables bacteria to assume a microcolony mode of growth in which the bacteria remain firmly attached to host tissues while being protected from host immune products, phagocytic cells, and antibiotics (36). A useful example of the role of the bacterial glycocalyx in colonization of mucosal surfaces is provided by the ubiquitous pathogen *P. aeruginosa*. Although fimbrial adhesins of non-mucoid *P. aeruginosa* are involved in adherence to respiratory tissues, mucoid strains of *P. aeruginosa* rely heavily on their production of mucoid exopolysaccharide (glycocalyx) for specific adhesion to the ciliated tracheal epithelium and for formation of microcolonies (36, 129, 165). Recently Ramphal et al. have shown that this exopolysaccharide also mediates adhesion to tracheobronchial mucin (164).

Bacteria capable of colonizing mucosal surfaces frequently express multiple adhesins simultaneously or sequentially as colonization progresses. Like the nonfimbrial protein adhesins discussed above, many carbohydrate and lipid adhesins act as complex bridging polymers which contribute to bacterial microcolony formation and adhesion to epithelial surfaces (30). Lipoteichoic acid, a component of streptococcal and staphylococcal cell walls, binds to a broad range of eucaryotic cells by interacting with a fibronectin receptor (38). It also contributes to adhesion of *Streptococcus mutans* to tooth enamel and dental plaque. It has binding affinity for hydroxyapatite of teeth, the glucosyltransferase enzyme secreted by *S. mutans*, and insoluble glucan polymers formed by the action of glucosyltransferase on sucrose (30, 74, 127, 209). Therefore, adhesion of *S. mutans* to teeth probably involves the complex interaction of multiple adhesins with a variety of receptors associated with tooth enamel and salivary pellicles (74, 209).

Expression of Bacterial Adhesins

The phenotypic expression of bacterial adhesins is largely determined by the conditions of growth both in vitro and in vivo (71, 79, 107, 111). Many bacterial pathogens that rely on adhesins for colonization of mucosal surfaces cease production of adhesins when grown on conventional culture media. Expression of many fimbrial adhesins is subject to qualitative phase variation and quantitative variation (107). Qualitative phase variation is the on-off switch for adhesin production. Such phase variation of type 1 fimbriation is under transcriptional control, with the transition between fimbriate and nonfimbriate phenotypes occurring at the rate of about 10^{-3} per bacterium per generation (51). Guerina et al. have shown that when rats are fed either fimbriated or nonfimbriated *E. coli* expressing K1 capsular antigen, most of the rats develop bacteremia and colonization of the oral cavity (79). Only fimbriated bacteria are subsequently isolated from the oral cavity, and only nonfimbriated bacteria are isolated from blood. Other studies of bacterial pathogenesis also support the concept that fimbrial adhesins are expressed by bacteria on mucosal surfaces in vivo, but extension of infection to the lamina propria or bloodstream requires a shift to the nonfimbriated phase. The shift to the nonfimbriated phase may increase bacterial survival in deep tissues, since many fimbriae enhance ingestion by phagocytic cells (7, 15, 22, 188, 189). Also, because production of fimbriae requires up to 2% of the protein-synthetic capacity of the bacterial cell, fimbriated bacteria have a growth disadvantage unless the fimbriae contribute to adhesion, colonization, or acquisition of substrates (111).

The quantity of adhesin produced by individual bacterial cells also varies with the bacterial environment. The temperature-dependent production of adhesins by several bacterial pathogens is probably a reflection of the different growth requirements in vivo and in the animal's environment. The K99 and K88 adhesins of enterotoxigenic E. coli are expressed in the small intestine and at 37°C in culture, but neither adhesin is produced in significant amounts at 18°C (71, 95). Type 1 fimbriae are readily produced by Salmonella typhimurium and E. coli grown in static broth culture beyond the logarithmic growth phase, but are poorly expressed by bacteria grown on solid media (25, 151). In contrast, E. coli K99 fimbriae are produced best in the logarithmic growth phase of well-aerated (shaken) broth culture (94).

Production of bacterial adhesins is either enhanced or inhibited by a variety of compounds in the microenvironment (44, 95). A number of antibiotics disrupt adhesin production in much the same way that they disrupt other bacterial functions (52, 95, 187). Both Neisseria meningitidis and N. gonorrhoeae cease production of fimbriae and adhere poorly to human cells when grown in low concentrations of tetracycline and penicillin (196). The synthesis, expression, and adhesive function of type 1 fimbriae of an E. coli strain isolated from urine are inhibited by the synergistic activity of trimethoprim and sulfamethoxazole used at 1/32 of the MIC of each drug (183).

Mucosal Receptors for Bacterial Adhesins

The epithelial cell membrane, glycocalyx, and mucous layer contain a diverse group of glycoproteins and glycolipids which act as receptors for growth factors, hormones, and a variety of other molecules in the extracellular milieu (41, 135, 194). These glycoconjugates are anchored in the phospholipid bilayer of the cell membrane by hydrophobic regions of the molecule, and oligosaccharide side chains project from the cell surface to function as potential receptor molecules (23, 149). Unfortunately, a variety of infectious agents have evolved mechanisms to utilize mucosal surface receptors to enhance their colonization. Carbohydrate receptors of the mucosal surface commonly provide binding sites for bacterial

adhesins and toxins (50, 107).

Because of the molecular diversity provided by glycoconjugates, these substances are ideally suited for specific recognition of proteinaceous adhesins (117). The repertoire of receptor molecules of a mucosal surface is a major determinant for the number and kinds of bacteria capable of infecting the tissue. The requirement for specific receptor-bacterial interaction dictates tissue tropism (73, 140), genetic specificity (185), age susceptibility (176), and species susceptibility (16) characteristic of many mucosal infections. Sellwood et al. found that intestinal brush borders from some of their experimental pigs were genetically resistant to adhesion by K88-positive E. coli (185). Through breeding studies they showed that expression of the K88 receptor in brush borders was coded for by autosomal dominant genes.

Since the discovery that D-mannose inhibits the agglutination of erythrocytes by bacteria expressing type 1 fimbriae (150), identification of receptor molecules has depended heavily on adhesion inhibition studies involving a battery of carbohydrates. Putative receptor molecules are mixed in excess with the bacterial inoculum, and the bacterial suspension is then added to a suitable target cell system. Inhibition of adhesion indicates that the putative receptor may be similar to the binding site of the natural receptor. Most putative receptors have proven to be carbohydrates composed of three or fewer monosaccharides of the D configuration. Only L-fucose, a putative receptor for the V. cholerae adhesin, is an exception.

Few receptors have been characterized beyond a corresponding list of minimal inhibitory compounds, nor has their distribution in tissue been determined (107). Using a rabbit model, Dean and Isaacson have determined the location of receptors in the intestinal mucosa for the 987P adhesin of E. coli (42). The 987P receptor was restricted to goblet cells in neonatal pigs and rabbits, but in adult rabbits the receptor was shown to exist both in goblet cells and along the entire villous surface. As receptors for mucosal bacterial pathogens are further characterized (43, 118, 166), it becomes apparent that many putative receptors are located both on epithelial cell surfaces and in the overlying mucous layer.

INVASION

Why are many bacterial pathogens content to colonize mucosal surfaces, while others extend their habitat to the intracellular environment? Although intracellular colonization may provide a new source of nutrients and protection from many host defenses, it also presents intracellular bacteria with several new problems. Successful intracellular pathogens must have mechanisms to enter host cells, avoid being killed, multiply, and provide for the escape and translocation of their progeny to new host cells (144).

In early studies of bacillary dysentery, penetration of the colonic epithelium by *Shigella flexneri* was recognized as the major event in the pathogenesis of this mucosal infection (116). The Sereny test was developed to determine the pathogenicity of *Shigella* isolates (186). A suspension of bacteria was applied to the conjunctival sacs of guinea pigs, and the animals were observed for signs of ocular disease. In the Sereny test, pathogenic *Shigella* strains cause purulent conjunctivitis progressing to keratitis and corneal ulceration. Morphologic studies showed that pathogenic shigellae invade the corneal epithelium and multiply intracellularly, whereas salmonellae and most other invasive bacteria invade the cornea only transiently and are then cleared from the eye.

Many of the morphological changes associated with bacterial invasion are similar regardless of the bacterial pathogen and eucaryotic cell involved. The ultrastructural pathology of salmonellosis in guinea pigs as described by Takeuchi illustrates many of the cellular lesions associated with invasive bacteria (202). Close proximity of *Salmonella typhimurium* to the epithelial brush border initiates the following sequence of events: (i) degeneration of subjacent microvilli, (ii) invagination of the cell membrane, (iii) degeneration of cell junctions and cellular organelles, (iv) engulfment of the bacterium in a membrane-bound vacuole (endocytosis), (v) development of electron-dense material around bacteria in vacuoles, (vi) bacterial multiplication, (vii) translocation to the subnuclear region of cytoplasm, and (viii) possible expulsion of bacteria from the infected cell (Fig. 5). Endocytic vacuoles may contain one or more bacteria, or bacteria may be free within the cytoplasm. In contrast to salmonellae, shigellae readily escape from endocytic vacuoles by disrupting the cell membrane (82, 181).

Most facultative and obligate intracellular parasites, including viruses, protozoa, and bacteria, enter eucaryotic cells by endocytosis, a process that is comparable to phagocytosis by

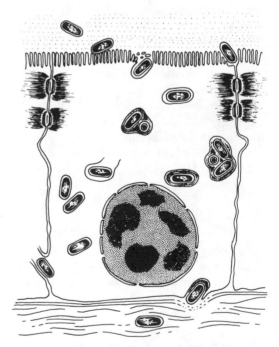

FIGURE 5. Bacterial invasion of the intestinal epithelium. Bacteria attach to the microvillus border after penetration of the mucous layer. Invasive bacteria stimulate endocytosis by the host cell and are delivered to the cytoplasm within a membrane-bound vacuole. Some bacteria remain and multiply within the vacuole while resisting effects of lysosomal enzymes, whereas other bacteria escape from the vacuole to replicate free in the cytoplasm. Bacteria spread from the infected cell by destruction of the cell membrane or by exocytosis from a vacuole.

macrophages and neutrophils. The processes require the function of contractile proteins (microfilaments) and energy provided through glycolytic and oxidative metabolic pathways. Once inside an endocytic vacuole, bacteria must have a mechanism to avoid being killed by the bactericidal products deposited by fusion of lysosomes with bacterium-containing vacuoles. *Shigella flexneri* escapes to the cytoplasm after causing lysis of the endocytic vacuole (82, 181), whereas *Legionella pneumophila* (152) and *Brucella abortus* (5) are routed to the rough endoplasmic reticulum, where multiplication occurs. Uptake of *Shigella flexneri* and *Salmonella typhimurium* by eucaryotic cells is reduced by treatment of host cells with cytochalasin B (disrupts microfilaments) or inhibitors of glycolytic and oxidative metabolism (26, 82). In contrast, endocytosis of *Chlamydia psittaci* elementary bodies is not inhibited by cytochalasin B. It appears that *C. psittaci* may utilize a unique mechanism of entry resembling receptor-mediated endocytosis (88). This process is used by eucaryotic cells for internalization of nutrients and polypeptide hormones that bind to membrane receptors within clathrin-coated pits (23). Other, less common, mechanisms of bacterial invasion are summarized in Table 2.

The genetic and molecular basis of invasion is most thoroughly characterized for enteric bacterial pathogens (65). Large plasmids are required for full expression of the invasive phenotype in *Shigella* spp. (81, 179, 180), *Salmonella typhimurium, Salmonella gallinarum, Yersinia enterocolitica,* and enteroinvasive *E. coli* (14, 33, 65). Loss of the plasmids is accompanied by loss of invasiveness, and the invasive phenotype is restored by reintroduction of the virulence-associated plasmid into plasmid-free avirulent strains. Antigenic characterization of seven polypeptides encoded by the 140-MDa virulence-associated plasmids of *Shigella flexneri* and enteroinvasive *E. coli* O143 revealed cross-reactivity among four of them (83). The similarities of these polypeptides among invasive enteric bacteria suggest that they may be determinants of the invasive phenotype (83). In contrast to the plasmid-mediated mechanisms described above, it appears that invasiveness of *Aeromonas hydrophila* and *Yersinia pseudotuberculosis* is mediated by genes located on the bacterial chromosome (101, 119).

COLONIZATION STRATEGIES OF SELECTED BACTERIAL PATHOGENS

In the overview of bacterial colonization and invasion, well-established mechanisms of human and animal bacterial pathogens were used to illustrate major concepts of pathogenesis. A

TABLE 2
Potential mechanisms of cellular invasion

Mechanism	Organism	References
Endocytosis	*Shigella flexneri*	82
	Neisseria spp.	138
	Listeria monocytogenes	163
	Salmonella spp.	167, 202
	Chlamydia psittaci	88
	Bartonella bacilliformis	19
Disruption by cytotoxins	*Clostridium perfringens*	147
	Salmonella spp.	170
Direct penetration (diacytosis)	*Bdellovibrio* spp.	144
Uptake by antigen sampling sites	*Salmonella* spp.	28, 89, 92

risk of this approach is that it is possible to lose sight of the complexity of mucosal infection, the significant gaps in our understanding of pathogenic mechanisms, and the contribution of multiple virulence factors functioning simultaneously or sequentially to promote mucosal infection and disease. In this section several diseases of humans, livestock, and poultry are discussed and compared, emphasizing potential contributions of multiple virulence factors. Because the next three chapters focus on virulence mechanisms of enteric bacteria in detail, nonenteric pathogens have been selected here to illustrate other mechanisms of colonization and invasion. Therefore, in the following section, bordetellosis is discussed to illustrate mechanisms of a strict respiratory pathogen and the similarities of these mechanisms among *Bordetella* species and their specific hosts. *Moraxella bovis* and *Bacteriodes nodosus* were chosen because they illustrate examples of both adhesion and invasion of epithelial surfaces distinct from those discussed above.

Bordetellosis

Bacteria of the genus *Bordetella* have a strict tropism for cilia of the respiratory epithelium (Fig. 2 and 6) (9, 17, 32, 136, 206, 207). Only the cilia-associated respiratory bacillus of rats has a more intimate association with cilia of tracheal epithelial cells (72). As noninvasive pathogens of the respiratory mucosa, bordetellae are strict aerobes that grow best at ca. 35°C, the approximate temperature of the respiratory mucosa (10, 77). Colonization of the respiratory epithelium, persisting for several weeks, is associated with ciliostasis (18), localized injury to the epithelium and subjacent mesenchymal tissues (9, 9a, 49, 76, 148) and systemic clinical signs of intoxication (159, 212).

Adhesion of *B. pertussis* to cilia is mediated by filamentous hemagglutinin and pertussis toxin (TOX) (205). Filamentous hemagglutinin appears not to be a filamentous adhesin after all (12), but instead is a heterogeneous surface protein composed of several high-molecular-weight subunits (2, 39). TOX

is a polymeric protein exotoxin which conforms to the A-B model of bacterial toxins (50). Mutants lacking either filamentous hemagglutinin or TOX have a reduced capacity to adhere to cilia, but these mutants regain their adhesive capacity when preincubated with purified filamentous hemagglutinin or TOX (205). These sticky surface proteins appear to function as bivalent adherence bridges between cilia and bacteria. Several other pathogenic bacteria are also able to utilize the adhesins to bind to cilia (203).

Two types of fimbriae, agglutinogen serotypes 2 and 6, have been isolated from *B. pertussis* (40). Fimbrial serotypes 2 and 6 are filaments (diameter, 5 to 6 nm) composed of a single protein subunit of 22 and 21.5 kDa, respectively (197, 216, 217). Compared with filamentous hemagglutinin and TOX, fimbriae apparently have a minor role in adhesion of *B. pertussis* to the respiratory epithelium (39, 208). Both filamentous hemagglutinin and TOX cause HA, but the *B. pertussis* fimbriae do not (39).

The ciliary receptor for *B. pertussis* appears to be a glycoconjugate (204). Pretreatment of ciliated cells with sodium periodate abolishes adhesion, indicating that the receptor is probably a polysaccharide (206). Receptor analogs containing variations of galactose N-acetylglucosamine strongly inhibit adhesion of *B. pertussis* (204).

Adhesion of *B. bronchiseptica* to cilia is influenced by phenotypic phase variation between smooth (phase I) and rough (phase IV) colony morphologies (160, 215). Smooth-colony isolates adhere readily to swine nasal epithelial cells in vitro and to hamster lung fibroblasts; however, rough-colony isolates adhere poorly to the nasal epithelium. Plotkin and Bemis have suggested that at least two colony-phase-associated, adhesive mechanisms are utilized by *B. bronchiseptica* (160). Binding of smooth-colony organisms to hamster lung fibroblasts is strongly inhibited by N-acetylglucosamine, whereas binding of the less adherent rough-colony organisms is inhibited by chelators of cations. Adhesion of rough-colony organisms is enhanced by addition of Ca^{2+}, Mn^{2+},

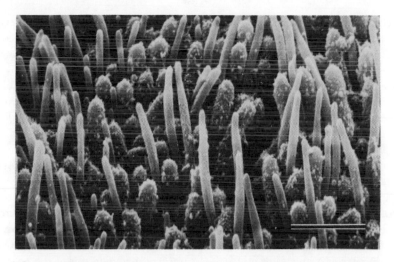

FIGURE 6. Microcolony of *B. avium* among the cilia of a tracheal epithelial cell from a young turkey. Bacteria are closely associated with cilia, possibly by the numerous knoblike structures on their surface. Bar, 2 μm.

Cd^{2+}, or Sr^{2+} to the system (160). More recently, Ishikawa and Isayama (100) have found that sialyl glycoconjugates inhibit adhesion to isolated nasal epithelial cells of pigs. Several types of fimbriae have also been isolated from *B. bronchiseptica* (122). Bacteria from smooth colonies of *B. bronchiseptica* are heavily fimbriated, whereas bacteria from rough colonies contain few fimbriae. The fimbriae are 3 to 4 nm in diameter and are composed of antigenically related subunits with a molecular size of 21 to 24 kDa. There is also a degree of cross-reactivity between fimbriae of *B. bronchiseptica* and serotype 2 fimbriae of *B. pertussis*. Although stringlike or fibrillar appendages between *B. bronchiseptica* cells and cilia have been observed by electron microscopy (17, 215), a role for fimbriae in the adhesion of *B. bronchiseptica* has not been definitely established.

B. avium sp. nov. (109), the species most recently proposed for inclusion in the *Bordetella* genus, specifically colonizes ciliated cells of the turkey respiratory tract and agglutinates guinea pig erythrocytes (9a, 103; L. H. Arp, R. D. Leyh, and R. W. Griffith, Am. J. Vet. Res., in press). Delicate fimbriae (diameter, 2 nm) have been observed on negatively stained *B. avium* cells, and preliminary evidence suggests

that the fimbriae may be involved in attachment to the tracheal mucosa in vitro (102). The fimbriae are composed of 13.1-kDa subunits and have no HA activity (102). Numerous knoblike structures cover the surface of *B. avium* cells colonizing ciliated cells of turkey tracheas (Fig. 6) (9a). In parallel with the observation that sialyl glycoconjugates may function as mucosal receptors for *B. bronchiseptica* (100), workers in our laboratory have recently found that sialogangliosides inhibit HA and in vivo adhesion of *B. avium* (L. H. Arp, D. R. Hellwig, and E. L. Huffman, manuscript in preparation).

Infectious Bovine Keratoconjunctivitis

Moraxella bovis is the principal cause of keratoconjunctivitis (pinkeye) in cattle, although ocular exposure to UV irradiation (91, 210) and *Mycoplasma bovoculi* (173) contribute to infection. Studies of the experimental infection of gnotobiotic calves show that colonization of the conjunctival and corneal epithelium is followed by invasion of the cornea. Bacterial invasion quickly progresses through the corneal epithelium into the stroma, resulting in ulcerative keratitis and visual impairment (171a).

Therefore, mechanisms of bacterial adhesion, colonization, and invasion are involved in the pathogenesis of pinkeye.

At least two virulence factors are required for pathogenicity of *Moraxella bovis:* fimbriae for adhesion and a pitting factor for penetration of the cornea (29, 158). The term pitting factor comes from the ultrastructural observation that the bacteria produce pitlike depressions in corneal epithelial cells (29, 210). Pathogenic strains also cause hemolysis on bovine blood agar (161), but any relationship between the hemolysin and pitting factor is unclear. Several different types of fimbriae have been isolated from *Moraxella bovis,* and fimbriated organisms have HA and autoagglutination activity (75). The fimbriae are about 6 nm in diameter (6, 190) and are composed of subunits ranging in size from 17 to 19 kDa (123, 124). Many of the fimbrin subunits are antigenically related (123). Although *Moraxella bovis* strains carry a variety of plasmids, fimbrial proteins are encoded by the chromosome (131).

In vitro models have been developed for the study of *Moraxella bovis* adhesion mechanisms (6, 84, 101). These studies have shown that the fimbriated phenotype exhibits the greatest adhesion to the corneal epithelium and tissue culture cells, but nonfimbriated cells also exhibit a minimal level of adhesiveness. Therefore, adhesins other than fimbriae may contribute to adhesion by *Moraxella bovis* (6, 101). Although putative target cell receptors for the adhesins of *Moraxella bovis* have not been identified, neither D-mannose nor D-galactose inhibits HA (75).

Mechanisms of invasion used by *Moraxella bovis* have not been clarified; however, virulent strains are hemolytic and produce a variety of hydrolytic enzymes including hyaluronidase, fibrinolysin, aminopeptidase, phosphoamidase, and phosphatase (66, 156). In the fimbriated phenotype, *Moraxella bovis* develops flat, rough, agar-corroding colonies on bovine blood agar (158). Ultrastructural studies of infected corneal epithelium indicate that *Moraxella bovis* bacteria form pits on the cell surface before being taken into the cell by endocytosis (Fig. 7). In the early infection many bacteria are found within membrane-bound vacuoles; however, as infection progresses many bacteria are found free in the cytoplasm, apparently by escape from endocytic vacuoles (171a). Hydrolytic enzymes may play a role in the escape from vacuoles and extension of bacteria to adjacent cells and stroma.

Ovine Footrot

Studies of the pathogenesis of severe ovine footrot have shown that exposure to wet environments and opportunistic bacteria enables the anaerobe *Bacteroides nodosus* to colonize the uncornified epidermis of the hoof, culminating in separation of the overlying horn. Full expression of virulence by this obligate parasite requires the production of fimbrial adhesins and extracellular proteases. Vaccines containing suspensions of *Bacteroides nodosus* or purified fimbriae protect against challenge by serologically related strains (121, 198).

Fimbriae of *Bacteroides nodosus* have a central role in pathogenesis and immunity to ovine footrot. The fimbriae have a polar location on the cell and contribute to twitching motility (47). They are straight filaments, about 6 nm in diameter and several micrometers long. Purified fimbriae are composed of two polypeptide antigens, a structural subunit with a molecular mass of 17 kDa and a basal protein of about 80 kDa (4). At least eight serologically distinct subunits (A through H) have been characterized (4). The fimbriae of *Bacteroides nodosus* conform to the category of type 4, as proposed by Ottow (157). Type 4 fimbriae, found on *Bacteroides nodosus, Moraxella bovis, N. gonorrhoeae,* and *P. aeruginosa,* appear to be closely related structurally, functionally, and evolutionarily (131, 137). These fimbriae share a high degree of sequence homology in the N-terminal region and have the modified amino acid methylphenylalanine as the first residue. Cloning of the *Bacteroides nodosus* gene for the fimbrial subunits into *E. coli* resulted in localization of subunits along the inner membrane, but no expression of fimbriae (3, 53). However,

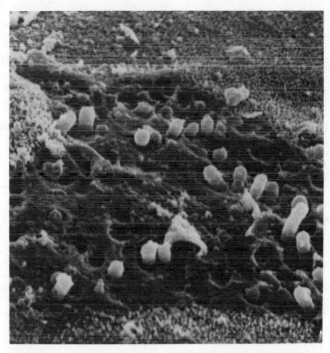

FIGURE 7. Numerous pits in the surface of a conjunctival epithelial cell colonized by *Moraxella bovis*. The photograph was kindly provided by D. G. Rogers, National Animal Disease Center, Ames, Iowa.

when the gene was instead cloned into a more closely related organism, *P. aeruginosa*, fimbriae were expressed on the bacterial surface (54, 137). Production of large amounts of *Bacteroides nodosus* fimbrial protein for vaccine purposes may now be possible by using recombinant *P. aeruginosa* (137).

Analysis of extracellular proteinases has been used to distinguish between virulent and benign isolates of *Bacteroides nodosus*. Virulent and benign isolates produce a distinct profile of five or six proteinases, respectively, with molecular masses ranging from 8 to 43 kDa (78, 113). Although the precise role of the extracellular proteinases is unclear, vaccines made from proteinase preparations have not prevented ovine footrot (139).

LITERATURE CITED

1. Allweiss, B., J. Dostal, K. E. Carey, T. F. Edwards, and R. Freter. 1977. The role of chemotaxis in the ecology of bacterial pathogens of mucosal surfaces. *Nature* (London) 266:448–450.

2. An Der Lan, B., J. L. Cowell, D. G. Burstyn, C. R. Manclark, and A. Chrambach. 1986. Characterization of the filamentous hemagglutinin from *Bordetella pertussis* by gel electrophoresis. *Mol. Cell. Biochem.* 70:31–55.

3. Anderson, B. J., M. M. Bills, J. R. Egerton, and J. S. Mattick. 1984. Cloning and expression in *Escherichia coli* of the gene encoding the structural subunit of *Bacteroides nodosus* fimbriae. *J. Bacteriol.* 160:748–754.

4. Anderson, B. J., C. L. Kristo, J. R. Egerton, and J. S. Mattick. 1986. Variation in the structural subunit and basal protein antigens of *Bacteroides nodosus* fimbriae. *J. Bacteriol.* 166:453–460.

5. Anderson, T. D., N. F. Cheville, and V. P. Meador. 1986. Pathogenesis of placentitis in the goat inoculated with *Brucella abortus*. II. Ultrastructural studies. *Vet. Pathol.* 23:227–239.

6. Annuar, B. O., and G. E. Wilcox. 1985. Adherence of *Moraxella bovis* to cell cultures of bovine origin. *Res. Vet. Sci.* 39:241–246.

7. Arp, L. H. 1985. Effect of antibodies to type 1 fimbriae on clearance of fimbriated *Escherichia coli* from the bloodstream of turkeys. *Am. J. Vet. Res.* 46:2644–2647.

8. **Arp, L. H., and E. E. Brooks.** 1986. An *in vivo* model for the study of *Bordetella avium* adherence to tracheal mucosa in turkeys. *Am. J. Vet. Res.* 47:2614–2617.

9. **Arp, L. H., and N. F. Cheville.** 1984. Tracheal lesions in young turkeys infected with *Bordetella avium*. *Am. J. Vet. Res.* 45:2196–2200.

9a. **Arp, L. H., and J. A. Fagerland.** 1987. Ultrastructural pathology of *Bordetella avium* infection in turkeys. Vet. Pathol. 24:411–418.

10. **Arp, L. H., and S. M. McDonald.** 1985. Influence of temperature on the growth of *Bordetella avium* in turkeys and in vitro. *Avian Dis.* 29:1066–1077.

11. **Ashworth, L. A. E., A. B. Dowsett, L. I. Irons, and A. Robinson.** 1985. The location of surface antigens of *Bordetella pertussis* by immuno-electron microscopy. *Dev. Biol. Stand.* 61:143–151.

12. **Ashworth, L. A. E., L. I. Irons, and A. B. Dowsett.** 1982. Antigenic relationship between serotype-specific agglutinogen and fimbriae of *Bordetella pertussis. Infect. Immun.* 37:1278–1281.

13. **Attridge, S. R., and D. Rowley.** 1983. The role of the flagellum in the adherence of *Vibrio cholerae. J. Infect. Dis.* 147:864–872.

14. **Barrow, P. A., J. M. Simpson, M. A. Lovell, and M. M. Binns.** 1987. Contribution of *Salmonella gallinarum* large plasmid toward virulence in fowl typhoid. *Infect. Immun.* 55:388–392.

15. **Bar-Shavit, Z., R. Goldman, I. Ofek, N. Sharon, and D. Mirelman.** 1980. Mannose-binding activity of *Escherichia coli*: a determinant of attachment and ingestion of the bacteria by macrophages. *Infect. Immun.* 29:417–424.

16. **Beachey, E. H.** 1981. Bacterial adherence: adhesin-receptor interactions mediating the attachment of bacteria to mucosal surfaces. *J. Infect. Dis.* 143:325–345.

17. **Bemis, D. A., H. A. Greisen, and M. J. G. Appel.** 1977. Pathogenesis of canine bordetellosis. *J. Infect. Dis.* 135:753–762.

18. **Bemis, D. A., and S. A. Wilson.** 1985. Influence of potential virulence determinants on *Bordetella bronchiseptica*-induced ciliostasis. *Infect. Immun.* 50:35–42.

19. **Benson, L. A., S. Kar, G. McLaughlin, and G. M. Ihler.** 1986. Entry of *Bartonella bacilliformis* into erythrocytes. *Infect. Immun.* 54:347–353.

20. **Bibel, D. J., R. Aly, L. Lahti, H. R. Shinefield, and H. I. Maibach.** 1987. Microbial adherence to vulvar epithelial cells. *J. Med. Microbiol.* 23:75–82.

21. **Blake, M. S., and E. C. Gotschlich.** 1983. Gonococcal membrane proteins: speculation on their role in pathogenesis. *Prog. Allergy* 33:298–313.

22. **Blumenstock, E., and K. Jann.** 1982. Adhesion of piliated *Escherichia coli* strains to phagocytes: differences between bacteria with mannose-sensitive pili and those with mannose-resistant pili. *Infect. Immun.* 35:264–269.

23. **Bretscher, M. S.** 1985. The molecules of the cell membrane. *Sci. Am.* 253:100–108.

24. **Brinton, C. C., Jr.** 1959. Non-flagellar appendages of bacteria. *Nature* (London) 183:782–786.

25. **Brinton, C. C., Jr.** 1965. The structure, function, synthesis and genetic control of bacterial pili and a molecular model for DNA and RNA transport in gram negative bacteria. *Trans. N.Y. Acad. Sci.* 27:1003–1054.

26. **Bukholm, G.** 1984. Effect of cytochalasin B and dihydrocytochalasin B on invasiveness of entero-invasive bacteria in HEp-2 cell cultures. *Acta Pathol. Microbiol. Immunol. Scand. Sect. B* 92:145–149.

27. **Burrows, M. R., R. Sellwood, and R. A. Gibbons.** 1976. Haemagglutinating and adhesive properties associated with the K99 antigen of bovine strains of *Escherichia coli. J. Gen. Microbiol.* 96:269–275.

28. **Carter, P. B., and F. M. Collins.** 1974. The route of enteric infection in normal mice. *J. Exp. Med.* 139:1189–1203.

29. **Chandler, R. L., K. Smith, and B. A. Turfrey.** 1985. Exposure of bovine cornea to different strains of *Moraxella bovis* and to other bacterial species in vitro. *J. Comp. Pathol.* 95:415–423.

30. **Christensen, G. D., W. A. Simpson, and E. H. Beachey.** 1985. Adhesion of bacteria to animal tissues: complex mechanisms, p. 279–305. *In* D. C. Savage and M. Fletcher (ed.), *Bacterial Adhesion Mechanisms and Physiological Significance.* Plenum Publishing Corp., New York.

31. **Clegg, H., N. Guerina, S. Langermann, T. W. Kessler, V. Guerina, and D. Goldmann.** 1984. Pilus-mediated adherence of *Escherichia coli* K-1 to human oral epithelial cells. *Infect. Immun.* 45:299–301.

32. **Collier, A. M., L. P. Peterson, and J. B. Baseman.** 1977. Pathogenesis of infection with *Bordetella pertussis* in hamster tracheal organ culture. *J. Infect. Dis.* 136:S196–S203.

33. **Cornelis, G., Y. Laroche, G. Balligand, and M.-P. Sory.** 1987. *Yersinia enterocolitica*, a primary model for bacterial invasiveness. *Rev. Infect. Dis.* 9:64–87.

34. **Costerton, J. W., and R. T. Irvin.** 1981. The bacterial glycocalyx in nature and disease. *Annu. Rev. Microbiol.* 35:299–324.

35. **Costerton, J. W., R. T. Irvin, and K.-J. Cheng.** 1981. The role of bacterial surface structures in pathogenesis. *Crit. Rev. Microbiol.* 8:303–338.

36. **Costerton, J. W., J. Lam, K. Lam, and R. Chan.** 1983. The role of the microcolony mode of growth in the pathogenesis of *Pseudomonas aeruginosa* infections. *Rev. Infect. Dis.* 5:S867–S873.

37. Costerton, J. W., T. J. Marrie, and K.-J. Cheng. 1985. Phenomena of bacterial adhesion, p. 3–43. *In* D. C. Savage and M. Fletcher (ed.), *Bacterial Adhesion Mechanisms and Physiological Significance.* Plenum Publishing Corp., New York.

38. Courtney, H. S., I. Ofek, W. A. Simpson, D. L. Hasty, and E. H. Beachey. 1986. Binding of *Streptococcus pyogenes* to soluble and insoluble fibronectin. *Infect. Immun.* 53:454–459.

39. Cowell, J. L., A. Urisu, J. M. Zhang, A. C. Steven, and C. R. Manclark. 1986. Filamentous hemagglutinin and fimbriae of *Bordetella pertussis:* properties and roles in attachment, p. 55–58. *In* L. Leive (ed.), *Microbiology—1986.* American Society for Microbiology, Washington, D.C.

40. Cowell, J. L., J. M. Zhang, A. Urisu, A. Suzuki, A. C. Steven, T. Liu, T.-Y. Liu, and C. R. Manclark. 1987. Purification and characterization of serotype 6 fimbriae from *Bordetella pertussis* and comparison of their properties with serotype 2 fimbriae. *Infect. Immun.* 55:916–922.

41. Dautry-Varsat, A., and H. F. Lodish. 1984. How receptors bring proteins and particles into cells. *Sci. Am.* 250:52–58.

42. Dean, E. A., and R. E. Isaacson. 1985. Location and distribution of a receptor for the 987P pilus of *Escherichia coli* in small intestines. *Infect. Immun.* 47:345–348.

43. Dean, E. A., and R. E. Isaacson. 1985. Purification and characterization of a receptor for the 987P pilus of *Escherichia coli. Infect. Immun.* 47:98–105.

44. de Graaf, F. K., P. Klaasen-Boor, and J. E. Van Hees. 1980. Biosynthesis of the K99 surface antigen is repressed by alanine. *Infect. Immun.* 30:125–128.

45. de Graaf, F. K., P. Klemmm, and W. Gaastra. 1981. Purification, characterization, and partial covalent structure of *Escherichia coli* adhesive antigen K99. *Infect. Immun.* 33:877–883.

46. de Graaf, F. K., and I. Roorda. 1982. Production, purification, and characterization of the fimbrial adhesive antigen F41 isolated from calf enteropathogenic *Escherichia coli* strain B41M. *Infect. Immun.* 36:751–758.

47. Depiazzi, L. J., and R. B. Richards. 1985. Motility in relation to virulence of *Bacteroides nodosus. Vet. Microbiol.* 10:107–116.

48. Duguid, J. P., I. W. Smith, G. Dempster, and P. N. Edmunds. 1955. Non-flagellar filamentous appendages ("fimbriae") and haemagglutinating activity in *Bacterium coli. J. Pathol. Bacteriol.* 70:335–348.

49. Duncan, J. R., R. F. Ross, W. P. Switzer, and F. K. Ramsey. 1966. Pathology of experimental *Bordetella bronchiseptica* infection in swine: atrophic rhinitis. *Am. J. Vet. Res.* 27:457–466.

50. Eidels, L., R. L. Proia, and D. A. Hart. 1983. Membrane receptors for bacterial toxins. *Microbiol. Rev.* 47:596–620.

51. Eisenstein, B. I. 1981. Phase variation of type 1 fimbriae in *Escherichia coli* is under transcriptional control. *Science* 214:337–339.

52. Eisenstein, B. I., I. Ofek, and E. H. Beachey. 1979. Interference with the mannose binding and epithelial cell adherence of *Escherichia coli* by sublethal concentrations of streptomycin. *J. Clin. Invest.* 63:1219–1228.

53. Elleman, T. C., P. A. Hoyne, D. L. Emery, D. J. Stewart, and B. L. Clark. 1986. Expression of the pilin gene from *Bacteroides nodosus* in *Escherichia coli. Infect. Immun.* 51:187–192.

54. Elleman, T. C., P. A. Hoyne, D. J. Stewart, N. M. McKern, and J. E. Peterson. 1986. Expression of pili from *Bacteroides nodosus* in *Pseudomonas aeruginosa. J. Bacteriol.* 168:574–580.

55. Espersen, F., and I. Clemmensen. 1982. Isolation of a fibronectin-binding protein from *Staphylococcus aureus. Infect. Immun.* 37:526–531.

56. Evans, D. G., and D. J. Evans, Jr. 1978. New surface-associated heat-labile colonization factor antigen (CFA/II) produced by enterotoxigenic *Escherichia coli* of serogroups O6 and O8. *Infect. Immun.* 21:638–647.

57. Evans, D. G., R. P. Silver, D. J. Evans, Jr., D. G. Chase, and S. L. Gorbach. 1975. Plasmid-controlled colonization factor associated with virulence in *Escherichia coli* enterotoxigenic for humans. *Infect. Immun.* 12:656–667.

58. Evans, D. J., Jr., D. G. Evans, and H. L. DuPont. 1979. Hemagglutination patterns of enterotoxigenic and enteropathogenic *Escherichia coli* determined with human, bovine, chicken, and guinea pig erythrocytes in the presence and absence of mannose. *Infect. Immun.* 23:336–346.

59. Evans, D. J., Jr., D. G. Evans, L. S. Young, and J. Pitt. 1980. Hemagglutination typing of *Escherichia coli:* definition of seven hemagglutination types. *J. Clin. Microbiol.* 12:235–242.

60. Fader, R. C., L. K. Duffy, C. P. Davis, and A. Kurosky. 1982. Purification and chemical characterization of type 1 pili isolated from *Klebsiella pneumoniae. J. Biol. Chem.* 257:3301–3305.

61. Faris, A., M. Lindahl, and T. Wadström. 1980. GM_2-like glycoconjugate as possible erythrocyte receptor for the CFA/I and K99 haemagglutinins of enterotoxigenic *Escherichia coli. FEMS Microbiol. Lett.* 7:265–269.

62. Feutrier, J., W. W. Kay, and T. J. Trust. 1986. Purification and characterization of fimbriae from *Salmonella enteritidis. J. Bacteriol.* 168:221–227.

63. Ficken, M. D., J. F. Edwards, J. C. Lay, and D. E. Tveter. 1986. Tracheal mucus transport rate in normal turkeys and in turkeys infected with *Bor-*

detella avium (Alcaligenes faecalis). Avian Dis. 30:154–159.

64. Folkhard, W., and D. A. Marvin. 1981. Structure of polar pili from *Pseudomonas aeruginosa* strains K and O. *J. Mol. Biol.* 149:79–93.

65. Formal, S. B., T. L. Hale, and P. J. Sansonetti. 1983. Invasive enteric pathogens. *Rev. Infect. Dis.* 5:S702–S707.

66. Frank, S. K., and J. D. Gerber. 1981. Hydrolytic enzymes of *Moraxella bovis. J. Clin. Microbiol.* 13:269–271.

67. Freter, R. 1981. Mechanisms of association of bacteria and mucosal surfaces, p. 36–55. *In* K. Elliott, M. O'Connor, and J. Whelan (ed.), *Adhesion and Microorganism Pathogenicity*. CIBA Foundation Symposium 80. Pitman Medical Ltd., London.

68. Freter, R., B. Allweiss, P. C. M. O'Brien, S. A. Halstead, and M. S. Macsai. 1981. Role of chemotaxis in the association of motile bacteria with intestinal mucosa: in vitro studies. *Infect. Immun.* 34:241–249.

69. Freter, R., and G. W. Jones. 1983. Models for studying the role of bacterial attachment in virulence and pathogenesis. *Rev. Infect. Dis.* 5:S647–S658.

70. Freter, R., P. C. M. O'Brien, and M. S. Macsai. 1981. Role of chemotaxis in the association of motile bacteria with intestinal mucosa: in vivo studies. *Infect. Immun.* 34:234–240.

71. Gaastra, W., and F. K. de Graaf. 1982. Host-specific fimbrial adhesins and noninvasive enterotoxigenic *Escherichia coli* strains. *Microbiol. Rev.* 46:129–161.

72. Ganaway, J. R., T. H. Spencer, T. D. Moore, and A. M. Allen. 1985. Isolation, propagation, and characterization of a newly recognized pathogen, cilia-associated respiratory bacillus of rats, an etiological agent of chronic respiratory disease. *Infect. Immun.* 47:472–479.

73. Gibbons, R. J., and J. Van Houte. 1971. Selective bacterial adherence to oral epithelial surfaces and its role as an ecological determinant. *Infect. Immun.* 3:567–573.

74. Gibbons, R. J., and J. Van Houte. 1975. Bacterial adherence in oral microbial ecology. *Annu. Rev. Microbiol.* 29:19–44.

75. Gil-Turnes, C., and G. A. Ribeiro. 1985. *Moraxella bovis* hemagglutinins: effect of carbohydrates, heating and erythrocytes. *Can. J. Comp. Med.* 49:112–114.

76. Goldman, W. E. 1986. *Bordetella pertussis* tracheal cytotoxin: damage to the respiratory epithelium, p. 65–69. *In* L. Leive (ed.), *Microbiology—1986*. American Society for Microbiology, Washington, D.C.

77. Goodnow, R. A. 1980. Biology of *Bordetella bronchiseptica. Microbiol. Rev.* 44:722–738.

78. Gordon, L. M., W. K. Yong, and C. A. M. Woodward. 1985. Temporal relationships and characterisation of extracellular proteases from benign and virulent strains of *Bacteroides nodosus* as detected in zymogram gels. *Res. Vet. Sci.* 39:165–172.

79. Guerina, N. G., T. W. Kessler, V. J. Guerina, M. R. Neutra, H. W. Clegg, S. Langermann, F. A. Scannapieco, and D. A. Goldmann. 1983. The role of pili and capsule in the pathogenesis of neonatal infection with *Escherichia coli* K1. *J. Infect. Dis.* 148:395–405.

80. Guyot, G. 1908. Ueber die bakterielle Hämagglutination (Bakterio-haemoagglutination). *Zentralbl. Bakteriol. Abt. 1 Orig. B* 67:640–653.

81. Hale, T. L., and S. B. Formal. 1986. Genetics of virulence in *Shigella. Microb. Pathogenesis* 1:511–518.

82. Hale, T. L., R. E. Morris, and P. F. Bonventre. 1979. Shigella infection of Henle intestinal epithelial cells: role of the host cell. *Infect. Immun.* 24:887–894.

83. Hale, T. L., E. V. Oaks, and S. B. Formal. 1985. Identification and antigenic characterization of virulence-associated, plasmid-coded proteins of *Shigella* spp. and enteroinvasive *Escherichia coli. Infect. Immun.* 50:620–629.

84. Hanamatsu, K. 1985. Adherence of *Moraxella bovis* to tissue culture cells. *Kitasato Arch. Exp. Med.* 58:97–103.

85. Hayashi, A., R. Yanagawa, and H. Kida. 1985. Adhesion of *Corynebacterium renale* and *Corynebacterium pilosum* to epithelial cells of bovine vulva. *Am. J. Vet. Res.* 46:409–411.

86. Henrici, A. T. 1933. Studies of freshwater bacteria. I. A direct microscopic technique. *J. Bacteriol.* 25:277–286.

87. Heukelekian, H., and A. Heller. 1940. Relation between food concentration and surface for bacterial growth. *J. Bacteriol.* 40:547–558.

88. Hodinka, R. L., and P. B. Wyrick. 1986. Ultrastructural study of mode of entry of *Chlamydia psittaci* into L-929 cells. *Infect. Immun.* 54:855–863.

89. Hohmann, A. W., G. Schmidt, and D. Rowley. 1978. Intestinal colonization and virulence of *Salmonella* in mice. *Infect. Immun.* 22:763–770.

90. Honda, E., and R. Yanagawa. 1978. Pili-mediated attachment of *Corynebacterium renale* to mucous membrane of urinary bladder of mice. *Am. J. Vet. Res.* 39:155–158.

91. Hughes, D. E., G. W. Pugh, Jr., and T. J. McDonald. 1965. Ultraviolet radiation and *Moraxella bovis* in the etiology of bovine infectious keratoconjunctivitis. *Am. J. Vet. Res.* 26:1331–1338.

92. Inman, L. R., J. R. Cantey, and S. B. Formal. 1986. Colonization, virulence, and mucosal interaction of an enteropathogenic *Escherichia coli* (strain

RDEC-1) expressing shigella somatic antigen in the rabbit intestine. *J. Infect. Dis.* 154:742–751.

93. Isaacson, R. E. 1977. K99 surface antigen of *Escherichia coli:* purification and partial characterization. *Infect. Immun.* 15:272–279.

94. Isaacson, R. E. 1980. Factors affecting expression of the *Escherichia coli* pilus K99. *Infect. Immun.* 28:190–194.

95. Isaacson, R. E. 1983. Regulation of expression of *Escherichia coli* pilus K99. *Infect. Immun.* 40:633–639.

96. Isaacson, R. E. 1985. Pilus adhesins, p. 307–336. In D. C. Savage and M. Fletcher (ed.), *Bacterial Adhesion Mechanisms and Physiological Significance.* Plenum Publishing Corp., New York.

97. Isaacson, R. E., P. C. Fusco, C. C. Brinton, and H. W. Moon. 1978. In vitro adhesion of *Escherichia coli* to porcine small intestinal epithelial cells: pili as adhesive factors. *Infect. Immun.* 21:392–397.

98. Isaacson, R. E., B. Nagy, and H. W. Moon. 1977. Colonization of porcine small intestine by *Escherichia coli:* colonization and adhesion factors of pig enteropathogens that lack K88. *J. Infect. Dis.* 135:531–539.

99. Isaacson, R. E., and P. Richter. 1981. *Escherichia coli* 987P pilus: purification and partial characterization. *J. Bacteriol.* 146:784–789.

100. Ishikawa, H., and Y. Isayama. 1987. Evidence for sialyl glycoconjugates as receptors for *Bordetella bronchiseptica* on swine nasal mucosa. *Infect. Immun.* 55:1607–1609.

101. Jackman, S. H., and R. F. Rosenbusch. 1984. In vitro adherence of *Moraxella bovis* to intact corneal epithelium. *Curr. Eye Res.* 3:1107–1112.

102. Jackwood, M. W., and Y. M. Saif. 1987. Pili of *Bordetella avium:* expression, characterization, and role in in vitro adherence. *Avian Dis.* 31:277–286.

103. Jackwood, M. W., Y. M. Saif, P. D. Moorhead, and R. N. Dearth. 1985. Further characterization of the agent causing coryza in turkeys. *Avian Dis.* 29:690–705.

104. Johanson, W. G., Jr., D. E. Woods, and T. Chaudhuri. 1979. Association of respiratory tract colonization with adherence of gram-negative bacilli to epithelial cells. *J. Infect. Dis.* 139:667–673.

105. Jones, G. W. 1977. The attachment of bacteria to the surfaces of animal cells, p. 141–176. In J. L. Reissing (ed.), *Microbial Interactions.* Chapman & Hall, Ltd., London.

106. Jones, G. W., G. D. Abrams, and R. Freter. 1976. Adhesive properties of *Vibrio cholerae:* adhesion to isolated rabbit brush border membranes and hemagglutinating activity. *Infect. Immun.* 14:232–239.

107. Jones, G. W., and R. E. Isaacson. 1983. Proteinaceous bacterial adhesins and their receptors. *Crit. Rev. Microbiol.* 10:229–260.

108. Jones, G. W., and J. M. Rutter. 1972. Role of the K88 antigen in the pathogenesis of neonatal diarrhea caused by *Escherichia coli* in piglets. *Infect. Immun.* 6:918–927.

109. Kersters, K., K.-H. Hinz, A. Hertle, P. Segers, A. Lievens, O. Siegmann, and J. De Ley. 1984. *Bordetella avium* sp. nov. isolated from the respiratory tracts of turkeys and other birds. *Int. J. Syst. Bacteriol.* 34:56–70.

110. Klemm, P. 1982. Primary structure of the CFA1 fimbrial protein from human enterotoxigenic *Escherichia coli* strains. *Eur. J. Biochem.* 124:339–348.

111. Klemm, P. 1985. Fimbrial adhesins of *Escherichia coli. Rev. Infect. Dis.* 7:321–340.

112. Knutton, S., D. R. Lloyd, D. C. A. Candy, and A. S. McNeish. 1985. Adhesion of enterotoxigenic *Escherichia coli* to human small intestinal enterocytes. *Infect. Immun.* 48:824–831.

113. Kortt, A. A., J. E. Burns, and D. J. Stewart. 1983. Detection of the extracellular proteases of *Bacteroides nodosus* in polyacrylamide gels: a rapid method of distinguishing virulent and benign ovine isolates. *Res. Vet. Sci.* 35:171–174.

114. Kudo, Y., R. Yanagawa, and T. Hiramune. 1987. Isolation and characterization of monoclonal antibodies against pili of *Corynebacterium renale* and *Corynebacterium pilosum. Vet. Microbiol.* 13:75–85.

115. Kumazawa, N., and R. Yanagawa. 1972. Chemical properties of the pili of *Corynebacterium renale. Infect. Immun.* 5:27–30.

116. Labrec, E. H., H. Schneider, T. J. Magnani, and S. B. Formal. 1964. Epithelial cell penetration as an essential step in the pathogenesis of bacillary dysentery. *J. Bacteriol.* 88:1503–1518.

117. Lark, D. L. 1986. *Protein-Carbohydrate Interations in Biological Systems.* Academic Press, Inc., New York.

118. Laux, D. C., E. F. McSweegan, T. J. Williams, E. A. Wadolkowski, and P. S. Cohen. 1986. Identification and characterization of mouse small intestine mucosal receptors for *Escherichia coli* K-12(K88ab). *Infect. Immun.* 52:18–25.

119. Lawson, M. A., V. Burke, and B. J. Chang. 1985. Invasion of HEp-2 cells by fecal isolates of *Aeromonas hydrophila. Infect. Immun.* 47:680–683.

120. Lee, A., S. M. Logan, and T. J. Trust. 1987. Demonstration of a flagellar antigen shared by a diverse group of spiral-shaped bacteria that colonize intestinal mucus. *Infect. Immun.* 55:828–831.

121. Lee, S. W., B. Alexander, and B. McGowan. 1983. Purification, characterization, and serologic characteristics of *Bacteroides nodosus* pili and use of a purified pili vaccine in sheep. *Am. J. Vet. Res.* 44:1676–1681.

122. Lee, S. W., A. W. Way, and E. G. Osen. 1986. Purification and subunit heterogeneity of pili of

Bordetella bronchiseptica. Infect. Immun. 51:586–593.

123. Lehr, C., H. G. Jayappa, and R. A. Goodnow. 1985. Serologic and protective characterization of *Moraxella bovis* pili. *Cornell Vet.* 75:484–492.

124. Lepper, A. W. D., and L. R. Hermans. 1986. Characterisation and quantitation of pilus antigens of *Moraxella bovis* by ELISA. *Aust. Vet. J.* 63:401–405.

125. Levine, M. M., P. Ristaino, G. Marley, C. Smyth, S. Knutton, E. Boedeker, R. Black, C. Young, M. L. Clements, C. Cheney, and R. Patnaik. 1984. Coli surface antigens 1 and 3 of colonization factor antigen II-positive enterotoxigenic *Escherichia coli*: morphology, purification, and immune responses in humans. *Infect. Immun.* 44:409–420.

126. Lewin, R. 1984. Microbial adhesion is a sticky problem. *Science* 224:375–377.

127. Loesche, W. J. 1986. Role of *Streptococcus mutans* in human dental decay. *Microbiol. Rev.* 50:353–380.

128. Lowe, M. A., S. C. Holt, and B. I. Eisenstein. 1987. Immunoelectron microscopic analysis of elongation of type 1 fimbriae in *Escherichia coli*. *J. Bacteriol.* 169:157–163.

129. Marcus, H., and N. R. Baker. 1985. Quantitation of adherence of mucoid and nonmucoid *Pseudomonas aeruginosa* to hamster tracheal epithelium. *Infect. Immun.* 47:723–729.

130. Mårdh, P.-A., and L. Weström. 1976. Adherence of bacteria to vaginal epithelial cells. *Infect. Immun.* 13:661–666.

131. Marrs, C. F., G. Schoolnik, J. M. Koomey, J. Hardy, J. Rothbard, and S. Falkow. 1985. Cloning and sequencing of a *Moraxella bovis* pilin gene. *J. Bacteriol.* 163:132–139.

132. Marshall, K. C. 1985. Mechanisms of bacterial adhesion at solid-water interfaces, p. 133–161. *In* D. C. Savage and M. Fletcher (ed.), *Bacterial Adhesion Mechanisms and Physiological Significance.* Plenum Publishing Corp., New York.

133. Marshall, K. C. (ed.). 1984. Glossary, p. 397–399. *Microbial Adhesion and Aggregation.* Springer-Verlag, New York.

134. Marshall, K. C., R. Stout, and R. Mitchell. 1971. Mechanism of the initial events in the sorption of marine bacteria to surfaces. *J. Gen. Microbiol.* 68:337–348.

135. Marx, J. L. 1985. A potpourri of membrane receptors. *Science* 230:649–651.

136. Matsuyama, T., and T. Takino. 1980. Scanning electron microscopic studies of *Bordetella bronchiseptica* on the rabbit tracheal mucosa. *J. Med. Microbiol.* 13:159–161.

137. Mattick, J. S., M. M. Bills, B. J. Anderson, B. Dalrymple, M. R. Mott, and J. R. Egerton. 1987. Morphogenetic expression of *Bacteroides no-*

dosus fimbriae in *Pseudomonas aeruginosa. J. Bacteriol.* 169:33–41.

138. McGee, Z. A., D. S. Stephens, L. H. Hoffman, W. F. Schlech III, and R. G. Horn. 1983. Mechanisms of mucosal invasion by pathogenic *Neisseria. Rev. Infect. Dis.* 5:S708–S714.

139. Merritt, G. C., and J. R. Egerton. 1978. IgG$_1$ and IgG$_2$ immunoglobulins to *Bacteroides (Fusiformis) nodosus* protease in infected and immunized sheep. *Infect. Immun.* 22:1–4.

140. Moon, H. W., R. E. Isaacson, and J. Pohlenz. 1979. Mechanisms of association of enteropathogenic *Escherichia coli* with intestinal epithelium. *Am. J. Clin. Nutr.* 32:119–127.

141. Moon, H. W., B. Nagy, R. E. Isaacson, and I. Ørskov. 1977. Occurrence of K99 antigen on *Escherichia coli* isolated from pigs and colonization of pig ileum by K99+ enterotoxigenic *E. coli* from calves and pigs. *Infect. Immun.* 15:614–620.

142. Morris, J. A., C. Thorns, A. C. Scott, W. J. Sojka, and G. A. Wells. 1982. Adhesion in vitro and in vivo associated with an adhesive antigen (F41) by a K99 mutant of the reference strain *Escherichia coli* B41. *Infect. Immun.* 36:1146–1153.

143. Morris, J. A., C. J. Thorns, and W. J. Sojka. 1980. Evidence for two adhesive antigens on the K99 reference strain *Escherichia coli* B41. *J. Gen. Microbiol.* 118:107–113.

144. Moulder, J. W. 1985. Comparative biology of intracellular parasitism. *Microbiol. Rev.* 49:298–337.

145. Mouricout, M. A., and R. A. Julien. 1987. Pilus-mediated binding of bovine enterotoxigenic *Escherichia coli* to calf small intestinal mucins. *Infect. Immun.* 55:1216–1223.

146. Mullany, P., A. M. Field, M. M. McConnell, S. M. Scotland, H. R. Smith, and B. Rowe. 1983. Expression of plasmids coding for colonization factor antigen II (CFA/II) and enterotoxin production in *Escherichia coli. J. Gen. Microbiol.* 129:3591–3601.

147. Niilo, L. 1980. *Clostridium perfringens* in animal disease: a review of current knowledge. *Can. Vet. J.* 21:141–148.

148. Novotny, P., A. P. Chubb, K. Cownley, and J. A. Montaraz. 1985. Adenylate cyclase activity of a 68,000-molecular-weight protein isolated from the outer membrane of *Bordetella bronchiseptica. Infect. Immun.* 50:199–206.

149. Ofek, I., H. Lis, and N. Sharon. 1985. Animal cell surface membranes, p. 71–88. *In* D. C. Savage and M. Fletcher (ed.), *Bacterial Adhesion Mechanisms and Physiological Significance.* Plenum Publishing Corp., New York.

150. Old, D. C. 1972. Inhibition of the interaction between fimbrial haemagglutinins and erythrocytes by D-mannose and other carbohydrates. *J. Gen.*

Microbiol. 71:149–157.

151. Old, D. C., and J. P. Duguid. 1970. Selective outgrowth of fimbriate bacteria in static liquid medium. *J. Bacteriol.* 103:447–456.

152. Oldham, L. J., and F. G. Rodgers. 1985. Adhesion, penetration and intracellular replication of *Legionella pneumophilia:* an *in vitro* model of pathogenesis. *J. Gen. Microbiol.* 131:697–706.

153. Ørskov, I., and F. Ørskov. 1983. Serology of *Escherichia coli* fimbriae. *Prog. Allergy* 33:80–105.

154. Ørskov, I., F. Ørskov, H. W. Smith, and W. J. Sojka. 1975. The establishment of K99, a thermolabile, transmissible *Escherichia coli* K antigen, previously called "Kco," possessed by calf and lamb enteropathogenic strains. *Acta Pathol. Microbiol. Scand. Sect. B* 83:31–36.

155. Ørskov, I., F. Ørskov, W. J. Sojka, and J. M. Leach. 1961. Simultaneous occurrence of *E. coli* B and L antigens in strains from diseased swine. *Acta Pathol. Microbiol. Scand. Sect. B* 53:404–422.

156. Ostle, A. G., and R. F. Rosenbusch. 1984. *Moraxella bovis* hemolysin. *Am. J. Vet. Res.* 45:1848–1851.

157. Ottow, J. C. G. 1975. Ecology, physiology, and genetics of fimbriae and pili. *Annu. Rev. Microbiol.* 29:79–108.

158. Pedersen, K. B., L. O. Frøholm, and K. Bøvre. 1972. Fimbriation and colony type of *Moraxella bovis* in relation to conjunctival colonization and development of keratoconjunctivitis in cattle. *Acta Pathol. Microbiol. Scand. Sect. B* 80:911–918.

159. Pittman, M. 1979. Pertussis toxin: the cause of the harmful effects and prolonged immunity of whooping cough. A hypothesis. *Rev. Infect. Dis.* 1:401–412.

160. Plotkin, B. J., and D. A. Bemis. 1984. Adherence of *Bordetella bronchiseptica* to hamster lung fibroblasts. *Infect. Immun.* 46:697–702.

161. Pugh, G. W., and D. E. Hughes. 1968. Experimental bovine infectious keratoconjunctivitis caused by sunlamp irradiation and *Moraxella bovis* infection: correlation of hemolytic ability and pathogenicity. *Am. J. Vet. Res.* 29:835–839.

162. Punsalang, A. P., Jr., and W. D. Sawyer. 1973. Role of pili in the virulence of *Neisseria gonorrhoeae.* *Infect. Immun.* 8:255–263.

163. Rácz, P., K. Tenner, and E. Mérö. 1972. Experimental Listeria enteritis. I. An electron microscopic study of the epithelial phase in experimental listeria infection. *Lab. Invest.* 26:694–700.

164. Ramphal, R., C. Guay, and G. B. Pier. 1987. *Pseudomonas aeruginosa* adhesins for tracheobronchial mucin. *Infect. Immun.* 55:600–603.

165. Ramphal, R., and G. B. Pier. 1985. Role of *Pseudomonas aeruginosa* mucoid exopolysaccharide in adherence to tracheal cells. *Infect. Immun.* 47:1–4.

166. Ramphal, R., and M. Pyle. 1983. Evidence for mucins and sialic acid as receptors for *Pseudomonas aeruginosa* in the lower respiratory tract. *Infect. Immun.* 41:339–344.

167. Reed, W. M., H. J. Olander, and H. L. Thacker. 1985. Studies on the pathogenesis of *Salmonella heidelberg* infection in weanling pigs. *Am. J. Vet. Res.* 46:2300–2310.

168. Reed, W. P., and R. C. Williams, Jr. 1978. Bacterial adherence: first step in pathogenesis of certain infections. *J. Chronic Dis.* 31:67–72.

169. Reid, G., and J. D. Sobel. 1987. Bacterial adherence in the pathogenesis of urinary tract infections: a review. *Rev. Infect. Dis.* 9:470–487.

170. Reitmeyer, J. C., J. W. Peterson, and K. J. Wilson. 1986. *Salmonella* cytotoxin: a component of the bacterial outer membrane. *Microb. Pathogenesis* 1:503–510.

171. Robins-Browne, R. M. 1987. Traditional enteropathogenic *Escherichia coli* of infantile diarrhea. *Rev. Infect. Dis.* 9:28–53.

171a. Rogers, D. G., N. F. Cheville, and G. W. Pugh. 1987. Pathogenesis of corneal lesions caused by *Moraxella bovis* in gnotobiotic calves. Vet. Pathol. 24:287–295.

172. Rolfe, R. D. 1984. Interactions among microorganisms of the indigenous intestinal flora and their influence on the host. *Rev. Infect. Dis.* 6:S73–S79.

173. Rosenbusch, R. F. 1983. Influence of mycoplasma preinfection on the expression of *Moraxella bovis* pathogenicity. *Am. J. Vet. Res.* 44:1621–1624.

174. Rosenthal, L. 1943. Agglutinating properties of *Escherichia coli*. Agglutination of erythrocytes, leucocytes, thrombocytes, spermatozoa, spores of molds, and pollen by strains of *E. coli*. *J. Bacteriol.* 14:545–550.

175. Runnels, P. L., and H. W. Moon. 1984. Capsule reduces adherence of enterotoxigenic *Escherichia coli* to isolated intestinal epithelial cells of pigs. *Infect. Immun.* 45:737–740.

176. Runnels, P. L., H. W. Moon, and R. A. Schneider. 1980. Development of resistance with host age to adhesion of K99+ *Escherichia coli* to isolated intestinal epithelial cells. *Infect. Immun.* 28:298–300.

177. Rutter, P. R., and B. Vincent. 1984. Physicochemical interactions of the substratum, microorganisms, and the fluid phase, p. 21–38. *In* K. C. Marshall (ed.), *Microbial Adhesion and Aggregation.* Springer-Verlag, New York.

178. Salit, I. E., and E. C. Gotschlich. 1977. Hemagglutination by purified type 1 *Escherichia coli* pili. *J. Exp. Med.* 146:1169–1181.

179. Sansonetti, P. J., D. J. Kopecko, and S. B. Formal. 1981. *Shigella sonnei* plasmids: evidence that a large plasmid is necessary for virulence. *In-*

fect. Immun. 34:75–83.

180. **Sansonetti, P. J., D. J. Kopecko, and S. B. Formal.** 1982. Involvement of a plasmid in the invasive ability of *Shigella flexneri. Infect. Immun.* 35:852–860.

181. **Sansonetti, P. J., A. Ryter, P. Clerc, A. T. Maurelli, and J. Mounier.** 1986. Multiplication of *Shigella flexneri* within HeLa cells: lysis of the phagocytic vacuole and plasmid-mediated contact hemolysis. *Infect. Immun.* 51:461–469.

182. **Sato, H., R. Yanagawa, and H. Fukuyama.** 1982. Adhesion of *Corynebacterium renale, Corynebacterium pilosum,* and *Corynebacterium cystitidis* to bovine urinary bladder epithelial cells of various ages and levels of differentiation. *Infect. Immun.* 36:1242–1245.

183. **Schifferli, D. M., S. N. Abraham, and E. H. Beachey.** 1986. Influence of trimethoprim and sulfamethoxazole on the synthesis, expression, and function of type 1 fimbriae of *Escherichia coli. J. Infect. Dis.* 154:490–496.

184. **Schoolnik, G. K., R. Fernandez, J. Y. Tai, J. Rothbard, and E. C. Gotschlich.** 1984. Gonococcal pili. Primary structure and receptor binding domain. *J. Exp. Med.* 159:1351–1370.

185. **Sellwood, R., R. A. Gibbons, G. W. Jones, and J. M. Rutter.** 1975. Adhesion of enteropathogenic *Escherichia coli* to pig intestinal brush borders: the existence of two pig phenotypes. *J. Med. Microbiol.* 8:405–411.

186. **Serény, B.** 1957. Experimental keratoconjunctivitis shigellosa. *Acta Microbiol. Acad. Sci. Hung.* 4:367–376.

187. **Shibl, A. M.** 1985. Effect of antibiotics on adherence of microorganisms to epithelial cell surfaces. *Rev. Infect. Dis.* 7:51–65.

188. **Silverblatt, F. J., J. S. Dreyer, and S. Schauer.** 1979. Effect of pili on susceptibility of *Escherichia coli* to phagocytosis. *Infect. Immun.* 24:218–223.

189. **Silverblatt, F. J., and I. Ofek.** 1978. Influence of pili on the virulence of *Proteus mirabilis* in experimental hematogenous pyelonephritis. *J. Infect. Dis.* 138:664–667.

190. **Simpson, C. F., F. H. White, and T. S. Sandhu.** 1976. The structure of pili (fimbriae) of *Moraxella bovis. Can. J. Comp. Med.* 40:1–4.

191. **Smith, H. W., and J. E. T. Jones.** 1963. Observations on the alimentary tract and its bacterial flora in healthy and diseased pigs. *Pathol. Bacteriol.* (*J. Pathol. Bacteriol.*) 86:387–412.

192. **Smith, H. W., and M. A. Linggood.** 1972. Further observations on *Escherichia coli* enterotoxins with particular regard to those produced by atypical piglet strains and by calf and lamb strains: the transmissible nature of these enterotoxins and of a K antigen possessed by calf and lamb strains. *J. Med. Microbiol.* 5:243–250.

193. **Smyth, C. J.** 1982. Two mannose-resistant haemagglutinins on enterotoxigenic *Escherichia coli* of serotype O6:K15:H16 or H⁻ isolated from travellers' and infantile diarrhoea. *J. Gen. Microbiol.* 128:2081–2096.

194. **Snyder, S. H.** 1985. The molecular basis of communication between cells. *Sci. Am.* 253:132–141.

195. **Stanislawski, L., W. A. Simpson, D. Hasty, N. Sharon, E. H. Beachey, and I. Ofek.** 1985. Role of fibronectin in attachment of *Streptococcus pyogenes* and *Escherichia coli* to human cell lines and isolated oral epithelial cells. *Infect. Immun.* 48:257–259.

196. **Stephens, D. S., J. W. Krebs, and Z. A. McGee.** 1984. Loss of pili and decreased attachment to human cells by *Neisseria meningitidis* and *Neisseria gonorrhoeae* exposed to subinhibitory concentrations of antibiotics. *Infect. Immun.* 46:507–513.

197. **Steven, A. C., M. E. Bisher, B. L. Trus, D. Thomas, J. M. Zhang, and J. L. Cowell.** 1986. Helical structure of *Bordetella pertussis* fimbriae. *J. Bacteriol.* 167:968–974.

198. **Stewart, D. J.** 1978. The role of various antigenic fractions of *Bacteroides nodosus* in eliciting protection against footrot in vaccinated sheep. *Res. Vet. Sci.* 24:14–19.

199. **Svanborg Edén, C., and H. A. Hansson.** 1978. *Escherichia coli* pili as possible mediators of attachment to human urinary tract epithelial cells. *Infect. Immun.* 21:229–237.

200. **Swanson, J.** 1983. Gonococcal adherence: selected topics. *Rev. Infect. Dis.* 5:S678–S684.

201. **Swanson, J., S. J. Kraus, and E. C. Gotschlich.** 1971. Studies on gonococcus infection. I. Pili and zones of adhesion: their relation to gonococcal growth patterns. *J. Exp. Med.* 134:886–906.

202. **Takeuchi, A.** 1967. Electron microscope studies of experimental salmonella infection. I. Penetration into the intestinal epithelium by *Salmonella typhimurium. Am. J. Pathol.* 50:109–136.

203. **Tuomanen, E.** 1986. Piracy of adhesins: attachment of superinfecting pathogens to respiratory cilia by secreted adhesins of *Bordetella pertussis. Infect. Immun.* 54:905–908.

204. **Tuomanen, E.** 1986. Adherence of *Bordetella pertussis* to human cilia: implications for disease prevention and therapy, p. 59–64. *In* L. Leive (ed.), *Microbiology—1986.* American Society for Microbiology, Washington, D.C.

205. **Tuomanen, E., and A. Weiss.** 1985. Characterization of two adhesins of *Bordetella pertussis* for human ciliated respiratory-epithelial cells. *J. Infect. Dis.* 152:118–125.

206. **Tuomanen, E. I., and J. O. Hendley.** 1983. Adherence of *Bordetella pertussis* to human respiratory epithelial cells. *J. Infect. Dis.* 148:125–130.

207. **Tuomanen, E. I., J. Nedelman, J. O. Hendley, and E. L. Hewlett.** 1983. Species specificity of *Bordetella* adherence to human and animal ciliated

respiratory epithelial cells. *Infect. Immun.* 42:692–695.

208. **Urisu, A., J. L. Cowell, and C. R. Manclark.** 1986. Filamentous hemagglutinin has a major role in mediating adherence of *Bordetella pertussis* to human WiDr cells. *Infect. Immun.* 52:695–701.

209. **Van Houte, J.** 1983. Bacterial adherence in the mouth. *Rev. Infect. Dis.* 5:3659–3669.

210. **Vogelweid, C. M., R. B. Miller, J. N. Berg, and D. A. Kinden.** 1986. Scanning electron microscopy of bovine corneas irradiated with sun lamps and challenge exposed with *Moraxella bovis. Am. J. Vet. Res.* 47:378–384.

211. **Watt, P. J., and M. E. Ward.** 1980. Adherence of *Neisseria gonorrhoeae* and other *Neisseria* species to mammalian cells, p. 253–288. *In* E. H. Beachey (ed.), *Bacterial Adherence.* Chapman & Hall, New York.

212. **Weiss, A. A., G. A. Myers, J. K. Crane, and E. L. Hewlett.** 1986. *Bordetella pertussis* adenylate cyclase toxin: structure and possible function in whooping cough and the pertussis vaccine, p. 70–74. *In* L. Leive (ed.), *Microbiology—1986.* Amer-ican Society for Microbiology, Washington, D.C.

213. **Wicken, A. J.** 1985. Bacterial cell walls and surfaces, p. 45–70. *In* D. C. Savage and M. Fletcher (ed.), *Bacterial Adhesion Mechanisms and Physiological Significance.* Plenum Publishing Corp., New York.

214. **Yanagawa, R., and K. Otsuki.** 1970. Some properties of the pili of *Corynebacterium renale. J. Bacteriol.* 101:1063–1069.

215. **Yokomizo, Y., and T. Shimizu.** 1979. Adherence of *Bordetella bronchiseptica* to swine nasal epithelial cells and its possible role in virulence. *Res. Vet. Sci.* 27:15–21.

216. **Zhang, J. M., J. L. Cowell, A. C. Steven, P. H. Carter, P. P. McGrath, and C. R. Manclark.** 1985. Purification and characterization of fimbriae isolated from *Bordetella pertussis. Infect. Immun.* 48:422–427.

217. **Zhang, J. M., J. L. Cowell, A. C. Steven, and C. R. Manclark.** 1985. Purification of serotype 2 fimbriae of *Bordetella pertussis* and their identification as a mouse protective antigen. *Dev. Biol. Stand.* 61:173–185.

218. **ZoBell, C. E.** 1943. The effect of solid surfaces upon bacterial activity. *J. Bacteriol.* 46:39–56.

Chapter 2

Molecular and Genetic Basis of Adherence for Enteric *Escherichia coli* in Animals

RICHARD E. ISAACSON

Department of Immunology and Infectious Diseases
Pfizer, Incorporated
Central Research Division
Groton, Connecticut 06340

INTRODUCTION

The initiation of most bacterial infections, whether they are invasive or not, depends on the ability of the organism to colonize a mucosal site. Several factors contribute to the ability of an organism to colonize a site; however, the net result is characterized by the maintenance of a stable or increasing population that is larger than normal. In general, colonization is facilitated by an association of bacteria with mucosal surfaces. The mechanism by which enterotoxigenic *Escherichia coli* (ETEC) colonize small intestines is direct attachment to the brush border membranes on enterocytes. In experimental infections in neonatal pigs, virulent ETEC may achieve mucosal populations of 10^9 cells per cm (29, 57, 82). Animals thus infected exhibit severe weight loss (as much as 25% of their body weight) and die within 24 h of challenge. Normally the *E. coli* population in neonatal pigs is less than 10^4 cells per cm. Although the ability to attach to enterocytes is necessary for colonization, it is not always sufficient. Other surface characteristics including capsules and outer membranes frequently are important to the colonization process.

For ETEC as well as several other *E. coli* pathogens, mucosal attachment is mediated by bacterial structures called pili. The following discussion briefly describes the evidence that pili are important adhesins (also called pilus adhesins) and then focuses on the molecular and genetic basis of pilus-mediated attachment. Several reviews have been written on these subjects (19, 29, 39, 43).

PILI AS ADHESINS

The initial identification of factors associated with ETEC colonization was based on epidemiologic studies. The observation in 1966 of association of an antigen called K88 with virulent ETEC led to the conclusion that this antigen promoted the colonization of small intestines of neonatal pigs (66). Experiments by Smith and Linggood (82) demonstrated that K88$^+$ ETEC intensively colonized small intestines of pigs. During the initial characterization of K88, it was recognized that K88 was encoded on a transmissible plasmid (4, 66). This observation allowed Smith and Linggood (82) to construct a series of K88$^+$ and K88$^-$ ETEC strains to be used as experimental challenges to infect neonatal pigs. Only K88$^+$ ETEC were virulent and colonized the small intestines of the pigs. A K88$^-$ ETEC strain that was made K88$^+$, by reintroduction of the K88 plasmid, regained its ability to colonize small intestines, and therefore its virulence was restored. The mucosal surfaces of tissues obtained from pigs challenged with K88$^+$ ETEC were heavily covered with E. coli, which is characteristic of the colonization process (3, 5, 58). The bacteria appeared to attach directly to the tissue surface on the basis of direct observation after staining with Giemsa or after staining with specific fluorescent labeled antibodies. Purification of K88 led to the observation that the physical organization of K88 was a filamentous structure resembling pili (or fimbriae) (84, 85). The fact that K88 was filamentous made it an ideal candidate as an adhesin on the basis of the predictions of the Derjaguin-Landau-Verwey-Overbeek (DLVO) theory (69, 72, 88, 91) (see Chapter 1 of this volume).

Additional pilus structures were ultimately identified as relevant adhesins by similar techniques and by using in vitro procedures. The current list of structures includes K88, K99, 987P, F41, FY, CFA/I, CFA/II, and AFR-1. CFA/II has subsequently been divided into three antigenically distinct groups: CS1, CS2, and CS3 (55). Classically, these adhesins have shown restricted species specificity (K88 and 987P pili are specific for pigs; K99 and F41 pili are specific for pigs, calves, and lambs; FY pili are specific for calves; CFA/I and CFA/II pili are specific for humans; and AFR-1 pili are specific for rabbits). Type 1 pili (also called common or somatic pili or fimbriae) are frequently found on ETEC and have been shown to recognize mannose-containing structures as receptors (16, 61), although no in vivo role has been ascribed to this structure. However, type 1 pili have been extensively studied, and since they may function as adhesins and certainly can serve as a prototypic structure of pili, they will be included in the following discussion.

The use of genetically constructed strains provides powerful evidence that certain pili are important colonization factors. As further evidence supporting this role, experiments were performed to show that these structures were produced in vivo. Segments of small intestines colonized by piliated ETEC have a characteristic fluorescent layer covering the mucosal surface when stained with pilus-specific fluorescent antibodies and observed by fluorescence microscopy, demonstrating that these structures are indeed produced in vivo (33, 51). Furthermore, supporting these observations, it is known that pilus-specific antibodies can be used to prevent colonization of small intestines and thus to prevent disease (2, 38, 56, 59, 70). Vaccination of pregnant pigs or calves with purified pili stimulates the production of antibodies against pili. Piglets, for example, that suckle vaccinated dams receive pilus-specific antibodies in colostrum and milk and consequently are protected against diarrheal disease caused by ETEC.

Although the results of in vivo experiments support a role for pili in the colonization of small intestines, they may not be used to draw conclusions about the specific role(s) of pili. The best evidence supporting the hypothesis that some pili are adhesins was derived from in vitro adhesion experiments. Piliated E. coli producing K88, K99, 987P, or type 1 pili adhere to slices of small intestines (40), to intact enterocytes (43, 58, 94), and to brush border membranes (71, 76) isolated from piglets, whereas isogenic, nonpiliated strains do not. CFA/I- and CFA/II-producing E. coli strains adhere to human intestinal cells and to transformed human intestinal cell lines (48). AFR-1-producing cells adhere to rabbit enterocytes (8). Nonagglutinating antibodies (Fab fragments) prepared against purified pili inhibit the attachment of piliated bacteria to enterocytes (32). However, Fab fragments against surface antigens other than pili do not affect attachment in vitro, demonstrating a specific role of pili as adhesins.

The results of competitive inhibition experiments with purified pili as the competitor demonstrate the high degree of specificity of the adhesive properties of *E. coli* pili (32). Purified pili competitively inhibit the attachment of bacteria producing the same pili for sites on enterocytes, but do not compete with bacteria producing different pili. Therefore, it can be concluded that pili bind to enterocytes, that the pili on *E. coli* cells mediate the attachment of the cells to the enterocyte, and the binding is specific (i.e., each pilus has a unique binding site or receptor).

STRUCTURE AND BIOCHEMISTRY OF PILI

Pili are defined as filamentous, hairlike surface structures of bacteria. The term fimbriae is a synonym. The pili on *E. coli* cells are peritrichous and are polymers composed of identical protein subunits called pilin (29, 39). Each type of pilus is composed of unique pilin molecules. The numer of pilin units and the manner of pilin association dictate the length, diameter, and molecular weight of an intact pilus. On any given cell there is an array of pilus lengths; however, the diameter is fixed. The forces holding pilin molecules together are unknown but do not include covalent bonds. It is known that intrachain disulfide bonds in K99, 987P, and type 1 pili are important for the molecular conformations of these pili (31, 34, 37, 47). Two models of subunit association have been put forth and can be used to describe two morphologically distinct pilus structures (29). The first group is defined as having a rigid structure. This group is exemplified by 987P and type 1 pili. These structures typically have uniform cross-sectional diameters and an axial hole (6, 34). 987P and type 1 pili are both 7 nm in diameter. The subunits appear to be organized as a helical structure with subunit interactions at the ends and sides (Fig. 1). Owing to this manner of association, the movement of the subunits is constrained, generating the overall rigid structure with well-defined cross-sectional diameter. For type 1 pili, the helix has been shown

to be right-handed, having 3 1/8 subunits per revolution (6). Pili of this class readily aggregate into highly ordered, parallel bundles. This suggests a highly precise interaction between subunits from individual pili. The pilus bundles also can associate with other bundles to form angle-layered crystals. The angle between the bundles is related to the subunit pitch in the pilus helix (6). The second group of pili appears morphologically to be flexible and is exemplified by K88 and K99. These structures have also been called fibrillae. The model for this class is also helical, but the pilin molecules do not have side-side interactions (Fig. 1). This type of structure is less ordered, which is consistent with the electron micrographs of K99, for which the cross-sectional diameter (2 to 8.4 nm) (13, 26, 90) appears to be much less precise than that of 987P (26, 90). K99 also forms parallel bundles; however, like the model of the K99 pilus structure, these bundles are less

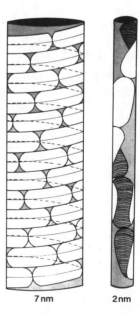

FIGURE 1. Schematic diagram of pili. The left structure is representative of type 1 pili with 3 1/8 subunits per revolution. The diameter is 7 nm. The right structure is a possible configuration of K99. K99 as drawn would be more flexible than type 1 pili. These diagrams are from reference 29, reprinted with permission of Plenum Publishing Corp.

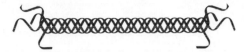

FIGURE 2. Model showing a possible helical association of K99 pili.

ordered. The K99 bundles appear to wrap around each other to form a loose, helical bundle (Fig. 2).

Pili readily dissociate into free subunits in the presence of sodium dodecyl sulfate, guanidine, or dilute acid. They may be separated electrophoretically or by other physical means. Free 987P (73) or type 1 (18) pilin obtained by treatment of intact pili with guanidine assembles into pili upon removal of the guanidine by dialysis. This assembly process in vitro is slow. Therefore, it is suggested that assembly in vivo is catalyzed by other cellular components. Consistent with this, it is now known that the in vivo expression and assembly of pili appear to be highly regulated and quite complex processes, requiring several different polypeptides (see below).

Pilin molecules are composed primarily of protein (29, 39). The molecular weights of some of the E. coli pilin molecules are shown in Table 1. Several non-amino acid substitutions have been detected on certain pili and include phosphate (6, 86), simple sugars (6, 34), and phospholipid (unpublished data). Whether these substituents are integral parts of the pilin mol-

ecules or simply contaminants left during purification is not known. However, when the hexosamine of 987P is cleaved by periodate, the pilus loses its ability to bind to its eucaryotic receptor, suggesting that the carbohydrate is important for the recognition of the 987P receptor (E. A. Dean, Ph.D. thesis, University of Michigan, Ann Arbor, 1984). This property is not unique to 987P, since the treatment of pili from Neisseria gonorrhoeae with periodate or galactosidase also abolishes its receptor-binding activity (22).

The amino acid compositions of several pilin molecules are shown in Table 2. Each contains about 50% nonpolar amino acids. The relative hydrophobicity of these pilin molecules has been calculated by using the values of amino acid hydrophobicity derived by Nozaki and Tanford (60). Values range from -511 to -648 cal/mol per amino acid ($-2,138$ to $-2,711$ J/mol per amino acid). All of these pilin molecules are less hydrophobic than human serum albumin (-769 cal/mol per amino acid [$-3,217$ J/mol per amino acid]). Nonetheless, the presence of pili on bacterial cells markedly increases their overall hydrophobicity. Type 1 pili reduce the electrophoretic mobility of E. coli cells and alter the phase partitioning of cells in polyethylene glycol-dextran (6). All of the E. coli pili promote the adsorption of cells to hydrophobic gels such as phenyl- or octyl-Sepharose (83, 90). The hydrophobic binding properties of pili have been successfully exploited as a potential target for anti-infective therapy by preventing colonization of small intestines by ETEC. The oral administration of hydrophobic gels to pigs reduces adherence and thus virulence of ETEC in vivo (90). Thus, one can conclude that hydrophobic interactions are promoted by pili and that these interactions may play a significant role in the attachment of bacterial cells to mucosal surfaces.

Charge interactions between bacteria and target cells, as predicted by the DLVO theory, also play a particularly significant role in the attachment process. The charge of the pilus

TABLE 1
Properties of various E. coli pilin molecules

Pilus	Pilin mol wt	pI (non-amino acid substitution)
K88ab	26,200	4.2
K88ad	26,000	ND[a]
K99	18,200	10.1
		(phosphatidylethanolamine)
987P	20,000	3.7
		(hexosamine)
F41	29,500	ND
CFA/I	14,500	ND
Type 1	17,100	3.9

[a]ND, Not determined.

TABLE 2
Amino acid composition of *E. coli* pilin molecules

Amino acid	Composition in:						
	K88ab	K88ab	K99	987P	Type 1	F41	CFA/I
Lysine	12	8	9	10	3	12	8
Arginine	7	8	4	2	3	6	3
Histidine	0	2	0	0	2	4	1
Aspartic	28	30	25	34	20	27	18
Threonine	27	23	20	28	20	18	13
Serine	16	20	12	23	10	33	11
Glutamic	16	20	7	16	13	24	12
Proline	6	9	3	8	2	11	4
Glycine	35	34	15	26	17	39	11
Alanine	27	27	46	26	34	16	16
Cysteine	0	0	2	2	2	ND[a]	0
Valine	18	22	14	15	13	17	13
Methionine	2	4	3	1	0	3	2
Isoleucine	10	13	13	12	4	10	6
Leucine	18	20	7	17	10	14	11
Tyrosine	8	9	0	1	0	13	4
Phenylalanine	10	10	0	3	8	9	3
Tryptophan	ND	4	3	1	0	ND	ND
Hydroxylysine	0	0	3	0	0	10	0
% Nonpolar	52.5	52.8	54.7	48.4	54.6	48.1	48.5
Hydrophobicity (J/mol per amino acid)	−2,548	−2,771	−2,414	−1,920	−2,138	−2,163	−2,489

[a]ND, Not determined.

therefore contributes to the overall attractive and repulsive forces between the bacterial cell and its target cell. Most pili are negatively charged structures, which should act to increase the repulsive forces. K99 is an exception, with an isoelectric point of pI 10 (26). This property makes K99 a particularly interesting adhesin, since it could promote attachment to mucosal surfaces solely on the basis of charge. Many of the in vitro adhesion data provide support for the conclusion that pilus-mediated attachment to musosal surfaces is highly specific. On the basis of the repulsive charge interactions predicted for most pili, the presence of highly specific receptors is necessary for colonization by most ETEC strains. It is likely that the positive charge of K99 serves to stabilize the interaction between bacterium and target. However, the establishment of specific, irreversible attachment is ultimately dependent on interactions with K99-specific receptors.

SEROLOGIC ANALYSIS OF PILI

The proteinaceous nature of pili makes them good antigens. This feature, coupled with the central role that certain pili play in virulence, has been successfully exploited to produce efficacious vaccines for ETEC-induced diarrhea (2, 3, 5, 56, 59, 70). However, to achieve broad-spectrum protection against the various potential ETEC pathogens, it has been necessary to mix various pili (30, 52), because antigenic cross-reactions among pili are limited. Antigenic relatedness among the different *E. coli* pilus adhesins has not been detected, with the sole exception of the K88 group. To date, three antigenic variants of K88 have been detected. Each contains a common *a* epitope(s) and a *b*, *c*, or *d* epitope (23, 24). Fortunately, the *a* epitope is protective, and therefore broad-spectrum protection against K88[+] ETEC strains is conferred by vaccination with a single variant of K88. By generating hydrophobicity plots to predict potential epitopes, it has been possible to locate regions in the K88 primary structure that are likely to represent the *a* sites as well as the variant *b*, *c*, and *d* sites (Fig. 3) (20).

Antigenic relatedness has been detected among a large group of structures classified as type 1 pili (38). This group initially was defined as pili that were mannose-sensitive hemagglutinins (a property known to be associated with type 1 pili). Type 1 pili also fall into a group of structures having similar morphology and amino acid sequence homolgy. There are members of this large type 1 pilus group, such as the F7 pilus, that have significant aminoterminal amino acid sequence homology with type 1 pili and yet are serologically unrelated (44, 67).

Recent studies with monoclonal antibodies have been used to map the locations of specific epitopes and correlate these sites with function. Monoclonal antibodies have, for example, been prepared against 987P pili and, on the basis of their reactivities, can be divided into three groups (73; unpublished data). Members of the first group of monoclonal antibodies prevent adhesion of 987P to mucosal target cells, cross-link the pili (or cause agglutination of piliated cells), and recognize dissociated pilin molecules (i.e., can be used in Western blots [immunoblots]). Members of the second group also recognize a site involved in adhesion, but this site is destroyed when pili are dissociated into pilin subunits. Members of the third group recognize only pilin subunits and prevent pilin from assembling into intact pili. Presumably, members of the third group recognize sites involved in subunit interactions which are exposed only when subunits are separated. Since this monoclonal antibody also recognizes the tips of 987P pili (identification of these monoclonal antibodies was by enzyme-linked immunosorbent assay with intact pili, and therefore they must recognize an epitope that resides on the pilus tip) and yet does not interfere with adhesion, it can be concluded that the pilus receptor interacts with a site located along the pilus side. Members of the second group of monoclonal antibodies demonstrate the presence of epitopes generated by quaternary structure, since recognition of the epitope is abolished upon disaggregation of the pilus structure into pilin. This is potentially significant in that any analysis of pilus funtion is complicated by the need to include sites generated by pilin-pilin interactions. When analyzing hydrophobicity plots, we must consider not only secondary and tertiary structure, but also quaternary structure. Preliminary experiments with monoclonal antibodies to K99 reveal a similar array of epitopes.

GENETICS OF PILUS ADHESINS

Considerable progress has been made toward the understanding of the genetic basis of pilus adhesins. Elegant studies, involving a variety of techniques, have been carried out to identify the genetic loci of pilus adhesins (K88 is on a 50-megadalton (MDa) plasmid; K99 is on a 58-MDa plasmid; CFA/I and CFA/II are on a 60-MDa plasmid; and 987P, F41, and type 1 are on the chromosome) and to understand the expression of these virulence factors.

The gene locus for type 1 pili was first identified by classical genetics (7). Various Hfr

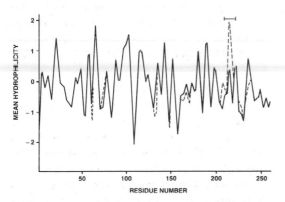

Figure 3. Plot of calculated hydrophilicity of the K88ab (-----) and K88ad (———) primary structures. The area in brackets indicates a major difference between the two and may represent the *d* epitope. Other hydrophilic regions may represent the *a* epitope.

strains were used in mating experiments with a stably nonpiliated recipient. Initial experiments showed a linkage with *ara*. In experiments involving interrupted matings, the type 1 pilus locus was ultimately assigned a map position of 98 min. The recent molecular cloning of type 1 pilus genes has provided evidence confirming that the type 1 pilus is encoded on the chromosome (64). Complementation analyses were performed by construction of double mutants with one mutation residing on the chromosome and the other on an F′ plasmid, F101 (87). F101 was used in these experiments since it contains the markers *thr*, *leu*, and *ara* and also specifies production of type 1 pili. Three complementation groups were identified and were designated *pilA*, *pilB*, and *pilC*.

The molecular cloning of the 987P (11, 53) and F41 (54) genes and subsequent DNA-DNA hybridization experiments have provided evidence that these pilus adhesins are encoded on the chromosome.

The genes encoding several other *E. coli* pilus adhesins have been associated with plasmids. Bak et al. (4) demonstrated that K88 was plasmid encoded. Smith and Linggood (82) later showed that in some cases K88 was self-transmissible. Subsequently it was shown that K88 was associated with a 50-MDa nonconjugative plasmid or with larger conjugative plamids (78). Frequently the ability to ferment raffinose also is encoded on the K88 plasmid. The genes encoding K99 also have been associated with a plasmid having a molecular mass of 58 MDa (35, 89). The genes for CFA/I (46, 81) and CFA/II (68) have been associated with different plasmids of 60 MDa. Also encoded on the CFA/II plasmid is the gene for heat-stable enterotoxin. Confirmation of plasmid loci for this group of pilus adhesins has been established by molecular cloning.

Genetic Organization of Pili

The genetic organization of K88, K99, 987P and type 1 pili has been determined by recombinant DNA technology.

K88 Pili

K88ab (49) and K88ac (77) have both been individually cloned from naturally occurring plasmids. Each is encoded on a 6.5-kilobase-pair (kb) *Hin*dIII-*Eco*RI restriction fragment, with a second *Eco*RI site located in the K88 structural gene (Fig. 4). Minicell-producing *E. coli* organisms containing either of the K88 recombinant plasmids were used to determine the number and size of polypeptides encoded by the cloned K88 fragments. Each encodes polypeptides of 81, 27.5, 27, 26, and 17 kDa for K88ab and 70, 29, 26, 23.5, and 17 kDa for K88ac. The 26- and 23.5-kDa polypeptides are the K88ab and the K88ac structural genes, respectively. The organization and locations of the specific cistrons on the cloned fragments were determined by deletion mapping (50) and insertional mutagenesis (15, 41) and are shown in Fig. 4. The organizations of both are nearly identical. A major difference between the two is that K88ab appears to be encoded by a single transcriptional unit that utilizes a promoter on the cloning vector for expression (50), while K88ac is encoded by two transcriptional units (41).

The functions of the various polypeptides, other than the K88 structural genes, have been deduced by a variety of techniques. For K88ab (50), the 81-kDa polypeptide is believed to be involved in subunit translocation from the periplasm to the outer membrane; the 17-kDa polypeptide modifies the subunit such that it is functional when assembled. A role for the 27.5-kDa polypeptide has not been determined.

The K88ac polypeptides are assumed to function in the following manner (15, 41). The 70-kDa polypeptide, like the large 81-kDa polypeptide for K88ab, is assumed to be an anchor for K88 in the outer membrane. The 29- and 17-kDa polypeptides are probably involved in polymerization of the pilin subunits into intact K88, even though the 17-kDa

FIGURE 4. Genetic maps of cloned pilus genes along with assignments of the locations of the various polypeptides encoded by these DNA segments.

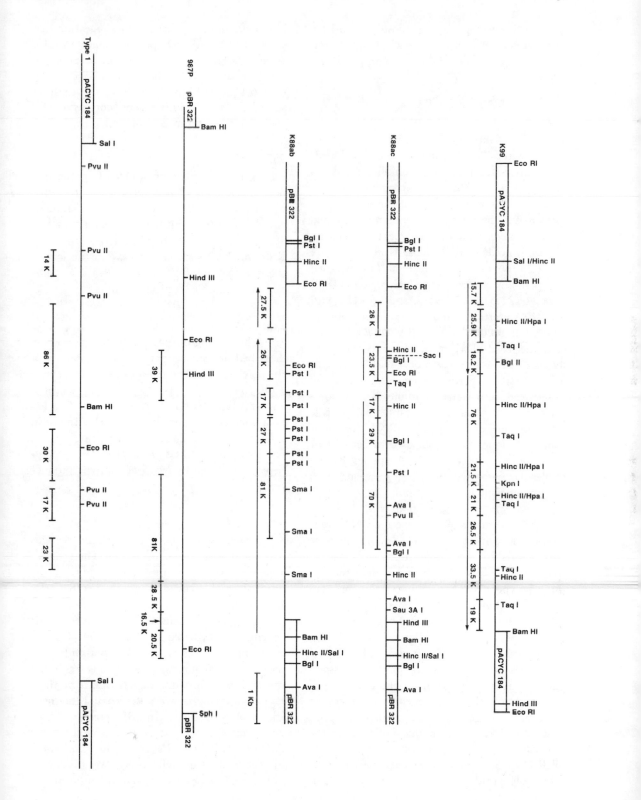

polypeptide was previously considered to be a positive regulator of the K88ac subunit cistron (41). The role of the 26-kDa polypeptide is not known.

K99 Pili

A 7.15-kb *Bam*HI restriction fragment from a naturally occurring plasmid was cloned, and cells containing the recombinant plasmid produced K99 (35, 89). Recombinants produced 4- to 40-fold-greater amounts of assembled K99. The recombinant plasmids specified between seven and nine polypeptides ranging in size from 15.7 to 76 kDa. Using a series of deletion mutants, de Graaf et al. (14) assigned the positions of seven of the polypeptides (18.2, 19, 21, 21.5, 65.5, 33.5, and 76 kDa [Fig. 4]). By insertional mutagenesis (unpublished data), the region between the left *Bam*HI site and the 18.2-kDa polypeptide was shown to be required for expression of K99. On the basis of expression experiments involving the use of insertional mutations in minicells, the locations of a 15.7- and a 25.5-kDa polypeptide were assigned (Fig. 4). DNA-RNA hybridization techniques have been used to detect four separate K99-specific mRNA species having molecular sizes of 9.15, 2.37, 1.47, and 0.76 kb (manuscript in preparation). The most predominant species is the 0.76-kb mRNA, which hybridizes with a K99 pilin-specific DNA probe and therefore must encode K99 pilin, while the largest mRNA species hybridizes with a DNA probe that covers the region encoding the 76-kDa polypeptide. Subcloning techniques can be used to divide the K99 genes into two complementation groups. The deduced functions of the polypeptides are as follows. The 18.2-kDa polypeptide is the K99 pilin gene. The 19- and 26.5-kDa polypeptides are physically associated with the K99 pilin on the basis of immunoprecipitation experiments and therefore have been suggested to be required for pilus assembly. Strains containing mutations in the 19-kDa polypeptide produce the normal array of K99-specific polypeptides (except for the 19-kDa polypeptide) but do not produce assem-

bled structures, supporting the suggestion that the role of the 19-kDa polypeptide is in pilus assembly. The roles of the remaining polypeptides are unknown, although the large size of the 76-kDa polypeptide is similar to the presumed 81- and 70-kDa anchor proteins of K88 and may serve a similar function.

987P Pili

A 12-kb chromosomal DNA fragment has been molecularly cloned and encodes the ability to produce 987P pili (11). This fragment encodes five polypeptides: 16.5, 20.5, 28.5, 39, and 81 kDa. Methods similar to those for K88 and K99 were used to assign the loci of the five cistrons (Fig. 4). The 20.5-kDa polypeptide is the 987P pilin subunit.

Type 1 Pili

The cloning of type 1 pili, like the others described above, has permitted an analysis of the polypeptides required for expression of type 1 pili (64, 65). Five polypeptides are required: 14, 17, 23, 30, and 86 kDa (Fig. 4). The 17-kDa polypeptide (encoded by *pilA*) is the pilin subunit, and the 23-kDa polypeptide plays a regulatory role. Mutations in the 23-kDa polypeptide (encoded by *hyp*) lead to hyperproduction of the *pilA* gene.

CFA/I Pili

Fewer details are known about the genetics and organization of CFA/I. The genetics appear to be more complex than those of the other plasmid-encoded pilus adhesins (81, 93). Genetically, CFA/I production is dependent on two noncontiguous DNA fragments. This conclusion was based on the results of insertional mutagenesis of a CFA/I plasmid. Mutations at two nonadjacent regions abolished the ability to produce CFA/I. Each of these regions was cloned: a 7.8-kb *Hin*dIII fragment and a 2.1-kb *Eco*RI-*Hin*dIII fragment (93). Alone, neither was capable of specifying production of CFA/I. However, when both were present in the same cell, CFA/I was produced. When each was introduced into minicells, it was shown that the smaller, 2.1-kb, fragment encoded three polypeptides (25.7, 14.9, and 13.9 kDa), while the larger, 7.8-kb, fragment encoded six polypeptides (13.3, 24.6, 26.9, 29.4, 38.8, and 85 kDa) (92). The 13.3-kDa polypeptide is believed to be the CFA/I pilin gene on the basis of its ability to react with anti-CFA/I.

Pilus Adhesin Production

The expression of pili can be divided into two general categories. The first is a qualitative process called phase variation (6, 62, 63). This is an all-or-none reversible process, with the rates of conversion from one phase to the other being greater than mutation rates and being characteristic of the organism, adhesin, and culture conditions. Not all pili are subject to phase variation. A second process is quantitative variation. As the name implies, this process governs the actual number of pili produced.

Pilus Phase Variation

E. coli type 1 and 987P pili undergo phase variation. In the laboratory, depending upon the method of culture, cultures containing cells in either phase can be grown. In general, aerobic growth selects for the nonpiliated phase, whereas growth at reduced levels of oxygen selects for the piliated phase (6, 62, 63). Growth of 987P-producing *E. coli* organisms in pigs results in the selection of cells in the piliated phase, suggesting that piliation in vivo is advantageous compared with the nonpiliated phase (58). Accompanying the change from one phase to the other is a corresponding change of the morphology of colonies growing on semisolid media (6, 58). Colonies containing piliated cells tend to be translucent, small, and cohesive, whereas colonies containing nonpiliated cells are the opposite.

The mechanism of pilus phase variation is believed to be similar to the mechanism of *Salmonella* flagellar phase variation, in which the switching between phenotypes results from the precise inversion of a DNA sequence (79). Several lines of evidence support this hypothesis. The first is based on results from Mu d*lac* fusions with type 1 pilus genes (17). The Mu bacteriophage contains the gene encoding β-galactosidase (*lacZ*); however, this gene is not expressed because it lacks a promoter. When the phage integrates into a gene near a promoter, the *lacZ* gene may be expressed by using the host promoter to initiate transcription. If the bacteria used for the fusion are Lac$^-$, such fusions will result in a Lac$^+$ phenotype. Fusions of Mu phage to *pil* genes were constructed, and expression of *lacZ* was shown to be regulated by the *pil* gene promoter. Lac$^+$ and Lac$^-$ clones were isolated; each was shown to undergo a transition to the other phenotype. Since promoters control transcription, it was concluded that phase variation was controlled at the transcriptional level. Orndorff et al. (65) confirmed these results by creating independent *pilA-lacZ* fusions and demonstrating that the expression of *lacZ* was now controlled by a *pilA* region and was subject to phase variation. The kinetics of the *lacZ* phase variation were of a similar magnitude to those obtained for pilus phase variation (ca. 4×10^{-4} per cell per generation). The Mu-*pil* fusions were cloned into a lambda phage and used to construct merodiploids in *pil*-positive cells (17). The switching phase was found to be *cis*-active.

However, the best evidence to support this hypothesis is based on direct observation of an invertible element adjacent to the type 1 structural gene (*pilA*) (1). Using well-characterized Mu-*pilA* fusions, Abraham et al. showed that upstream from *pilA* was a 314-base-pair region that was capable of inverting (1). In one orientation *pilA* was expressed, while in the other orientation *pilA* was not expressed.

Quantitative Pilus Variation

Pili such as K88, K99, and CFA/I do not appear to be subject to phase variation. Most, if not all, pili are, however, subject to quantitative variation. The most extensively studied example of quantitative variation pertains to K99.

Environmental factors known to influence K99 production include aeration, glucose, L-alanine, growth rate, and temperature of incubation (6, 12, 25, 27, 28, 36, 90). K99$^+$ *E. coli* incubated at 37°C produce pili on the surface (i.e., assembled K99) exclusively during the exponential phase of growth (27, 28, 36). The degree of aeration affects the number of pili on the cell surface. Vigorous shaking increases aeration, which results in increased piliation; poor aeration results in the opposite effect. This result may be explained by alteration of growth rates in response to various degrees of aeration. Glucose added to the growth medium suppresses piliation, the degree of suppression being correlated with the amount of glucose and the basal medium. Glucose in a rich medium such as tryptic soy broth results in a high degree of K99 suppression. Cyclic AMP alleviates the glucose-mediated repression. Interestingly, glucose in minimal medium does not significantly reduce piliation.

More extensive studies have confirmed that K99 genes are subject to glucose-mediated catabolite repression. The K99 plasmid was transferred to a mutant in which the enzyme adenylate cyclase (*cya*) was not produced (28). This strain produced normal quantities of cell-surface-associated K99, suggesting that the glucose effect observed with rich medium was not related to the K99 genes. However, when the actual synthesis of K99 subunits was measured, rather than the degree of piliation (i.e., measuring subunits and not the amount of assembled pilus on the cell surface), the *cya* mutation effected a dramatic reduction on subunit synthesis (ca. 33-fold). The synthesis of subunits was also determined during various phases of bacterial growth and compared with the amount of K99 on the cell surface. While K99 appeared to be assembled on the cell surface exclusively during the exponential phase, subunits were synthesized continuously during all phases of growth. It was concluded, therefore, that K99 expression could be divided into two interactive but independent steps: subunit synthesis, which is subject to catabolite repression, and pilus assembly.

In experiments to further profile the physiology of K99 expression, the effect of inhibiting protein synthesis on K99 expression was determined (28). Chloramphenicol added to actively growing K99$^+$ cultures stopped subunit synthesis, while assembly proceeded normally. Therefore, assembly does not require active protein synthesis and probably draws on a pool of subunits known to exist in the outer membrane of the cell. The results from the *cya* mutant experiments indicate that a 33-fold reduction of the subunit pool does not affect assembly. Thus, a substantial pool must normally exist which, even when subunit synthesis is inhibited, is still ample for pilus assembly. In wild-type strains, K99 subunits are synthesized in great excess and stored in the outer membrane. A small fraction is ultimately assembled into functional pili. An interesting question that remains to be addressed is that of why cells would produce such an excess of K99 subunits.

The facts that K99 is a membrane protein synthesized with a 3-kDa leader sequence (14) and that an outer membrane subunit pool exists (28) suggest that the membrane(s) plays an integral role in expression. Cells grown at 18°C fail to synthesize and assemble the pilus. Likewise, cells grown at 37°C in the presence of excess L-alanine also fail to synthesize and assemble the pilus. Both conditions result in altered cell membranes, which are therefore presumed to be necessary for K99 expression. Interestingly, most other *E. coli* pili also are not produced when cells are incubated at 18°C.

Genetic Relatedness of Pilus Adhesins

Homologies among the DNA sequences of various pilin genes have been sought. It was previously believed that there was a limited degree of homology between K88 and K99 (42); however, attempts to confirm these results have not been successful (54; unpublished data). A small *Hin*fI DNA probe that encodes the entire K99 pilin gene failed to hybridize with DNA from K88$^+$ and 987P$^+$ ETEC (Fig. 5). This probe did hybridize to DNA from K99$^+$

strains. In similar experiments, K88- and F41-specific gene probes hybridized only with DNA from K88- or F41-producing cells, respectively. Moseley et al. (54) did show, however, that there was DNA homology between the coding regions of F41 and K88 as measured by Southern DNA-DNA hybridization, although this homogy was localized to accessory polypeptide sequences and not the pilin genes.

Among ETEC strains producing K99, the plasmids encoding K99 have been highly conserved. The screening of a battery of K99$^+$ ETEC showed that K99 plasmids retained a similar size (58 MDa [Fig. 5]). Furthermore, restriction endonuclease analysis demonstrated that with a single exception, K99 remained encoded on a 7.15-kb BamHI fragment.

ADHESIN RECEPTORS

The interaction between adhesin and receptor must be specific and result in selective adhesion of the bacterium to a surface. Direct evidence for the existence of specific receptors has been derived in part from studies on the pathogenesis of K88$^+$ ETEC. In particular, it has been shown that some pigs are resistant to disease caused by K88$^+$ ETEC and that K88$^+$ strains fail to attach to the brush border membranes of these pigs (71, 78). These results suggest that the resistant pigs lack the receptor for K88. The results of in vitro adhesion experiments, particularly those demonstrating competitive inhibition by purified pili, also strongly support the existence of specific receptors for K88, K99, 987P, and type 1 pili (32). Receptors on the target cells provide the apparent selectivity to the adhesive process. The distribution of receptors on animal cells may be diverse. Some adhesins specific for the gastrointestinal tract, for example, also recognize receptors on certain erythrocytes. In some instances the receptor is distributed on nontarget cells. This property has been particularly useful in the identification of strains that are potentially adhesive pathogens. The early evaluation of the adhesiveness of type 1 pili and several other pilus adhesins was based on hemagglutination properties. Most receptors appear to be glycoconjugates, with the sugar residues providing an essential recognition site. Interaction of adhesins with substrates containing correct carbohydrates, although not the natural support, may occur and appear to be selective. Type 1 pili recognize free mannose as well as mannose on erythrocytes and on the yeast cell polymer mannan (16, 61). Other receptors are

A a b c d e f g h i j k l m n o p q r s   B a b c d e f g h i j k l m n o p q r s

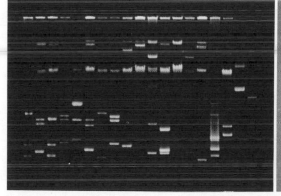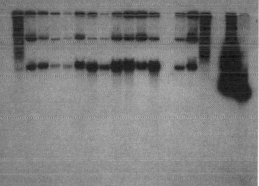

FIGURE 5. (A) Agarose gels of plasmids obtained from K99$^+$ (lanes a to l and n to p), K88$^+$ (lane m), and 987P$^+$ (lane q) E. coli and stained with ethidium bromide. Lane r, Recombinant K99 plasmid; lane s, the pure BamHI restriction fragment encoding K99. (B) Autoradiogram from a Southern hybridization with the plasmids in panel A and a small HinfI DNA probe encoding the entire K99 pilin gene.

discussed below. The relevance of any receptor is therefore dependent upon the demonstration of biological activity.

K88 Receptor

The hemagglutinating activity of K88 can be inhibited by glycoprotein obtained from porcine colostrum (21). Treatment of the glycoproteins to remove terminal β-D-galactose residues results in the loss of inhibitor activity. β-D-Galactose also prevents the attachment of purified K88 to neonatal porcine brush borders (74). Other experiments have suggested that N-acetylglucosamine, N-acetylgalactosamine, and D-galactosamine may also be important sugars in the K88 receptor (75). Recent attempts to isolate the receptor from mouse mucus and brush borders has resulted in the identification of 57- and 64-kDa proteins that possess K88 receptor activity (45).

987P Receptor

The adult rabbit small intestine has been used as a model for studying 987P pilus-receptor interactions as well as 987P receptor structure (9). Although $987P^+$ ETEC are not pathogens of adult rabbits, several properties of the rabbit make it well suited to such studies. First, there is age specificity. Infant rabbits lack the receptor and thus may be used as mutants. Second, the interaction is specific in that purified 987P pili prevent in vitro attachment of piliated cells to the epithelium of the small intestine. Third, other piliated *E. coli* cells do not adhere to adult rabbit small intestine, except for the rabbit pathogen RDEC. The rabbit receptor has been purified from brush border membranes by methanol-chloroform extraction and gel filtration chromatography (10). The receptor can be stained with periodic acid-Schiff reagent, demonstrating that it contains carbohydrate groups. Treatment with periodate, pronase, or proteinase K abolishes receptor activity. Several lipases, phospholipases, and boiling, however, have no effect on receptor activity. Thus, it was concluded that the receptor was a glycoprotein. The lectin

soybean agglutinin, which recognizes D-galactose and N-acetylgalactosamine, also prevents pilus-receptor interaction, suggesting that one of these sugars is important for receptor activity.

K99 Receptor

Smit et al. (80) isolated and identified a receptor from equine erythrocytes that was specific for K99. Although equine erythrocytes are not the natural target cells for K99, the purified receptor competitively inhibited the attachment of $K99^+$ cells to porcine small intestinal epithelial cell receptor. The receptor was characterized as a glycolipid having the structure N-acetylneuraminic $\alpha(2\rightarrow3)$-galactose $\beta(1\rightarrow4)$-glucose $\beta(1\rightarrow1)$-ceramide.

AFR-1 Receptor

The rabbit receptor for the AFR-1 pilus of the rabbit enteric pathogen RDEC has been partially purified and appears to be associated with the isomaltase enzyme complex (8).

CONCLUSIONS

The understanding of bacterial adhesion has been stimulated by the recognition of the importance of this process in the pathogenesis of diseases caused by bacteria. The most thoroughly studied examples have been the ETEC strains that infect livestock. Such investigations were greatly facilitated, since these organisms are natural pathogens of animals and therefore relevant infection models, primarily in pigs, were developed. Although our understanding of ETEC adhesion is well advanced, compared with other bacterial species, it is obvious that we still lack a precise understanding of the molecular and genetic processes involved. The expression of pilus structures is a complex process that requires accessory proteins. These proteins are likely to be required as gene regulators and aids in assembly and structure transport. Pilus-adhesin-specific receptors also are beginning to be isolated and characterized.

The adhesive characteristics of other enteric *E. coli* pathogens such as classical enteropathogenic, enteroadherent, enteroeffacing, and invasive strains, as well as those causing weanling diarrhea, are poorly, if at all, understood. As more information is obtained regarding these pathogens, rational strategies similar to those currently being used for ETEC will be developed to control these pathogens. In addition to the development of vaccines, an understanding of the interaction(s) between adhesin and receptor should lead to novel modes to prevent or intervene in the infectious-disease process.

LITERATURE CITED

1. Abraham, J. M., C. S. Freitag, J. R. Clements, and B. I. Eisenstein. 1985. An invertible element of DNA controls phase variation of type 1 fimbriae of *Escherichia coli*. *Proc. Natl. Acad. Sci. USA* 82:5724–5727.

2. Acres, S. D., R. E. Isaacson, L. A. Babiuk, and R. A. Kapitany. 1979. Immunization of calves against enterotoxigenic colibacillosis by vaccinating dams with purified K99 antigen and whole cell bacterins. *Infect. Immun.* 25:121–126.

3. Arbuckle, J. B. R. 1970. The location of *Escherichia coli* in the pig intestine. *J. Med. Microbiol.* 3:333–340.

4. Bak, A. L., G. Christiansen, C. Christiansen, A. Stenderup, I. Ørskov, and F. Ørskov. 1972. Circular DNA molecules controlling synthesis and transfer of the surface antigen (K88) in *Escherichia coli*. *J. Gen. Microbiol.* 73:373–385.

5. Bertschinger, H. U., and H. W. Moon. 1972. Association of *Escherichia coli* with the small intestinal epithelium. I. Comparison of enteropathogenic and nonenteropathogenic porcine strains in pigs. *Infect. Immun.* 5:595–605.

6. Brinton, C. C. 1965. The structure, function, synthesis and genetic control of bacterial pili and a molecular model for DNA and RNA transport in gram negative bacteria. *Trans. N.Y. Acad. Sci.* 27:1003–1054.

7. Brinton, C. C., P. Gemski, S. Falkow, and L. S. Baron. 1961. Location of the piliation factor on the chromosome of *Escherichia coli*. *Biochem. Biophys. Res. Commun.* 5:293–298.

8. Cheney, C. P., and E. C. Boedecker. 1984. Appearance of host intestinal receptors for pathogenic *E. coli* with age, p. 157–166. *In* E. C. Boedecker (ed.), *Attachment of Organisms to the Gut Mucosa*, vol. 2. CRC Press, Inc., Boca Raton, Fla.

9. Dean, E. A., and R. E. Isaacson. 1982. In vitro adhesion of piliated *Escherichia coli* to small intestinal villous epithelial cells from rabbits and the identification of a soluble 987P pilus receptor-containing factor. *Infect. Immun.* 36:1192–1198.

10. Dean, E. A., and R. E. Isaacson. 1985. Purification and characterization of a receptor for the 987P pilus of *Escherichia coli*. *Infect. Immun.* 47:98–105.

11. de Graaf, F. K., and P. Klaasen. 1986. Organization and expression of genes involved in the biosynthesis of 987P fimbriae. *Mol. Gen. Genet.* 204:75–81.

12. de Graaf, F. K., P. Klaasen-Boor, and J. E. vanHess. 1980. Biosynthesis of the K99 surface antigen is repressed by alanine. *Infect. Immun.* 30:125–128.

13. de Graaf, F. K., P. Klemm, and W. Gaastra. 1981. Purification, characterization, and partial covalent structure of *Escherichia coli* adhesive antigen K99. *Infect. Immun.* 33:877–883.

14. de Graaf, F. K., B. E. Krenn, and P. Klaasen. 1984. Organization and expression of genes involved in the biosynthesis of K99 fimbriae. *Infect. Immun.* 43:508–514.

15. Dougan, G., G. David, and M. Kehoe. 1983. Organization of K88ac encoded polypeptides in the *Escherichia coli* cell envelope: use of minicells and outer membrane protein mutants for studying assembly of pili. *J. Bacteriol.* 153:364–370.

16. Duguid, J. P., and D. C. Old. 1980. Adhesive properties of Enterobacteriaceae, p. 185–217. *In* E. H. Beachy (ed.), *Bacterial Adherence*. Chapman & Hall, Ltd., London.

17. Eisenstein, B. 1981. Phase variation of type 1 fimbriae in *Escherichia coli* is under transcriptional control. *Science* 214:337–339.

18. Eshdat, Y., F. J. Silverblatt, and N. Sharon. 1981. Dissociation and reassembly of *Escherichia coli* type 1 pili. *J. Bacteriol.* 148:308–314.

19. Gaastra, W., and F. K. de Graaf. 1982. Host-specific fimbrial adhesins of noinvasive enterotoxigenic *Escherichia coli* strains. *Microbiol. Rev.* 46:129–161.

20. Gaastra, W., P. Klemm, and F. K. de Graaf. 1983. The nucleotide sequence of the K88ad protein subunit of porcine enterotoxigenic *Escherichia coli*. *FEMS Microbiol. Lett.* 18:177–183.

21. Gibbons, R. A., G. W. Jones, and R. Sellwood. 1975. An attempt to identify the intestinal receptor for the K88 adhesin by means of a haemagglutination inhibition test using glycoproteins and fractions from sow colostrum. *J. Gen. Microbiol.* 86:228–240.

22. Gubish, E. R., K. D. S. Chen, and T. M. Buchanan. 1982. Attachment of gonococcal lectrin-resistant clones of Chinese hamster ovary cells. *Infect. Immun.* 37:189–194.

23. Guinee, P. A. M., and W. H. Jansen. 1979. Be-

havior of *Escherichia coli* antigens K88ab, K88ac, and K88ad in immunoelectrophoresis, double diffusion, and hemagglutination. *Infect. Immun.* 23:700–705.

24. Guinee, P. A. M., F. R. Mooi, and W. H. Jansen. 1980. Preparation of specific *Escherichia coli* K88 antisera by means of purified K88ab and K88ad antigens. *Zentralbl. Bakteriol. Parasitenkd. Infekionskr. Hyg. Abt. 1 Orig. Reihe A* 248:182–89.

25. Guinee, P. A. M., J. Velkamp, and W. H. Hansen. 1977. Improved Minca medium for the detection of K99 antigen in calf enterotoxigenic strains of *Escherichia coli. Infect. Immun.* 15:676–678.

26. Isaacson, R. E. 1977. K99 surface antigen of *Escherichia coli*: purification and partial characterization. *Infect. Immun.* 15:272–279.

27. Isaacson, R. E. 1980. Factors affecting the expression of the *Escherichia coli* pilus K99. *Infect Immun.* 28:190–194.

28. Isaacson, R. E. 1983. Regulation of the *Escherichia coli* pilus K99. *Infect Immun.* 40:633–639.

29. Isaacson, R. E. 1985. Pilus adhesins, p. 307–336. In D. C. Savage and M. Fletcher (ed.), *Bacterial Adhesion.* Plenum Publishing Corp., New York.

30. Isaacson, R. E. 1985. Development of vaccines for bacterial diseases using recombinant DNA technology. *Avian Dis.* 30:28–36.

31. Isaacson, R. E., J. Colmenero, and P. Richter. 1981. *Escherichia coli* K99 pili are composed of one subunit species. *FEMS Microbiol. Lett.* 12:229–232.

32. Isaacson, R. E., P. C. Fusco, C. C. Brinton, and H. W. Moon. 1978. In vitro adhesion of *Escherichia coli* to porcine small intestinal epithelial cells: pili as adhesive factors. *Infect. Immun.* 21:392–397.

33. Isaacson, R. E., H. W. Moon, and R. A. Schneider. 1978. Distribution and virulence of *Escherichia coli* in the small intestines of calves with and without diarrhea. *Am. J. Vet. Res.* 39:1750–1755.

34. Isaacson, R. E., and P. Richter. 1981. *Escherichia coli* 987P pilus: purification and partial characterization. *J. Bacteriol.* 146:784–789.

35. Isaacson, R. E., and P. Richter. 1983. Molecular and genetic analysis of K99 plasmids, p. 179–190. In S. Acres (ed.), *Fourth International Symposium on Neonatal Diarrhea.* Veterinary Infectious Disease Organization, Saskatoon, Sask., Canada.

36. Jacobs, A. A. C., and F. K. de Graaf. 1985. Production of K88, K99, and F41 fibrillae in relation to growth phase, and a rapid procedure for adhesin purification. *FEMS Microbiol. Lett.* 26:15–19.

37. Jann, K., B. Jann, and G. Schmidt. 1981. SDS polyacrylamide gel electrophoresis and serological analysis of pili from *Escherichia coli* of different pathogenic origin. *FEMS Microbiol. Lett.* 11:21–25.

38. Jayappa, H. G., J. G. Strayer, R. A. Goodnow, P. C. Fusco, S. W. Wood, P. Haneline, H.-J. Cho, and C. C. Brinton. 1983. Experimental infection and field trial evaluations of a multiple-pilus

phase-cloned bacterin for the simultaneous control of neonatal colibacillosis and mastitis in swine, p. 518–547. In S. Acres (ed.), *Fourth International Symposium on Neonatal Diarrhea.* Veterinary Infectious Disease Organization, Saskatoon, Sask., Canada.

39. Jones, G. W., and R. E. Isaacson. 1983. Proteinaceous bacterial adhesins and their receptors. *Crit. Rev. Microbiol.* 10:229–260.

40. Jones, G. W., and J. M. Rutter. 1974. Role of the K88 antigen. Protection against disease by neutralizing the adhesive properties of K88 antigen. *Infect. Immun.* 6:918–927.

41. Kehoe, M., R. Sellwood, P. L. Shipley, and G. Dougan. 1981. Genetic analysis of K88-mediated adhesion of enterotoxigenic *Escherichia coli. Nature* (London) 291:122–126.

42. Kehoe, M., M. Winther, G. Dowd, P. Morrissey, and D. Dougan. 1982. Nucleotide sequence homology between the K88 and K99 adhesion system of enterotoxigenic *Escherichia coli. FEMS Microbiol. Lett.* 14:129–132.

43. Klemm, P. 1985. Fimbrial adhesins of *Escherichia coli. Rev. Infect. Dis.* 7:321–340.

44. Klemm, P., I. Ørskov, and F. Ørskov. 1982. F7 and type 1-like fimbriae from three *Escherichia coli* strains isolated from urinary tract infections: protein, chemical, and immunological aspects. *Infect. Immun.* 36:462–468.

45. Laux, D. C., E. F. McSweegan, T. J. Williams, E. A. Wadolkowski, and P. S. Cohen. 1986. Identification and characterization of mouse small intestine mucosal receptors for *Escherichia coli* K-12(K88ab). *Infect. Immun.* 52:18–25.

46. McConnell, M. M., H. R. Smith, G. A. Willshaw, A. M. Field, and B. Rowe. 1981. Plasmids coding for colonization factor antigen I and heat stable enterotoxin production isolated from enterotoxigenic *Escherichia coli*: comparison of their properties. *Infect. Immun.* 32:927–936.

47. McMichael, J. C., and J. T. Ou. 1979. Structure of common pili from *Escherichia coli. J. Bacteriol.* 138:969–975.

48. McNeish, A. S., P. Turner, J. Fleming, and N. Evans. 1975. Mucosal adherence of human enteropathogenic *Escherichia coli. Lancet* ii:946–948.

49. Mooi, F. R., F. K. de Graaf, and J. D. A. van Embden. 1979. Cloning, mapping and expression of the genetic determinant that encodes for the K88ab antigen. *Nucleic Acids Res.* 6:849–865.

50. Mooi, F. R., N. Harms, D. Bakker, and F. K. de Graaf. 1981. Organization and expression of genes involved in the production of the K88ab antigen. *Infect. Immun.* 32:1155–1163.

51. Moon, H. W., E. M. Kohler, R. A. Schneider, and S. C. Whipp. 1980. Prevalence of pilus antigens, enterotoxin types, and enteropathogenicity among K88-negative enterotoxigenic *Escherichia coli*

from neonatal pigs. *Infect. Immun.* 27:222–230.

52. Morgan, R. L., R. E. Isaacson, H. W. Moon, C. C. Brinton, and C. C. To. 1978. Immunization of suckling pigs against enterotoxigenic *Escherichia coli*-induced diarrheal disease by vaccinating dams with purified 987 or K99 pili: protection correlates with pilus homology of vaccine and challenge. *Infect. Immun.* 22:771–777.

53. Morrissey, P. M., and G. Dougan. 1986. Expression of a cloned 987P adhesion-antigen fimbrial determinant in *Escherichia coli* K-12 strain. *Gene* 43:79–84.

54. Moseley, S. L., G. Dougan, R. A. Schneider, and H. W. Moon. 1986. Cloning of chromosomal DNA encoding the F41 adhesin of enterotoxigenic *Escherichia coli* and genetic homology between adhesins F41 and K88. *J. Bacteriol.* 167:799–804.

55. Mullany, P., A. M. Field, M. M. McConnell, S. M. Scotland, and B. Rowe. 1983. Expression of plamids coding for colonization factor antigen II (CFA/II) and enterotoxin production in *Escherichia coli*. *J. Gen Microbiol.* 129:3591–3601.

56. Nagy, B. 1980. Vaccination of cows with a K99 extract to protect newborn calves against experimental enterotoxic colibacillosis. *Infect. Immun.* 27:21–24.

57. Nagy, B., H. W. Moon, and R. E. Isaacson. 1976. Colonization of porcine small intestines by *Escherichia coli*: ileal colonization and adhesion by pig enteropathogens that lack K88 antigen and by some acapsular mutants. *Infect. Immun.* 13:1214–1220.

58. Nagy, B., H. W. Moon, and R. E. Isaacson. 1977. Colonization of porcine small intestines by enterotoxigenic *Escherichia coli*: selection of piliated forms in vivo, adhesion of piliated forms to epithelial cells in vitro, and incidence of a pilus antigen among porcine enteropathogenic *Escherichia coli*. *Infect. Immun.* 16:344–352.

59. Nagy, B., H. W. Moon, R. E. Isaacson, and C. C. Brinton. 1978. Immunization of suckling pigs against enterotoxigenic *Escherichia coli* infection by vaccinating dams with purified pili. *Infect. Immun.* 21:269–274.

60. Nozaki, L., and C. Tanford. 1971. The solubility of amino acid and two glycine peptides in aqueous ethanol and dioxane solutions. *J. Biol. Chem.* 246:2211–2217.

61. Old, D. C. 1972. Inhibition of the interaction between fimbrial hemagglutinins and erythrocytes by D-mannose and other carbohydrates. *J. Gen. Microbiol.* 71:149–157.

62. Old, D. C., and J. P. Duguid. Selective outgrowth of fimbriate bacteria in static medium. *J. Bacteriol.* 103:447–456.

63. Old, D. C., I. Cornell, L. F. Gibson, A. D. Thomson, and J. P. Duguid. 1968. Fimbriation pellicle formation and the amount of growth of *Salmonella* in broth. *J. Gen. Microbiol.* 51:1–16.

64. Orndorff, P. E., and S. Falkow. 1984. Organization and expression of genes responsible for type 1 piliation in *Escherichia coli*. *J. Bacteriol.* 159:736–744.

65. Orndorff, P. E., P. A. Spears, D. Schauer, and S. Falkow. 1985. Two modes of control of *pilA*, the gene encoding type 1 pilin in *Escherichia coli*. *J. Bacteriol.* 164:321–330.

66. Ørskov, I., and F. Ørskov. 1966. Episome-carried surface antigen K88 of *Escherichia coli*. I. Transmission of the determinant of the K88 antigen and influence on the transfer of chromosomal markers. *J. Bacteriol.* 91:69–75.

67. Ørskov, I., F. Ørskov, and A. Birch-Andersen. 1980. Comparison of *Escherichia coli* fimbrial antigen F7 with type 1 fimbriae. *Infect. Immun.* 27:657–666.

68. Penaranda, M. E., G. G. Evans, B. E. Murray, and D. J. Evans. 1983. ST:LT:CFA/II plasmids belonging to serogroups O6, O8, O85, and O139. *J. Bacteriol.* 154:980–983.

69. Pethica, B. A. 1980. Microbial and cell adhesion, p. 9–45. *In* R. C. W. Berkeley, J. M. Lynch, J. Melling, P. R. Rutter, and B. Vincent (ed.), *Microbial Adhesion to Surfaces.* Ellis Horwood, Chichester, England.

70. Runnels, P. L., S. L. Moseley, and H. W. Moon. 1987. F41 pili as protective antigens of enterotoxigenic *Escherichia coli* that produce F41, K99, or both pilus antigens. *Infect. Immun.* 55:555–558.

71. Rutter, J. M., M. R. Burrows, R. Sellwood, and R. A. Gibbons. 1975. A genetic basis for resistance to enteric disease caused by *E. coli*. *Nature* (London) 257:135–136.

72. Rutter, P. R., and B. Vincent. 1980. The adhesion of microorganisms to surfaces: physico-chemical aspects, p. 79–92. *In* R. C. W. Berkeley, J. M. Lynch, J. Melling, P. R. Rutter, and B. Vincent (ed.), *Microbial Adhesion to Surfaces.* Ellis Horwood, Chichester, England.

73. Schifferli, D. M., A. N. Abraham, and E. H. Beachey. 1987. Use of monoclonal antibodies to probe subunit- and polymer-specific epitopes of 987P fimbriae of *Escherichia coli*. *Infect. Immun.* 55:923–930.

74. Sellwood, R. 1980. The interaction of the K88 antigen with porcine intestinal epithelial cell brush-borders. *Biochim. Biophys. Acta* 632:326–335.

75. Sellwood, R. 1984. An intestinal receptor for the K88 antigen of porcine enterotoxigenic *Escherichia coli*, p. 167–175. *In* E. C. Boedecker (ed.), *Attachment of Organisms to the Gut Mucosa*, vol. 2. CRC Press, Inc., Boca Raton, Fla.

76. Sellwood, R., R. A. Gibbons, G. W. Jones, and J. M. Rutter. 1975. Adhesions of enteropathogenic *Escherichia coli* to pig intestinal brush-borders: the existence of two pig phenotypes. *J. Med. Microbiol.* 8:405–411.

77. Shipley, P. L., G. Dougan, and S. Falkow. 1981. Identification and cloning of the genetic determinant

that encodes for the K88ac adherence antigen. *J. Bacteriol.* 145:920–925.

78. Shipley, P. L., C. L. Gyles, and S. Falkow. 1978. Characterization of plasmids that encode the K88 colonization antigen. *Infect. Immun.* 20:559–566.

79. Silverman, M., and M. Simon. 1980. Phase variation: genetic analysis of switching mutants. *Cell* 19:845–854.

80. Smit, H., W. Gaastra, J. P. Kamerling, J. F. G. Vliengenthart, and F. K. de Graaf. 1984. Isolation and structural characterization of the equine erythrocyte receptor for enterotoxigenic *Escherichia coli* K99 fimbrial adhesin. *Infect. Immun.* 46:578–584.

81. Smith H. R., G. A. Willshaw, and B. Rowe. 1982. Mapping of a plasmid, coding for colonization factor antigen I and heat-stable enterotoxin production, isolated from an enterotoxigenic strain of *Escherichia coli. J. Bacteriol.* 149:264–275.

82. Smith, H. W., and M. A. Linggood. 1971. Observations on the pathogenic properties of *K88, Hly,* and *Ent* plasmids of *Escherichia coli* with particular reference to porcine diarrhea. *J. Med. Microbiol.* 4:467–485.

83. Smyth, C., P. Jonsson, E. Soderlund, J. Rosengren, S. Hjerten, and T. Wadstrom. 1978. Differences in hydrophobic surface characteristics of porcine enteropathogenic *Escherichia coli* with and without K88 antigen as revealed by hydrophobic interaction chromatography. *Infect. Immun.* 22:462–472.

84. Spears, P. A., D. Schauer, and P. E. Orndorff. 1986. Metastable regulation of type 1 piliation in *Escherichia coli* and isolation and characterization of a phenotypically stable mutant. *J. Bacteriol.* 168:179–185.

85. Stirm, S., F. Ørskov, I. Ørskov, and A Birch-Anderson. 1967. Episome-carried surface antigen K88 of *Escherichia coli.* III. Morphology. *J. Bacteriol.* 93:740–748.

86. Stirm, S., F. Ørskov, I. Ørskov, and B. Mansa. 1967. Episome-carried surface antigen K88 of *Escherichia coli.* II. Isolation and chemical analysis. *J. Bacteriol.* 93:731–739.

87. Swaney, L. M., Y.-P. Liu, K. Ippen-Ihler, and C. C. Brinton. 1977. Genetic complementation analysis of *Escherichia coli* type 1 somatic pilus mutants. *J. Bacteriol.* 130:506–511.

88. Tadros, T. F. 1980. Particle-surface adhesion, p. 93–116. *In* R. C. W. Berkeley, J. M. Lynch, J. Melling, P. R. Rutter, and B. Vincent (ed.), *Microbial Adhesion to Surfaces.* Ellis Horwood, Chichester, England.

89. van Embden, J. D. A., F. K. de Graaf, L. M. Schouls, and J. S. Teppema. 1980. Cloning and expression of a deoxyribonucleic acid fragment that encodes the adhesive antigen K99. *Infect. Immun.* 29:1125–1133.

90. Wadstrom, T., C. J. Smyth, A. Faris, P. Jonsson, and J. H. Freer. 1978. Hydrophobic absorptive and hemagglutinating properties of enterotoxigenic *Escherichia coli* with different colonizing factors: K88, K99, and colonization factor antigens and adherence factor, p. 29–45. *In* S. Acres (ed.), *Second International Symposium on Neonatal Diarrhea.* Veterinary Infectious Disease Organization, Saskatoon, Sask., Canada.

91. Weiss, L., and J. P. Harlos. 1972. Short term interations between cell surfaces. *Prog. Surf. Sci.* 1:355–405.

92. Willshaw, G. A., H. R. Smith, M. M. McConnell, and B. Rowe. 1985. Expression of cloned plasmid regions encoding colonization factor antigen I (CFA/I) in *Escherichia coli. Plasmid* 13:8–16.

93. Willshaw, G. A., H. R. Smith, and B. Rowe. 1983. Cloning of regions encoding colonisation factor antigen I and heat-stable enterotoxin in *Escherichia coli. FEMS Microbiol. Lett.* 16:101–106.

94. Wilson, M. R., and A. W. Hohmann. 1974. Immunity to *Escherichia coli* in pigs: adhesion of enteropathogenic *Escherichia coli* to isolated intestinal epithelial cells. *Infect. Immun.* 10:766–786.

Chapter 3

Mechanisms of Bacterial Colonization of the Mucosal Surfaces of the Gut

Rolf Freter

Department of Microbiology and Immunology
The University of Michigan
Ann Arbor, Michigan 48109

INTRODUCTION

One of the oldest fields of study in medical and veterinary microbiology is concerned with the nature, the functions, and the control of the intestinal microflora. It is therefore surprising to realize that although considerable progress has been made with respect to defining the nature of the intestinal microflora and understanding many of its functions, we still know very little about the mechanisms that control its nature, i.e., the mechanisms that control which bacteria will colonize certain areas of the gastrointestinal tract and which bacteria will be excluded. At the present state of our understanding, the question of what characteristics are needed to enable a bacterium to become a part of the indigenous microflora is identical to the question of what virulence mechanisms a pathogen will need to carry out the first step of pathogenicity, namely, to colonize the host. For this reason, no distinction will be made in the present article between evidence obtained with bacteria of the indigenous microflora and data from studies with pathogens.

As has been reviewed by several authors, a considerable number of ecological studies are now available which describe the bacterial populations in various regions of the human and animal intestine. Nevertheless, much remains to be done along these lines (35). The numerous functions of the intestinal microflora also have been explored extensively. Gnotobiotic techniques have been the most valuable for such studies. It appears that there are very few physiological parameters of the human or animal body that are not in some way affected by the presence of the indigenous microflora (16). Functions of the intestinal microflora that are of greatest interest to veterinarians certainly include (i) its possible influence on nutrition and feed utilization and (ii) the protection it gives against colonization by pathogens. The latter phenomenon has been discovered and rediscovered many times since the early days, when Metchnikoff (37) thought that the ingestion of lactobacilli would suppress the growth of "putrefactive" bacteria in the gut. Terms such as bacterial antagonism (12), bacterial interference (7), or colonization resistance (51) have been used to describe this protective activity.

In view of the economic importance to the livestock industry of weight gain, feed utilization, and protection against infections, a number of empirical measures are commonly taken in an attempt to optimize the above-mentioned two activities of the intestinal microflora. One of these measures is the use of subtherapeutic doses of antibiotics as feed supplements. There can be no doubt that such regiments are effective in stimulating weight gain and feed utilization, especially in young animals (3, 10, 52). Nevertheless, this practice is highly controversial because of the demonstrated spread of antibiotic-resistant pathogens such as salmonellae to the human population and because of the possible spread to humans of resistance genes which reside in nonpathogens and which later could be transferred to human pathogens. The mechanisms by which antibiotic feed supplements exert their desirable effects are still subject to speculation (10), except that they appear to be mediated via the indigenous microflora. The most convincing type of evidence supporting this conclusion is the absence of a growth-enhancing effect of antibiotics in germfree animals (52). Because of the possible detrimental side effects and because of the lack of a sound theoretical foundation, continued administration of subtherapeutic doses of antibiotics is not practiced in human medicine.

A second measure that is used with increasing frequency in veterinary practice is the feeding of bacterial supplements to livestock in the hope of optimizing the protective functions of the indigenous microflora. This practice shares with that of feeding subtherapeutic doses of antibiotics the lack of a sound theoretical basis. It differs, however, in that it also lacks a sound basis of data showing practical effectiveness. The impetus for bacterial supplements can be traced back to the above-mentioned ideas of Metchnikoff (37), which were further developed by workers such as Rettger et al. (42). In contrast to the use of subtherapeutic doses of antibiotics, the ingestion of milk fermented by lactobacilli is widely practiced among human populations. In commenting upon this practice, Tannock (50) writes: "For every article in the scientific literature that claims beneficial results from the ingestion of fermented milk, another article will provide evidence to the contrary. Most of the reported studies have not been adequately controlled, statistical analysis of the results is rarely made, and the conclusions are largely subjective."

Inspired, perhaps, by the popularity of *Lactobacillus* preparations among human populations, increasing attention has been paid in recent years to the feeding of preparations containing live bacteria to mammals and birds of commercial interest. These preparations usually contain viable cultures of lactobacilli or streptococci or both. This practice, called probiotics in the trade, is said by some to contribute to the establishment of a beneficial microflora in the intestinal tracts of the animals and to result in increased weight gain and resistance to infections. Unfortunately, the above-quoted remarks by Tannock (50) seem to apply here also. Some of the published studies were done with pure cultures in vitro or with gnotobiotic animals associated with only a few bacterial species (40). As will be discussed below, neither of these methods duplicates the bacterial interactions that occur in a conventional animal. Moreover, many commercial probiotic preparations contain other additives, such as vitamins, which may be responsible wholly or in part for any observed beneficial effects. Often an effect of feeding bacterial supplements is noted on certain groups of indigenous bacteria, such as coliforms (see, e.g., references 1 and 38), but it is usually not clear whether the observed reduction actually affects the coliform populations that inhabit areas of the gut where pathogenic coliforms localize (e.g., the small intestine), or whether the reduction affects the indigenous coliforms in the large intestine. It should be noted that increases in fecal lactobacillus counts and decreases in coliform counts have been seen after feeding *Lactobacillus* supplements, without a correspondingly increased resistance to challenge with enteropathogenic *Escherichia coli* (38). The current emphasis on high counts of lactobacilli and low counts of coliforms as the most desirable situation is curious in light of the classical attempts at promoting human intestinal "eubiosis" by giving oral supplements of viable *E. coli* strains (39). Such *E. coli*-containing preparations are still used medically (29, 44, 45) and are thought to increase patients' resistance by stimulating nonspecific immunity via unknown mechanisms. The clinical evidence is not strong, however (45). To my knowledge, there are no proper double-blind studies available which test the effect of bacterial dietary supplements in animals. In human medicine, double-blind refers to studies, overseen by a third party, in which neither the attending physician nor the volunteer patient knows whether the patient receives a placebo or the treatment under study. In tests on animals the caretaker certainly would have to be included among the "blind" to make a study valid. This precaution is especially important in view of the relatively small differences between control and experimental groups that are usually observed in tests of probiotics (41). It remains to be demonstrated, therefore, whether the "healthy" balance of intestinal flora that is one of the desired aims of many probiotic regimens (e.g., high *Lactobacillus* and low *E. coli* populations) is indeed causally related to robust health and resistance to infection. Alternatively, such a balance may be merely the indicator of a properly functioning ecosystem in which the predominant (anaerobic) bacteria create conditions that limit the populations of coliforms more severely than they limit the populations of lactobacilli. If the latter were true, then attempts to change such a balance by feeding the indicator microorganisms would be the equivalent of trying to cure a fever by shaking the thermometer to a lower reading.

Lee (35), in discussing the subject, points out that lactobacilli and bifidobacteria (and one may include here streptococci as well) are still used in dietary supplements for historical reasons and because of their ease of culture. However, these organisms are not the logical choice for these purposes, because they are not the dominant organisms in the intestinal micro flora. As is detailed below, there is considerable evidence that the predominant strict anaerobes of the large intestine are of major importance in bringing about the bacterial antagonism that protects the host against colonization by pathogens. To be sure, there are reports in the literature of the feeding of single strains of bacteria which successfully inhibited colonization of the host by pathogens. These involved the use of avirulent bacterial antagonists which are taxonomically closely related to the pathogen to be inhibited (8, 55). A theory supporting this approach is discussed below.

As is apparent from the above discussion, the deliberate manipulation of the indigenous microflora for the benefit of the host is still in its infancy and lacks a solid scientific foundation. This is very unfortunate, because the protective function of the indigenous microflora against colonization by pathogens is a well-established phenomenon which is no less important to the human or animal host than the conventional, antibody-based or cellular immune mechanisms (15). As noted above, the reason why no reliable practical means exist for harnessing this type of immunity is obvious: namely, the fact that very little is known about the mechanisms that control the composition of the indigenous microflora. A better understanding of these mechanisms is therefore not only of theoretical interest in defining the virulence mechanisms that pathogens must possess to be able to colonize, but is also important for human and veterinary medicine and for the economics of livestock husbandry. The present article, therefore, will present a brief review of the subject with some emphasis on recent work from my laboratory. Accordingly, most of the following pages will deal with the flora of the large intestine, but the principles to be discussed are likely to apply as well to bacterial populations colonizing other body surfaces.

MICROHABITATS AND THE ROLE OF THE MUCUS GEL

When bacterial populations colonize mucosal surfaces, it is often difficult to determine with certainty whether their habitat is the mucus gel itself or whether they are more intimately associated with the epithelial cell surfaces. The main reason for this difficulty is the collapse of the highly hydrated mucus gel that occurs during preparation of specimens for electron microscopy. The gel may either coalesce into isolated strands or collapse into the epithelial cells, carrying entrapped bacteria with it, thereby yielding a preparation which may give the impression that the bacteria in the original specimen were also located adjacent to the epithelial surface (30, 43). Rozee et al. (43) developed a method whereby the mucosa was first exposed to antimucus antibody before the dehydration step. This method yielded preparations of mouse ileum for electron microscopy in which a continuous mucus blanket was preserved, which contained large entrapped bacterial populations. Without the preliminary antibody step, a collapsed mucus blanket was seen which had withdrawn from the epithelium, thus giving the impression that the epithelial surface was free of bacteria. Bollard et al. (2) confirmed that antimucus antibody pretreatment stabilized the mucus blanket as a continuous sheet. In their preparations of the rat mid-colon, there were few bacteria present in the stabilized mucus gel (which was presumably in its natural configuration), whereas in the absence of stabilization the mucus collapsed onto the epithelial surface, apparently drawing with it bacteria which normally were located in the lumen, above the mucus blanket. Thus, the unstabilized preparation gave the impression that large populations of bacteria were originally located adjacent to the epithelium. Consequently, artifacts due to the collapse of the mucus gel either may remove bacteria normally located adjacent to the epithelium or, conversely, may draw to the epithelial surface bacteria that are normally located in the lumen. Thus, unless distinct attachment mechanisms such as fimbriae or more intimate "hold-fast" mechanisms (4) can be demonstrated by eletron microscopy, it is often difficult to decide whether bacteria seen adjacent to the epithelial surface are indeed attached to it or whether they form a part of a population that extends throughout the mucus

gel. Light microscopy of frozen sections, especially when these are stabilized with agents such as methyl cellulose or stained quickly without fixation (18), often gives a more realistic estimate of the natural distribution of bacteria on a mucosal surface, but, unfortunately, does not provide the resolution necessary to detect specialized attachment structures.

With the above reservations, it may be useful to distinguish three main microhabitats along the gastrointestinal tract. The first of these comprise bacteria that colonize the deep layers of the mucus gel. Most frequently these are spiral bacteria, which populate the crypts of the ileum, cecum, and colon. Lee and co-workers have contributed much to the understanding of these populations (reviewed in references 34 and 35) and have shown that these consist of very different bacteria in various regions of the gut. The common feature of spiral morphology is thought to contribute to the ability to traverse viscous media, such as mucus gel (35). In this view the bacteria withstand removal with the mucus flow by active motility directed, perhaps by chemotactic stimuli, toward the bottom of the crypts. In such a situation, special means of attachment to the epithelial surface would not be required for successful colonization. Spiral bacteria also inhabit areas below the mucus layer in the stomachs of humans (27) and animals (11, 35).

The second intestinal habitat for bacterial populations is the surface of the epithelial cells. Thus, lactobacilli attach to the stomachs of mammals and the crops of chicken in a very specific manner; i.e., strains isolated from chickens will not attach to and colonize rats, and vice versa. As mentioned above, some indigenous bacteria of the small and large intestine have developed rather complex and intimate attachment mechanisms to epithelial cells (34, 35). Attachment to the epithelial cells of the small intestine is also the mechanism by which some of the classical enteric pathogens, such as enterotoxigenic *E. coli*, manage to evade removal by the peristaltic activity of the jejunum and ileum and thus are able to colonize.

This subject is discussed in Chapters 1 and 2 of this volume and is not detailed further here.

Except in acute diarrheal diseases, the first two types of microhabitat discussed above contain relatively sparse populations consisting of one or only a few different kinds of bacteria. There is, however, a third type, which is distinguished by the presence of a dense and complex flora that consists of a large number of different kinds of bacteria. Such habitats include dental plaque, the gingival crevice, the crops of birds, the throat, the lower ileum, the cecum, and the colon. Bacterial populations in the last three areas of the intestine form thick layers which are embedded in the mucus gel. It is well known that many of the indigenous species are able to degrade mammalian mucus (14), and it is therefore uncertain whether the material that surrounds the bacterial populations is indeed entirely of host origin, whether it is partially degraded material of host origin, or whether it represents in part, or entirely, material produced by the bacteria.

The role of mucus gel in promoting or inhibiting bacterial colonization has been the subject of much debate (14). Some earlier workers considered mucus gel to be a "particle and macromolecule proof coating for cell surfaces" through which bacteria must "bore a channel" by means of special virulence mechanisms. This view has persisted until recent times (9), although it had been shown for some time that spermatozoa move in cervical mucus along planes of stress created by stretching of the gel (24). Likewise, cholera vibrios moved along lines of strain created by stretching mucus gel from rabbit small intestine. In contrast, when the same mucus gel was simply deposited on a microscope slide, vibrios penetrated poorly, presumably because there were no parallel lines of stress (33). It is possible that similar lines of stress are formed by the natural strain that is created when mucus gel is extruded by intestinal goblet cells. Such lines of stress may be expected to parallel the flow of mucus and thereby to form channels for bacterial penetration that lead from the lumen to the epithelium and into the crypts. Studies in

my laboratory (19–21) have implicated the chemotactic attraction of motile bacteria into the mucus gel as a major force aiding such microorganisms in the penetration of the intestinal mucus layer. Penetration was rapid, requiring less than 15 min when intestinal slices were incubated in bacterial suspensions in vitro or when the bacteria were injected into intestinal loops of mice or rabbits. Yeast cells or inert polystyrene particles in the size range of bacteria also penetrated mucus gel, but at a much lower rate. Interestingly, the rate of penetration of inert particles was inversely related to their size (unpublished data), a finding that is consistent with the idea that channels of limited diameter allow particles to enter the mucus gel. Taxins (e.g., mucosal extracts), when present on the lumenal side of the mucosa, prevented the active penetration of the mucus layer by motile bacteria, presumably by blocking the taxin receptors on the bacterial surface and thereby preventing chemotaxis. Superior ability to penetrate mucus gel was correlated with superior ecological fitness: nonchemotactic mutants were rapidly outgrown by their chemotactic parents in rabbit intestinal loops and in gnotobiotic mice. Interestingly, nonmotile mutants rapidly outgrew normally motile but nonchemotactic vibrios in gnotobiotic mice. Consequently, motility appeared to confer an ecological burden on the bacteria in vivo, unless the motility was also guided by chemotactic stimuli, in which case motility was strikingly advantageous.

More recent unpublished studies from my laboratory have extended the work on chemotaxis of vibrios (which populate the small intestine) to bacteria of the predominant strictly anaerobic flora of the large intestine. When the ceca of mice are removed under strict anaerobiosis in an anaerobic chamber and their contents are observed through a microscope located in that chamber, a large majority of the bacteria present show a high rate of motility, with a velocity which resembles that of the most rapidly moving types of bacteria, such as cholera vibrios. A highly motile gram-positive bacterium (probably of the genus *Clostridium*) was isolated from the mouse cecum, and a non-chemotactic but normally motile (smooth-swimming) mutant was selected. This mutant showed significantly reduced ability to enter the mucosa of the mouse cecum and was not able to colonize the mouse large intestine when the chemotactic parent was also present. Interestingly, no evidence of positive chemotaxis could be demonstrated with the parent strain, nor with a number of other strictly anaerobic bacteria isolated from the mouse cecum. Testing of these anaerobes for positive chemotaxis was difficult because they did not maintain motility in buffers that lacked an energy source. For this reason, small amounts of either amino acids or glucose had to be added to the buffers. Any such energy sources in the buffer are themselves possible taxins, and their presence in the chemotaxis assay may have obscured weaker chemotactic responses to the large number of other carbohydrates and amino acids that were tested for possible taxin activity. For this reason, the possibility of false-negative results in testing for positive chemotaxis cannot be excluded entirely. On the other hand, all anaerobes tested showed strong negative chemotaxis when tested on semisolid agar with short-chain fatty acids (e.g., acetic, butyric, and propionic acids) as the negative taxins. It is therefore entirely possible that many anaerobes that populate the large intestine are indeed incapable of positive chemotaxis and that they are driven toward the mucosa, their natural habitat, by a gradient of negative taxins such as the short-chain fatty acids which accumulate in the lumen as the metabolic end products of many indigenous microbial species.

In an interesting series of reports, Cohen et al. (5, 6) have shown that the ability of enteric bacteria such as *E. coli* and salmonellae to colonize the mouse intestine correlated with the ability of the bacteria to adhere to mucus gel that is immobilized in polystyrene wells. They found that mucus gel may contain sequences that resemble receptors for bacterial adhesins located on the epithelial cell surface. Consequently, adhesion of bacteria to the mucus gel in an in vitro test may simply be an indicator of the presence of receptors for these bacteria on the epithelial surface, a circumstance which could explain the correlation with colonizing ability. On the other hand, colonization may involve the trapping of the bacteria in the mucus layer by means of the receptors present on the mucus molecule. Alternatively, under conditions different from those prevailing in the experiments of Cohen et al., receptors in the mucus gel may competitively inhibit bacterial adhesion to the analogous receptor sequences on the epithelial surface (13). It is obvious, then, that the precise details of bacterial association with the mucus gel must await further investigation. For this reason, the discussion below will simply take for granted the amply demonstrated fact that the terminal ileum and cecum contain large populations of bacteria in the mucus gel, without making additional assumptions about the mechanisms of retention involved. The term "association with the mucosa" is sufficiently noncommittal to describe such a situation and is used hereafter in that sense. For reasons of convenience, the term "adhesion" is also used, especially in discussions of mathematical models, but its meaning in this article should be taken as synonymous with association. The only (intuitively obvious) assumption that is made is that the association of bacteria with the mucosa reduces the rate of their removal by the peristaltic movements of the bowel, analogous to the effect that would be seen with true adhesion of bacteria to the epithelial cell surface.

INTERACTIONS IN THE LARGE INTESTINE AMONG BACTERIA AND BETWEEN BACTERIA AND HOST

Experimental Models

It is well known that most bacteria, even species not indigenous to the intestinal flora, are able to colonize germfree animals, whereas colonization of conventional animals or of humans is usually difficult (15). One must conclude, therefore, that some of the major mechanisms that control the composition of the indigenous microflora of the large intestine are based on the interactions among the numerous microbial species present. Since it is difficult to study such interactions in intact animals, in which homeostatic mechanisms necessary for survival of the host limit the range of feasible experimental manipulations, most early (and even contemporary) investigators resorted to working with in vitro models of bacterial interactions. This approach creates a serious problem, because in vitro models cannot a priori be relied upon to reflect the mechanisms by which microorganisms interact in vivo. This is a consequence of the well-known ecological principle that the nature of interactions among different populations—whether these be microorganisms or higher forms—depends to a large extent on the nature of the habitat in which these interactions take place. Many instances have been recorded in the literature that document the lack of correlation between microbial interactions among different kinds of bacteria observed in vitro and the interactions among these same bacteria in the guts of intact animals. An early study, which has considerably influenced my thinking, demonstrated that the interactions between *Shigella flexneri* and a number of other bacteria differed widely depending on the in vitro culture system used for testing these interactions. Only continuous-flow (CF) cultures were able to simulate the dynamics of interactions among these bacteria as they occurred in the mouse intestine (28). Somewhat later, Maier et al. showed that *S. flexneri* was strongly inhibited by *Bacteroides* strains in vitro, whereas these anaerobes had no effect on *S. flexneri* growth in the mouse intestine (36). In another example, early studies on the possible in vivo role of bacteriocins had shown a strong correlation between in vitro colicin production by *E. coli* strains isolated from patients with bacillary dysentery and the time during the course of the disease at which these strains had been isolated. In other words, *E. coli* strains isolated during the recovery phase, when *Shigella* populations declined in the patients, showed significantly higher in vitro colicin ac-

tivity against shigellae than did *E. coli* strains isolated from patients in the early phases of dysentery, when the *Shigella* populations in the feces were high (23, 26). Unfortunately, later experimental studies by this and other groups failed to correlate in vitro colicin production with intestinal antagonistic activity (23, 31, 47). Interestingly, a good correlation between in vitro production of colicins active against shigellae and the inhibitory action of the same *E. coli* strains against the same shigellae in an unnatural in vivo habitat, namely, the peritoneal cavity, has been reported (23). In a classic study, Shinefield et al. showed that the deliberate colonization of newborn babies with an avirulent strain of *Staphylococcus aureus* protected them against nosocomial infections by virulent staphylococci (48). The interactions of these strains could be duplicated in various experimental models, such as broth cultures, allantoic fluid, and embryonated eggs. In each of these models the *S. aureus* strain that had antagonized the colonization of infants by other staphylococci would also antagonize the in vitro growth of the latter. Unfortunately, the mechanisms of these interactions differed in each experimental model, thus allowing no conclusions about the mechanisms that had actually operated on the surface of the infants' bodies. Consequently, the fact that the final outcome of bacterial interactions in each model had duplicated the final event occurring in infants was simply a coincidence (reviewed in reference 48). It should be noted in this context that even some seemingly ideal in vivo models, namely, gnotobiotic animals that are associated with only a few bacterial species, do not necessarily duplicate bacterial interactions that occur in a conventional animal harboring a complete indigenous microflora. Implanting a number of known bacteria usually redresses some, but rarely all, of the abnormalities that distinguish germfree animals from their conventional counterparts, and the contents of the intestines of germfree animals are entirely different from those of the intestines of conventional animals (reviewed in reference 49). Consequently, studies of bacterial interactions conducted in gnotobiotic animals associated with only a few bacterial species are no more significant than similar studies conducted with in vitro cultures, unless independent evidence is available to show that the mechanisms of interaction are indeed similar to those in conventional animals. One must conclude, therefore, that a major reason for current ignorance of the mechanisms that control bacterial populations in the intestine is the difficulty in finding appropriate experimental models and the resulting use of inappropriate models in studies concerned with this question.

Candidate Control Mechanisms

Despite the points made in the preceding paragraph, it is important to realize that the study of bacterial interactions in vitro or in gnotobiotic animals serves one important function, namely, to identify mechanisms of bacterial interaction which *potentially* might be involved in the control of bacterial populations in the gut. In this manner a large number of mechanisms have been identified by which one bacterium may inhibit the growth of another under physiological conditions which, when realized in the intestine, would not be incompatible with life of the animal. These include changes in oxidation-reduction potential and acidity; the presence of inhibitory substances such as bacteriocins, fatty acids, hydrogen sulfide, and deconjugated bile salts; competition for nutrients and adhesion sites; and local immunity (reviewed in reference 46). In attempting to evaluate this range of possibilities and the likelihood that any one of these is important in controlling the microbial populations in the gut, it will be useful to first mention some of the details of intestinal microecology which any putative control mechanism must be able to explain. These are described in the next three paragraphs.

Most important here is the fact that the flora of the lower ileum and large intestine consists of several hundred bacterial species and strains, with an even distribution of dominant species; i.e., all of these coexist without one or

a few displacing the others. The dominant species are mostly strict anaerobes, which reach densities of 10^9 to 10^{11}/g of feces, but there are also constant populations of low density (in the order of 10^6/g) of other species, such as *E. coli* and other members of the family *Enterobacteriaceae* (35). Considering this high diversity, it is impossible to conceive of a single mechanism that would be sufficient to bring about such a complex equilibrium. For example, it is obvious that any bacterium that forms a population of constant size in the intestine must maintain a rate of multiplication which exactly equals its rate of elimination from the gut. For this reason, it is theoretically impossible to account for the presence of constant low populations of a sensitive species (e.g., *E. coli*) solely on the basis of growth inhibitors (such as fatty acids) that are produced by the predominant indigenous species. If this were the case, either too much inhibitor would be present and would eliminate the sensitive species, or too little inhibitor would be present, in which case the population of the sensitive species would increase until it became limited by some other mechanism (e.g., lack of nutrients). Constant populations of a sensitive species could be maintained at only one precise inhibitor concentration, i.e., that which reduces the potentially high growth rate of the sensitive species to the point at which it equals the rate of excretion of the bacteria. Such precise control of inhibitor concentrations is not likely to be maintained in natural systems. Additional mechanisms must therefore participate in the control of populations. As pointed out previously (22), one such mechanism is the association of the bacteria with the wall of the intestine; others will be discussed below. It is apparent, then, that the lack of substantial progress in identifying the mechanisms that control microbial populations in the gut can be attributed in part to the predilection of scientists to experiment with only a single mechanism at a time.

A second important property of the intestinal microflora that must be considered here is its stability. As mentioned above, stability implies that microorganisms (including pathogens) that enter the gut from the environment are prevented from colonizing it. Even if the invader strain is of a type indigenous to the gut (e.g., a recently isolated *E. coli* strain), its ingestion will rarely result in colonization of the host (reviewed in reference 15). Nevertheless, the same *E. coli* strain will usually colonize well and become a part of the indigenous flora when it is introduced *first*, i.e., as a monocontaminant into germfree mice, and the indigenous microflora is implanted *afterwards*. In this type of experiment the implanted indigenous flora functioned normally, i.e., it did inhibit the colonization of bacteria that were ingested later. Nevertheless, the *E. coli* strain that was introduced first maintained a constant population at a density typical of indigenous *E. coli* in conventional mice (18).

The third and last important feature of intestinal microecology that must be considered here concerns the dynamics of bacterial growth in the large intestine. The optimal growth rate of *E. coli* in a monoassociated mouse is similar to that in a broth culture, with a doubling time of approximately 20 min (22). In contrast, the mean retention time of intestinal contents in the large intestine of the mouse is much longer, on the order of 3 h (22), and bacteria with a doubling time of less than 3 h would soon form populations of infinite size in the gut. Consequently, most and possibly all bacteria inhabiting the gut appear to multiply at a rate that is considerably lower than the maximum rate which they could sustain in a monoassociated animal or in vitro. One must conclude, therefore, that the physiological conditions of the large intestine are much less than optimal for bacterial multiplication: a shortcoming which may be due to the lack of nutrients, the presence of inhibitors, or both.

Results with an Experimental Model

As mentioned above, CF cultures appeared to be promising in vitro models of bacterial interactions in the large intestine. Considerable evidence has now been accumulated

in my laboratory that anaerobic CF cultures can simulate at least many of the interactions of bacteria as they occur in the cecum of mice. The CF culture must be strictly anaerobic and must be inoculated with cecal contents of conventional mice which had been autopsied in an anaerobic chamber to avoid exposure of the inoculum to oxygen. The types of evidence for similarities between bacterial interactions in such CF cultures and the mouse intestine include the following (17). (i) The balance among the numerous indigenous anaerobes in CF cultures is similar to that in the large intestine of mice. (ii) The short-chain fatty acids that are the major metabolic end products of many indigenous anaerobes are similar in quality and concentration in both systems. (iii) When effluent from 2-month-old CF cultures of conventional mouse flora was fed to germfree mice, it reversed the germfree abnormalities. This is a stringent test, because such a reversal has not been achieved to date by feeding complex mixtures of pure cultures of mouse-indigenous bacteria. This shows that the CF cultures had maintained at least the more important bacterial species responsible for the normal functions of the indigenous flora. (iv) Proper balance in the CF culture ecosystem depends on the development of thick layers of bacterial growth associated with the wall. As mentioned above, such layers are also typical of the mammalian large intestine. If these adherent layers are removed, CF cultures no longer resemble the mouse intestine and, for example, will no longer resist colonization by newly introduced bacteria. (v) Like the guts of conventional animals, CF cultures of mouse cecal flora resist colonization by bacteria that are introduced into the system. As discussed above, bacteria that are introduced first as monoassociates into gnotobiotic mice usually become a part of the indigenous flora when a conventional flora is introduced later. This phenomenon is also reproduced in CF cultures.

Although the above data do not provide an absolute proof that the control of bacterial populations in CF cultures involves at least the more important mechanisms among those actually operating in the mouse large intestine, the evidence points strongly to that conclusion, because it is difficult to imagine two different sets of mechanisms that fortuitously would bring about exactly similar steady-state balances among populations of the degree of complexity as those in the mammalian large intestine. It therefore appeared appropriate to study the relevant mechanisms in some detail. For this purpose, an apparatus was devised which permits the installation of a diffusion chamber that is completely submersed in the CF culture of mouse cecal flora. The chamber is separated from the culture proper by a cellophane membrane. When the chamber was filled with sterile filtrate of effluent from a CF culture, bacteria inoculated into the chamber were inhibited in their growth and underwent the same length of lag as if they were inoculated directly into the CF culture. Experimental manipulation of the contents of the diffusion chamber made it possible to identify a number of mechanisms that control the growth and colonization of bacteria in CF cultures of mouse cecal flora (18). These include (i) the presence of H_2S, which appears to restrict the utilization of certain nutritional substrates by the bacteria; (ii) competition for nutrients of the kind which can be used as carbon and energy sources under the prevailing conditions of strict anaerobiosis and in the presence of H_2S; (iii) adhesion of the indigenous microflora to the wall; and (iv) the prolonged lag phase that invading bacteria entering the environment of the CF culture or of the large intestine must undergo. Under the prevailing physiological conditions in the large intestine, lag phases of newly introduced bacteria may extend over several days, and for this reason, newly introduced bacteria may be washed out of a CF culture before they can begin multiplication.

Analysis by a Mathematical Model and Development of Hypotheses

Although the above analysis of control mechanisms in CF cultures has identified several that are likely to operate also in the mouse intestine, there is no indication of the relative importance of these mechanisms to the overall balance. It is likely, furthermore, that the relative importance of various mechanisms changes in different circumstances. For example, inhibitors of growth rates of bacteria are likely to have a less decisive impact on populations that adhere to the wall than on populations residing in the lumen (18). The role of adhesion in the large intestine also needs further explanation. As described above, CF cultures failed to simulate bacterial interactions in the mouse large intestine when adhesion of the flora to the wall of the culture vessel was prevented. This is surprising, because of the slow mean retention time of contents in the large intestine. It is well known that the peristaltic movements in the small intestine are so rapid that bacteria can colonize only by adhering to the gut wall. That is not the case in the large intestine, however, and bacterial populations could well compensate for the slow washout rate by their potentially much faster rates of multiplication. Why, then, the need for adherent bacterial populations in the large intestine?

To evaluate the above-mentioned questions, a mathematical model was developed which describes the fate of an invader strain that is being swallowed (or inoculated into an established CF culture of the indigenous microflora) and competes with an already established resident strain that may or may not belong to the same species. In this approach, the rest of the indigenous flora is not described in detail, but is regarded as a part of the intestinal environment (which, as described above, is indeed defined to a large extent by the activities of the indigenous flora). The mathematical model has the following properties (15). (i) Resident and invader strains have exactly the same physiological characteristics. (ii) Residents and invaders compete for the same adhesion sites on the wall of the gut or CF culture. (iii) Residents and invaders compete for the same limiting nutrient. (iv) Offspring of adherent bacteria occupy additional adhesion sites until most sites are filled. Thereafter, daughter cells of adherent bacteria are shed into the lumen.

(v) Adhesion of bacteria is reversible and is governed by rate constants for adhesion and elution in a mass action type of relation.

Application of this model to the ecology of mouse large-intestinal flora in CF cultures led to the hypothesis (15) that the populations of most indigenous bacteria of the large intestine are controlled by substrate competition; i.e., that each indigenous species is more efficient than the rest in utilizing one (or a few) of the many nutritional substances that are present in the gut. Such substrates may be components of the diet as well as mucopolysaccharides and cell debris of host origin, all of which may be partially modified by some components of the flora. The hypothesis further holds that the function of the system is modified by the presence of inhibitors (such as H_2S). A colonizing species or strain is successful when it can realize the highest rate of multiplication at the lowest concentration of a particular nutrient compared with all of its actual and potential competitors. The hypothesis finally postulates that the regulation described above is modified further by the effects of bacterial adhesion to the wall. Residents (which are already adhering to the wall) are washed out of the system at a rate which is much lower than that for freely suspended material. Consequently, the population of adherent residents expands until the concentration of the limiting nutrient is reduced to the point at which it will support a rate of multiplication of the residents which just balances their rate of elution. For this reason residents can form constant populations at nutrient concentrations which are too low to support a growth rate that would be adequate to maintain a constant population of the invaders, which, at least initially, are all suspended and therefore are washed out more rapidly. Consequently, invaders are at a relative disadvantage with respect to residents even if the two populations have identical physiological properties. This resolves the apparent paradox mentioned above, namely, the necessity for adhesion in the large intestine, where the rate of bacterial elimination is much lower than the maximal growth rate of the bacteria.

The mathematical model shows that association of the indigenous microflora with the mucosa is necessary for stability by creating conditions adverse to colonization by invaders. An invader, therefore, can colonize only if it is able to rapidly find sites for association with the mucosa. This may be possible if the invader can adhere to sites different from those occupied by the resident or if it is more efficient in associating at the same sites, i.e., if its rate constant of adhesion is higher or if its rate constant of elution is lower than that of the resident. These interactions among nutrient concentrations, growth rates, and rates of adhesion and elution also explain the observed phenomenon that a bacterium which cannot colonize a CF culture harboring an established indigenous flora can nevertheless become a resident strain if it is implanted *before* the indigenous flora. In the latter case, the bacterium can colonize the adhesion sites for which it has an affinity, but these sites apparently are occupied by residents when it attempts to invade an already colonized ecosystem (15).

In more recent experiments (unpublished data), the rate constants for adhesion and elution of an invading *E. coli* strain were estimated in CF cultures. Small glass cover slips were suspended in these cultures for a minimum of 2 weeks to allow colonization of the surfaces by indigenous flora. The invader was then introduced into the CF culture. In the experiment illustrated in Fig. 1, the slides were transferred 12 h later to a second CF culture of mouse intestinal flora which had not been inoculated with invaders. At appropriate intervals cover slips were removed and homogenized, and the number of adherent invaders was determined by quantitative culture. Computer analysis indicated that the data could be explained only by assuming that there were at least two types of adhesion sites for the invader strain, respectively mediating weak and strong adhesion (Fig. 1). When the rate constants of adhesion and elution determined from this and similar experiments were used in the mathematical model, it became apparent that the weak adhesion did not contribute much to coloni-

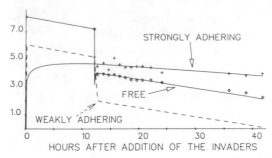

FIGURE 1. Association of an invading *E. coli* strain with glass surfaces (cover slips) that had been suspended for 3 weeks in a CF culture of conventional mouse flora. At 12 h after introduction of the invader, the cover slips were transferred to a second CF culture of conventional mouse flora (note the precipitous drop of free invaders at the time). The data points are experimental, and the lines were generated by a computer program that optimized the rate constants of adhesion and elution to obtain the best fit to the experimental points. For the duration of this experiment the invaders were unable to commence multiplication and, consequently, were slowly washed out of the culture.

zation by the invader. Strong adhesion alone would have allowed the invader to colonize (albeit at low population levels), which is contrary to the experimental observations described above (in which the invader was unable to colonize). The mathematical model indicated, therefore, that additional mechanisms were important and had to be considered. For this reason, a lag phase of growth was introduced into the mathematical model to cause the invader to delay multiplication for several days (as had been observed experimentally [Fig. 1]). After this additional feature was introduced, the model did indeed improve its reproduction of the experimental findings; i.e., the invader could colonize only at very low population densities. Complete elimination of the invader was predicted by the mathematical model when the assumption was made that fewer daughter cells of the invader, which presumably adheres only to the superficial bacterial layers on the gut wall, would find new adhesion sites than daughter cells of residents, which presumably colonize deeper layers, where more daughter cells are retained. The mathematical model therefore indicates that the prevention

of colonization of invaders by the indigenous flora in CF cultures is a complex phenomenon which cannot be explained on the basis of a single mechanism. As a minimum, all four mechanisms discussed above (competition for adhesion sites and for nutrients, the long lag phase, and the fate of daughter cells of bacteria located in the superficial layers of the mucosa-associated flora) appear to be involved.

Similar experiments as described above for CF cultures were also carried out with conventional mice harboring a complete indigenous microflora. Invader *E. coli* strains were introduced into the stomach of each mouse, and their fate throughout the various parts of the gastronintestinal tract was determined by culture of adherent and free bateria. Mathematical analysis of the experimental data obtained to date has shown that the *E. coli* strain used as the invader reacted in a similar manner in the mouse as it had previously in CF cultures. Exceptions found were that (i) there were fewer strong adhesion sites for this *E. coli* strain in the mouse than in CF cultures, and (ii) the lag phase of growth in vivo was only approximately 36 h, i.e., somewhat shorter than in CF cultures. This was the first instance of a discrepancy between the two systems, which, as reviewed above, had been found to be remarkably similar. Another discrepancy between the interaction of *Clostridium difficile* with conventional cecal hamster flora in vivo versus that observed in CF cultures was reported by Wilson and Freter (54). Only CF cultures containing a medium supplemented with extract of fecal pellets from germfree mice reproduced the suppression of *C. difficile* that occurred in vivo. The authors speculated on the basis of this and other evidence that elements of the hamster-indigenous microflora that are important for controlling *C. difficile* populations fail to colonize CF cultures unless some required nutrients (possibly mucopolysaccharides) are supplied by the fecal extract. Undoubtedly, additional differences will be found when future studies delve into ever finer details of bacterial interactions in these systems. Future investigations of the causes of such discrepancies may be expected to shed further light on the function and relative importance in intestinal microecology of the various mechanisms of bacterial interactions.

DISCUSSION AND CONCLUSIONS

Two features of the experimental approach described in this article have proven very useful in my laboratory, namely, the use of an in vitro model which appears to duplicate at least many of the more important characteristics of the large intestinal ecosystem and the development of a mathematical model that can provide an analysis of the interactions among the various mechanisms that control the bacterial populations. The experiments had identified several mechanisms of potential importance in the ecology of the large intestine, but had given no hint of the manner in which these might interact to bring about the observed gross phenomena. The hypotheses concerning the mechanisms controlling the flora of the mouse large intestine outlined above could not have been formulated, therefore, without a close coordination between experimental studies and an evaluation of the experimental data by the mathematical model. The hypotheses still incorporate a number of assumptions, and the details will almost certainly have to be modified as more evidence becomes available. Nevertheless, they do provide a unified picture of this complex ecosystem which heretofore had not been available and which explains what is known of the behavior of the system. It is possible that a similar dual (i.e., experimental and mathematical) approach may also be useful in gaining a better understanding of other in vivo environments that harbor a complex microflora.

What can these hypotheses contribute to an understanding of the practical problems discussed in the introduction to this chapter? If each type of bacterium in the ecosystem depends for its presence in the system on its ability to associate with the mucosa and on its ability to be most efficient in utilizing one

limiting nutrient, then the development of an effective resistance to colonization by pathogens requires that the resident populations collectively are able to react with *all* available adhesion sites and that they are able to utilize *all* available nutrients (at least all sites and nutrients which potential pathogens could use for growth). Since no single bacterial strain can be expected to monopolize the efficient utilization of all nutrients, the establishment of resistance to infections is likely to require the presence of a complex flora. It is unlikely, therefore, that the deliberate administration of single bacterial cultures to animals of commercial interest will significantly decrease the establishment of undesirable microorganisms in the intestine. Theoretically, the administration of a complex flora would be much more promising, and this approach has already been shown to be effective in chickens given either fecal suspensions from healthy animals or a defined complex mixture of bacterial isolates from the indigenous microflora (reviewed in reference 32). There is one possible exception from this rule, namely, when a single strain is introduced which physiologically closely resembles the pathogen to which one wants to impart resistance. In this case the introduced strain will compete with the particular pathogen for the same adhesion sites and the same limiting nutrients. Thus, if such a strain is administered in sufficiently large concentrations of viable cells, or if it is able to colonize on its own, it may be able to reduce the rate of multiplication of that particular pathogen sufficiently to prevent infection. Indeed, instances have been described in the literature in which administration of an avirulent mutant protected experimental animals against infection with the virulent parent strain. For example, Wilson and Sheagren (55) have shown that cefoxitin-treated hamsters could be protected against colitis from an experimental infection with *C. difficile* when the animals were first associated with a nontoxigenic strain of *C. difficile*. Interestingly, and as expected by the hypotheses developed in this article, there was no protection when the antibiotic-treated animals were challenged simultaneously with a mixture of the toxigenic and nontoxigenic strains. In another example, Duval-Iflah et al. (8) showed that plasmid-free strains of *E. coli* could prevent the colonization of gnotobiotic mice by isogenic strains bearing resistance plasmids. Here again, effective antagonism depended on the plasmid-free antagonist's being introduced first. In addition, and again as would be predicted by the above theories, these workers found that physiological adaptation of the invading *E. coli* strain to the intestinal microenvironment conferred an advantage which was lost upon subculture in broth.

A considerably less well established possibility of beneficial effects is thought by some to be mediated by the metabolic activities of large quantities of viable bacteria administered per os. Thus, Goldin and Gorbach (reviewed in reference 25) noted a reduction in fecal enzymes that have been suspected of being associated with the risk of large-bowel cancer, but Whitt and Savage (53) found no effect of lactobacilli on host enzymes in gnotobiotic mice.

In conclusion, then, pathogens that must colonize body surfaces face a formidable range of obstacles provided by the host and its indigenous flora. As the topics covered in this volume demonstrate, only two of the many types of virulence mechanisms that pathogens need to overcome these obstacles are understood at least to some extent, namely, mechanisms of adhesion to the wall of the small intestine and mechanisms of penetration of the intestinal epithelium. A study of the mechanisms of colonization used by the indigenous microflora can serve, therefore, as an example of what one may look for in studying the colonization potential of pathogens and, on the other hand, can define the nature of one of the most important barriers that the virulence mechanisms of pathogens must overcome.

ACKNOWLEDGMENTS.   Recent work from my laboratory reviewed here was supported by Public Health Service grant AI 20387 from the National Institute of Allergy and Infectious Diseases.

LITERATURE CITED

1. Barrow, P. A., B. E. Brooker, R. Fuller, and M. J. Newport. 1980. The attachment of bacteria to the gastric epithelium of the pig and its importance in the microecology of the intestine. *J. Appl. Bacteriol.* 48:147–154.

2. Bollard, J. E., M. A. Vanderwee, G. W. Smith, C. Tasman-Jones, J. B. Gavin, and S. P. Lee. 1986. Location of bacteria in the mid-colon of the rat. *Appl. Environ. Microbiol.* 51:604–608.

3. Burg, R. W. 1982. Fermentation products in animal health. *ASM News* 48:460–463.

4. Chase, D. G., and S. L. Erlandsen. 1976. Evidence for a complex life cycle and endospore formation in attached, filamentous, segmented bacterium from mouse ileum. *J. Bacteriol.* 127:572–583.

5. Cohen, P. S., and D. C. Laux. 1985. Fractionation and characterization of mouse small intestine mucus and brush border receptors for the K88ab adhesin. *Microecol. Ther.* 15:71–83.

6. Cohen, P. S., E. A. Wadolkowski, and D. C. Laux. 1986. Adhesion of a human fecal Escherichia coli strain to a 50.5 KDal glycoprotein receptor present in mouse colonic mucus. *Microecol. Ther.* 16:231–241.

7. Dubos, R. 1963. Staphylococci and infection immunity. *Am J. Dis. Child.* 105:643–645.

8. Duval-Iflah, Y., P. Raibaud, and M. Rousseau. 1981. Antagonism among isogenic strains of *Escherichia coli* in the digestive tracts of gnotobiotic mice. *Infect. Immun.* 34:957–969.

9. Edwards, P. A. W. 1978. Is mucus a selective barrier to macromolecules? *Br. Med. Bull.* 34:55–56.

10. Feighner, S. D., and M. P. Dashkevicz. 1987. Subtherapeutic levels of antibiotics in poultry feeds and their effects on weight gain, feed efficiency, and bacterial cholyltaurine hydrolase activity. *Appl. Environ. Microbiol.* 53:331–336.

11. Fox, J. G., B. M. Edvise, N. Cabot, C. Beaucage, and J. C. Murphy. 1986. Isolation of Campylobacter-like organisms from gastric mucosa in the ferret. *Am. J. Vet. Res.* 47:236–239.

12. Freter, R. 1956. Experimental enteric Shigella and Vibrio infections in mice and guinea pigs. *J. Exp. Med.* 104:411–418.

13. Freter, R. 1980. Prospects for preventing the association of harmful bacteria with host mucosal surfaces, p. 441–458. *In* E. H. Beachey (ed.), *Bacterial Adherence.* Chapman & Hall, Ltd., London.

14. Freter, R. 1982. Bacterial association with the mucus gel system of the gut, p. 278–281. *In* D. Schlessinger (ed.), *Microbiology—1982.* American Society for Microbiology, Washington, D.C.

15. Freter, R. 1983. Mechanisms that control the microflora in the large intestine, p. 33–54. *In* D. J. Hentges (ed.), *Human Intestinal Flora in Health and*

Disease. Academic Press, Inc., Boca Raton, Fla.

16. Freter, R. 1986. Gnotobiotic and germfree animal systems, p. 205–227. *In* E. R. Leadbetter and J. S. Poindexter (ed.), *Bacteria in Nature, a Treatise on the Interaction of Bacteria and Their Habitats*. Plenum Publishing Corp., New York.

17. Freter, R., H. Brickner, M. Botney, D. Cleven, and A. Aranki. 1983. Mechanisms which control bacterial populations in continuous flow culture models of mouse large intestinal flora. *Infect. Immun.* 39:676–685.

18. Freter, R., H. Brickner, J. Fekete, and M. M. Vickerman. 1983. Survival and implantation of *Escherichia coli* in the intestinal tract. *Infect. Immun.* 39:686–703.

19. Freter, R., and P. C. M. O'Brien. 1981. The role of chemotaxis in the association of motile bacteria with intestinal mucosa: chemotactic responses of *Vibrio cholerae* and description of motile non-chemotactic mutants. *Infect. Immun.* 34:215–221.

20. Freter, R., and P. C. M. O'Brien. 1981. The role of chemotaxis in the association of motile bacteria with intestinal mucosa: fitness and virulence of nonchemotactic *Vibrio cholerae* mutants in infant mice. *Infect. Immun.* 34:222–233.

21. Freter, R., and P. C. M. O'Brien. 1981. The role of chemotaxis in the association of motile bacteria with intestinal mucosa: in vitro studies. *Infect. Immun.* 34:234–240.

22. Freter, R., E. Stauffer, C. Cleven, L. V. Holdeman, and W. E. C. Moore. 1983. Continuous flow cultures as in vitro models of the ecology of large intestinal flora. *Infect. Immun.* 39:666–675.

23. Friedman, D. R., and S. P. Halbert. 1960. Mixed bacterial infections in relation to antibiotic activities. *J. Immunol.* 84:11–19.

24. Gibbons, R. A., and R. Sellwood. 1973. The macromolecular biochemistry of cervical secretions, p. 251–265. *In* R. J. Blandau and K. Moghissi (ed.), *The Biology of the Cervix*. University of Chicago Press, Chicago.

25. Gorbach, S. L. 1982. The intestinal microflora and its colon cancer connection. *Infection* 10:379–384.

26. Halbert, S. P. 1948. The relation of antagonistic coliform organisms to Shigella infections. II. Observations in acute infections. *J. Immunol.* 60:359–381.

27. Hazell, S. A., A. Lee, L. Brady, and W. Hennessy. 1986. Campylobacter pyloridis and gastritis: association with intercellular spaces and adaptation to an environment of mucus as important factors in colonization of the gastric epithelium. *J. Infect. Dis.* 153:658–663.

28. Hentges, D. J., and R. Freter. 1962. In vivo and in vitro antagonism of intestinal bacteria against Shigella flexneri. I. Correlation between various tests. *J. Infect. Dis.* 110:30–37.

29. Herget, H. F., and E. Weinrauch. 1979. Criteria and application of microbiological therapy of the gastrointestinal tract in the department of anaesthesia and intensive medicine of Justus-Liebig-University. *Microecol. Ther.* 9:63–73. (In German with English summary.)

30. Hill, R. H. 1985. Prevention of adhesion by indigenous bacteria to rabbit cecum epithelium by a barrier of microvesicles. *Infect. Immun.* 47:540–543.

31. Ikari, N. S., D. M. Kenton, and V. M. Young. 1969. Interaction in the germfree mouse intestine of colicinogenic and colicin-sensitive microorganisms. *Pro. Soc. Exp. Biol. Med.* 130:1280–1284.

32. Impey, C. S., G. C. Mead, and S. M. George. 1982. Competitive exclusion of salmonellas from the chick caecum using a defined mixture of bacterial isolates from the caecal microflora of an adult bird. *J. Hyg.* 89:479–490.

33. Jones, G. W., and R. Freter. 1976. Adhesive properties of *Vibrio cholerae*. *Infect. Immun.* 14:232–245.

34. Lee, A. 1980. Normal flora of animal intestinal surfaces, p. 145–173. *In* G. Bitton and K. C. Marshall (ed.), *Adsorption of Microorganisms to Surfaces*. John Wiley & Sons, Inc., New York.

35. Lee, A. 1985. Neglected niches, the microbial ecology of the gastrointestinal tract. *Adv. Microb. Ecol.* 8:115–162.

36. Maier, B. R., A. B. Onderdonk, R. C. Baskett, and D. J. Hentges. 1972. Shigella, indigenous flora interactions in mice. *J. Clin. Nutr.* 25:1433–1440.

37. Metchnikoff, E. 1907. *The Prolongation of Life. Optimistic Studies*, p. 151–183. Heinemann, London.

38. Muralidhara, K. S., G. G. Sheggeby, P. R. Elliker, D. C. England, and W. E. Sandine. 1977. Effect of feeding lactobacilli on the coliform and Lactobacillus flora of intestinal tissue and feces from piglets. *J. Food Prot.* 40:288–295.

39. Nissle, A. 1916. Ueber die Grundlagen einer neuen ursaechlichen Bekaempfung der pathologischen Darmflora. *Dtsch. Med. Wochenschr.* 42:1181–1184.

40. Olentine, C. 1983. Microbial cultures: vodoo or can do? *Anim. Nutr. Health* 38:8–10.

41. Peo, E. R., Jr., J. D. Crenshaw, and A. H. Lewis. 1984. Probiotics—are they here to stay? *Nebraska Swine Report*, p. 24–25. EC. 84–219. Nebraska Cooperative Extension Service.

42. Rettger, L. F., M. N. Levy, L. Weinstein, and J. E. Weiss. 1935. *Lactobacillus acidophilus & Its Therapeutic Applications*. Yale University Press, New Haven, Conn.

43. Rozee, K. R., D. Cooper, K. Lam, and J. W. Costerton. 1982. Microbial flora of the mouse ileum mucous layer and epithelial surface. *Appl. Environ. Microbiol.* 43:1451–1463.

44. Rusch, V. 1980. Medicine and the microbial world. *Microecol. Ther.* 10:163–172. (In German with English summary.)

45. Rusch, V., R. M. Hyde, and T. D. Luckey. 1980. Documentation on the identity, manufacture, saftey, efficacy, and stability of SYMBIOFLOR products. *Microecol. Ther.* 10:173–203.

46. Savage, D. C. 1977. Microbial ecology of the gastrointestinal tract. *Annu. Rev. Microbiol.* 31:107–133.

47. Sears, H. J., I. Brownlee, and J. K. Uchigama. 1949. Persistence of individual strains of *Escherichia coli* in the intestinal tract of man. *J. Bacteriol.* 59:293–301.

48. Shinefield, H. R., J. C. Ribble, M. Boris, and H. F. Eichenwald. 1972. Bacterial interference, p. 503–515. *In* J. O. Cohen (ed.), *The Staphylococci.* John Wiley & Sons, Inc., New York.

49. Syed, S. A., G. D. Abrams, and R. Freter. 1970. The efficiency of various intestinal bacteria in assuming normal functions of enteric flora after association with germfree mice. *Infect. Immun.* 2:376–386.

50. Tannock, G. W. 1984. Control of gastrointestinal pathogens by normal flora, p. 374–382. *In* M. J. Klug and C. A. Reddy (ed.), *Current Perspectives in Microbial Ecology.* American Society for Microbiology, Washington, D.C.

51. van der Waaij, D., J. M. Berghuis de Vries, and J. E. C. Lekkerkerk. 1971. Colonization resistance of the digestive tract in conventional and antibiotic-treated mice. *J. Hyg.* 69:405–411.

52. Visek, W. J. 1978. The mode of growth promotion by antibiotics. *J. Anim. Sci.* 46:1447–1469.

53. Whitt, D. E., and D. C. Savage. 1987. Lactobacilli as effectors of host functions: no influence on the activities of enzymes in enterocytes of mice. *Appl. Environ. Microbiol.* 53:325–330.

54. Wilson, K. H., and R. Freter. 1986. Interactions of *Clostridium difficile* and *Escherichia coli* with microfloras in continuous flow cultures and gnotobiotic mice. *Infect. Immun.* 54:354–358.

55. Wilson, K. H., and J. N. Sheagren. 1983. Antagonism of toxigenic Clostridium difficile by nontoxigenic Clostridium difficile. *J. Infect Dis.* 147:733–736.

Chapter 4

Virulence Mechanisms of Enteroinvasive Pathogens

THOMAS LARRY HALE AND SAMUEL B. FORMAL

Department of Enteric Infections
Walter Reed Army Institute of Research
Washington, DC 20307-5100

INTRODUCTION

Enteroinvasive bacterial pathogens which cause disease in animals include members of the genera *Salmonella, Yersinia,* and *Shigella. Salmonella* infections in cattle, sheep, swine, and horses are usually manifested as acute or chronic enteritis, but acute bacteremia accompanied by abortion and death can also result from ingestion of these organisms. *Yersinia pseudotuberculosis* is a common cause of epizootic disease of birds and rodents, and this organism can also cause enteritis and septic abortions in domestic animals. Humans are the natural reservoirs of *Shigella* species, but *Shigella* infections often occur in captive monkey populations.

LABORATORY MODELS

Several laboratory models have been useful in the study of enteroinvasive enteric diseases, and a brief description of these will provide the background for a discussion of the pathogenesis of the infections. The least stringent model is an in vitro system which uses cultured mammalian cells as surrogates of intestinal epithelial cells. Since virulent *Shigella, Salmonella,* and *Yersinia* strains invade these cells by a process which appears to be analogous to the invasion of enterocytes in vivo, this model has been useful in evaluating one aspect of the virulence of individual bacterial strains and in studying the mechanism of bacterial invasion. Although the tissue culture model can assess the ability of an enteroinvasive strain to initiate infection, it does not address other determinants of virulence. For example, the organisms must overcome host defense mechanisms in the intact intestine which are not present in vitro. Therefore, various animal models have been used in the study of enteroinvasive pathogens. The ability of shigellae to invade corneal epithelial cells and elicit keratoconjunctivitis in the eyes of rabbits, guinea pigs, or mice (Sereny test) assesses both invasiveness and resistance to mucosal defense mechanisms. The ligated rabbit ileal loop model has been used to assess the ability of shigellae or salmonellae to invade the intestinal mucosa and elicit inflammation and fluid secretion. Oral challenge of starved and opiated guinea pigs measures the lethality of these organisms in a compromised host, whereas oral challenge of monkeys can reproduce the enteritis of *Salmonella* infections or the dysentery commonly seen with shigellosis.

OVERVIEW OF PATHOGENIC MECHANISMS OF *SHIGELLA* SPP.

Ingestion

In humans, as few as 10 shigellae can cause dysentery, whereas the 50% infective dose in monkeys is approximately 10^{10}. The basis of the relative resistance of monkeys to *Shigella* infection is unknown. Shigellae do not colonize or invade the small intestine unless peristaltic motion is inhibited by opiates or ligation. The lack of chemotactic motility may be one mitigating factor which discourages colonization of the small intestine by shigellae, but recent data indicate that pancreatic enzymes may also protect the mucosa from invasion by shigellae. Pretreatment of a virulent culture of *Shigella flexneri* 5 with trypsin or chymotrypsin causes the loss of invasive potential as measured by the ability of these organisms to invade HeLa cell monolayers in vitro. Suspension of the organisms in fresh culture medium allows the complete regeneration of the invasive phenotype after two rounds of cell division (T. L. Hale, manuscript in preparation). These data suggest that outer membrane proteins which are necessary for adherence and invasion are cleaved as shigellae pass through the duodenum and jejunum. Presumably these outer membrane proteins are regenerated in time to facilitate invasion of the colonic epithelium, which is the target tissue of shigellae.

Diarrheal Stage

Although they do not actually invade the mucosa, shigellae often elicit abnormal fluid secretion when traversing the small intestine. For example, there is net fluid secretion in the jejunum when rhesus monkeys ingest virulent *S. flexneri*. In combination with inhibited colonic absorption, this abnormal fluid flux is manifested as diarrhea. If the shigellae are injected directly into the cecum, however, the only transport abnormality is the inhibition of fluid absorption, and the clinical manifestation is dysentery (36). These data suggest that an enterotoxin is elaborated by shigellae during

transit through the ileum, and the obvious candidates for such a toxin are the Shiga toxin produced by *Shigella dysenteriae* 1 or the Shiga-like toxin produced by both *S. dysenteriae* 1 and the other *Shigella* spp. (32). The latter toxin is neutralizable by antibody raised against the classical Shiga toxin, but the Shiga-like toxin genes share only about 50% homology with the Shiga toxin genes. Arguing against a role for these toxins in the diarrheal stage of disease is the experimental finding that ingestion of a noninvasive strain of *S. dysenteriae* 1 does not cause diarrhea in monkeys, even though this strain is highly toxigenic (9). In the final analysis, invasion of the intestinal mucosa seems to be the essential step in the pathogenesis of shigellosis, and the additional role of *Shigella* toxins remains unclear.

Once shigellae have traversed the upper digestive tract, they encounter fatty acids and reducing conditions in the colonic lumen. These by-products of the metabolic activity of fusiform anaerobes are toxic for shigellae. In addition, chemostat experiments designed to simulate the luminal environment in vitro indicate that the most serious obstacle facing members of the family *Enterobacteriaceae* attempting to colonize the bowel is the competition of the resident flora for carbon sources utilizable under low-pH and reducing conditions (19). These environmental pressures have apparently selected and maintained the invasive phenotype in the genus *Shigella*. The evolution of this phenotype has allowed shigellae to escape from the fully occupied niche of the lumen and to occupy the extreme environment represented by the cytosol of the colonic epithelial cells (28). By occupying this unique environmental niche, shigellae also avail themselves of an inexhaustible carbon source—glucose from the host blood stream.

Colonic Invasion and Dysentery

The intestinal mucus layer is the first barrier encountered by shigellae which are invading the colonic mucosa. The effectiveness of mucus as a barrier can be readily demonstrated in vitro by using cultured explants of monkey colon. These explants, which are characteristically blanketed by a layer of mucus, cannot be infected by a pure culture of *S. flexneri* (G. Dinari and T. L. Hale, unpublished observations). Since solubilized monkey mucus does not inhibit the invasion of epithelial cells by shigellae (5), the mucus on the explants probably acts as a mechanical barrier. Other investigators have found that *S. flexneri* will not attach to intestinal slices obtained from gnotobiotic mice; however, these organisms do attach to slices which have been treated with extracts of normal mouse feces (34). Thus, it appears that glycosidases produced by the normal intestinal flora may indirectly facilitate *Shigella* invasion by digesting colonic mucus.

Once they have breached the mucus layer, shigellae apparently induce endocytic activity in the normally nonphagocytic enterocytes. The tissue culture model involving the use of HeLa cells has been used to characterize this phenomenon. The first step of this process involves adherence of shigellae to the HeLa cell membrane. This adherence is mediated by components which can be cleaved by trypsin treatment of intact bacteria, so that it is apparently different from the lipopolysaccharide-mediated adherence to guinea pig enterocytes which has previously been reported (21).

Shigellae invade HeLa cells by an endocytic process which does not rupture the plasma membrane and which requires both host cell energy production and microfilament function (13). Ultrastructurally, the invasion process is characterized by the formation of areas of close apposition between the surface of the bacterium and the surface of the host cell (13). These areas of close apposition may represent localized binding of bacterial surface ligands to receptors on the host cell membrane. Occasionally a thin section reveals a number of areas of close apposition around the circumference of an attached organism (13, 17), and this morphology gives the impression that the shigellae are "zippered up" into an endocytic vacuole by sequential receptor-ligand binding.

When shigellae are internalized by HeLa cells, they are initially contained within endocytic vacuoles. Within 30 min, however, these vacuoles disappear (13, 41). A similar dissolution of endocytic vacuoles apparently occurs within infected colonic epithelial cells, because membrane-bound shigellae are rarely observed in vivo (44). Organisms which are unable to lyse these endocytic vacuoles are less virulent because they are less able to spread to contiguous epithelial cells (41). Another intracellular event which accompanies the endocytosis of virulent shigellae is the inhibition of host cell protein synthesis (41). The cytotoxic manifestation of Shiga-like toxins probably inhibits macromolecular synthesis (14), but the lysis of microsomal membranes may also be involved (41). Glucose and amino acid transport continue in infected HeLa cells, but these nutrients support bacterial multiplication rather than host cell functions (14, 31). Presumably a similar parasitic relationship allows shigellae to survive and propagate within the colonic epithelium, and, as mentioned above, this is probably the powerful selective advantage which has allowed the evolution and conservation of the invasive phenotype.

A secondary result of this parasitism of the colonic mucosa is the tissue destruction which is the underlying cause of the symptoms of bacillary dysentery. The inflammation elicited by mucosal destruction is accompanied by increased peristaltic motion and goblet cell evacuation. These abnormal bowel functions have the effect of sweeping shigellae that have been released from degenerating enterocytes out of the intestinal tract, and this discourages the establishment of new foci of infection.

GENETICS OF VIRULENCE IN SHIGELLAE

Chromosomal Virulence Genes

The virulence-associated regions of the chromosome in *S. flexneri* 2a have been extensively studied. These studies, which involve the conjugal transfer of chromosomal material from *Escherichia coli* K-12 to *S. flexneri* by uninterrupted matings, show that replacement of three *Shigella* chromosomal regions with homologous regions from *E. coli* has an effect upon the virulence of the *Shigella* recipient in animal models. For example, incorporation of a large chromosomal region including the *xyl* (79 min) and *rha* (88 min) genes is associated with loss of ability to cause a fatal infection in orally challenged guinea pigs (7), and replacement of the *his* locus (45 min) is associated with loss of the ability to cause a positive Sereny test (8). Transduction of the *purE* locus (12 min) from *E. coli* to *S. flexneri* also results in both a Sereny-negative phenotype and a decrease in virulence in the guinea pig model (6). Since none of these avirulent *E. coli-S. flexneri* hybrids lost the ability to invade mammalian cells in vitro, it appears that the chromosomal regions replaced by *E. coli* genes are necessary for the survival of shigellae in the lumen of the bowel or in the tissues.

Potential virulence determinants have been identified in two of these *Shigella* chromosomal regions. The *xyl-rha* region encodes an aerobactin iron-binding system in *S. flexneri* (11); however, recent analysis of aerobactin-negative *Shigella* mutants indicates that this phenotype is not necessary for virulence (26). The ability to elicit fluid accumulation in the ligated rabbit ileal loop model is associated with the chromosomal region including *mtl* (80 min) and *arg* (90 min) (39). The genes encoding a Shiga-like toxin have been localized in this chromosomal region in *S. dysenteriae* 1 (46), and the virulence determinant encoded by this region in *S. flexneri* may be a toxin (32). The *his* genes are linked to the *rfb* gene cluster in *E. coli,* and this chromosomal region is necessary for synthesis of the complete somatic antigen in either *E. coli* or *S. flexneri*. Although the somatic antigen is probably the key virulence determinant encoded by the *his* region in *Shigella* species, an additional determinant(s) may also be expressed (8). In contrast to the *xyl-rha* and the *his* regions, a virulence determinant encoded by the *purE* region has not been identified. Nonetheless, this region has been given a genetic epitaph based on the Sereny test phenotype, i.e., *kcp,* denoting keratoconjictivitis provocation (6).

Plasmid Virulence Genes

Virtually all selectable chromosomal markers can be conjugally transferred from *S. flexneri* to *E. coli* K-12 without altering the avirulent phenotype of the recipient. This observation suggests that extrachromosomal elements are also necessary for expression of virulence. About 5 years ago it was shown that a 120-megadalton (MDa) plasmid was indeed necessary for expression of both the group D somatic antigen and the invasive phenotype in *Shigella sonnei* (40). Later it was found that expression of the latter phenotype was associated with a 140-MDa plasmid in other *Shigella* species and in enteroinvasive strains of *E. coli* (38). These plasmids are at least 80% homologous and are functionally interchangeable in their ability to confer the invasive phenotype (38). A 6-MDa plasmid, which is unrelated to the invasive plasmids, is necessary for synthesis of the complete somatic antigen in *S. dysenteriae* 1 (49).

Genetic analysis of the large plasmids of *S. flexneri* and *S. sonnei* has revealed at least four loci which influence various aspects of virulence. For example, a 22-MDa fragment of the 140-MDa plasmid of *S. flexneri* 5 can confer the invasive phenotype upon a *Shigella* strain which has lost the 140-MDa plasmid (27). Transposon mutagenesis indicates that this region of *Shigella* invasion plasmids carries at least two invasion loci, designated *ipa* (invasion plasmid antigen) (3) and *invA* (48). Two other loci, which are apparently located outside the 22-MDa invasion region, may also be necessary for expression of the virulent phenotype. These include the *virF* genes, which are necessary for the binding of Congo red (37), and the *virG* locus, which is necessary for expression of a positive Sereny phenotype (42).

Three *ipa* gene protein products have been designated *b* (57 kDa), *c* (43 kDa), and *d* (37 kDa) (3, 15). Additional products which are also encoded by *ipa*-linked genes include polypeptides designated *a* (78 kDa), *f* (25 kDa), and *g* (20 kDa) (15). *ipa* gene products *a* through *d* are immunodominant protein antigens which elicit serum and mucosal antibody during *Shi-*

gella infections in monkeys (4, 30) and humans (16). Four *inv* gene products, of 81, 47, 41, and 38 kDa, have been identified in minicells (48). These proteins, which are immunologically distinct from the *ipa* gene products, do not induce antibody in convalescent-monkey antisera (T. L. Hale and H. Watanabe, unpublished data). The *virF* region expresses three polypeptides, of 21, 27, and 30 kDa (42). The products of *virG* have not yet been identified.

Possible Roles of Plasmid Gene Products in Virulence

Anucleate minicells isolated from *S. flexneri* can invade HeLa cells (15). Since minicells contain no chromosomal DNA, the 140-MDa plasmid apparently carries all the genetic information necessary for expression of the invasive phenotype. As discussed above, a 22-MDa fragment of this plasmid has now been shown to carry the genes necessary for the invasion step, and some of the protein products of these genes have been identified. The functions of these proteins have not been rigorously defined, but preliminary data suggest that the *ipa* gene polypeptides designated *b* and *c* are probably the bacterial proteins which actually trigger the uptake of shigellae. When extracted under nondenaturing conditions, these polypeptides have a proclivity for the surface of HeLa cells. It is our current hypothesis that this interaction triggers endocytic activity, which results in the ingestion of the attached bacterium. The *invA* locus seems to function as a transport system, allowing insertion of *ipa* polypeptides into the outer membrane in a functional orientation (T. Pal and T. L. Hale, unpublished data).

OVERVIEW OF PATHOGENIC MECHANISMS OF *SALMONELLA* AND *YERSINIA* SPP.

Ingestion

In humans the infective dose of *Salmonella typhimurium* is approximately 10^5, while ingestion of 10^{10} organisms can cause gastroenteritis in monkeys. Rough *Salmonella* strains are avirulent, and the underlying cause of avirulence probably involves the loss of chemotactic motility as well as diminished resistance to gastric acidity (29). Smooth strains, which are more actively motile than rough strains, are attracted to damaged HeLa cells in vitro by a gradient of the amino acid glycine (47). It has been proposed that *S. typhimurium* organisms are attracted to the dying cells on the villus tips of the ileal epithelium and that this chemotactic response facilitates the establishment of a *Salmonella* infection (47). The action of pancreatic enzymes may also enhance the invasiveness of the salmonellae. Pretreatment of *S. typhimurium* with trypsin causes these organisms to invade HeLa cells much more avidly than do untreated control cultures (Hale, unpublished data). Thus, the enzymatic environment of the small intestine may activate the invasive phenotype by modifying protein components of the outer membrane. The possible roles of mannose-resistant hemagglutinins and mannose-sensitive hemagglutinins (type 1 fimbriae) in mediating the adherence of *S. typhimurium* to cultured epithelial cells in vitro has been documented, but there is no clear evidence that these adhesins play a role in attachment to the intestinal epithelium (45).

Once the salmonellae have penetrated the mucus layer of the small intestine, the microvilli on epithelial cells in the immediate vicinity degenerate. Invaginations then form in the apical cytoplasm of enterocytes, and the organisms are taken up within endocytic vacuoles (43). The morphological and biochemical aspects of this invasion process have been studied in the HeLa cell model, and the general pattern is similar to that observed with shigellae. The organisms adhere to the plasma membrane and develop areas of close apposition which may represent sequential receptor-ligand binding (23). Ingestion of attached organisms requires host cell energy production and microfilament contraction (24). Unlike shigellae, however, the ingested salmonellae remain enveloped within endocytic vacuoles in the cytoplasm of HeLa cells (23) or enterocytes (43). Indeed, many

Salmonella species seem to be transported across the intestinal epithelium without harming the epithelial cells. These organisms then enter the lymphatic system and become distributed throughout many tissues in the host (43).

Like salmonellae, *Yersinia pseudotuberculosis* invades epithelial cells by an endocytic process which leaves endocytic vacuoles intact (1), and these organisms are also often transported into the mesenteric lymph nodes. Since *Y. pseudotuberculosis* is not actively motile at 37°C, chemotactic activity is apparently not involved in adherence or invasion in vivo. Outer membrane proteins mediate the adherence of *Y. pseudotuberculosis* to HeLa cells (2), and an outer membrane protein which mediates the invasion of these cell has also been recently identified (20). Additional studies with *Y. enterocolitica* have indicated that a plasmid-encoded cytotoxin is produced by internalized organisms, but such cytotoxic effects have not been reported in cells infected with *Y. pseudotuberculosis*.

Diarrheal Stage

When ingested by rhesus monkeys, *S, typhimurium* invades mucosa of the jejunum, ileum, and colon. This infection is accompanied by the net secretion of fluids in all three portions of the intestine (35). The physiological basis of this transport abnormally may involve the activation of adenlyate cyclase, which is mediated by a choleralike enterotoxin produced by *S. typhimurium* (33). However, it is interesting that some fully invasive strains of *S. typhimurium* do not elicit significant mucosal inflammation, and these strains do not cause diarrhea (10). Therefore, it has been suggested that prostaglandins synthesized as a result of the acute inflammation associated with *Salmonella* enteritis may also activate mucosal adenylate cyclase (10). A role for a Shiga-like cytotoxin in eliciting this mucosal inflammation has been postulated (25). Arguing against this hypothesis, however, is the finding that HeLa cells infected with a toxin-producing strain of *S. typhimurium* continue to synthesize protein

at a normal rate (13, 25). In addition to the determinants of the invasive phenotype, it is obvious that other virulence determinants are necessary for *Salmonella* enteritis, but the contribution of *Salmonella* toxins to this disease process remains a matter for conjecture.

GENETICS OF VIRULENCE IN *SALMONELLA* AND *YERSINIA* SPP.

Salmonella spp.

In contrast to localized *Shigella* infections, the disease process in salmonellosis involves invasion of the intestinal epithelium, spread of organisms to the mesenteric lymph nodes, and systemic dissemination. The genetic basis of this complex pathogenesis is not well understood. Nontyphoid *Salmonella* serotypes uniformly harbor large plasmids which are necessary for virulence in animal models (18), but the virulence determinant(s) encoded by the plasmids has not been characterized. Although it has been suggested that a 60-MDa plasmid is necessary for invasion of epithelial cells by *S. typhimurium* (22), current reports indicate that this plasmid is probably more closely associated with serum resistance and survival within macrophages (12, 18). *Salmonella dublin* also harbors a large plasmid (80 MDa), which is necessary for fatal systemic infections in mice, but is not involved in the initiation of infection at the level of the gut (D. Guiney, J. Fierer, G. Chikami, and P. Beninger, *Abstr. UCLA Symp. Mol. Cell. Biol., J. Cell. Biochem.* 11B:109, 1987). These observations suggest that the invasive phenotype is encoded by chromosomal genes in *Salmonella* species, but, like the genes encoding enterotoxins and cytotoxins, this marker has not been mapped.

Yersinia spp.

The gene encoding the invasive phenotype in *Y. pseudotuberculosis* is also located on the chromosome, but unlike the invasion genes of *Salmonella* spp., this gene has been cloned into *E. coli* and its protein product has been char-

TABLE 1
Summary of pathogenesis and virulence determinants of enteroinvasive pathogens

Organism	Target organ	Chemotactic motility	Adhesion	Endocytic protein	Intracellular fate	Additional virulence determinants
Shigella spp.	Colon	None	Plasmid-encoded, OMP(s)[a]	Plasmid-encoded *ipa* gene products	Escape from vacuoles, bacterial growth, and host cell death	Shiga and Shiga-like toxin, plasmid-encoded contact hemolysin
Salmonella spp.	Small intestine and colon	Yes	Chromosomal hemagglutinins	Unknown	Limited growth within vacuoles and translocation to basement membrane	Cholera-like enterotoxin, Shiga-like toxin, and plasmid-encoded survival mechanism for serum and RES[b]
Yersinia spp.	Small intestine	None at 37°C	Chromosomal OMP	Invasin	Same as for *Salmonella* spp.	Cytotoxin in *Y. enterocolitica*

[a] OMP, Outer membrane protein.
[b] RES, Reticuloendothelial system.

acterized (20). The ability to invade tissue culture cells is conferred by a 3.2-kDa chromosomal region carrying a gene designated *inv*, and this gene expresses a 108-kDa outer membrane protein, which has been designated invasin. When bound to a solid matrix, invasin facilitates the adherence of HEp-2 cells. Therefore, it has been proposed that this protein causes *Y. pseudotuberculosis* to bind to the surface of epithelial cells in a way that induces endocytic uptake (R. R. Isberg, *Abstr. UCLA Symp. Mol. Cell. Biol., J. Cell. Biochem.* 11B:108, 1987). Since site-directed mutagenesis of the *inv* gene causes the loss of virulence in the orally challenged mouse, it would appear that invasin probably plays a role in the initation of intestinal infections in vivo (R. R. Isberg, submitted for publication).

SUMMARY OF PATHOGENIC MECHANISMS OF ENTEROINVASIVE ORGANISMS

In the previous sections we have attempted to give a survey and synthesis of recent experimental observations as they relate to the pathogenesis of invasive enteric disease. Table 1 summarizes some of the salient points

of comparison between the genera *Shigella, Salmonella,* and *Yersinia.* It should be remembered, however, that each of these genera elicits a range of clinical manifestations and that their underlying pathogenic mechanisms vary with both the host and the tissue. Nonetheless, we hope that the basic characteristics of these infections have been accurately recounted and that future research with the genetic tools which are revolutionizing the study of bacterial pathogenesis will allow the characterization of these disease processes on a molecular level.

LITERATURE CITED

1. Bovallius, A., and G. Nilsson. 1975. Infestion and survival of *Y. pseudotuberculosis* in HeLa cells. *Can. J. Microbiol.* 21:1997–2007.
2. Brunius, G., and I. Bolin. 1983. Interaction between *Yersinia pseudotuberculosis* and the HeLa cell surface. *J. Med. Microbiol.* 16:245–261.
3. Buysse, J. M., C. K. Stover, E. V. Oaks, M. Venkatesan, and D. J. Kopecko. 1987. Molecular cloning of invasion plasmid antigen (*ipa*) genes from *Shigella flexneri*: analysis of *ipa* gene products and genetic mapping. *J. Bacteriol.* 169:2561–2569.
4. Dinari, G., T. L. Hale, S. Austin, and S. B. Formal. 1987. Local and systemic antibody response to shigella infection in rhesus monkeys. *J. Infect. Dis.* 155:1065–1069.

5. Dinari, G., T. L. Hale, O. Washington, and S. B. Formal. 1986. Effect of guinea pig or monkey mucus on *Shigella* aggregation and invasion of HeLa cells by *Shigella flexneri* 1b and 2a. *Infect. Immun.* 51:975–978.

6. Formal, S. B., P. Gemski, L. S. Baron, and E. H. LaBrec. 1971. A chromosomal locus which controls the ability of *Shigella flexneri* to evoke keratoconjunctivitis. *Infect. Innum.* 3:73–79.

7. Formal, S. B., E. H. LaBrec, T. H. Kent, and S. Falkow. 1965. Abortive intestinal infection with an *Escherichia coli-Shigella flexneri* hybrid strain. *J. Bacteriol.* 89:1374–1382.

8. Gemski, P., D. G. Sheahan, O. Washington, and S. B. Formal. 1972. Virulence of *Shigella flexneri* hybrids expressing *Escherichia coli* somatic antigens. *Infect. Immun.* 6:104–111.

9. Gemski, P., Jr., A. Takeuchi, O. Washington, and S. B. Formal. 1972. Shigellosis due to *Shigella dysenteriae* 1: relative importance of mucosal invasion versus toxin production in pathogenesis. *J. Infect. Dis.* 126:523–530.

10. Giannella, R. A., R. E. Gots, A. N. Charney, W. B. Greenough III, and S. B. Formal. 1975. Pathogenesis of salmonella-mediated intestinal fluid secretion. *Gastroenterology* 69:1238–1245.

11. Griffiths, E., P. Stevenson, T. H. Hale, and S. B. Formal. 1985. Synthesis of aerobactin and a 76,000-dalton iron-regulated outer membrane protein by *Escherichia coli* K-12–*Shigella flexneri* hybrids and by enteroinvasive strains of *Escherichia coli*. *Infect. Immun.* 49:67–71.

12. Hackett, J., I. Kotlarski, V. Mathan, K. Franki, and D. Rowley. 1986. The colonization of Peyer's patches by a strain of *Salmonella typhimurium* cured of the cryptic plasmid. *J. Infect. Dis.* 153:1119–1125.

13. Hale, T. L. 1986. Invasion of epithelial cells by shigellae. *Ann. Inst. Pasteur Microbiol.* 137A:311–314.

14. Hale, T. L., and S. B. Formal. 1981. Protein synthesis in HeLa or Henle 407 cells infected with *Shigella dysenteriae* 1, *Shigella flexneri* 2a, or *Salmonella typhimurium* W118. *Infect. Immun.* 32:137–144.

15. Hale, T. L., E. V. Oaks, and S. B. Formal. 1985. Identification and antigenic characterization of virulence-associated, plasmid-coded proteins of *Shigella* spp. and enteroinvasive *Escherichia coli*. *Infect. Innum.* 50:620–629.

16. Hale, T. L., E. V. Oaks, S. B. Formal, G. Dinari, and P. Echeverria. 1986. Immune response to *Shigella* infections and to *Shigella* vaccines, p. 181–185. *In* F. Brown, R. M. Chanock, and R. A. Lerner (ed.), *Vaccines 86.* Cold Spring Harbor Laboratory, Cold Spring Harbor, N.Y.

17. Hale, T. L., P. A. Schad, and S. B. Formal. 1983. The envelope and tissue invasion, p. 87–108. *In* E. F. Easmon (ed.), *Medical Microbiology,* vol. 3. Academic Press, Inc. (London), Ltd., London.

18. Helmuth, R., R. Stephan, C. Bunge, B. Hoog, A. Steinbeck, and E. Bulling. 1985. Epidemiology of virulence-associated plasmids and outer membrane protein patterns within seven common *Salmonella* serotypes. *Infect. Immun.* 48:175–182.

19. Hentges, D. L. 1975. Resistance of the indigenous intestinal flora to the establishment of invading microbial populations, p. 116–119. *In* D. Schlessinger (ed.), *Microbiology—1975.* American Society for Microbiology, Washington, D.C.

20. Isberg, R. R., and S. Falkow. 1985. A single genetic locus encoded by *Yersinia pseudotuberculosis* permits invasion of cultured animal cells by *Escherichia coli* K-12. *Nature (London)* 317:262–264.

21. Izhar, M., Y. Nuchamowitz, and D. Mirelman. 1982. Adherence of *Shigella flexneri* to guinea pig intestinal cells is mediated by a mucosal adhesin. *Infect. Immun.* 35:1110–1118.

22. Jones, G. W., D. K. Rabert, D. M. Svinarich, and H. J. Whitfield. 1982. Association of adhesive, invasive, and virulent phenotypes of *Salmonella typhimurium* with autonomous 60-Mdal plasmids. *Infect. Immun.* 38:476–486.

23. Kihlstrom, E., and S. Latkovic. 1978. Ultrastructural studies on the interaction between *Salmonella typhimurium* 395 M and HeLa cells. *Infect. Immun.* 22:804–809.

24. Kihlstrom, E., and L. Nilsson. 1977. Endocytosis of *Salmonella typhimurium* 395 MS and MR10 by HeLa cells. *Acta Pathol. Microbiol. Scand. Sect. B* 85:322–328.

25. Koo, F. C. W., J. W. Peterson, C. W. Houston, and N. C. Molina. 1984. Pathogenesis of experimental salmonellosis: inhibition of protein synthesis by cytotoxin. *Infect. Immun.* 43:93–100.

26. Lawlor, K. M., P. A. Daskaleros, R. E. Robinson, and S. M. Payne. 1987. Virulence of iron transport mutants of *Shigella flexneri* and utilization of host iron compounds. *Infect. Immun.* 55:594–599.

27. Maurelli, A. T., B. Baudry, H. d'Hauteville, T. L. Hale, and P. J. Sansonetti. 1985. Cloning of plasmid DNA sequences involved in invasion of HeLa cells by *Shigella flexneri*. *Infect. Immun.* 49:164–171.

28. Moulder, J. W. 1974. Intracecellular parasitism: life in an extreme environment. *J. Infect. Dis.* 130:300–306.

29. Nevola, J. J., B. A. D. Stocker, D. C. Laux, and P. S. Cohen. 1985. Colonization of the mouse intestine by an avirulent *Salmonella typhimurium* strain and its lipopolysaccharide-defective mutants. *Infect. Immun.* 50:152–159.

30. Oaks, E. V., T. L. Hale, and S. B. Formal. 1986. Serum immune response to shigella protein antigens in rhesus monkeys and humans infected with *Shigella* spp. *Infect. Immun.* 53:57–63.

31. Oaks, E. V., M. E. Wingfield, and S. B. Formal.

1985. Plaque formation by virulent *Shigella flexneri*. *Infect. Immun.* 48:124–129.

32. O'Brien, A. D., M. R. Tompson, P. Gemski, B. P. Doctor, and S. B. Formal. 1977. Biological properties of *Shigella flexneri* 2a toxin and its serological relationship to *Shigella dysenteriae* 1 toxin. *Infect. Immun.* 15:796–798.

33. Peterson, J. W., and P. D. Sandefur. 1979. Evidence of a role for permeability factors in the pathogenesis of salmonellosis. *Am. J. Clin. Nutr.* 32:197–209.

34. Prizont, R. 1982. Degradation of intestinal glycoproteins by pathogenic *Shigella flexneri*. *Infect. Immun.* 36:615–620.

35. Rout, W. R., S. B. Formal, G. J. Dammin, and R. A. Gianella. 1974. Pathophysiology of *Salmonella* diarrhea in the rhesus monkey: intestinal transport, morphological and bacteriological studies. *Gastroenterology* 67:59–70.

36. Rout, W. R., S. B. Formal, R. A. Giannella, and G. J. Dammin. 1975. The pathophysiology of *Shigella* diarrhea in the rhesus monkey: intestinal transport, morphology and bacteriological studies. *Gastroenterology* 68:270–278.

37. Sakai, T., C. Sasakawa, S. Makino, and M. Yoshikawa. 1986. DNA sequence and product analysis of the *virF* locus responsible for Congo red binding and cell invasion in *Shigella flexneri* 2a. *Infect. Immun.* 54:395–402.

38. Sansonetti, P. J., H. d'Hauteville, C. Ecobichon, and C. Pourcel. 1983. Molecular comparison of virulence plasmids in *Shigella* and enteroinvasive *Escherichia coli*. *Ann. Inst. Pasteur Microbiol.* 134A:295–318.

39. Sansonetti, P. J., T. L. Hale, G. J. Dammin, C. Kapfer, H. H. Collins, Jr., and S. B. Formal. 1983. Alterations in the pathogenicity of *Escherichia coli* K-12 after transfer of plasmid and chromosomal genes from *Shigella flexneri*. *Infect. Immun.* 39:1392–1402.

40. Sansonetti, P. J., D. J. Kopecko, and S. B. Formal. 1982. *Shigella sonnei* plasmids: evidence that a large plasmid is necessary for virulence. *Infect. Immun.* 34:852–860.

41. Sansonetti, P. J., A. Ryter, P. Clerc, A. T. Maurelli, and J. Mounier. 1986. Multiplication of *Shigella flexneri* within HeLa cells: lysis of the phagocytic vacuole and plasmid-mediated contact hemolysis. *Infect. Immun.* 51:461–469.

42. Sasakawa, C., S. Makino, K. Kamata, and M. Yoshikawa. 1986. Isolation, characterization, and mapping of Tn5 insertions into the 140-megadalton invasion plasmid defective in the mouse Sereny test in *Shigella flexneri* 2a. *Infect. Immun.* 54:32–36.

43. Takeuchi, A. 1967. Electron microscope studies of experimental salmonella infection. I. Penetration into the intestinal epithelium by *Salmonella typhimurium*. *Am. J. Pathol.* 50:109–136.

44. Takeuchi, A., S. B. Formal, and H. Sprinz. 1968. Experimental acute colitis in the rhesus monkey following peroral infection with *Shigella flexneri*. *Am. J. Pathol.* 52:503–520.

45. Tavendale, A., C. K. H. Jardine, C. Old, and J. P. Duguid. 1983. Haemagglutinins and adhesion of *Salmonella typhimurium* to HEp2 and HeLa cells. *J. Med. Microbiol.* 16:371–380.

46. Timmis, K. N., C. L. Clayton, and T. Sekizaki. 1985. Localization of Shiga toxin gene in the region of *Shigella dysenteriae* 1 specifying virulence functions. *FEMS Microbiol. Lett.* 30:301–305.

47. Uhlman, D. L., and G. W. Jones. 1982. Chemotaxis as a factor in interactions between HeLa cells and *Salmonella typhimurium*. *J. Gen. Microbiol.* 128:415–418.

48. Watanabe, H., and A. Nakamura. 1986. Identification of *Shigella sonnei* form I plasmid genes necessary for cell invasion and their conservation among *Shigella* species and enteroinvasive *Escherichia coli*. *Infect. Immun.* 53:352–358.

49. Watanabe, H., A. Nakamura, and K. Timmis. 1984. Small virulence plasmid of *Shigella dysenteriae* 1 strain W30864 encodes a 41,000-dalton protein involved in formation of specific lipopolysaccharide side chains of serotype 1 isolates. *Infect. Immun.* 46:55–63.

Section II: Bacterial Resistance to Humoral Defense Mechanisms

Chapter 5

Bacterial Resistance to Humoral Defense Mechanisms: an Overview

JOHN B. WOOLCOCK

Department of Veterinary Pathology and Public Health
University of Queensland
St. Lucia, Queensland 4067
Australia

INTRODUCTION

Once an organism has breached the integrity of a body surface, the host responds to its presence by making conditions unfavorable for survival of the invader. These conditions may develop actively or passively, specifically or nonspecifically, immediately or more slowly. The combination of the various processes involved is in most cases successful in eliminating the organism. Pathogens by definition have the capacity to thwart one or more of the host defense mechanisms and are able to do so by a variety of means. Humoral defense mechanisms are encountered initially, and pathogens may evade them by rendering them impotent, by avoiding their effect, or by withstanding their action.

HUMORAL DEFENSE MECHANISMS

The two humoral factors which play the most important roles in host defense against bacterial pathogens are immunoglobins and complement. There are other serum factors which should also be considered in this con-

text, including fibronectin, C-reactive protein (CRP), lysozyme, and transferrin.

Immunoglobulins

An extensive review of such well-characterized serum components as immunoglobulins is unwarranted here. However, some mention should be made of the main characteristics of the major classes of antibody as they relate to antibacterial defense. Immunoglobulins A, G, and M (IgA, IgG, and IgM) are vital to this task and fulfill their functions optimally in different bodily locations. Thus, IgA is found predominantly in mucosal secretions, after complexing with secretory component during its transepithelial passage (13). Although this immunoglobulin does not perform with the efficiency of IgG and IgM in opsonic and bactericidal activity, it is most effective at mucosal surfaces in restricting bacterial adhesion (51). The ability of secretory IgA to resist proteolytic digestion is clearly advantageous in the milieu of the intestinal tract.

IgG functions both in the bloodstream and in the tissues into which it diffuses after injury or damage. Its small size allows this extravascular location, which ensures its widespread availability for host defense. The key antibacterial functions of IgG are opsonization and killing. Both functions may be mediated by complement which is fixed by IgG. Additionally the immunoglobulin may opsonize directly by facilitating bacterium-phagocyte contact via the Fc receptors on the phagocytes. In ruminant animals, serum IgG1 is selectively transported across mucosal surfaces, so that the antibody content in colostrum, milk, and intestinal juice is dominated by this immunoglobulin class and not by IgA (121). Significantly, bovine IgG1 shows the same resistance to proteolysis as does secretory IgA.

IgM is the dominant immunoglobulin early in the primary response to an antigen before the appearance of specific IgG. Because of its size it is confined largely to the intravascular spaces, where it protects against blood-borne organisms. This immunoglobulin is highly efficient at fixing complement and is predominant in what is called natural antibody in normal serum (144). Such antibody presumably arises by stimulation mainly from intestinal flora, which would account for its wide range of cross-reacting specificity and potential to react with a number of antigens present on invasive pathogens. The selective transport mechanism for IgA across mucosal surfaces may also operate for IgM (19). It can therefore be found in pulmonary, intestinal, and mammary secretions.

Complement

The complement system plays a crucial role in humoral defense against microbial pathogens and has been recently reviewed (55). This series of serum proteins which are sequentially activated produces two major effects in terms of host defense: (i) deposition onto the microbial surface of an opsonic protein (C3b), which promotes phagocytosis by interacting with specific receptors on phagocytic cells, and (ii) assembly of a membrane attack complex (MAC) (C5b-9) capable of lysing susceptible gramnegative bacteria. The latter effect of direct bacterial killing is known as the serum bactericidal reaction. Complement activation may take place by either of two pathways, resulting in activation of the vital third component of complement, C3. Thereafter the sequence is common to both pathways.

The classical pathway of complement activation normally follows interaction between antibody and antigen, with C1q (part of the C1 complex) binding to the Fc portion of the antibody-antigen complex. More recently the interaction of bacteria directly with C1q and without the need for antibody has also been shown to participate in initiating this pathway (3, 100). Activation of the alternative pathway may occur with, or more commonly without, antibody, and this pathway assumes great importance in the nonimmune host, when bacterial components such as capsular polysaccharides, lipopolysaccharides (LPS), and other cell wall constituents may be activating factors (43).

The terminal sequence of complement activation is unable to effect changes in grampositive bacteria, because although it forms on the cell walls, it cannot penetrate the thick peptidoglycan layer to produce bactericidal lesions in the cytoplasmic membrane (80). However, both gram-positive and gram-negative organisms may act as effective surfaces for deposition of C3b. This deposition is vital for its activity as an opsonin and may be modulated by antibody, which can optimize its opsonizing effect, e.g., by increasing the extent of C3b deposition (72). However, because the presence of antibody is not an absolute requirement for C3b attachment to bacterial surfaces, a nonimmune host is provided with an effective form of protection early in an infection as C3b deposition occurs. This deposition determines the ensuing interaction with appropriate receptors on phagocytic cells. It follows that deficiency in host C3 levels is accompanied by susceptibility to recurrent, severe infections (2).

Other Humoral Factors

CRP

CRP appears in serum at high levels during inflammatory conditions or following tissue damage in humans and other mammals. Trace quantities can be found in normal blood but may rise to 1,000 times normal levels during the acute phase of an inflammatory response. The name derives from its ability to precipitate with the C-polysaccharide of the pneumococcal cell wall after specific interaction with phosphate esters, especially phosphocholine. CRP may bind not only to pathogenic bacteria (90) but also to damaged tissue and cells at sites of inflammation (37). Many in vitro activities of CRP have been described (50), including its ability to activate complement and act with complement as an opsonin. However, its role in vivo is uncertain. CRP does enhance opsonization (as measured by chemiluminescence) in serum with markedly decreased immunoglobulin levels (40) and has been shown to protect mice from pneumococcal infection (181). Animals infected with a *Salmonella typhimurium* strain which does not bind CRP are not protected by treatment with CRP (119).

CRP shares the binding specificity and opsonic activity of IgM antibody to phosphocholine and can afford protection against pneumococcal infection in animals lacking antibody to phosphocholine (110). Such antibody is normally protective against this type of infection (17). To assess both the importance of this serum protein in host defense and the factors influencing bacterial resistance to its effect, one must therefore ask how widespread among bacteria are binding sites for CRP.

Fibronectin (Opsonic Glycoprotein)

Another serum protein with nonimmunological opsonic activity is fibronectin. Along its length are sites which allow binding both to a range of circulating target particles that include bacteria and to phagocytic cells of the reticuloendothelial system. Thus, particles opsonized by fibronectin may be removed by the reticuloendothelial system. Because fibronectin can bind not only to microorganisms but also to tissue debris and fibrin aggregates, various clinical conditions in which there is failure of reticuloendothelial system function are fre-

quently associated with a drop in the level of circulating fibronectin (98).

Although fibronectin has been shown to bind to several species of bacteria, both gram positive and gram negative, there is no evidence that it promotes the uptake of these organisms by phagocytic cells (165). A heat-labile serum opsonin is apparently necessary for binding and uptake, but this is unrelated to the presence or absence of plasma fibronectin. If this protein, then, does not behave as a proper opsonin for bacterial phagocytosis, its beneficial effects in such situations as trauma and sepsis may be attributable to its role in clearance of tissue debris and of complement-bound materials.

For streptococci there is evidence that the glycolipid moiety of lipoteichoic acid binds to fatty acid-binding sites on plasma fibronectin (33). For staphylococci the fibronectin receptor is a protein distinct from protein A, which binds to other serum proteins including fibrinogen and immunoglobulin (139). The effect of this binding may be negated by localized or circulating proteases, some of which may be microbial in origin. They are able to split fibronectin, thus making it functionally ineffective (20).

Lysozyme

Lysozyme is one of the components of the heat-stable serum bactericidal complex to which the name β-lysin was originally applied (29). In vitro the purified product is effective against gram-positive cells, and saprophytic bacteria are especially susceptible (148). With gram-negative organisms lysozyme operates independently of other serum bactericidal factors but may facilitate the action of the terminal components of complement on the cytoplasmic membrane (105). Although the antibacterial action of lysozyme is undisputed, its importance in host defense in different animal species is ill defined.

Lactoferrin and Transferrin

The iron-binding protein lactoferrin is found in milk and many other secretions including nasal, bronchial, salivary, lachrymal, intestinal, seminal, and cervical secretions (59). In serum, transferrin performs the same function, which, in the present context, is withholding of iron necessary for microbial multiplication in the host. Normally the host environment is iron-restricted, and this state also prevails in sites of inflammation owing to the combined effects of serum transferrin and lactoferrin, together with lactoferrin from polymorphonuclear leukocytes. Iron levels in serum drop during infection, and it is lactoferrin from this source that is responsible for the decrease (166). The fact that pathogens can multiply in locations of iron deprivation indicates that they have developed mechanisms to overcome this host defense mechanism. Alternatively, the host environment may alter in its availability of iron, thus creating conditions whereby bacterial growth is encouraged or restricted. Such a situation prevails in the bovine mammary gland, which when dry has high levels of lactoferrin and lysozyme and is resistant to experimental infusion with *Escherichia coli*. At or following parturition, these levels, together with other conditions affecting iron binding by lactoferrin, alter and the lactating gland then allows multiplication of the coliforms (133).

Conglutinin

Bovine serum contains a high-molecular-weight protein which can aggregate antigen-antibody complexes to which complement is bound. Levels of this nonimmunoglobulin protein drop during severe infections, which could suggest that it plays a role in host defense (75). In cattle, and many other animal species, another type of conglutination is recognized in which antibodies of the IgG, IgM, or IgA class interact with antigenic determinants of complement proteins during complement activation. These immunoconglutinins appear following infection and are able to augment the normal defense mechanisms of complement fixation, serum bactericidal activity, and phagocytosis.

BACTERIAL RESISTANCE MECHANISMS

Resistance to Complement

Gram-Negative Organisms

Rowley (137) found that as a general rule, rough, gram-negative bacteria were sensitive to the bactericidal activity of serum, even though their parent, smooth strains were resistant. This finding indicated that differences in cell wall structure determined differences in serum sensitivity. The importance of serum resistance as a determinant of virulence has been emphasized by examination of strains recovered from a variety of infections in both humans and animals. Thus, Roantree and Rantz (135) recovered serum-resistant organisms more frequently from blood cultures of patients with bacteremia due to gram-negative bacteria. Nearly all gonococci recovered from the blood in gonococcal bacteremic disease are serum resistant (143). *E. coli* strains causing acute urinary tract infection in children are significantly more serum resistant than strains from the feces of healthy children (125). The capacity of coliforms to cause bovine mastitis is related to their ability to resist bovine serum bactericidal activity (27, 28). The response of smooth strains of *Salmonella cholerae-suis* to serum bactericidal activity usually gives an indication of the virulence of these strains for pigs (57). Howard (73) examined the variation in the susceptibility of bovine mycoplasmas to killing by the alternative complement pathway in bovine serum and concluded that resistance to killing may be considered a virulence determinant of mycoplasmas.

These examples confirm the association between bacterial structure and complement activation. Bacterial resistance to complement activation may therefore function by preventing or diminishing complement activation or by rendering the MAC impotent. Various surface antigens have been identified which render bacterial cells resistant to complement activity. These include the LPS component of the outer membrane layer of the gram-negative cell wall, capsules, and cell wall proteins. The recognition of smooth and rough forms of gram-negative bacteria and the associated observation that these forms differ in their pathogenic potential has long pointed to the importance of LPS in relation to serum bactericidal activity. More recently, some of the factors delineating that importance have been defined.

LPS and complement resistance. LPS has the capacity to activate complement by both the classical and alternative pathways (81). Interaction of LPS with specific antibody can be the activating factor in both situations, while complete LPS alone may activate the alternative pathway. The capacity of LPS to act in the latter manner is determined by its structure. Liang-Takasaki et al. (103) used *Salmonella* strains genetically constructed so that only their O-antigen side chains differed. These differences were reflected in differential complement consumption and were associated with variations in polysaccharide structure of the LPS, not with the length of the O antigen; i.e., complement activation is not affected by wide variations in LPS length (64), but rather by subtle changes in O-antigen structure. These changes affect the rate of complement deposition and thus opsonization and phagocytosis (141).

The importance of the LPS in relation to serum sensitivity can also be illustrated with *E. coli*, in which susceptibility to serum can be related to the degree to which the bacterial surface is covered by LPS (65). When the compositions of the outer membranes of a serum-sensitive strain and a serum-resistant mutant strain were compared, there was no difference in the protein and phospholipid contents. However, the mutant strain had twice as much LPS as the sensitive strain did. Leptospirae also have LPS as the main component of their cell envelopes. Decreasing the content of this LPS is associated with increasing susceptibility to the bactericidal activity of serum (76). With *Neisseria gonorrhoeae*, sensitivity to normal human serum is affected by the core polysaccharide of the gonococcal LPS (149), and resis-

tance to serum has been associated with the presence of a 3.6-kilodalton lipooligosaccharide (142). The O antigen of the LPS of *Klebsiella pneumoniae* is the major determinant of resistance to serum bactericidal activity (163), while loss of the O antigen of *Klebsiella aerogenes* is associated with a marked sensitivity to complement-mediated serum killing (175). The virulence of *Haemophilus ducreyi* is associated with resistance to serum killing, and virulent and avirulent strains differ in their LPS profiles (123). It seems, then, that one mechanism by which some organisms may resist the important host defense of complement is to modify their LPS to affect its action. Indeed, it has been shown that the extent of alternative pathway activation in *Salmonella* spp. is determined by the nature of the O antigen in the LPS, which affects the rate and extent of C3b deposition (63).

Resistance to complement-mediated killing may result not only from failure or limitation of complement activation but also from failure of activated complement to exert its effect. Thus, the O antigen of *Salmonella minnesota* thwarts the action of complement by preventing insertion of the MAC (C5b-9) into critical membrane sites of the bacterial cell (84). Bacteriolysis occurs when the MAC is inserted into the lipid bilayer of the bacterial membranes. This insertion may be impeded by the presence of O-polysaccharide side chains, even though the terminal complement components are activated, bound, and properly formed. However, this binding may not be stable, so that the components are shed from the bacterial surface in a nonfunctional state. In smooth, serum-resistant organims, fixation of C3b may occur in association with the longest O-polysaccharide side chains of the LPS (83). Since C3b focuses the formation of the MAC, it is possible that the MAC does not insert in smooth organisms because it forms too far from the critical components of the bacterial cell (82). This proposal would satisfactorily explain the serum resistance of mutants of *E. coli* O111 which contain increased amounts of LPS and more extensive coverage of the lipid A core with O antigen (54). It would also explain how polymyxin B nonapeptide, which interferes with the organization of the gram-negative outer membrane, may render serum-resistant strains of *E. coli* serum sensitive, i.e., by allowing the MAC access to the vulnerable deeper parts of the bacterial cell (164).

Capsules and complement resistance. Bacterial capsules are the most external components of the cell surface and as such make first contact with the host defenses. That most bacteria associated with invasive infections are encapsulated highlights the importance of the capsule in resisting these defenses. This is not to say, however, that possession of a capsule is invariably a virulence factor. There are some cases in which this is indeed true, and in these situations it would appear that the role of the capsule in pathogenesis is to prevent opsonization (136). In the same way that LPS structure affects complement activation, capsular composition is equally critical; e.g., although there are in excess of 100 capsular types of *E. coli,* only a few are associated with pathogenic strains. Unrelated organisms may have capsular polysaccharides of the same composition, further supporting the existence of a restricted range of polysaccharides affecting virulence.

The K1 capsule of *E. coli* and the capsule of group B meningococci are similar chemically and immunologically and are polymers of N-acetylneuraminic acid. In *E. coli* the K1 capsule probably covers underlying components which would normally effect complement activation and in addition is poorly immunogenic. A number of investigations have convincingly demonstrated the capacity of the K1 capsule to protect organisms from the bactericidal action of serum (36, 49, 126). It appears to act in this way by impeding activation of the alternative complement pathway (130), as do other sialosylglycolipids, by enhancing the proteolytic cleavage of C3b (124). The different capsular polysaccharides of *E. coli* have different abilities to activate complement, and those found during invasive infections are gen-

erally poor activators (158). Similarly, the sialic acid capsule of group B meningococci inhibits alternative-pathway activation in an unprotected host (78).

Although the effect of serum on *K. pneumoniae* is not affected by the presence of the capsular polysaccharide (163), both K and O antigens are involved in determining the resistance of *K. aerogenes* to killing by serum (175). Simoons-Smit et al. (153) confirmed that although isogenic K^+ and K^- *Klebsiella* strains differed in their resistance to serum-mediated killing, factors other than the capsular antigens are also involved. This conclusion was drawn because of the recognition of K variants which remained serum resistant. What chemical and conformational characteristics of polysaccharides, whether in O antigens or in capsules, determine the capacity of some to initiate and of others to inhibit alternative-pathway activation is not known (101).

Outer membrane proteins and complement resistance. Other components of the gram-negative cell envelope which may contribute to serum resistance and which are recognized by serum bactericidal antibody are the outer membrane proteins. Some of these proteins may be determined by plasmids and only function in this way when associated with a complete set of O antigens (161). Moll et al. (111) identified a major outer membrane protein in *E. coli* as the product of a conjugative multiple-antibiotic resistance plasmid. This plasmid (R6-5) was able to confer serum resistance, but only when interacting with other surface components of the bacterial cell. The combined effect may be to prevent the functioning of the MAC (162). Another plasmid, ColV, is found in many invasive strains of *E. coli* and is associated with the production of an outer membrane protein which confers resistance to serum (11). Similarly, the cryptic plasmid of *Salmonella typhimurium* codes for a 11-kilodalton outer membrane protein which mediates serum resistance (66).

When serum-sensitive strains of *N. gonor-*

rhoeae are transformed by DNA from serum-resistant strains (which are recovered during disseminated gonococcal infection), there are simultaneous changes in outer membrane protein composition of the transformants (69). Furthermore, there is a strong association between the presence of protein I (principal outer membrane protein) and serum resistance in gonococci (21). Indeed, serum sensitivity in *N. gonorrhoeae* may be altered by very small changes in protein I structure combined with small differences in lipooligosaccharide composition (86). The components of the gonococcal surface to which MAC is bound differ between serum-resistant and serum-sensitive strains, and this difference in configuration affects the capacity of MAC to insert into the gonococcal membranes (85). It should be understood, however, that although there may be an association between outer membrane proteins and serum resistance for some gram-negative bacteria, these proteins have not yet been shown to be the sole mediator of that resistance.

Gram-Positive Organisms

Complement resistance. Bacterial resistance to complement among gram-positive organisms may operate in a number of ways. As with the capsular material of gram-negative bacteria, capsular material of organisms such as *Staphylococcus aureus* prevents the opsonic activity of C3 by functionally masking it; i.e., the capsule prevents interaction between the wall-associated C3 molecules and receptors on the plasma membrane of the polymorphonuclear cells (174). Similarly, the pneumococcal capsule may act as a barrier between fixed C3b and phagocytic cells (177). The capsules of type III group B streptococci act against complement not by masking, but rather by preventing activation of the alternative complement pathway (41). Critical to this activity is the sialic acid component of the capsule, and in particular its tertiary molecular confirmation. By acting as a nonactivating surface for one of the primary recognition systems of nonimmune hosts, the capsule will thus confer an advantage on the infecting organism.

A major virulence factor in group A streptococci is the M protein. The presence of this fibrillar surface antigen decreases the ability of the streptococcal surface to fix C3 (12), which becomes restricted to patches (77). The effect of the M protein could be steric hindrance, as with the capsules of *S. aureus* and *Streptococcus pneumoniae,* and there are other possible explanations, e.g., the C3 which is bound to the M^+ surface is not opsonically active, or the M protein masks sites which are necessary for the activation of the alternative complement pathway. This masking may occur in association with fibrinogen which binds to the M protein (170). Degradation products of fibrinogen and fibrin exert the same effect as intact fibrinogen (171). The effect of M protein in combination with fibrinogen would seem to be prevention of access of complement to underlying cell wall structures. Although the identity of these structures has not been determined, it is known that streptococcal peptidoglycan activates complement very effectively by the alternative pathway (56). Streptococcal cellular components other than M protein may also bind fibrinogen, with the same effect of inhibiting complement fixation (31).

Complement destruction. Resistance to complement may be exerted by interfering with the formation of functional activity of complement components. Group A streptococci produce a cell-associated peptidase which inactivates C5a (122, 169). This cleavage product of C5 is a chemotaxin which interacts with polymorphonuclear leukocytes and is unable to act in this way when chemically altered by the C5a peptidase (168). The surface location of the enzyme would optimize its effect on the complement system, whose activation also occurs at the bacterial surface (116).

Resistance to the inflammatory response. Since the acute inflammatory response is a key defense mechanism by which the host attempts to localize foreign material, any capacity of a microorganism to restrict this response will clearly work in favor of the organism. Agarwal (1) suggested that virulent staphylococci possess some factor(s) which acts in just such a way by inhibiting leukocyte migration and edema exudation at the lesion site. From the cell walls of mouse-virulent *S. aureus,* Hill (70) extracted material which inhibited the accumulation of edema fluid at the infection site. He used the term aggressin to describe the activity of this material, which was composed predominantly of mucopeptide, together with some protein. When used to immunize mice, this aggressin material gave protection against homologous challenge and a number of heterologous strains (71). No protection was afforded by the cell wall fraction derived from a nonvirulent strain. These fractions were obtained by extracting cell walls with deoxycholate, and the residue was also called impedin, to indicate its role in inhibiting a normal host defense mechanism. The same relationship between virulence and impedin activity established between strains virulent for humans was also demonstrated for two strains virulent for animals and isolated from animals with bovine mastitis (30). Easmon et al. (38) hypothesized that impedin exerts its effect by preventing activation of Hageman factor and thus release of kinins.

S. aureus may also resist the inflammatory response by consuming complement. Lew et al. (102) reported that such consumption could be extensive at the site of infection, leaving only complement breakdown products and minimal opsonic activity. This complement-consuming capacity has been attributed to the existence of an extracellular substance designated decomplementation antigen (8). Bhakdi and Muhly (8) showed that immune complex formation between decomplementation antigen and IgG is a powerful activator of complement primarily via the classical pathway, thus consuming the early-reacting complement components and making them unavailable for opsonization. Decomplementation antigen appears to be extracellular teichoic acid, which can readily precipitate with naturally occurring human IgG antibodies (9). Decomplementation of serum

may also occur in pneumococcal infection (53). The capsular polysaccharide of *Streptococcus pneumoniae* is able to activate the alternative complement pathway, and during a bacteremia there may be sufficient antigen to induce an associated serum opsonic deficiency.

Resistance to Immunoglobulin

Immunoglobulin Binding

Staphylococcal cell walls are composed predominantly of peptidoglycan, teichoic acid, and protein A. Protein A combines with human IgG via the Fc fragment (47), and this complex can activate both the classical and alternative pathways of complement (157). However, there are two ways in which protein A can provide resistance to host defenses. First, the binding to the Fc portion of IgG interferes with the attachment of the immunoglobulin, and thus the opsonized bacteria, to the Fc receptors of phagocytic cells. Second, protein A, which may be either bound to the cell wall or released extracellularly, can interfere with complement activity. Bound protein A can block activation of complement by the alternative pathway (156). It may do this by covering underlying peptidoglycan, the cell wall constituent most responsible for complement activation via the alternative pathway (167). Extracellular protein A, released during staphylococcal replication, is capable of activating complement, and this effectively diminishes the availability of complement for activation at the critical locus of the bacterial surface (128). Nevertheless, there is very little difference in pathogenicity between protein A-deficient mutants and protein A-rich cells when compared by their abilities to initiate either local or generalized infection (46).

Most group A, C, and G streptococci also possess Fc receptors for IgG (93). These receptors differ from, but are closely related to, those on protein A (117), one difference being the capacity of the receptor of *Streptococcus zooepidemicus* to react with animal immunoglobulins

(118). The group C and G streptococcal surface structures are proteinaceous (132), and the capacity of these streptococcal components for negating the opsonizing effect of mammalian immunoglobulins may provide an organism with a means of survival within a host.

Some group B streptococci may bind IgA, and in this situation the streptococcal receptor has been shown to be a detergent-extractable surface protein with a molecular weight of 130,000 (138). IgA may also be bound to group A and G streptococci, and human serum albumin is another serum protein similarly bound by these organisms (96). This capacity of streptococci, to bind a number of host serum proteins, e.g., fibrinogen (95), aggregated β_2-microglobulin (94), and haptoglobin (91), in addition to IgG and IgA and serum albumin, may suggest that these organisms could escape host defenses by avoiding recognition in this camouflaged state.

Nonimmune immunoglobulin binding has most frequently been described as a feature of some gram-positive organisms. Recently a gram-negative pathogen, *Taylorella equigenitalis*, has been shown to exhibit the same capacity (173). This organism binds equine IgG most strongly, IgM to a lesser extent, and IgA not at all. The immunoglobulin binding shows species specificity, which may have implications for host species specificity of the pathogen and for the ability of *T. equigenitalis* to persist in the genital tract despite a local immune response (172).

Immunoglobulin Degradation

One of the means by which pathogenic bacteria can resist the activity of antibody is the production of trypsinlike enzymes which cleave that antibody, rendering it nonfunctional. Those enzymes which have been described are mainly human IgA1 proteases, and their properties and production have been reviewed most recently by Mulks (113). The microbial proteases have the following characteristics: (i) they are produced by organisms of the genera *Neisseria*, *Haemophilus*, and *Streptococcus*; (ii) they are large, extracellular products, de-

tectable in culture supernatants and in cell-free fluids of infected patients; (iii) their synthesis is not determined by any extrachromosomal genetic material, including plasmids; (iv) because of their mode of action, they are effective only against human IgA1; and (v) they are strongly antigenic, and antibodies which can negate their activity can be detected in human secretions and serum (129).

Although an organism which can produce enzymes capable of cleaving antibody would appear to be at a distinct advantage in the encounter between host and parasite, the role of proteases in disease pathogenesis is not known. That they are involved is suggested by the following evidence (114): (i) the proteases are produced by pathogens which infect mucosal surfaces protected by secretory IgA; (ii) nonpathogenic *Haemophilus* and *Neisseria* species are non protease producers; (iii) the secretions of infected patients exhibit protease activity; and (iv) the inhibition by secretory IgA of bacterial adherence to tissue is reduced by the activity of proteases.

Using an IgA1 protease-deficient mutant of *Haemophilus influenzae* in an experimental model of human nasopharyngeal tissue in organ culture and comparing its capacity for attachment, colonization, and invasion with that of its IgA1 protease-producing parent, Farley et al. (42) were unable to show that the enzyme was essential for any of these pathogenic events. Studies of this kind need to be extended, although it is unlikely that further studies will indicate either that protease production is a sole determinant of virulence or that it has no role at all in disease genesis. This conclusion is based partly on evidence which shows that although IgA protease production is a characteristic which can distinguish pathogenic from nonpathogenic species of the genus *Neisseria*, it cannot differentiate between disease-associated and harmless members of the same *Neisseria* species (115). Furthermore, clinical isolates of *Branhamella catarrhalis*, which may be a nasopharyngeal commensal or an opportunistic pathogen, do not produce IgA1 protease (106).

When animal pathogens have been examined, many do not exhibit proteolytic activity against IgA derived from various animal species (92). These organisms include *Bordetella bronchiseptica, Pasteurella multocida,* and *Pasteurella pneumotropica*. However, *Haemophilus pleuropneumoniae,* recovered from the lungs of fatally infected pigs, produces an IgA protease which cleaves porcine secretory IgA but not human IgA proteins (89). This finding was not confirmed (113), but extension of this type of study may indicate whether the ability of host-specific organisms to cleave only IgA of their specific hosts provides an insight into the basis of host specificity in some microbial infections.

Cleavage of immunoglobulins other than IgA has been described for proteases produced by *Pseudomonas aeruginosa* and *Serratia marcescens*. In the former case, an IgG protease is produced by both mucoid and nonmucoid strains (R. B. Fick, R. S. Baltimore, J. B. L. Gee, and H. Y. Reynolds, Program Abstr. 22nd Intersci. Conf. Antimicrob. Agents Chemother., abstr. no. 374, 1982), which, if functional in vivo, may aid in the disease process. Similarly, *Serratia marcescens* can degrade IgG3 (and IgA1) by production of an extracellular protease (112). This protease can also degrade other humoral proteins involved in host defense, including lysozyme and fibronectin, as well as tissue constituents including fibroblasts.

In addition to immunoglobulin degradation by organisms associated with pneumonia and meningitis, the same capacity has been demonstrated for some bacteria associated with human periodontal disease (88). A variety of *Bacteroides* and *Capnocytophaga* species are able to degrade IgA1, IgA2, and IgG. Some streptococci associated with dental plaque formation also produce IgA1 proteases (92). The IgA1 proteases of *Bacteroides* and *Capnocytophaga* species have the same cleavage site, and each species of the former genus produces an antigenically distinct protease (48). The capacity to produce such enzymes would seem to be highly advantageous to a potential periodontal pathogen.

Avoidance of Humoral Defense Mechanisms

So far we have considered active means by which bacteria can resist humoral defense mechanisms. Resistance may also be achieved passively; i.e., organisms may simply avoid an encounter with host defenses. They may do this by taking what Smith (154) calls "sanctuary in immunologically deficient sites," i.e., places protected from humoral and cellular defenses. Smith gives as examples of such places the epithelial cells lining the respiratory, alimentary, and urogenital tracts, the mammary gland, and the gall bladder. These nonprofessional phagocytic cells are able to internalize a number of bacterial pathogens. These organisms may persist in this protected environment, and such a situation could account for the asymptomatic carriage state which is a feature of some infectious diseases.

Certain locations in the body appear to be immunologically deprived and may provide a haven for any microorganisms which find their way there. Thus, the kidney exhibits a primary complement deficiency by virtue of its normal metabolic activity, which generates ammonia (6). This is an anticomplementary agent, and any organism which has the capacity to generate more of it through urease activity will clearly exacerbate this anticomplementary state. Another site which may provide a sanctuary for avoidance of host defenses is the area within blood vessel walls (15). *P. aeruginosa* has a proclivity for vascular tissue and, once ensconced there, is untouched by defense mechanisms.

Antigenic Strategies

Antigenic Similarity

If an organism possesses antigenic similarity with the host tissue, it is possible that the organism will be tolerated and may thus escape the host defenses. The capsular polysaccharides of meningococci are important components in the pathogenesis of meningococcal disease, and vaccination is directed against them. The group B polysaccharide is poorly immu-

RESISTANCE TO HUMORAL DEFENSE MECHANISMS   83

nogenic, even when conjugated with protein
carriers (79). The capsule of *E. coli* K1 is an
immunochemically identical polysaccharide (87),
and both organisms are important causes of
neonatal meningitis. Glycoproteins of human
and rat brain contain oligosaccharide side chains
which are antigenically similar to the capsular
polysaccharides of the two pathogens (45). Such
cross-reactivity must significantly limit the nature of the immune response to these organisms and must be considered a means by which
some pathogens can avoid normal defense
mechanisms. A further consideration is that
there may be hazards associated with attempts
to increase the immunogenicity of these polysaccharides for purposes of vaccination. One such
danger is the possiblity of inducing an autoimmune reaction. Indeed, the demonstration of
shared antigenic determinants between the *E.
coli* K1 capsule and human gangliosides (155)
would suggest that such a reaction could occur. However, this fear may be groundless, because in humans there are naturally occurring
autoantibodies against common glycolipids
which are not apparently associated with any
adverse effects (134).

Antigenic Shift

   Microorganisms may resist the effect of
specific immune responses mounted against
them by altering the antigens against which
those responses are directed. In this way pathogens may survive within a host, and antigenic
variation may account for microbial persistence
and chronicity of infection. Such a phenomenon has been recognized for some time in certain viral and protozoal diseases, most notably
influenza and malaria, respectively. Antigenic
variation does occur in some bacterial infections and is not just a matter of laboratory interest.

   Campylobacter fetus subsp. *intestinalis,* found
in the intestinal tracts of cattle and sheep, may
cause enzootic abortion in sheep and sporadic
abortion in cattle. In an experimental infection
of the reproductive tracts of cattle with this
organism, *C. fetus* was found to persist for many

weeks postinfection, and associated with this
persistence was an alteration in the serotype of
the infecting strain (145). It was considered
possible that antibodies present in the genital
secretions and directed against the infecting
strain could have induced these changes to the
superficial antigens of *C. fetus.* This possibility
was confirmed by studies which monitored both
the antigenic composition of isolates recovered
over a period following infection with *C. fetus*
subsp. *venerealis* and the specificity of antibody
in cervicovaginal mucus (32). These studies
suggested that animals could become asymptomatic carriers of the organism in the cervi
covaginal mucus, despite the presence of antibody. Similarly, vaccinated animals may harbor
antigenic variants induced by antibodies to the
vaccine antigens (146). We have here a beau-
tiful example of how both host and parasite respond dynamically to a situation which threat-
ens the health of both. Antigenic variation in
C. fetus subsp. *venerealis* has also been shown to
occur in bulls (10), but the phenomenon does
not pose a threat to the success of vaccination
for control of the infection in either cows or
bulls.

   The antigenic structure of *Vibrio cholerae*
adjusts in vivo to immunological pressure, as
has been shown with gnotobiotic mice (140) in
which a persistent asymptomatic infection could
be established. In these mice the rough form
of the organism emerged as the final stage of
this adaptive process. When one of these rough
colonies was propagated in fresh gnotobiotic
mice, smooth organisms similar to the original
culture developed. Indeed, when a rough strain
was passed serially in gnotobiotic mice, smooth
strains could be recovered which were more
virulent than the original human isolate (109).
The implications of these studies are (i) that
rough *V. cholerae* strains from convalescent carriers could, in the right circumstances, become
typical smooth *V. cholerae* strains and (ii) that
serotypic changes to *V. cholerae* may occur in a
community, resulting in the occurrence of strains
not affected by the prevailing type-specific antibody.

   Leptospiras may undergo serotypic conversion in vitro in the presence of homologous immune serum (24, 179). Antigenic variants have also been recovered from mice experimentally infected with *Leptospira interrogans* serovar *copenhageni* (178). These variants were isolated from the renal cortex by using media containing immune serum against the parent strain. If the same phenomenon occurs in the field, it is conceivable that such variants could infect other animals via the urine. These animals, although vaccinated, may not be protected against the new antigenic types. Although this situation remains a theoretical possibility, there has been no demonstration that it represents a threat to the efficacy of vaccination.

The colonization of gonotobiotic rats by *Streptococcus mutans* is associated with the emergence over time of antigenic variants which arise in the face of developing salivary IgA (52). These variants are less virulent than the parent strain and emerge more quickly when the animals are vaccinated orally prior to colonization. Antigenic variation may occur when populations of *Streptococcus mutans* colonize not only the oral cavity but also the intestinal tract (14). *Streptococcus salivarius* also exhibits changes in its antigenic composition while resident in the human mouth (74).

Antigenic shift in bacteria is well recognized but not as well defined in biochemical terms as with trypanosomes. The most detailed studies in bacteria have been with *Borrelia* species which cause a disease characterized by relapses at regular intervals. These relapses are associated with the appearance of organisms having a different antigenic composition from that of organisms causing the preceding episode. Antigenic conversion takes place continuously, independently of the relapses and at a rate unaffected by antibody production (159). Indeed, a single *Borrelia hermsii* organism injected into a mouse may be the progenitor of 24 different serotypes. It would seem likely, then, that antibody acts to select variants and eliminate the predominant serotype. This antigenic variation is associated with DNA rearrangements within the genome (107), which mediate differential expression of a major sur-face protein which also confers serotypic specificity (5). A similarly located protein varies in the Lyme disease spirochete (*Borrelia burgdorferi*), although antigenic variation in vivo has not been demonstrated for this organism (4).

In humans, the best studied example of antigenic variation is that associated with gonococcal infection, in which the organism can persist in the host in the face of an immune response. Over the course of a natural infection there is extensive antigenic variation in both pili and outer membrane protein II (182). Such variations have been recognized in laboratory cultures of *N. gonorrhoeae*, and in the natural host various influences may induce antigenic diversity, e.g., hormonal factors, tissue affinity, and immune response. The last factor is considered to be significant, since there is much variation in the host antibody response to the variant proteins. The ability of meningococci to vary the expression of major outer membrane proteins and pili may suggest that antigenic changes also occur in this infection (131).

Nutritional Strategies

Iron and Infection

Since iron is essential for bacterial growth and survival, an important host defense mechanism is to make this metal unavailable to invading bacteria (23). Conversely, pathogenic bacteria may grow and survive in the low-iron environment of the tissues by possessing mechanisms for obtaining iron. Pathogens must do this because although there is plenty of iron in the body, most of it is unavailable. Therefore, to obtain the metal, these organisms must be able either to assimilate protein-bound iron or to acquire it from heme-containing compounds. They do this in the following ways (22): (i) production of high-affinity iron-chelating agents which, by competing directly with host iron-binding proteins (essentially transferrin and lactoferrin), claim iron for the organisms; (ii) direct removal of iron from iron-binding proteins by interaction with bacterial surface receptors; and (iii) degradation of iron-binding and heme-containing proteins. Furthermore, iron may become freely available to an organism following trauma in which there is hemolysis and/or a drop in tissue oxidation-reduction potential (22). In the latter situation, transferrin may release iron for acquisition by infecting organisms. Some organisms which produce a hemolysin in vivo may thus liberate heme, which could then be utilized as a source of iron (104).

The direct competition with transferrin in serum and lymph and lactoferrin in external secretions and milk takes place by way of bacterial siderophores (120). These iron-sequestering compounds, which are produced only under conditions of low iron supply, are either phenolate compounds such as enterochelin (enterobactin) of enteric bacteria or hydroxamates such as aerobactin, also of enteric organisms. That siderophores provide a mechanism whereby organisms can overcome the capacity of the host to withhold iron and thus restrict bacterial growth and survival has been supported by evidence which demonstrates enterochelin secretion by *E. coli* during fatal infections (60) and enterochelin production as necessary for the growth in serum of *Salmonella typhimurium* and its high virulence for mice (180). In the latter studies it was shown that the addition of enterochelin to an inoculum of a mutant lacking the capacity to produce this siderophore reduced the 50% lethal dose to that of the wild-type strain of *Salmonella typhimurium*. Aerobactin production is involved in the virulence of *E. coli* isolated during avian septicemia (97) and human and animal bacteremia (176). Nevertheless, the relationship between siderophore production and virulence is not absolute. In murine models of typhoid and cholera, for example, lethality and infection are independent of siderophore production (7, 151), while aerobactin production is not essential for invasion or intracellular multiplication of *Shigella flexneri* (99). With some *Campylobacter jejuni* strains, siderophore synthesis is not the only factor determining virulence (44).

Siderophores are not used by all bacteria as a means of sequestering iron. Iron may be taken directly from an iron-binding protein, following interaction between that protein, e.g., transferrin, and receptors on the bacterial cell surface, as in *Neisseria meningitidis* (152). This interaction may precede enzymatic degradation of transferrin at the cell surface and subsequent release of iron for assimilation by the bacteria. By manipulating the pH and availability of iron to *N. meningitidis*, Brener et al. (16) were able to show changes both in virulence and in outer membrane protein profile. They were attempting to simulate conditions of an inflammatory reaction, i.e., low pH and iron limitation, and it is possible that the concomitant changes observed may be related. That is, inhospitable host conditions may induce an adaptive response in the invading organism, whereby it can now procure iron from serum transferrin and even from lactoferrin derived from neutrophilic granules. The changed outer membrane profile may reflect this adaptation and may include the receptor(s) for iron-binding proteins.

Some microorganisms can make iron available by freeing it from iron-binding or heme-containing proteins. *Listeria monocytogenes* does this by producing a soluble reductant (34). *Bacteroides* species and *H. influenzae* may degrade transferrin as well as the hemoglobin-binding serum protein haptoglobin and the heme-binding proteins hemopexin and albumen (25, 68, 160). This may be significant in mixed anaerobic infections involving *Bacteroides* species. *Yersinia pseudotuberculosis*, *Yersinia enterocolitica*, and *Yersinia pestis* can all utilize hemin as a sole source of iron, and accumulation takes place via a cell-bound transport system operating independently of siderophores (127). Many *Neisseria* species can acquire iron from hemin, and some can obtain it from hemoglobin (108). Furthermore, although commensal *Neisseria* species are inhibited by transferrin, all gonococci, as well as meningococci, can utilize this protein as an iron source, which may well assist their survival in the host. *Vibrio vulnificus* produces hemolysins, which could be expected to result in an increase in hemoglobin levels in plasma. Serum haptoglobin can bind hemoglobin (39), thus making the iron in the hemoglobin unavailable to bacteria. However, *V. vulnificus* can acquire iron from the haptoglobin-hemoglobin complex (67).

Integral to the capacity of bacteria for uptake of iron by siderophores is the production of protein receptors and enzymes in the outer membrane (58). Virulence in the fish pathogen *Vibrio anguillarum* is associated with a plasmid which mediates an iron uptake system and codes for an outer membrane protein (35), and in *Yersinia* species there is a correlation between virulence and the presence of certain iron-regulated outer membrane proteins (26). Changes in the outer membrane protein profile of *N. meningitidis* grown under simulated in vivo conditions have been noted previously (16), and further evidence confirms that these iron-regulated outer membrane proteins are produced in vivo by *P. aeruginosa* (18), *E. coli* (62), *V. cholerae* (147), and urinary tract pathogens 150. In these situations, then, we see environmental conditions inducing iron-regulated phenotypic changes in organisms. These changes represent a response of pathogens whereby they are able to counter the important host defense mechanism of iron deprivation. How these iron-regulated changes to outer membrane protein composition relate to other changes in the behavior of an organism has not been established (58). Recent experiments, however, indicate that a chromosomal segment associated with virulence of *Shigella flexneri* and extraintestinal strains of *E. coli* codes for the production of both aerobactin and an iron-regulated outer membrane protein (61).

CONCLUSION

Bacterial pathogens may adapt in a variety of ways to the adverse environmental conditions provided by the host. Many of those bacterial adaptations are recognized by examination of the behavior of an organism in an in vitro system. How this relates to infection in vivo is frequently difficult to prove, and in many cases a strong association between possession of a particular determinant and virulence is the most that can be claimed. Even so, such evidence may be sufficient to suggest effective strategies to overcome infections caused by organisms with one or more of these determinants.

LITERATURE CITED

1. Agarwal, D. S. 1967. Subcutaneous staphylococcal infection in mice. I. The role of cotton-dust in enhancing infection. *Br. J. Exp. Pathol.* 48:436–449.
2. Alper, C. A., N. Abramson, R. B. Johnston, J. H. Jandl, and F. S. Rosen. 1970. Increased susceptibility to infection associated with abnormalities of complement-mediated functions and of the third component of complement (C3). *N. Engl. J. Med.* 282:349–358.
3. Baker, C. J., M. S. Edwards, B. J. Webb, and D. L. Kasper. 1982. Antibody-independent classical pathway mediated opsonophagocytosis of type 1a group B streptococcus. *J. Clin. Invest.* 69:394–404.
4. Barbour, A. G., S. L. Tessier, and S. F. Hayes. 1984. Variation in a major surface protein of Lyme disease spirochetes. *Infect. Immun.* 45:94–100.
5. Barbour, A. G., S. L. Tessier, and H. G. Stoenner. 1982. Variable major proteins of *Borrelia hermsii. J. Exp. Med.* 156:1312–1324.
6. Beeson, P. B., and D. Rowley. 1959. The anticomplementary effect of kidney tissue. Its association with ammonia production. *J. Exp. Med.* 110:685–697.
7. Benjamin, W. H., C. L. Turnbough, B. S. Posey, and D. E. Briles. 1985. The ability of *Salmonella typhimurium* to produce the siderophore enterobactin is not a virulence factor in mouse typhoid. *Infect. Immun.* 50:392–397.
8. Bhakdi, S., and M. Muhly. 1985. Decomplementation antigen: a possible determinant of staphylococcal pathogenicity. *Infect. Immun.* 47:41–46.
9. Bhakdi, S., and M. Muhly. 1985. Isolation and partial characterization of staphylococcal decomplementation antigen. *Infect. Immun.* 47:47–51.
10. Bier, P. J., C. E. Hall, J. R. Duncan, and A. J. Winter. 1977. Experimental infections with *Campylobacter fetus* in bulls of different ages. *Vet. Microbiol.* 2:13–27.
11. Binns, M. M., F. P. A. Carr, and R. P. Levine. 1981. Plasmids and phages and complement resistance, p. 583. *In* S. B. Levy, R. C. Clowes, and E. L. Koenig (ed.), *Molecular Biology, Pathogenicity and Ecology of Bacterial Plasmids.* Plenum Publishing Corp., New York.
12. Bisno, A. L. 1979. Alternate complement pathway activation by group A streptococci: role of M-pro-

tein. *Infect. Immun.* 26:1172–1176.

13. Brandtzaeg, P., and K. Baklien. 1977. Intestinal secretion of IgA and IgM: a hypothetical model, p. 77–108. *In Immunology of the Gut.* CIBA Foundation Symposium no. 46. Elsevier Scientific Publishing Co., Amsterdam.

14. Bratthall, D., and R. J. Gibbons. 1975. Antigenic variation of *Streptococcus mutans* colonizing gnotobiotic rats. *Infect. Immun.* 12:1231–1236.

15. Braude, A. I. 1981. Some reasons for clinical concern—Discussion, p. 13. *In* F. O'Grady and H. Smith (ed.), *Microbial Perturbation of Host Defences.* Academic Press, Inc. (London), Ltd., London.

16. Brener, D., I. W. Devoe, and B. E. Holbein. 1981. Increased virulence of *Neisseria meningitidis* after in vitro iron-limited growth at low pH. *Infect. Immun.* 33:59–66.

17. Briles, D. E., M. Nahm, K. Schroer, J. Davie, P. Baker, J. Kearney, and R. Barlette. 1981. Antiphosphocholine antibodies found in normal mouse serum are protective against intravenous infection with type 3 *Streptococcus pneumoniae*. *J. Exp. Med.* 153:694–705.

18. Brown, M. R. W., H. Anwar, and P. A. Lambert. 1984. Evidence that mucoid *Pseudomonas aeruginosa* in the cystic fibrosis lung grows under iron-restricted conditions. *FEMS Microbiol. Lett.* 21:113–117.

19. Brown, P. J., and F. J. Bourne. 1976. Distributions of immunoglobulin-containing cells in alimentary tract, spleen, and mesenteric lymph node of the pig demonstrated by peroxidase-conjugated antiserums to porcine immunoglobulins G, A, and M. *Am. J. Vet Res.* 37:9–14.

20. Brown, R. A. 1983. Failure of fibronectin as an opsonin in the host defence system: a case of competitive self inhibition. *Lancet* ii:1058–1060.

21. Buchanan, T. M., and J. F. Hildebrandt. 1981. Antigen-specific serotyping of *Neisseria gonorrhoeae*: characterization based upon principal outer membrane protein. *Infect. Immun.* 32:985–994.

22. Bullen, J. J. 1985. Iron and infection. *Eur. J. Clin. Microbiol.* 4:537–539.

23. Bullen, J. J., H. J. Rogers, and E. Griffiths. 1978. Role of iron in bacterial infection. *Curr. Top. Microbiol. Immunol.* 80:1–35.

24. Cacciapuoti, B., A. Pinto, and I. Silva. 1985. Antigenic population changes of *Leptospira biflexa* strains grown under the selective pressure of factorial antibodies. *J. Gen. Microbiol.* 131:521–526.

25. Carlsson, J., J. F. Hofling, and G. K. Sundquist. 1984. Degradation of albumen, haemopexin, haptoglobin, and transferrin by black-pigmented *Bacteroides* species. *J. Med. Microbiol.* 18:39–46.

26. Carniel, E., D. Mazigh, and H. H. Mollaret. 1987. Expression of iron-regulated proteins in *Yersinia* species and their relation to virulence. *Infect. Immun.* 55:277–280.

27. Carroll, E. J., N. C. Jain, O. W. Schalm, and J. Lasmanis. 1973. Experimentally induced coliform mastitis: inoculation of udders with serum-sensitive and serum-resistant organisms. *Am. J. Vet. Res.* 34:1143–1146.

28. Carroll, E. J., and D. E. Jasper. 1977. Bactericidal activity of standard bovine serum against coliform bacteria isolated from udders and the environment of dairy cows. *Am. J. Vet. Res.* 38:2019–2022.

29. Carroll, S. F., and R. J. Martinez. 1979. Role of rabbit lysozyme in in vitro serum and plasma serum bactericidal reactions against *Bacillus subtilis*. *Infect. Immun.* 25:810–819.

30. Chandler, R. L., K. Smith, and H. S. Anger. 1976. Observations of staphylococcal strains with respect to impedin and mastitis. *Br. Vet. J.* 132:647–648.

31. Chhatwal, G. S., I. S. Dutra, and H. Blobel. 1985. Fibrinogen binding inhibits the fixation of the third component of human complement on surface of groups A, B, C and G streptococci. *Microbiol. Immunol.* 29:973–980.

32. Corbeil, L. B., G. G. D. Schurig, P. J. Bier, and A. J. Winter. 1975. Bovine venereal vibriosis: antigenic variation of the bacterium during infection. *Infect. Immun.* 11:240–244.

33. Courtney, H. S., W. A. Simpson, and E. H. Beachey. 1983. Binding of streptococcal lipoteichoic acid to fatty acid-binding sites on human plasma fibronectin. *J. Bacteriol.* 153:763–770.

34. Cowart, R. E., and B. G. Foster. 1985. Differential effects of iron on growth of *Listeria monocytogenes*: minimum requirements and mechanism of acquisition. *J. Infect. Dis.* 151:721–730.

35. Crosa, J. H., and L. L. Hodges. 1981. Other membrane proteins induced under conditions of iron limitations in the marine fish pathogen *Vibrio anguillarum*. *Infect. Immun.* 31:223–227.

36. Cross, A. S., P. Gemski, J. C. Sadoff, F. Ørskov, and I. Ørskov. 1984. The importance of the K1 capsule in invasive infections caused by *Escherichia coli*. *J. Infect. Dis.* 149:184–193.

37. Du Clos, T. W., C. Mold, P. Y. Paterson, J. Alroy, and H. Gewurz. 1981. Localisation of C-reactive protein in inflammatory lesions of experimental allergic encephalomyelitis. *Clin. Exp. Immunol.* 43:565–573.

38. Easmon, C. S. F., I. Hamilton, and A. A. Glynn. 1973. Mode of action of a staphylococcal anti-inflammatory factor. *Br. J. Exp. Pathol.* 54:638–645.

39. Eaton, J. W., P. Brandt, J. R. Mahoney, and J. T. Lee. 1982. Haptoglobin: a natural bacteriostat. *Science* 215:691–693.

40. Edwards, K. M., C. Mold, T. F. Lint, and H. Gewurz. 1982. A role for C-reactive protein in the complement mediated stimulation of human neutrophils by type 27 *Streptococcus pneumoniae*. *J. Im-*

munol. 128:2493–2496.

41. **Edwards, M. S., D. L. Kasper, H. J. Jennings, C. J. Baker, and A. Nicholson-Weller.** 1982. Capsular sialic acid prevents activation of the alternative complement pathway by type III, group B, streptococci. *J. Immunol.* 128:1278–1283.

42. **Farley, M. M., D. S. Stephens, M. H. Mulks, M. D. Cooper, J. V. Bricker, S. S. Mirra, and A. Wright.** 1986. Pathogenesis of IgA1 protease-producing and -nonproducing *Haemophilus influenzae* in human nasopharyngeal organ cultures. *J. Infect. Dis.* 154:752–759.

43. **Fearon, D. T., and K. F. Austen.** 1980. The alternative pathway of complement—a system for host resistance to microbial infection. *N. Engl. J. Med.* 303:259–263.

44. **Field, L. H., V. L. Headley, S. M. Payne, and L. J. Berry.** 1986. Influence of iron on growth, morphology, outer membrane protein composition, and synthesis of siderophores in *Campylobacter jejuni*. *Infect. Immun.* 54:126–132.

45. **Finne, J., M. Leinonen, and P. H. Mäkelä.** 1983. Antigenic similarities between brain components and bacteria causing meningitis. *Lancet* ii:355–357.

46. **Forsgren, A., and K. Nordström.** 1974. Protein A from *Staphylococcus aureus:* the biological significance of its reaction with IgG. *Ann. N.Y. Acad. Sci.* 236:252–266.

47. **Forsgren, A., and J. Sjöquist.** 1966. Protein A from *Staphylococcus aureus.* I. Pseudoimmune reactions with human γ-globulin. *J. Immunol.* 97:822–827.

48. **Fransden, E. V. G., J. Reinholdt, and M. Kilian.** 1987. Enzymatic and antigenic characterization of immunoglobulin A1 proteases from *Bacteroides* and *Capnocytophaga* spp. *Infect. Immun.* 55:631–638.

49. **Gemski, P., A. S. Cross, and J. C. Sadoff.** 1980. K1 antigen-associated resistance to the bactericidal activity of serum. *FEMS Microbiol. Lett.* 9:193–197.

50. **Gewurz, H., C. Mold, J. Siegel, and B. Fiedel.** 1982. C-reactive protein and the acute phase response. *Adv. Intern. Med.* 27:345–372.

51. **Gibbons, R. J.** 1974. Bacterial adherence to mucosal surfaces and its inhibition by secretory antibodies, p. 315–325. *In* J. Mestecky and A. R. Lawton (ed.), *The Immunoglobulin A System.* Plenum Publishing Corp., New York.

52. **Gibbons, R. J., and J. V. Qureshi.** 1980. Virulence-related physiological changes and antigenic variation in populations of *Streptococcus mutans* colonizing gnotobiotic rats. *Infect. Immun.* 29:1082–1091.

53. **Giebink, G. S., J. V. Grebner, Y. Kim, and P. G. Quie.** 1978. Serum opsonic deficiency produced by *Streptococcus pneumoniae* and by capsular polysaccharide antigens. *Yale J. Biol. Med.* 51:527–538.

54. **Goldman, R. C., K. Joiner, and L. Leive.** 1984.

Serum-resistant mutants of *Escherichia coli* O111 contain increased lipopolysaccharide, lack an O-antigen-containing capsule, and cover more of their lipid A core with O antigen. *J. Bacteriol.* 159:877–882.

55. **Gordon, D. L., and M. K. Hostetter.** 1986. Complement and host defence against microorganisms. *Pathology* 18:365–375.

56. **Greenblatt, J., R. J. Boackle, and J. H. Schwab.** 1978. Activation of the alternate complement pathway by peptidoglycan from streptococcal cell wall. *Infect. Immun.* 19:286–303.

57. **Griffith, R. W., T. T. Kramer, and J. F. Pohlenz.** 1984. Relationship between the antibody-complement susceptibility of smooth *Salmonella cholerae-suis* var. *kunzendorf* strains and their virulence for mice and pigs. *Am. J. Vet. Res.* 45:1342–1348.

58. **Griffiths, E.** 1983. Adaptation and multiplication of bacteria in host tissues. *Philos. Trans. R. Soc. Lond. Ser. B* 303:85–96.

59. **Griffiths, E.** 1983. Availability of iron and survival of bacteria in infection, p. 153–177. *In* C. S. F. Easmon, J. Jeljaszewicz, M. R. W. Brown, and P. A. Lambert (ed.), *Medical Microbiology,* vol. 3. Academic Press, Inc. (London), Ltd., London.

60. **Griffiths, E., and J. Humphreys.** 1980. Isolation of enterochelin from the peritoneal washings of guinea pigs lethally infected with *Escherichia coli. Infect. Immun.* 28:286–289.

61. **Griffiths, E., P. Stevenson, T. L. Hale, and S. B. Formal.** 1985. Synthesis of aerobactin and a 76,000-dalton iron-regulated outer membrane protein by *Escherichia coli* K-12–*Shigella flexneri* hybrids and by enteroinvasive strains of *Escherichia coli. Infect. Immun.* 49:67–71.

62. **Griffiths, E., P. Stevenson, and P. Joyce.** 1983. Pathogenic *Escherichia coli* exposes new outer membrane proteins when growing in vivo. *FEMS Microbiol. Lett.* 16:95–99.

63. **Grossman, N., K. A. Joiner, M. M. Frank, and L. Leive.** 1986. C3b binding, but not its breakdown, is affected by the structure of the O-antigen polysaccharide in lipopolysaccharide from salmonellae. *J. Immunol.* 136:2208–2215.

64. **Grossman, N., and L. Leive.** 1984. Complement activation via the alternative pathway by purified *Salmonella* lipopolysaccharide is affected by its structure but not its O-antigen length. *J. Immunol.* 132:376–385.

65. **Guan, L. T., and G. K. Scott.** 1980. Analysis of outer membrane components of *Escherichia coli* ML308 225 and of a serum-resistant mutant. *Infect. Immun.* 28:387–392.

66. **Hackett, J., P. Wyk, P. Reeves, and V. Mathan.** 1987. Mediation of serum resistance in *Salmonella typhimurium* by an 11-kilodalton polypeptide

encoded by the cryptic plasmid. *J. Infect. Dis.* 155:540–549.

67. **Helms, S. D., J. D. Oliver, and J. C. Travis.** 1984. Role of heme compounds and haptoglobin in *Vibrio vulnificus* pathogenicity. *Infect. Immun.* 45:345–349.

68. **Herrington, D. A., and P. F. Sparling.** 1986. *Haemophilus influenzae* can use human transferrin as a sole source for required iron. *Infect. Immun.* 48:248–251.

69. **Hildebrandt, J. F., L. W. Mayer, S. P. Wang, and T. M. Buchanan.** 1978. *Neisseria gonorrhoeae* acquire a new principal outer membrane protein when transformed to resistance to serum bactericidal activity. *Infect. Immun.* 20:267–273.

70. **Hill, M. J.** 1969. A staphylococcal aggression. *J. Med. Microbiol.* 1:33–43.

71. **Hill, M. J.** 1969. Protection of mice against infection by *Staphylococcus aureus. J. Med. Microbiol.* 2:1–7.

72. **Hostetter, M. K.** 1986. Serotypic differences in covalently bound C3b and its degradation fragments among virulent pneumococci. I. Implications for phagocytosis and antibody production. *J. Infect. Dis.* 153:682–691.

73. **Howard, C. J.** 1980. Variation in the susceptibility of bovine mycoplasmas to killing by the alternate complement pathway in bovine serum. *Immunology* 41:561–568.

74. **Howell, T. H., D. M. Spinell, and R. J. Gibbons.** 1979. Antigenic variation in populations of *Streptococcus salivarius* isolated from the human mouth. *Arch. Oral Biol.* 24:389–397.

75. **Ingram, D. G.** 1982. Comparative aspects of conglutinin and immunoconglutinin, p. 1–23. *In* J. B. Hay (ed.), *Animal Models of Immunological Processes.* Academic Press, Inc., New York.

76. **Isogai, E., H. Isogai, and N. Ito.** 1986. Decreased lipopolysaccharide content and enhanced susceptibility of leptospiras to serum leptospiricidal action and phagocytosis after treatment with diphenylamine. *Zentralbl. Bakteriol. Mikrobiol. Hyg. Abt. 1 Orig. Reihe A* 262:438–447.

77. **Jacks-Weis, J., Y. Kim, and P. P. Cleary.** 1982. Restricted deposition of C3 on M$^+$ group A streptococci: correlation with resistance to phagocytosis. *J. Immunol.* 128:1897–1902.

78. **Jarvis, G. A., and N. A. Vedros.** 1987. Sialic acid of group B *Neisseria meningitidis* regulates alternative complement pathway activation. *Infect. Immun.* 55:174–180.

79. **Jennings, H. J., and C. Lugowski.** 1981. Immunochemistry of groups A, B and C meningococcal polysaccharide—tetanus toxoid conjugates. *J. Immunol.* 127:1011–1018.

80. **Joiner, K. A., E. Brown, C. Hammer, K. Warren, and M. Frank.** 1983. Studies of the mecha-
nism of bacterial resistance to complement-mediated killing. III. C5b-9 deposits stably on rough and type 7 *Streptococcus pneumoniae* without causing bacterial killing. *J. Immunol.* 130:845–849.

81. **Joiner, K. A., E. J. Brown, and M. M. Frank.** 1984. Complement and bacteria: chemistry and biology in host defence. *Annu. Rev. Immunol.* 2:461–491.

82. **Joiner, K. A., L. F. Fries, and M. M. Frank.** 1986/87. Studies of antibody and complement function in host defense against bacterial infection. *Immunol. Lett.* 14:197–202.

83. **Joiner, K. A., N. Grossman, M. Schmetz, and L. Leive.** 1986. C3 binds preferentially to long-chain lipopolysaccharide during alternative pathway activation by *Salmonella montevideo. J. Immunol.* 136:710–715.

84. **Joiner, K. A., C. H. Hammer, E. J. Brown, and M. M. Frank.** 1982. Studies on the mechanism of bacterial resistance to complement-mediated killing. II. C8 and C9 release C5b67 from the surface of *Salmonella minnesota* S218 because the terminal complex does not insert into the bacterial outer membrane. *J. Exp. Med.* 155:809–819.

85. **Joiner, K. A., K. A. Warren, C. Hammer, and M. M. Frank.** 1985. Bactericidal but not nonbactericidal C5b-9 is associated with distinctive outer membrane proteins in *Neisseria gonorrhoeae. J. Immunol.* 134:1920–1925.

86. **Judd, R. C., M. Tam, and K. Joiner.** 1987. Characterization of protein I from serum-sensitive and serum-resistant transformants of *Neisseria gonorrhoeae. Infect. Immun.* 55:273–276.

87. **Kasper, D. L., J. L. Winkelhake, W. D. Zollinger, B. L. Brandt, and M. S. Artenstein.** 1973. Immunochemical similarity between polysaccharide antigens of *Escherichia coli* O7:K1(L):NM and group B *Neisseria meningitidis. J. Immunol.* 110:262–268.

88. **Kilian, M.** 1981. Degradation of immunoglobulins A1, A2, and G by suspected principal periodontal pathogens. *Infect. Immun.* 34:757–765.

89. **Kilian, M., J. Mestecky, and R. E. Schrohenloher.** 1979. Pathogenic species of the genus *Haemophilus* and *Streptococcus pneumoniae* produce immunoglobulin A1 protease. *Infect. Immun.* 26:143–149.

90. **Kindmark, C. O.** 1971. Stimulating effect of C-reactive protein on phagocytosis of various species of pathogenic bacteria. *Clin. Exp. Immunol.* 8:941–948.

91. **Köhler, W., and O. Prokop.** 1978. Relationship between haptoglobin and *Streptococcus pyogenes* T4 antigens. *Nature* (London) 271:373.

92. **Kornfeld, S. J., and A. G. Plaut.** 1981. Secretory immunity and the bacterial IgA proteases. *Rev. Infect. Dis.* 3:521–534.

93. **Kronvall, G.** 1973. A surface component of group A, C and G streptococci with non-immune reactiv-

ity for immunoglobulin G. *J. Immunol.* 111:1401–1406.

94. Kronvall, G., E. Myrhe, L. Björck, and I. Berggard. 1978. Binding of aggregated human B$_2$-microglobulin to surface protein structure in group A, C, and G streptococci. *Infect. Immun.* 22:136–142.

95. Kronvall, G., C. Schönbeck, and E. Myrhe. 1979. Fibrinogen binding structures in β-haemolytic streptococci group A, C and G. Comparisons with receptors for IgG and aggregated β-microglobulin. *Acta Pathol. Microbiol. Scand. Sect. B* 87:303–310.

96. Kronvall, G., A. Simmons, E. B. Myrhe, and S. Jonsson. 1979. Specific absorption of human serum albumin, immunoglobulin A, and immunoglobulin G with selected strains of group A and G streptococci. *Infect. Immun.* 25:1–10.

97. Lafont, J.-P., M. Dho, H. M. D'Hauteville, A. Bree, and P. J. Sansonetti. 1987. Presence and expression of aerobactin genes in virulent avian strains of *Escherichia coli. Infect. Immun.* 55:193–197.

98. Lanser, M. E., and T. M. Saba. 1983. Correction of serum opsonic defects after burns and sepsis by opsonic fibronectin administration. *Arch. Surg.* 60:577–594.

99. Lawlor, K. M., P. A. Daskaleros, R. E. Robinson, and S. M. Payne. 1987. Virulence of iron transport mutants of *Shigella flexneri* and utilization of host iron compounds. *Infect. Immun.* 55:594–599.

100. Leist-Welsh, P., and A. B. Bjornson. 1982. Immunoglobulin-independent utilisation of the classical complement pathway in opsonophagocytosis of *Escherichia coli* by human peripheral leucocytes. *J. Immunol.* 128:2643–2651.

101. Leive, L. L., and V. E. Jimenez-Lucho. 1986. Lipopolysaccharide O-antigen structure controls alternative pathway activation of complement: effects on phagocytosis and virulence of salmonellae, p. 14–17. *In* L. Leive (ed.), *Microbiology—1986.* American Society for Microbiology, Washington, D.C.

102. Lew, P. D., R. Zubler, P. Vandaux, J. J. Farquet, F. A. Waldvogel, and P. H. Lambert. 1979. Decreased heat-labile opsonic activity and complement levels associated with evidence of C3 breakdown products in infected pleural effusions. *J. Clin. Invest.* 63:326–334.

103. Liang-Takasaki, C., N. Grossman, and L. Leive. 1983. Salmonellae activate complement differentially via the alternative pathway depending on the structure of their lipopolysaccharide O-antigen. *J. Immunol.* 130:1867–1870.

104. Linggood, M. A., and P. L. Ingram. 1982. The role of alpha haemolysin in the virulence of *Escherichia coli* for mice. *J. Med. Microbiol.* 15:23–30.

105. Martinez, R. J., and S. F. Carroll. 1980. Sequential metabolic expressions of the lethal process in human serum-treated *Escherichia coli:* role of lysozyme. *Infect. Immun.* 28:735–745.

106. McLeod, D. T., M. J. Croughan, F. Ahmad, R. P. Brettle, and M. A. Calder. 1986. Lack of immunoglobulin A1 protease production by *Branhamella catarrhalis. Infect. Immun.* 52:631–632.

107. Meier, J. T., M. I. Simon, and A. G. Barbour. 1985. Antigenic variation is associated with DNA rearrangements in a relapsing fever *Borrelia. Cell* 41:403–409.

108. Mickelsen, P. A., and P. F. Sparling. 1981. Ability of *Neisseria gonorrhoeae, Neisseria meningitidis,* and commensal *Neisseria* species to obtain iron from transferrin and iron compounds. *Infect. Immun.* 33:555–564.

109. Miller, C. E., K. H. Wong, J. C. Feeley, and M. E. Forlines. 1972. Immunological conversion of *Vibrio cholerae* in gnotobiotic mice. *Infect. Immun.* 6:739–742.

110. Mold, C., S. Nakayama, T. J. Holzer, H. Gewurz, and T. W. Du Clos. 1981. C-reactive protein is protective against *Streptococcus pneumoniae* infection in mice. *J. Exp. Med.* 154:1703–1708.

111. Moll, A., P. A. Manning, and K. N. Timmis. 1980. Plasmid-determined resistance to serum bactericidal activity: a major outer membrane protein, the *traT* gene product, is responsible for plasmid-specified serum resistance in *Escherichia coli. Infect. Immun.* 28:359–367.

112. Molla, A., K. Matsumoto, I. Oyamada, T. Katsuki, and H. Maeda. 1986. Degradation of protease inhibitors, immunoglobulins, and other serum proteins by *Serratia* protease and its toxicity to fibroblasts in culture. *Infect. Immun.* 53:522–529.

113. Mulks, M. 1985. Microbial IgA proteases, p. 81–104. *In* I. A. Holder (ed.), *Bacterial Enzymes and Virulence.* CRC Press, Inc., Boca Raton, Fla.

114. Mulks, M. H., S. J. Kornfeld, B. Frangione, and A. G. Plaut. 1982. Relationship between the specificity of IgA proteases and serotypes in *Haemophilus influenzae. J. Infect. Dis.* 146:266–274.

115. Mulks, M. H., and A. G. Plaut. 1978. IgA protease as a characteristic distinguishing pathogenic from harmless *Neisseriaceae. N. Engl. J. Med.* 299:973–976.

116. Muller-Eberhard, H. J. 1975. Complement. *Annu. Rev. Biochem.* 44:697–724.

117. Myhre, E. B., and G. Kronvall. 1977. Heterogeneity of nonimmune immunoglobulin Fc reactivity among gram-positive cocci: description of three major types of receptors for human immunoglobulin G. *Infect. Immun.* 17:475–482.

118. Myhre, E. B., and G. Kronvall. 1980. Demonstration of a new type of immunoglobulin G receptor in *Streptococcus zooepidemicus* strains. *Infect. Immun.* 27:808–816.

119. Nakayama, S., H. Gewurz, T. Holzer, T. W. DuClos, and C. Mold. 1983. The role of the spleen in the protective effect of C reactive protein in *Strep-*

tococcus pneumoniae infection. *Clin. Exp. Immunol.* 54:319–326.

120. Neilands, J. B. 1981. Microbial iron compounds. *Annu. Rev. Biochem.* 50:715 731.

121. Newby, T., and F. J. Bourne. 1976. The nature of the local immune system of the bovine small intestine. *Immunology* 31:475–480.

122. O'Connor, S. P., and P. P. Cleary. 1986. Localization of the streptococcal C5 peptidase to the surface of group A streptococci. *Infect. Immun.* 53:432–434.

123. Odumeru, J. A., G. M. Wiseman, and A. R. Ronald. 1987. Relationship between lipopolysaccharide composition and virulence of *Haemophilus ducreyi*. *J. Med. Microbiol.* 23:155 162.

124. Okada, N., T. Yasuda, and H. Okada. 1982. Restriction of alternative complement pathway activation by sialosylglycolipids. *Nature* (London) 299:261–263.

125. Olling, S. 1977. Sensitivity of Gram-negative bacilli to serum bactericidal activity: a marker of host-parasite relationship in acute and persisting infections. *Scand. J. Infect. Dis. Suppl.* 10:1–40.

126. Opal, S., A. Cross, and P. Gemski. 1982. K antigen and serum sensitivity of rough *Escherichia coli*. *Infect. Immun.* 37:956–960.

127. Perry, R. D., and R. R. Brubaker. 1979. Accumulation of iron by yersiniae. *J. Bacteriol.* 137:1290–1298.

128. Peterson, P. K., J. Verhoef, L. D. Sabath, and P. G. Quie. 1977. Effect of protein A on staphylococcal opsonization. *Infect. Immun.* 15:760–764.

129. Plaut, A. G. 1983. The IgA1 proteases of pathogenic bacteria. *Annu. Rev. Microbiol.* 37:603–622.

130. Pluschke, G., J. Mayden, M. Achtman, and R. P. Levine. 1983. Role of the capsule and the O antigen in resistance of O18:K1 *Escherichia coli* to complement-mediated killing. *Infect. Immun.* 42:907–913.

131. Poolman, J. T., C. T. P. Hopman, and H. C. Zanen. 1983. Immunogenicity of meningococcal antigens as detected in patient sera. *Infect. Immun.* 40:398–406.

132. Reis, K. J., H. F. Hansen, and L. Björck. 1986. Extraction and characterisation of streptococcal IgG Fc receptors from group C and G streptococci. *Mol. Immunol.* 23:425–431.

133. Reiter, B. 1978. Review of the progress of dairy science: antimicrobial systems in milk. *J. Dairy Res.* 45:131–147.

134. Richards, R. L., and C. Alving. 1980. Immune reactivities of antibodies against glycolipids. *ACS Symp. Ser.* 128:461–473.

135. Roantree, R. J., and L. A. Rantz. 1960. A study of the relationship of the normal bactericidal activity of human serum to bacterial infection. *J. Clin. Invest.* 39:72–81.

136. Robbins, J. B., R. Schneerson, W. B. Egan, W. Vann, and D. T. Lui. 1980. Virulence properties of bacterial capsular polysaccharides—unanswered questions, p. 115–132. *In* H. Smith, J. J. Skehel, and M. J. Turner (ed.), *The Molecular Basis of Microbial Pathogenicity*. Dahlem Conference. Verlag Chemie, Weinheim, Federal Republic of Germany.

137. Rowley, D. 1956. Some factors affecting the resistance of animals to bacterial infection. *Ann. N.Y. Acad. Sci.* 66:304–311.

138. Russell-Jones, G. J., E. C. Gotschlich, and M. S. Blake. 1984. A surface receptor specific for human IgA on group B streptococci possessing the Ibc protein antigen. *J. Exp. Med.* 160:1467–1475.

139. Ryden, C., K. Rubin, P. Speziale, M. Hook, M. Lindberg, and T. Wadström. 1983. Fibronectin receptors from *Staphylococcus aureus*. *J. Biol. Chem.* 258:3396–3401.

140. Sack, R. B., and C. E. Miller. 1969. Progressive changes of vibrio serotypes in germ-free mice infected with *Vibrio cholerae*. *J. Bacteriol.* 99:688–695.

141. Saxen, H., I. Reima, and P. H. Mäkelä. 1987. Alternative complement pathway activation by *Salmonella* O polysaccharide as a virulence determinant in the mouse. *Microb. Pathogenesis* 2:15–28.

142. Schneider, H., J. M. Griffiss, R. E. Mandrell, and G. A. Jarvis. 1985. Elaboration of a 3.6-kilodalton lipooligosaccharide, antibody against which is absent from human sera, is associated with serum resistance of *Neisseria gonorrhoeae*. *Infect. Immun.* 50:672–677.

143. Schoolnik, G. K., T. M. Buchanan, and K. K. Holmes. 1976. Gonococci causing disseminated gonococcal infections are resistant to the bactericidal action of normal human serum. *J. Clin. Invest.* 58:1163–1173.

144. Schoolnik, G. K., H. D. Ochs, and T. M. Buchanan. 1979. Immunoglobulin class responsible for gonococcal bactericidal activity of normal human sera. *J. Immunol.* 122:1771–1779.

145. Schurig, G. D., C. E. Hall, K. Burda, L. B. Corbeil, J. R. Duncan, and A. J. Winter. 1973. Persistent genital tract infection with *Vibrio fetus intestinalis* associated with serotypic alteration of the infecting strain. *Am. J. Vet. Res.* 34:1399–1403.

146. Schurig, G. G. D., C. E. Hall, L. B. Corbeil, J. R. Duncan, and A. J. Winter. 1975. Bovine venereal vibriosis: cure of genital infection in females by systemic immunization. *Infect. Immun.* 11:245–251.

147. Sciortino, C. V., and R. A. Finkelstein. 1983. *Vibrio cholerae* expresses iron-regulated outer membrane proteins in vivo. *Infect. Immun.* 42:990–996.

148. Selsted, M. E., and R. J. Martinez. 1978. Lysozyme: primary bactericidin in human plasma serum active against *Bacillus subtilis*. *Infect. Immun.* 20:782–791.

149. Shafer, W. M., K. Joiner, L. F. Guymon, M. S. Cohen, and P. F. Sparling. 1984. Serum sensitivity of *Neisseria gonorrhoeae:* the role of lipopolysaccharide. *J. Infect. Dis.* 149:175–183.

150. Shand, G. H., H. Anwar, J. Kadurugamuwa, M. R. W. Brown, S. H. Silverman, and J. Melling. 1985. In vivo evidence that bacteria in urinary tract infection grow under iron-restricted conditions. *Infect. Immun.* 48:35–39.

151. Sigel, S. P., J. A. Stoebner, and S. M. Payne. 1985. Iron-vibriobactin transport system is not required for virulence of *Vibrio cholerae. Infect. Immun.* 47:360–362.

152. Simonson, C., D. Brener, and I. W. DeVoe. 1982. Expression of a high-affinity mechanism for acquisition of transferrin iron by *Neisseria meningitidis. Infect. Immun.* 36:107–113.

153. Simoons-Smit, A. M., A. M. J. J. Verweij-van Vught, and D. M. Maclaren. 1986. The role of K antigens as virulence factors in *Klebsiella. J. Med. Microbiol.* 21:133–137.

154. Smith, H. 1984. Bacterial subversion rather than suppression of immune defences, p. 171–190. *In* G. Falcone, M. Campa, H. Smith, and G. M. Scott (ed.), *Bacterial and Viral Inhibition and Modulation of Host Defences.* Academic Press, Inc. (London), Ltd., London.

155. Söderström, T., G. Hansson, and G. Larson. 1984. The *Escherichia coli* K capsule shares antigenic determinants with the human gangliosides GM3 and GD3. *N. Engl. J. Med.* 310:726–727.

156. Spika, J. S., H. A. Verbrugh, and J. Verhoef. 1981. Protein A effect on alternative pathway complement activation and opsonization of *Staphylococcus aureus. Infect. Immun.* 34:455–460.

157. Stalenheim, G., O. Götze, N. R. Cooper, J. Sjöquist, and H. J. Müller-Eberhard. 1973. Consumption of human complement components by complexes of IgG with protein A of *Staphylococcus aureus. Immunochemistry* 10:501–507.

158. Stevens, P., L. S. Young, and S. Adamu. 1983. Opsonisation of various capsular (K) *E. coli* by the alternative complement pathway. *Immunology* 50:497–502.

159. Stoenner, H. G., T. Dodd, and C. Larsen. 1982. Antigenic variation of *Borrelia hermsii. J. Exp. Med.* 156:1297–1311.

160. Stull, T. L. 1987. Protein sources of heme for *Haemophilus influenzae. Infect. Immun.* 55:148–153.

161. Taylor, P. W., and M. K. Robinson. 1980. Determinants that increase the serum resistance of *Escherichia coli. Infect. Immun.* 29:278–280.

162. Timmis, K. N., P. A. Manning, C. Echarti, J. K. Timmis, and A. Moll. 1981. Serum resistance in *E. coli*, p. 133–144. *In* S. B. Levy, R. C. Clowes, and E. L. Koenig (ed.), *Molecular Biology, Pathogenicity, and Ecology of Bacterial Plasmids.* Plenum Publishing Corp., New York.

163. Tomas, J. M., V. J. Benedi, B. Ciurana, and J. Jofre. 1986. Role of capsule and O antigen in resistance of *Klebsiella pneumoniae* to serum bactericidal activity. *Infect. Immun.* 54:85–89.

164. Vaara, M., P. Viljanen, T. Vaara, and P. H. Mäkelä. 1984. An outer membrane-disorganising peptide PMBN sensitises *E. coli* strains to serum bactericidal action. *J. Immunol.* 132:2582–2589.

165. Van de Waters, L., A. T. Destree, and R. O. Hynes. 1983. Fibronection binds to some bacteria but does not promote their uptake by phagocytic cells. *Science* 220:201–204.

166. Van Snick, J. L., P. L. Masson, and J. F. Heremans. 1974. The involvement of lactoferrin in the hyposideraemia of acute inflammation. *J. Exp. Med.* 140:1068–1084.

167. Verbrugh, H. A., W. C. Van Dijk, R. Peters, M. E. Van Erne, M. R. Daha, P. K. Peterson, and J. Verhoef. 1980. Opsonic recognition of staphylococci mediated by cell wall peptidoglycan: antibody-independent activation of human complement and opsonic activity of peptidoglycan antibodies. *J. Immunol.* 124:1169–1173.

168. Wexler, D. E., D. E. Chenoweth, and P. P. Cleary. 1985. Mechanism of action of the group A streptococcal C5a inactivator. *Proc. Natl. Acad. Sci. USA* 82:8144–8148.

169. Wexler, D. E., R. D. Nelson, and P. P. Cleary. 1983. Human neutrophil chemotactic response to group A streptococci: bacteria-mediated interference with complement-derived chemotactic factors. *Infect. Immun.* 39:239–246.

170. Whitnack, E., and E. H. Beachey. 1982. Antiopsonic activity of fibrinogen bound to M protein on the surface of group A streptococci. *J. Clin. Invest.* 69:1042–1045.

171. Whitnack, E., and E. H. Beachey. 1985. Inhibition of complement-mediated opsonisation and phagocytosis of *Streptococcus pyogenes* by D fragments of fibrinogen and fibrin bound to cell surface M protein. *J. Exp. Med.* 162:1983–1997.

172. Widders, P. R., C. R. Stokes, J. S. E. David, and F. J. Bourne. 1986. Specific antibody in the equine genital tract following local immunisation and challenge infection with contagious equine metritis organism (*Taylorella equigenitalis*). *Res. Vet. Sci.* 40:54–58.

173. Widders, P. R., C. R. Stokes, T. J. Newby, and F. J. Bourne. 1985. Nonimmune binding of equine immunoglobulin by the causative organism of contagious equine metritis, *Taylorella equigenitalis. Infect. Immun.* 48:417–421.

174. Wilkinson, B. J., S. P. Sisson, Y. Kim, and P. K. Peterson. 1979. Localization of the third component of complement on the cell wall of encapsulated *Staphylococcus aureus* M: implications for

the mechanism of resistance to phagocytosis. *Infect. Immun.* **26**:1159–1163.

175. **Williams, P., P. A. Lambert, M. R. W. Brown, and R. J. Jones.** 1983. The role of the O and K antigens in determining the resistance of *Klebsiella aerogenes* to serum killing and phagocytosis. *J. Gen. Microbiol.* **129**:2181–2191.

176. **Williams, P. H.** 1979. Novel iron uptake system specified by Col V plasmids: an important component in the virulence of invasive strains of *Escherichia coli. Infect. Immun.* **26**:925–932.

177. **Winkelstein, J. A., A. S. Abramovitz, and A. Tomasz.** 1980. Activation of C3 via the alternative complement pathway results in fixation of C3b to the pneumococcal cell wall. *J. Immunol.* **124**:2502–2506.

178. **Yanagawa, R., and Y. Adachi.** 1978. Studies of antigenic variants of leptospira isolated from ex-

perimentally infected mice. *Zentralbl. Bakteriol. Mikrobiol. Hyg. Abt. 1 Orig. Reihe A* **240**:347–355.

179. **Yanagawa, R., and T. Takashima.** 1974. Conversion of serotype in *Leptospira* from *hebdomadis* to *kremastos. Infect. Immun.* **10**:1439–1442.

180. **Yancey, R. J., S. A. L. Breeding, and C. E. Lankford.** 1979. Enterochelin (enterobactin): virulence factor for *Salmonella typhimurium. Infect. Immun.* **24**:174–180.

181. **Yother, J., J. E. Volanakis, and D. E. Briles.** 1982. Human C-reactive protein is protective against fatal *Streptococcus pneumoniae* infection in mice. *J. Immunol.* **128**:2374–2376.

182. **Zak, K., J.-L. Diaz, D. Jackson, and J. E. Heckels.** 1984. Antigenic variation during infection with *Neisseria gonorrhoeae:* detection of antibodies to surface proteins in sera of patients with gonorrhoea. *J. Infect. Dis.* **149**:166–174.

Chapter 6

Bacterial Resistance to Antibody-Dependent Host Defenses

PHILLIP R. WIDDERS

Department of Veterinary Microbiology and Pathology
Washington State University
Pullman, Washington 99164-7040

INTRODUCTION

Successful microbial pathogens have developed an array of mechanisms that favor survival in the host. Just as the host can mobilize an arsenal of defensive measures for eliminating infectious and foreign agents, bacterial pathogens can summon an impressive range of strategies to evade host defense.

The aim of this review is to describe bacterial mechanisms that effectively evade antibody-dependent host effector functions. In considering the host-parasite relationship, it is important to recognize that the balance between eliminating infection and producing disease is precarious, and a range of factors affecting host defense can precipitate disease. Factors as apparently disparate as climate, nutrition, housing, transport, and concurrent infection can all depress host defense sufficiently to favor microbial multiplication and disease production.

Microbial virulence mechanisms are also important in limiting effective host defense. Since the host-parasite balance is delicate, microbial suppression of immunity need not be absolute for infection to ensue. Microbial survival depends on dislocation of host defenses only to the point at which bacterial multiplication is at least equivalent to bacterial death. Any less, and infection will be cleared. Thus, although some microbial virulence mechanisms devastate host defenses, other, more subtle mechanisms operate to disarm rather than destroy immune effectiveness.

However, although evasion of host defenses is important in pathogenesis, individual bacterial mechanisms affecting the immune system are unlikely to be the sole determinant of virulence. Successful pathogenesis generally depends on a multifactorial interaction between the host and the invading organism, often to the extent that identification of a role in pathogenesis for individual bacterial factors is difficult, if not impossible. Current research defining bacterial virulence mechanisms generally describes evasion of host effector functions in vitro, where complicating factors can be controlled or eliminated. To identify evasion of host effector functions associated with specific bacterial factors in vivo is a daunting task. This problem is well illustrated by analysis of the role of staphylococcal protein A in pathogenesis. As discussed below, in vitro studies demonstrate evasion of host defenses mediated by protein A, including an effect on opsonization and phagocytosis (22, 55, 79). However, numerous studies performed in vivo have failed to identify a significant role in' pathogenesis for protein A (27, 34, 40, 55).

Despite this problem, investigation of microbial virulence mechanisms has made a significant contribution to our understanding of the pathogenesis of infectious disease and can introduce new and imaginative approaches to enhancement of host resistance on the basis of techniques for overcoming evasive mechanisms.

Antibody-dependent protection against bacterial infection has primary significance in relation to extracellular pathogens. Protective function is dependent largely on the Fc portion of antibody, by way of interaction with accessory cells or complement. Other functions of antibody are also important in protection, particularly at mucosal surfaces. Bacterial agglutination by antibody limits colonization of a mucosal surface and enhances clearance within the mucus layer in the respiratory, reproductive, and gastrointestinal tracts. Antigen specificity inhibits receptor-mediated interaction between bacteria and host target cells systemically and at mucosal surfaces. In addition, specific antibody can neutralize bacterial toxins that are important in virulence.

Bacterial mechanisms that evade antibody-dependent effector functions include factors that influence antibody synthesis, antibody-antigen interaction, opsonization, and agglutination and binding in mucus.

BACTERIAL MECHANISMS AFFECTING ANTIBODY SYNTHESIS

Antibody synthesis may be affected by restricted immunogenicity of bacterial surface antigens and by suppression and modulation of the immune response. Bacterial factors that can influence antibody synthesis include polysaccharide capsules, mimicry of host antigens, and, possibly, mechanisms that mask bacterial surface antigens.

Bacterial capsules are considered essential for successful invasion and disease production by many bacterial pathogens (89). The role of the capsule in evasion of specific components of antibody activity is discussed below. An important role in virulence mediated by certain bacterial capsules involves an apparent restriction to the ability of the host to mount a specific humoral response.

The basis for the limited immunogenicity of many bacterial polysaccharide capsules is uncertain, but may involve mimicry of host antigens or active induction of T suppressor cells. The poor antibody response to the capsules of *Escherichia coli* K1 and *Neisseria meningitidis* group B (30, 108), which are polymers of sialic acid, may be due to the presence of sialic acid residues in mammalian cell membranes and glycoproteins (30, 97, 108, 124). In apparent contradiction to this hypothesis, however, is the finding that the group C meningococcal capsule, also a polymer of sialic acid but with a different structure, is highly immunogenic (33, 89). An alternative mechanism involves restricted antibody production in response to pneumococcal polysaccharide capsule, a function of antigen-specific suppressor T-cell induction (4, 107).

Bacterial cell wall antigens that limit induction of specific antibody have been described for *Haemophilus pleuropneumoniae* (86), *Haemophilus influenzae* (57), *Bordetella pertussis* (87), and *Serratia marcescens* (42), although the basis for this limited immunogenicity has not been defined.

Bacterial mimicry of host antigens has been described for noncapsular surface antigens in a range of pathogens including streptococci (19, 26, 50, 127) and mycoplasmas (122). The significance of this cross-reactivity as a determinant of microbial virulence has not been defined, although particularly with streptococci, its role in the etiology of postinfectious immunopathological sequelae in humans has been extensively studied. Surface-exposed epitopes of M proteins from different serotypes of rheumatogenic group A streptococci cross-react with sarcolemmal membrane proteins of human myocardium (19, 26, 50, 127). This cross-reactivity has been implicated in the etiology of poststreptococcal rheumatic fever (44, 128). Similarly, increased synthesis of autoantibody specific for mammalian cytoskeletal components has been correlated with the presence of shared epitopes on the mycoplasma surface and mammalian intermediate filaments (122).

Thus, host antigen mimicry by microbial surface components is implicated in the etiology of immunopathological conditions. It is also likely that antigenic mimicry inhibits or at least reduces the host response to epitopes that are recognized as self. Certainly, microbial mechanisms, such as capsules or antigenic mimicry, that limit the synthesis of antibody specific for surface antigens are likely to favor extracellular survival of microbial pathogens in vivo.

Induction of a specific antibody response can also be limited by microbial binding of host constituents. *Haemophilus somnus,* a gram-negative systemic and mucosal pathogen of cattle, expresses a receptor on the bacterial surface specific for the Fc region of the immunoglobulin molecule (P. R. Widders, J. W. Smith, M. Yarnall, T. C. McGuire, and L. B. Corbeil, submitted for publication; M. Yarnall, P. R. Widders, and L. B. Corbeil, submitted for publication). Bacterial proteins with molecular masses of approximately 350, 270, 120, and 41 kilodaltons (350K, 270K, 120K, and 41K proteins) have been identified that retain Fc receptor activity following electrophoresis in sodium dodecyl sulfate and transfer to nitrocellulose (Yarnall et al., submitted). The 41K antigen is a major constituent of the bacterial outer membrane (14, 32). However, this antigen is not recognized by the bovine immune response in calves convalescent after *H. somnus* pneumonia (32), in cows after *H. somnus*-induced abortion (14), or in cattle after hyperimmunization with whole bacteria emulsified in Freund incomplete adjuvant (unpublished data).

Thus, a major surface protein of *H. somnus* is apparently nonimmunogenic in its native configuration in whole bacteria. The immunological basis for the failure of this outer membrane protein to stimulate a humoral response is uncertain, but this specific immunosuppression may well be related to nonimmune immunoglobulin binding mediated by the 41K antigen. Since specific antibody to *H. somnus* protects against experimental pneumonia (32), failure to stimulate production of antibody specific for a major bacterial outer membrane protein must favor bacterial survival in vivo.

Comparable suppression of a specific immune response is suggested in studies of the local immune response in the equine genital tract (115, 116). *Taylorella equigenitalis,* the causative organism of contagious equine metritis, expresses a surface receptor specific for the constant region of equine immunoglobulin (117). Although local immunization with a protein antigen was effective in stimulating a local immunoglobulin G (IgG) and IgA response in the equine uterus (115), immunization and challenge infection with *T. equigenitalis* failed to stimulate a local IgG response, with uterine and vaginal antibody restricted to the IgA and IgM isotypes (116). The bacterial antigen used for immunization and challenge was cultured in equine serum-supplemented medium (116) and thus retained equine IgG bound to the bacterial cell surface (117). The role of this surface-bound IgG in limiting a specific immune response is unknown, and an association between bacterial binding of IgG and regulation of the immune response in vivo is at present only speculative. However, the survival advantage of a bacterial mechanism that limits induction of a specific IgG response to an extracellular pathogen is obvious.

A different form of modulation of a specific immune response has been studied in relation to the malarial parasite *Plasmodium falciparum* (3, 64). The high antigen load in malaria, coupled with the presence of repeat oligopeptides that produce complex cross-reactive epitopes, is considered the basis of a block to maturation in the humoral immune response (3). This maturational defect results in preservation of the bulk of activated B-cell clones (64) and may account for the large amounts of relatively low-affinity antibody in infected individuals (64).

Bacterial mechanisms that effect nonspecific modulation of the humoral immune system have also been described. In contrast to the specific immunosuppression correlated with Fc receptor activity in gram-negative bacteria, staphylococcal protein A is associated with increased lymphocyte activity. Soluble or cell-associated protein A has been shown to increase T- and B-cell mitogenesis (28, 94, 95, 101) and to stimulate immunoglobulin synthesis (65, 88, 98). Proliferation of B cells has been related to protein A interaction with B-cell surface immunoglobulin (88, 90), although other studies suggest that stimuli apparently unrelated to immunoglobulin binding are also involved (55, 73, 98, 101).

Other nonspecific suppressive mechanisms involve various constituents of group A streptococci, including exotoxin (37), teichoic acid (63), and a cytoplasmic constituent (59, 60), which suppress induction of an antibody response to unrelated antigens. Similar effects have been documented for a capsular polysaccharide of *Klebsiella pneumoniae* (74) and the cell membrane of *Mycoplasma arthritidis* (7). Lipopolysaccharide and lipid A have also been shown to effect nonspecific modulation of a humoral immune response (102).

EVASION OF ANTIBODY BINDING

Inhibition of antibody binding to the bacterial cell surface can enhance bacterial survival in vivo by limiting effective phagocytic cell function, evading classical pathway-mediated complement killing, or limiting antibody-mediated agglutination and clearance at mucosal surfaces.

Mechanisms that can limit antibody binding include the presence of bacterial capsules, nonimmune binding of host constituents, and variation in surface antigens.

The role of capsules as determinants of bacterial virulence has been extensively studied. Much of the evidence for capsule-mediated effects on antibody activity derives from studies of the antiphagocytic effects of capsules, and these findings are discussed below in relation to inhibition of opsonization. In most cases the basis for capsular inhibition of opsonization has not been defined, but is generally manifested only in the absence of specific anticapsular antibody (38, 39, 80, 89, 108, 119). Under these conditions, failure of opsonization is most probably related to limited interaction between phagocytic cells and opsonins deposited on the bacterial cell wall. Studies of *Staphylococcus aureus* demonstrate that the bacterial capsule does not present a barrier to cell wall deposition of complement or immunoglobulin (49, 77, 120). Conceptually, however, bacterial surface structures may also mask cell wall antigens targeted by antibody and complement and thereby protect against serum bactericidal activity or phagocytosis. Thus, the effect of the K1 capsule of *E. coli* in limiting susceptibility to serum (2) is considered to be related to decreased complement activation (108).

Binding of host constituents to the microbial cell surface may also limit host effector functions mediated by antibody or complement. Bacterial factors responsible for binding of host components, with well-characterized effects on antibody-dependent clearance mechanisms, include fibrinogen binding by the M protein of group A streptococci (113, 114) and immunoglobulin binding by protein A of *S. aureus* (55).

The M protein of streptococci is an important virulence determinant. Studies of antibody and complement deposition and phagocytosis in vitro suggest that the fibrinogen-binding capacity of streptococcal M protein is important in limiting these elements of host defense (113, 114). Streptococcal isolates lacking M protein are effectively opsonized by activating the alternative pathway of complement (10, 78), whereas bacteria expressing M protein do not activate complement efficiently (10, 41) and are less readily phagocytosed (113, 114). Opsonization and phagocytosis of M-positive streptococci was enhanced in serum compared with plasma, and this effect was abrogated by fibrinogen supplementation of serum (113, 114). The protective effect of fibrinogen was based on decreased complement deposition on fibrinogen-treated bacteria (113) and dose-dependent inhibition of specific antibody deposition (114). This block to antibody deposition could be overcome by increasing the concentration of antibody specific to M protein (114), probably by competitive inhibition of fibrinogen binding. Thus, inhibition of opsonization and phagocytosis of group A streptococci is mediated by binding of fibrinogen to the bacterial cell surface, limiting activation of the alternative pathway of complement and deposition of specific antibody.

Similar effects are mediated by nonimmune binding of immunoglobulin. Protein A from *S. aureus* has binding specificity for the Fc region of IgG from a range of mammalian species (55) and, by complexing with IgG, interferes with antibody-dependent effector functions. Cell-associated protein A is correlated with reduced antibody- or antibody- and complement-mediated opsonization and phagocytosis of bacteria in vitro (22, 79). This effect may indicate that bacterial surface antigens targeted by specific antibody or complement are masked by nonimmune binding of IgG (22), since complement-dependent opsonization of protein A-rich isolates is enhanced in the absence of IgG (22, 55, 79).

The demonstrated antiopsonic properties of bacterial binding of fibrinogen and IgG may reflect a similar contribution to virulence in other organisms for which comparable mechanisms have been described. Immunoglobulin binding by streptococci has been extensively studied, with four different types of IgG receptors characterized among group A, C, and G streptococci (11, 51, 69, 71, 72, 125, 126). In addition, binding of albumin and IgA on the surfaces of group B, C, and G streptococci has been demonstrated (53, 70, 92). Immunoglobulin binding on the surfaces of *Mycoplasma* spp. (56, 121) and *Coprococcus comes* (112) has been identified. For gram-negative bacteria, nonimmune immunoglobulin binding on

the surfaces of *Brucella abortus* (75, 76), *H. somnus* (Widders et al., submitted; Yarnall et al., submitted), and *T. equigenitalis* (117) has been described. The contribution of nonimmune binding to virulence has not been defined for gram-negative bacteria, but similar mechanisms enhance evasion of host defenses by streptococci (96), staphylococci (55), and herpesvirus (23). Immunoglobulin-Fc binding is also associated with pathogenicity among trypanosomes (25). A correlation between virulence and immunoglobulin binding by *T. equigenitalis* is suggested by the specificity of the Fc receptor for equine IgG. Immunoglobulin from other domestic animal species was not bound by this organism (117), reflecting the limited pathogenicity of this organism for nonequine species (109–111).

A reduction in antibody binding to bacteria can also result from variation in surface antigens. Among pathogenic bacteria, antigenic shift has been recognized in *Borrelia* spp. (5, 6, 61, 81, 105), in *Neisseria gonorrhoeae* (35), in *Vibrio cholerae* (62, 93), and in both subspecies of the bovine pathogen *Campylobacter fetus* (8, 15, 99). Variation in surface antigens for *Borrelia* spp. is plasmid mediated (81). Antigenic variation in gonococcal pili has been localized to specific regions of the bacterial chromosome (35). The role of antigenic shift in the pathogenesis of borreliosis is suggested by the correlation between the incidence of clinical disease and the isolation of a variant organism (6, 105). Since antibody to gonococcal pili enhances phagocytosis in vitro (85), the ability to vary the expression of surface antigens probably contributes to bacterial survival in vivo.

The source of variation in *C. fetus* is apparently the heat-labile surface antigens (15), although the surface structure and the biochemical basis for variation have not been characterized. Antibody is important in eliminating *C. fetus* infection in the genital tract and mediating opsonization for phagocytosis by polymorphonuclear leukocytes and macrophages (16). Thus, variation in surface antigens can be an effective bacterial strategy for evasion of antibody-dependent defenses in the genital tract and might be associated with the persistence of *C. fetus* in the face of detectable local antibody levels following infection (15) or systemic immunization (100).

INHIBITION OF OPSONIZATION

Bacterial evasion of antibody-dependent opsonization can be mediated by limiting antibody binding, restricting interaction between phagocytic cells and opsonized bacteria, or destroying opsonins. Both soluble bacterial Fc receptors and capsules can limit phagocytic cell binding to opsonin, and immunoglobulin proteases can cleave the Fc fragment of immunoglobulin involved in complement activation and binding to leukocyte Fc receptors.

Bacterial pathogens for which surface expression of immunoglobulin-Fc receptors has been characterized, including streptococci (125), *S. aureus* (55), and *H. somnus* (Yarnall et al., submitted), also elaborate Fc receptor in the soluble form into the bacterial cell-free culture supernatant. For *S. aureus,* many of the potentially evasive properties of protein A have been ascribed to the soluble rather than the cell-associated bacterial Fc receptor. Soluble protein A can inhibit antibody-dependent complement fixation (52, 54, 123), IgG catabolism (20, 36), binding to Fc receptor-bearing immune cells (1, 21, 106), and antibody-dependent cell-mediated cytoxicity (18, 45, 91).

Deposition of the first component of complement onto IgG bound in antigen-antibody complexes is inhibited by protein A (31, 54, 96). This inhibition is considered to be due to shared (54) or approximate (55) binding sites for C1q and protein A in the C_H2 and C_H2-C_H3 domains, respectively, of IgG. Although other studies demonstrate that protein A complexed with free IgG activates complement by both classical and alternative pathways (24, 52, 104, 123), this apparent contradiction can be resolved by considering the structural composition of complexes formed with free or antigen-bound IgG (54). In fact, it is likely that complement consumption by protein A complexed with free immunoglobulin may enhance bacterial virulence by depleting complement levels at an infection site (24).

Competition between C1q and protein A for binding to immunoglobulin-Fc is manifested in a reduction in opsonization (22,79,96). In addition, immunoglobulin binding by soluble protein A limits antibody interaction with Fc receptor-bearing immune cells, resulting in reduced phagocytosis (22, 55, 79) and antibody-dependent cell-mediated cytotoxicity (18, 45, 91). This effect is considered a function of steric hindrance rather than shared epitopes recognized by protein A and immune-cell Fc receptors (31), although reactivity of antibody to protein A with leukocyte Fc receptors (9) suggests some overlap.

Bacterial capsules can have an antiopsonic effect above and beyond a capacity to limit antibody deposition on the bacterial cell wall. Encapsulation of *S. aureus* cells, for example, does not limit bacterial deposition of opsonins (49, 77, 80, 119, 120), but apparently inhibits interaction between the phagocyte receptor and opsonin bound to the cell wall. Studies of complement depletion with encapsulated or unencapsulated *S. aureus* cells found similar rates of complement consumption (77). Immunochemical studies confirmed that for both variants complement C3 was deposited on the bacterial cell wall, despite the presence of an intact capsule (119, 120), demonstrating that the *S. aureus* capsule is not a barrier to components of the complement cascade. Although the capsule of *S. aureus* limits bacterial attachment of bacteriophages (118), it appears that immunoglobulin is not prevented from binding to the bacterial cell wall. Protein A-mediated immunoglobulin binding is comparable in encapsulated and unencapsulated strains (49), suggesting that the capsule is freely permeable to immunoglobulin. For *S. aureus,* then, it appears that the antiphagocytic effect of the bacterial capsule is mediated not by a block to the deposition of opsonins, but by limiting the interaction between the phagocytic cell and opsonins deposited on the bacterial cell wall.

A mechanism such as this, which limits

opsonization and phagocytosis in the absence of capsular-specific antibody, is also important in considering vaccine-induced immunity. For many pathogens, capsule production is suppressed or lost on growth in vitro (17, 103). Use of such laboratory-grown bacteria as vaccine antigen will stimulate production of antibody specific for the bacterial cell wall. However, capsule production may be regained or reexpressed on animal passage (17, 103). Antibody specific for bacterial cell wall antigens that is opsonic for unencapsulated strains has been shown in many studies to be ineffective in opsonizing encapsulated organisms (89, 119). However, antibody specific for the bacterial capsule will enhance in vivo clearance of encapsulated bacteria (89, 119). Therefore, in developing protective immunization regimes, it is important to consider the role of encapsulation in bacterial pathogenesis.

Finally, effective opsonization may be limited by the activity of microbial immunoglobulin proteases. Although the effect of specific proteases does not influence the deposition of antibody, unless by decreasing avidity consequent to reducing binding valence, cleavage of the Fc portion of IgG prevents interaction with phagocytes and complement. IgG proteases have been described for human pathogens in periodontal disease (109). Since IgA does not fix complement and has limited value opsonically, IgA proteases are unlikely to limit opsonization or complement fixation.

INHIBITION OF AGGLUTINATION AND CLEARANCE AT MUCOSAL SURFACES

An important component in the defense of mucosal surfaces is the prevention of colonization of epithelial cells by pathogenic bacteria. Mucus and mucous flow have an important role in protecting the respiratory, gastrointestinal, and reproductive tracts by trapping bacteria within the mucus layer and preventing contact with epithelial cells (12). Antibody, particularly of the IgA isotype, is

important in this form of mucosal protection through bacterial agglutination and binding to the gel phase of mucus (12, 58). Complementarity in the structure of IgA carbohydrate units and mucous glycoprotein has been proposed as the basis for the interaction between IgA and mucus (12). Thus, bacterial mechanisms that limit agglutination and antibody-mediated binding to mucus, such as immunoglobulin proteases or factors that inhibit antibody binding, can enhance bacterial colonization of a mucosal surface.

Some bacterial pathogens of mucosal surfaces produce extracellular enzymes that specifically cleave IgA (82, 83). IgA protease activity has been described for *N. gonorrhoeae* (83), *N. meningitidis* (83), *H. influenzae* (82), *Streptococcus pneumoniae* (82), *Streptococcus sanguis* (82), and *Ureaplasma urealyticum* (29, 43, 47). Among veterinary bacterial isolates, IgA protease activity has been demonstrated with *U. urealyticum* recovered from the canine urogenital tract (43) and with *H. pleuropneumoniae* (48), although subsequent studies have failed to duplicate the last result (67).

Although a role in virulence has not been confirmed, IgA protease activity is considered important in pathogenesis: cleavage of IgA by these enzymes results in a loss of functional integrity (68, 82, 84); protease activity is associated with species characterized as mucosal pathogens and not by related, nonpathogenic species (82); enzyme specificity is often restricted to cleavage of host, but not nonhost, IgA (43); protease activity has been recovered from infected secretions (82); and antiprotease antibody has been found in secretions obtained from convalescent patients (66, 82, 117). The association between IgA protease activity and bacterial virulence has been tested in vitro by measuring bacterial binding to explants of fallopian tube mucosa to estimate mucosal colonization (13). Although there was no correlation between protease activity and mucosal colonization (13), failure to demonstrate the presence of a specific IgA response suggests that the experimental conditions did not favor the identification of such an effect.

CONCLUSIONS

Pathogenic survival of microorganisms has depended on the evolution of a range of strategies for evasion of host defenses. Although such mechanisms are rarely the sole determinant of bacterial virulence, they are essential for pathogenicity. Analysis and characterization of these evasive mechanisms provide a fascinating insight into the microorganism-host interaction. More importantly, however, the results of these studies direct research toward developing techniques to enhance host immunity by overcoming microbial evasion. Thus, surface antigens of limited immunogenicity can be coupled to protein antigens to enhance the immune response. The effect of nonimmune binding of host constituents in evading humoral effectors may be overcome by stimulating production of high-affinity antibodies that effectively compete with receptor activity. In this respect, the effect of fibrinogen binding by the M protein of group A streptococci is abrogated, at least in vitro, by increasing concentrations of antibody specific for M protein (114). Evasion of host defenses mediated by variation in bacterial surface antigens might be overcome by identifying conserved surface antigens that stimulate a protective immune response.

LITERATURE CITED

1. Ades, E. W., D. J. Phillips, S. L. Shore, D. S. Gordon, M. P. LaVia, C. M. Black, and C. B. Reiner. 1976. Analysis of mononuclear cell surface with fluoresceinated staphylococcal protein A complexed with IgG antibody of heat aggregated gamma globulin. *J. Immunol.* 117:2119–2123.

2. Aguero, M. E., and F. C. Cabello. 1983. Relative contribution of Col V plasmid and K1 antigen to the pathenogenicity of *Escherichia coli. Infect. Immun.* 40:359–368.

3. Anders, R. F. 1986. Multiple cross-reactivities amongst antigens of *Plasmodium falciparum* impair the development of protective immunity against malaria. *Parasite Immunol.* 8:529–539.

4. Baker, P. J., D. F. Amsbaugh, P. W. Stashak, G. Caldes, and B. Prescott. 1981. Regulation of the antibody response to pneumococcal polysaccharide by thymus derived cells. *Rev. Infect. Dis.* 3:332–341.

5. Barbour, A. G., O. Barrera, and R. C. Judd. 1983. Structural analysis of the variable major proteins of Borrelia hermsii. *J. Exp. Med.* 158:2127–2140.

6. Barbour, A. G., and H. G. Stoenner. 1985. Antigenic variation of *Borrelia hermsii*, p. 123–135. *In* I. Herskowitz and M. I. Simon (ed.), *Genome Rearrangement*. Alan R. Liss, Inc., New York.

7. Bergquist, L. M., B. H. S. Lau, and C. E. Winter. 1974. Mycoplasma-associated immunosuppression: effect on hemagglutinin response to common antigens in rabbits. *Infect. Immun.* 9:410–415.

8. Bier, P. J., C. E. Hall, J. R. Duncan, and A. J. Winter. 1977. Experimental infections with Campylobacter fetus in bulls of different ages. *Vet. Microbiol.* 2:13–27.

9. Biguzzi, S. 1979. Interaction of anti-staphylococcal protein A antisera with Fc receptor-bearing human normal lymphocytes. *Eur. J. Immunol.* 9:52–60.

10. Bisno, A. L. 1979. Alternate complement pathway activation by group A streptococci: role of M protein. *Infect. Immun.* 26:1172–1176.

11. Bjorck, L., and G. Kronvall. 1980. Purification and some properties of streptococcal protein G, a novel IgG-binding reagent. *J. Immunol.* 133:969–974.

12. Clamp, J. R. 1984. The relationship between the immune system and mucus in the protection of mucous membranes. *Biochem. Soc. Trans.* 12:754–756.

13. Cooper, M. D., Z. A. McGhee, M. H. Mulks, J. M. Koomey, and T. L. Hindman. 1984. Attachment to and invasion of human fallopian tube mucosa by an IgA1 protease deficient mutant of Neisseria gonorrhoeae and its wild-type parent. *J. Infect. Dis.* 150:737–744.

14. Corbeil, L. B., J. E. Arthur, P. R. Widders, J. W. Smith, and A. F. Barbet. 1987. Antigenic specificity of convalescent serum from cattle with *Haemophilus somnus*-induced experimental abortion. *Infect. Immun.* 55:1381–1386.

15. Corbeil, L. B., G. G. D. Schurig, P. J. Bier, and A. J. Winter. 1975. Bovine venereal vibriosis: antigenic variation of the bacterium during infection. *Infect. Immun.* 11:240–244.

16. Corbeil, L. B., and A. J. Winter. 1978. Animal model for the study of genital secretory immune mechanisms: venereal vibriosis in cattle, p. 293–299. *In* G. F. Brooks, E. C. Gotschlich, K. K. Holmes, W. D. Sawyer, and F. E. Young (ed.), *Immunobiology of Neisseria gonorrhoeae*. American Society for Microbiology, Washington, D.C.

17. Costerton, J. W., and R. T. Irvin. 1981. The bacterial glycocalyx in nature and disease. *Annu. Rev. Microbiol.* 35:299–324.

18. Cowan, F. M., D. L. Klein, G. L. Armstrong, and J. W. Pearson. 1979. Neutralization of immune complex inhibition of antibody dependent

cellular cytotoxicity by S. aureus protein A. *Biomedicine* 30:23–27.

19. Dale, J. B., and E. H. Beachey. 1985. Multiple heart-cross-reactive epitopes of streptococcal M proteins. *J. Exp. Med.* 161:113–122.

20. Dima, S., C. Medesan, G. Mota, I. Moraru, J. Sjoquist, and V. Ghetie. 1983. Effect of protein A and its fragment B on the catabolism and Fc receptor sites of IgG. *Eur. J. Immunol.* 13:605–614.

21. Dorrington, K. J., and M. H. Klein. 1982. Binding sites for Fc receptors on immunoglobulin G and factors influencing their expression. *Mol. Immunol.* 19:1215–1221.

22. Dossett, J. H., G. Kronvall, R. C. Williams, and P. G. Quie. 1969. Antiphagocytic effects of staphylococcal protein A. *J. Immunol.* 103:1405–1410.

23. Dowler, K. W., and R. W. Veltri. 1984. In vitro neutralization of HSV-2: inhibition by binding of normal IgG and purified Fc to virion Fc receptor (FcR). *J. Med. Virol.* 13:251–259.

24. Espersen, F. 1985. Complement activation by clumping factor and protein A from Staphylococcus aureus strain E 2371. *Acta Pathol. Microbiol. Immunol. Scand. Sect C* 93:59–64.

25. Ferreira de Miranda-Santos, I. K., and A. Campos-Neto. 1981. Receptor for immunoglobulin Fc on pathogenic but not on non-pathogenic protozoa of the trypanosomatidae. *J. Exp. Med.* 154:1732–1742.

26. Ferretti, J. J., C. Shea, and M. W. Humphrey. 1980. Cross-reactivity of *Streptococcus mutans* antigens and human heart tissue. *Infect. Immun.* 30:69–73.

27. Forsgren, A. 1972. Pathogenicity of Staphylococcus aureus mutants in general and local infections. *Acta. Pathol. Microbiol. Immunol. Scand. Sect. B* 80:564–570.

28. Forsgren, A., A. Svedjelund, and H. Wigzell. 1976. Lymphocyte stimulation by protein A of Staphylococcus aureus. *Eur. J. Immunol.* 6:207–213.

29. Frandsen, E. V. G., J. Reinholdt, and M. Kilian. 1987. Enzymatic and antigenic characterization of immunoglobulin A1 proteases from *Bacteroides* and *Capnocytophaga* spp. *Infect. Immun.* 55:631–638.

30. Frosch, M., I. Gorgen, G. J. Boulnois, K. N. Timmis, and D. Bitter-Suerman. 1985. NZB mouse system for production of monoclonal antibodies to weak bacterial antigens: isolation of an IgG antibody to the polysaccharide capsules of Escherichia coli K1 and group B meningococci. *Proc. Natl. Acad. Sci. USA* 82:1194–1198.

31. Ghetie, V., G. Mota, M. A. Dobre-Ghetie, M. Laky, A. Olinescu, S. Dima, I. Moraru, and J. Sjoquist. 1986. Modulation of IgG effector functions by a monovalent fragment of staphylococcal protein A. *Mol. Immunol.* 23:377–384.

32. Gogolewski, R. P., S. A. Kania, T. J. Inzana, P. R. Widders, H. D. Liggitt, and L. B. Corbeil. 1987. Protective ability and specificity of convalescent serum from calves with Haemophilus somnus pneumonia. *Infect. Immun.* 55:1403–1411.

33. Gold, R. 1979. Immunogenicity of meningococcal polysaccharides in man, p. 121–151. *In* J. A. Rudbach and P. J. Baker (ed.), *Immunology of Bacterial Polysaccharides*. Elsevier/North Holland Publishing Co., Amsterdam.

34. Gross, G. N., S. R. Rehm, G. B. Toews, D. A. Hart, and A. K. Pierce. 1978. Lung clearance of *Staphylococcus aureus* strains with differing protein A content: protein A effect on in vivo clearance. *Infect. Immun.* 21:7–9.

35. Hagblom, P., E. Segal, E. Billyard, and M. So. 1985. Intragenic recombination leads to pilus antigenic variation in Neisseria gonorrhoeae. *Nature* (London) 315:156–158.

36. Hallgren, R., G. Stalenheim, and A. Bill. 1977. Elimination of protein A-IgG complexes from the blood circulation in rabbits: role of spleen and liver. *Acta Pathol. Microbiol. Immunol. Scand. Sect. C* 85:435–440.

37. Hanna, E. E., and D. W. Watson. 1968. Host-parasite relationships among group A streptococci. IV. Suppression of antibody response by streptococcal pyrogenic exotoxin. *J. Bacteriol.* 95:14–21.

38. Horwitz, M. A., and S. C. Silverstein. 1980. Influence of the Escherichia coli capsule on complement fixation and on phagocytosis and killing by human phagocytes. *J. Clin. Invest.* 65:82–94.

39. Howard, C. J., and A. A. Glynn. 1971. The virulence for mice of strains of Escherichia coli related to the effects of K antigens on their resistance to phagocytosis and killing by complement. *Immunology* 20:767–777.

40. Hsieh, S., E. Goldstein, W. Lippert, and L. Margulies. 1978. Effect of protein A on the antistaphylococcal defence mechanism of the murine lung. *J. Infect. Dis.* 138:754–759.

41. Jacks-Weis, J., Y. Kim, and P. P. Cleary. 1982. Restricted deposition of C3 on M+ group A streptococci: correlation with resistance to phagocytosis. *J. Immunol.* 128:1897–1902.

42. Jessop, H. L., and P. A. Lambert. 1985. Immunochemical characterization of the outer membrane complex of Serratia marcescens and identification of the antigens accessible to antibodies on the cell surface. *J. Gen. Microbiol.* 131:2343–2348.

43. Kapatais-Zoumbos, K., D. K. F. Chandler, and M. F. Barile. 1985. Survey of immunoglobulin protaese activity among selected species of Ureaplasma and Mycoplasma: specificity for host immunoglobulin A. *Infect. Immun.* 47:704–709.

44. Kaplan, M. H., R. Bolande, L. Rakita, and J. Blair. 1964. Presence of bound immunoglobulin and

complement in the myocardium in acute rheumatic fever. *N. Engl. J. Med.* 271:637–645.

45. Kay, D. H., G. D. Bonnard, W. H. West, and R. B. Herbermann. 1977. A functional comparison of human Fc receptor bearing lymphocytes active in natural cytotoxicity and antibody dependent cellular cytotoxicity. *J. Immunol.* 118:2058–2066.

46. Kilian, M. 1981. Degradation of immunoglobulins A1, A2, and G by suspected periodontal pathogens. *Infect. Immun.* 34:757–765.

47. Kilian, M., M. B. Brown, T. A. Brown, E. A. Freundt, and G. H. Cassel. 1984. Immunoglobulin A1 protease activity in strains of Ureaplasma urealyticum. *Acta Pathol. Microbiol. Immunol. Scand. Sect. B* 92:61–64.

48. Kilian, M., J. Mestecky, and R. E. Schrohenloher. 1979. Pathogenic species of the genus *Haemophilus* and *Streptococcus pneumoniae* produce immunoglobulin A1 protease. *Infect. Immun.* 26:143–149.

49. King, B. F., and B. J. Wilkinson. 1981. Binding of human immunoglobulin G to protein A in encapsulated *Staphylococcus aureus*. *Infect. Immun.* 33:666–672.

50. Krisher, K., and M. W. Cunningham. 1985. Myosin: a link between streptococci and heart. *Science* 227:413–415.

51. Kronvall, G. 1973. A surface component on group A, C and G streptococci with non-immune reactivity for immunoglobulin G. *J. Immunol.* 111:1401–1406.

52. Kronvall, G., and H. Gewerz. 1970. Activation and inhibition of IgG mediated complement fixation by staphylococcal protein A. *Clin. Exp. Immunol.* 7:211–220.

53. Kronvall, G., A. Simmons, E. B. Myhre, and S. Jonsson. 1979. Specific absorption of human serum albumin, immunoglobulin A, and immunoglobulin G with selected strains of group A and G streptococcus. *Infect. Immun.* 25:1–10.

54. Laky, M., J. Sjoquist, I. Moraru, and V. Ghetie. 1985. Mutual inhibition of the binding of C1q and protein A to rabbit IgG immune complexes. *Mol. Immunol.* 22:1297–1302.

55. Langone, J. J. 1982. Protein A of Staphylococcus aureus and related immunoglobulin receptors produced by streptococci and pneumococci. *Adv. Immunol.* 32:157–252.

56. Lemke, H. R. Krausse, J. Sorenzen, and B. Hausteen. 1985. Mycoplasma infection of cell lines can simulate the expression of Fc receptors by binding of the carbohydrate moiety of antibodies. *Eur J. Immunol.* 15:442–447.

57. Loeb, M. R., and D. H. Smith. 1982. Human antibody response to individual outer membrane proteins of *Haemophilus influenzae* type b. *Infect. Immun.* 37:1032–1036.

58. Magnusson, K.-E., and I. Stjernstrom. 1982.

Mucosal barrier mechanisms. Interplay between secretory IgA (SIgA), IgG and mucins on the surface properties and association of salmonellae with intestines and granulocytes. *Immunology* 45:239–248.

59. Malakien, A., and J. H. Schwab. 1968. Immunosuppressant from group A streptococci. *Science* 159:880–881.

60. Malakien, A. H., and J. H. Schwab. 1971. Biological characterization of an immunosuppressant from group A streptococci. *J. Exp. Med.* 134:1253–1265.

61. Meier, J. T., M. I. Simon, and A. G. Barbour. 1985. Antigenic variation is associated with DNA rearrangements in a relapsing fever Borrelia. *Cell* 41:403–409.

62. Miller, C. E., K. H. Wong, J. C. Feeley, and M. E. Forlines. 1972. Immunological conversion of *Vibrio cholerae* in gnotobiotic mice. *Infect. Immun.* 6:739–742.

63. Miller, G. A., and R. W. Jackson. 1973. The effect of a Streptococcus pyogenes teichoic acid on the immune response of mice. *J. Immunol.* 110:148–156.

64. Mitchell, G. F. 1986. Cellular and molecular aspects of host-parasite relationships, p. 798–808. *In* B. Cinader and R. G. Miller (ed.), *Progress in Immunology*, vol. VI. Academic Press, Inc., New York.

65. Moller, G., and P. Landwall. 1977. The polyclonal B-cell activating property of protein A is not due to its interaction with the Fc part of immunoglobulin receptors. *Scand. J. Immunol.* 6:357–366.

66. Mulks, M. H. 1985. Microbial IgA proteases, p. 81–104. *In* I. A. Holder (ed.), *Microbial Enzymes and Virulence*. CRC Press, Inc., Boca Raton, Fla.

67. Mulks, M. H., E. R. Moxon, J. Bricker, A. Wright, and A. G. Plaut. 1984. Examination of *Haemophilus pleuropneumoniae* for immunoglobulin A protease activity. *Infect. Immun.* 45:276–277.

68. Mulks, M. H., A. G. Plaut, and M. Lamm. 1980. Gonococcal IgA protease reduces inhibition of bacterial attachment by human secretory IgA, p. 217–220. *In* S. Normark and D. Danielsson (ed.), *Genetics and Immunobiology of Pathogenic Neisseria*. University of Umeå, Umeå, Sweden.

69. Myhre, E. B., and G. Kronvall. 1977. Heterogeneity of immunoglobulin Fc reactivity among gram-positive cocci: description of three major types of receptors for human immunoglobulin G. *Infect. Immun.* 17:475–482.

70. Myhre, E. B., and G. Kronvall. 1980. Demonstration of specific binding sites for human serum albumin in group C and G streptococci. *Infect. Immun.* 27:6–14.

71. Myhre, E. B., and G. Kronvall. 1980. Demonstration of a new type of immunoglobulin G receptor in *Streptococcus zooepidemicus* strains. *Infect. Immun.* 27:808–816.

72. **Myhre, E. B., and G. Kronvall.** 1981. Immunoglobulin specifications of defined types of streptococcal Ig receptors, p. 209–210. *In* S. E. Holm and P. Christenssen (ed.), *Basic Concepts of Streptococci and Streptococcal Diseases.* Reedbooks Ltd., Chertsey, England.

73. **Nakao, Y., M. Kishihara, Y. Baba, T. Fujita, and K. Fujiwara.** 1980. Mitogenic response of human and murine T lymphocytes to staphylococcal protein A: not mediated by binding to cell surface immunoglobulins. *Cell. Immunol.* 50:361–368.

74. **Nakashima, I., T. Kobayashi, and N. Kato.** 1971. Alterations in the antibody response to bovine serum albumin by polysaccharide of Klebsiella pneumoniae. *J. Immunol.* 107:1112–1121.

75. **Nielsen, K., and J. R. Duncan.** 1982. Demonstration that nonspecific bovine Brucella abortus agglutinin is EDTA-labile and not calcium-dependent. *J. Immunol.* 129:366–369.

76. **Nielsen, K., K. Stilwell, B. Stemshorn, and J. R. Duncan.** 1981. Ethylenediaminetetraacetic acid (disodium salt)-labile bovine immunoglobulin M Fc binding to *Brucella abortus:* a cause of nonspecific agglutination. *J. Clin. Microbiol.* 14:32–38.

77. **Peterson, P. K., Y. Kim, B. J. Wilkinson, D. Schmeling, A. F. Michael, and P. G. Quie.** 1978. Dichotomy between opsonization and serum complement activation by encapsulated staphylococci. *Infect. Immun.* 20:770–775.

78. **Peterson, P. K., D. Schmeling, P. P. Cleary, B. J. Wilkinson, Y. Kim, and P. G. Quie.** 1979. Inhibition of alternative complement pathway opsonization by group A streptococcal M protein. *J. Infect. Dis.* 139:575–585.

79. **Peterson, P. K., J. Verhoef, L. D. Sabath, and P. G. Quie.** 1977. Effect of protein A on staphylococcal opsonization. *Infect. Immun.* 15:760–764.

80. **Peterson, P. K., B. J. Wilkinson, Y. Kim, D. Schmeling, and P. G. Quie.** 1978. Influence of encapsulation on staphylococcal opsonization and phagocytosis by human polymorphonuclear leukocytes. *Infect. Immun.* 19:943–949.

81. **Plasterk, R. H. A., M. I. Simon, and A. G. Barbour.** 1985. Transposition of structural genes to an expression sequence on a linear plasmid causes antigenic variation in the bacterium Borrelia hermsii. *Nature* (London) 318:257–263.

82. **Plaut, A. G.** 1983. The IgA1 proteases of pathogenic bacteria. *Annu. Rev. Microbiol.* 37:603–622.

83. **Plaut, A. G., J. V. Gilbert, M. S. Artentstein, and J. D. Capra.** 1975. Neisseria gonorrhoeae and Neisseria meningitidis: extracellular enzyme cleaves human immunoglobulin A. *Science* 190:1103–1105.

84. **Plaut, A. G., J. V. Gilbert, and R. Wistar, Jr.** 1977. Loss of antibody activity in human immunoglobulin A exposed to extracellular immunoglobulin A proteases of *Neisseria gonorrhoeae* and *Strepto-*

coccus sanguis. Infect. Immun. 17:130–135.

85. **Punsalang, A. P., and W. D. Sawyer.** 1973. Role of pili in the virulence of *Neisseria gonorrhoeae. Infect. Immun.* 8:255–263.

86. **Rapp, V. J., and R. F. Ross.** 1986. Antibody response of swine to outer membrane components of *Haemophilus pleuropneumoniae* during infection. *Infect. Immun.* 54:751–760.

87. **Redhead, K.** 1984. Serum antibody responses to the outer membrane proteins of *Bordetella pertussis. Infect. Immun.* 44:724–729.

88. **Ringden, O.** 1985. Induction of immunoglobulin secretion by protein A from Staphylococcus aureus in human blood and bone marrow B cells. *Scand. J. Immunol.* 22:17–26.

89. **Robbins, J. B., R. Schneerson, W. B. Egan, W. Vann, and D. T. Liu.** 1980. Virulence properties of bacterial capsular polysaccharides—unanswered questions, p. 115–132. *In* H. Smith, J. J. Skehel, and M. J. Turner (ed.), *The Molecular Basis of Microbial Pathogenicity.* Dahlem Konferenzen 1980. Verlag Chemie GmbH, Weinhem, Federal Republic of Germany.

90. **Romagnani, S., M. G. Guidizi, R. Biagiotti, F. Almerigogna, E. Maggi, G. Del Prete, and M. Ricci.** 1981. Surface immunoglobulins are involved in the interaction of protein A with human cells and in the triggering of B cell proliferation induced by protein A containing Staphylococcus aureus. *J. Immunol.* 127:1307–1313.

91. **Rosenblatt, J., P. M. Zelzer, J. Portaro, and R. C. Seegar.** 1977. Inhibition of antibody dependent cellular cytotoxicity by protein A from Staphylococcus aureus. *J. Immunol.* 118:981–985.

92. **Russell-Jones, G. J., E. C. Gotschlich, and M. S. Blake.** 1984. A surface receptor specific for human IgA on group B streptococci possessing the Ibc protein antigen. *J. Exp. Med.* 160:1467–1475.

93. **Sack, R. B., and C. E. Miller.** 1969. Progressive changes of vibrio serotypes in germ-free mice infected with *Vibrio cholerae. J. Bacteriol.* 99:688–695.

94. **Saiki, O., and P. Ralph.** 1981. Induction of human immunoglobulin secretion. I. Synergistic effect of B cell mitogen Cowan I plus T cell mitogens or factors. *J. Immunol.* 127:1044–1047.

95. **Sakane, T., and I. Green.** 1978. Protein A from Staphylococcus aureus—a mitogen for human T lymphocytes and B lymphocytes but not L lymphocytes. *J. Immunol.* 120:302–311.

96. **Schalen, C., L. Truedsson, K. K. Christensen, and P. Christensen.** 1985. Blocking of antibody complement-dependent effector functions by streptococcal IgG Fc receptor and staphylococcal protein A. *Acta Pathol. Microbiol. Immunol. Scand. Sect. B* 93:395–400.

97. **Schauer, R.** 1982. Chemistry, metabolism and biological functions of sialic acids. *Adv. Carbohydr.*

Chem. Biochem. 40:131–234.

98. Scholten, P., R. Schuurman, and H. Ploegh. 1986. Activation of human B cells: involvement of surface immunoglobulin as evidenced by two biochemically distinct types of response to Staphylococcus aureus. *Hum. Immunol.* 16:1–13.

99. Schurig, G. D., C. E. Hall, K. Burda, L. B. Corbeil, J. R. Duncan, and A. J. Winter. 1973. Persistent genital infection with Vibrio fetus intestinalis associated with serotypic alteration of the infecting strain. *Am. J. Vet. Res.* 34:1399–1403.

100. Schurig, G. D., C. E. Hall, L. B. Corbeil, J. R. Duncan, and A. J. Winter. 1975. Bovine venereal vibriosis: cure of genital infection in females by systemic immunization. *Infect. Immun.* 11:245–251.

101. Schuurman, R. K. B., E. W. Gelfand, and H.-M. Dosch. 1980. Polyclonal activation of human lymphocytes in vitro. I. Characterization of the lymphocyte response to a T cell independent B cell mitogen. *J. Immunol.* 125:820–826.

102. Schwab, J. H. 1975. Suppression of the immune response by microorganisms. *Bacteriol. Rev.* 39:121–143.

103. Sima, G. L., M. S. Klempner, D. L. Kasper, and S. L. Gorbach. 1982. Alterations in opsonophagocytic killing by neutrophils of bacteroides fragilis associated with animal and laboratory passage: effect of capsular polysaccharide. *J. Infect. Dis.* 145:72–77.

104. Stalenheim, G., and J. Sjoquist. 1970. Protein A from Staphypococcus aureus. X. Complement fixing activity of complexes between protein A and myeloma IgG or papain fragments of IgG. *J. Immunol.* 105:944–948.

105. Stoenner, H. G., T. Dodd, and C. Larsen. 1982. Antigenic variation of Borrelia hermsii. *J. Exp. Med.* 156:1297–1311.

106. Sulica, A., C. Medesan, M. Laky, D. Onica, J. Sjoquist, and V. Ghetie. 1979. Effect of protein A of Staphylococcus aureus on the binding of monomeric and polymeric IgG to Fc receptor bearing cells. *Immunology* 38:173–179.

107. Taylor, C. E., P. W. Stashak, G. Caldes, B. Prescott, T. E. Cushed, A. Brooks, and P. J. Baker. 1983. Activation of antigen specific suppressor T-cells by B cells from mice immunized with type III pneumococcal polysaccharide. *J. Exp. Med.* 158:703–717.

108. Timmis, K. N., G. J. Boulnois, D. Bitter-Suerman, and F. C. Cabello. 1985. Surface components of Escherichia coli that mediate resistance to the bactericidal activities of serum and phagocytes. *Curr. Top. Microbiol. Immunol.* 118:197–218.

109. Timoney, P. J., V. P. Geraghty, P. B. Dillon, and J. F. McArdle. 1978. Susceptibility of laboratory animals to infection with Haemophilus equigenitalis. *Vet. Rec.* 103:563–564.

110. Timoney, P. J., P. J. O'Reilly, J. McArdle, and J. Ward. 1978. Attempted transmission of contagious equine metritis to other domestic animal species. *Vet. Rec.* 102:152.

111. Timoney, P. J., S. J. Shin, D. H. Lein, and R. H. Jacobsen. 1984. Transmissibility of the contagious equine metritis organism for the cat. *Comp. Immunol. Microbiol. Infect. Dis.* 7:131–140.

112. Van de Merwe, J. P., and J. H. Stegeman. 1985. Binding of Coprococcus comes to the Fc portion of IgG. A possible role in the pathogenesis of Crohn's disease? *Eur. J. Immunol.* 15:860–863.

113. Whitnack, E., and E. H. Beachey. 1982. Antiopsonic activity of fibrinogen bound to M protein on the surface of group A streptococci. *J. Clin. Invest.* 69:1042–1045.

114. Whitnack, E., J. B. Dale, and E. H. Beachey. 1984. Common protective antigens of group A streptococcal M proteins masked by fibrinogen. *J. Exp. Med.* 159:1201–1212.

115. Widders, P. R., C. R. Stokes, J. S. E. David, and F. J. Bourne. 1985. Specific antibody in the equine genital tract following systemic and local immunization. *Immunology* 54:763–769.

116. Widders, P. R., C. R. Stokes, J. S. E. David, and F. J. Bourne. 1986. Specific antibody in the equine genital tract following local immunization and challenge infection with contagious equine metritis organism (Taylorella equigenitalis). *Res. Vet. Sci.* 40:54–58.

117. Widders, P. R., C. R. Stokes, T. J. Newby, and F. J. Bourne. 1985. Nonimmune binding of equine immunoglobulin by the causative organism of contagious equine metritis (*Taylorella equigenitalis*). *Infect. Immun.* 48:417–421.

118. Wilkinson, B. J., and K. M. Holmes. 1979. *Staphylococcus aureus* cell surface: capsule as a barrier to bacteriophage adsorption. *Infect. Immun.* 23:545–548.

119. Wilkinson, B. J., P. K. Peterson, and P. G. Quie. 1979. Cryptic peptidoglycan and the antiphagocytic effect of the *Staphylococcus aureus* capsule: model for the antiphagocytic effect of bacterial cell surface polymers. *Infect. Immun.* 23:502–508.

120. Wilkinson, B. J., S. P. Sisson, Y. Kim, and P. K. Peterson. 1979. Localization of the third component of complement on the cell wall of encapsulated *Staphylococcus aureus* M: implications for the mechanisms of resistance to phagocytosis. *Infect. Immun.* 26:1159–1163.

121. Williams, M. H., J. Brostoff, and I. M. Roitt. 1970. Possible role of Mycoplasma fermentans in the pathogenesis of rheumatoid arthritis. *Lancet* ii:277–280.

122. Wise, K. S., and R. K. Watson. 1985. Antigenic mimicry of mammalian intermediate filaments by mycoplasmas. *Infect. Immun.* 48:587–591.

123. Wright, C. K., J. Willan, J. Sjodahl, D. R. Burton, and R. A. Dwek. 1977. The interaction of protein A and the Fc fragment of rabbit immunoglobulin G as probed by complement fixation and nuclear magnetic resonance. *Biochem. J.* 169:661–668.

124. Wyle, F. A., M. S. Artestein, B. L. Brandt, E. C. Tramont, D. L. Kasper, P. L. Altieri, S. L. Berman, and J. P. Lowenthal. 1972. Immunological response of man to group B meningococcal polysaccharide vaccines. *J. Infect. Dis.* 126:514–522.

125. Yarnall, M., and M. D. P. Boyle. 1986. Isolation and partial characterization of a type II Fc receptor from a group A streptococcus. *Mol. Cell. Biochem.* 70:57–66.

126. Yarnall, M., and M. D. P. Boyle. 1986. Evidence for a unique receptor for the Fc region of human IgG3. *J. Immunol.* 136:2670–2673.

127. Zabriskie, J. B., and E. H. Freimer. 1966. An immunological relationship between the group A streptococcus and mammalian muscle. *J. Exp. Med.* 124:661–676.

128. Zabriskie, J. B., K. C. Hsu, and B. C. Seegal. 1970. Heart-reactive antibody associated with rheumatic fever: characterization and diagnostic significance. *Clin. Exp. Immunol.* 7:147–159.

Chapter 7

Bacterial Resistance to Complement

Peter W. Taylor

CIBA-GEIGY Pharmaceuticals
Horsham, West Sussex RH12 4AB
United Kingdom

INTRODUCTION

The serum complement system was first recognized almost 100 years ago (11, 57) through its ability to bring about dissolution of gram-negative bacteria. Steady expansion of our knowledge has shown that complement features prominently in a range of biological activities including killing and phagocytosis of bacteria, neutralization of viruses, disposal of harmful immune complexes, and the induction and modulation of the inflammatory response. Complement may also play a role in immune regulation and surveillance. The importance of the complement system as a component of host defenses against infection is reflected both in its wide distribution within the animal kingdom (3) and in the frequently observed increased susceptibility to infection of individuals congenitally deficient in biosynthesis of individual complement components (1).

Although complement alone is unable to affect the viability of gram-positive bacteria to any significant extent, it is able, at suitable concentrations and under the right conditions, to effect very rapid and efficient killing of a wide variety of gram-negative bacteria (36, 74). If the complement source used is serum or plasma, complement-mediated killing is often accompanied by lysis of target bacteria owing to the presence of the peptidoglycan-degrading enzyme lysozyme; killing can, however, proceed at near-maximal rates in the absence of this enzyme (52, 77). Efficient killing of target bacteria can be mediated by either the classical or alternative pathway of complement following activation by antibody-dependent or antibody-independent mechanisms (38, 70). Removal of any of the late-acting components from serum results in complete loss of antibacterial activity, and it is now clear that killing is dependent upon the assembly at the bacterial surface of a multimolecular complex formed from five precursor complement proteins: C5, C6, C7, C8, and C9; stable insertion of these C5b-9 complexes into the target cell envelope initiates a series of poorly defined events culminating in the loss of bacterial viability (79).

Almost without exception, rough strains of gram-negative bacteria producing outer membrane-located lipopolysaccharide devoid of O-specific side chains are highly susceptible to C5b-9-mediated killing, whereas smooth strains synthesizing a complete lipopolysaccharide are frequently, but not invariably, resistant to the potentially lethal action of complement. Other cell surface components, including capsular polysaccharide and chromosome- and plasmid-determined outer membrane proteins, may also contribute to reduction in bacterial sensitivity by reducing or abolishing the capacity of C5b-9 complexes to form a stable association with the bacterial surface (42). Such complement-resistant strains have a distinct advantage over susceptible organisms regarding their ability to survive in sites in the body containing functionally effective concentrations of complement proteins. However, since other host defense systems such as phagocytosis also play a key role in determining the in vivo fate of potential pathogens, interpretation of the bulk of epidemiological data generated in attempts to establish causal relationships between complement resistance and infectivity has led to a certain degree of controversy about the relative importance of host defense mechanisms in preventing infectious disease. Thus, although the vast majority of strains causing septicemia or bacteremia in humans and animals have been found to be complement resistant (58), the situation is less clear for a variety of other infectious disease states (74).

Since it is likely that a clear understanding of the basis of complement resistance in gram-negative bacteria will emerge only from a full appreciation of the mechanism of complement-mediated bactericidal activity, the present contribution reviews current knowledge of the interactions of the key proteins of the complement cascade with the surfaces of susceptible bacteria and then considers the cell surface structures known to play a role in the determination of complement resistance. Finally, the role of complement resistance as a bacterial virulence factor in infections of humans and animals is assessed.

INTERACTION OF COMPLEMENT WITH SUSCEPTIBLE TARGET BACTERIA

Susceptible gram-negative bacteria can be killed by complement following activation of either the classical or the alternative pathway, and with some strains both pathways may be activated simultaneously. The main features of both pathways of activation are shown in Fig.

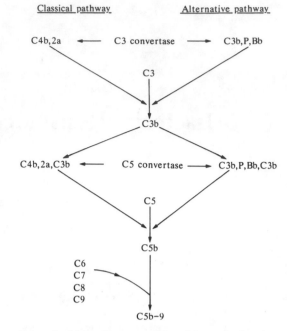

FIGURE 1. Schematic representation of the mechanisms by which microorganisms activate C3 and generate bactericidal C5b-9 membrane attack complexes. Modified from reference 88.

1. The complement system consists of a series of glycoproteins that circulate in the extracellular fluid compartment and interact in a precise sequence of reactions, resulting in the production of biologically active cleavage fragments that promote opsonization and phagocytosis as well as direct cell damage (2, 53). The classical pathway is normally activated by interaction of an antibody of the appropriate class and subclass with an antigen on the bacterial surface, although under certain conditions some bacteria can directly activate the classical pathway without the intervention of antibody (15). Binding of C1, the first classical-pathway component, to antigen-antibody complexes at the surface results in activation of the C1 molecule and the acquisition by C1s of serine esterase activity. This enzyme cleaves the next two components of the cascade, C4 and C2; the two larger cleavage fragments, C4b and C2a, constitute an enzymatically active complex that is covalently bound through the C4b molecule to the target membrane surface. This C3 conver-

tase generates two fragments from C3, and the larger, C3b, binds covalently to the bacterial surface and noncovalently to C4b to form a serine esterase complex (C4b, 2a, C3b) with C5-cleaving activity.

In contrast to the classical pathway, the alternative pathway can be activated on the surfaces of certain bacteria in the absence of specific antibody. Thus, factor D, a serine esterase present in active form in blood, cleaves molecules of factor B that are transiently associated with C3 or C3b on a bacterial surface. The complex formed can interact with factor P to form a stable C3-cleaving complex (C3b, P, Bb) that can bind another molecule of C3b and acquire C5-cleaving activity.

Following C5 cleavage by either the classical- or the alternative-pathway C5-converting enzyme complexes, the larger cleavage fragment, C5b, may spontaneously associate with native C6 and C7 to form a trimolecular C5b-7 complex that inserts itself into the hydrocarbon core of the target membrane (62). Binding of one C8 molecule to each C5b-7 complex gives rise to small transmembrane channels, of less than 1 nm in functional diameter (63), that may perturb the target membrane. However, the main role of C5b-8 appears to be that of a catalyst for the polymerization of C9 at the membrane attack site. Thus, binding of one molecule of C9 to a C5b-8 complex initiates a process of C9 oligomerization; if 16 to 18 C9 molecules are incorporated into the complex, a discrete channel structure is formed that appears as a short, hollow cylinder 15 to 16 nm in length with an internal diameter of 10 nm and rimmed at one end by an annulus of external diameter 20 to 22 nm. The terminus distal to the annulus bears an apolar surface 4 nm in length that is embedded in the hydrophobic interior of the target membrane (4).

Because the molar concentration of C9 in serum is only about twice that of C8, C5b-9 complexes generated on target membranes display a degree of heterogeneity with regard to C9 content (5, 9). However, individual C5b-9 complexes contribute to the killing of sus-

ceptible target bacteria even when they contain substantially less than 16 to 18 C9 molecules. For example, Bloch et al. (7) found that killing of *Escherichia coli* J5 occurred when C5b-9 complexes generated at the bacterial surface contained an average of three C9 molecules per complex. Furthermore, the deposition of as few as 50 to 100 C5b-9 complexes per target cell may be sufficient for rapid killing to occur (8). Further evidence that completion of the C5b-9 cylindrical structure is not essential to effect killing comes from observations with thrombin-cleaved C9 ($C9^n$) in serum bactericidal assays. $C9^n$ can bind to C5b-8, but is unable to form the classical cylindrical lesion (17); it is, however, as effective as native C9 in killing susceptible *E. coli* strains (18a).

Gram-negative bacteria that are rapidly killed by complement in the absence of lysozyme undergo no apparent gross morphological change and retain many of the structural features of viable cells. Although the mechanism of complement killing has not been precisely defined in molecular terms, it is clear that loss of viability is dependent upon irreversible damage to the cytoplasmic membrane. Feingold et al. (25, 26) found that the cytoplasmic membrane of a rough *E. coli* strain became permeable to the cryptic substrate β-D-galactopyranoside following exposure of the bacteria to lethal doses of lysozyme-free serum, and they and other workers (52, 89) found loss of crypticity to be strongly correlated with cell death. Active transport of sugars, amino acids, and monovalent cations are inhibited by serum treatment (19). However, damage to the cytoplasmic membrane in the absence of lysozyme appears to be restricted, since this membrane appears as a typical bilayer membrane when visualized by electron microscopy following bacterial killing (86), cytoplasmic enzymes such as β-galactosidase are retained by the cell and are not released into the reaction mixture (77, 89), and bacterial respiration remains relatively unaffected until late into the reaction sequence (71). Similarly, cessation of DNA, RNA, and protein synthesis late in the reaction appears to be a secondary event that reflects a decrease of cellular activity in bacteria that have already been rendered nonviable (79).

A number of groups (48, 52, 89) have observed that exposure of susceptible strains to complement results in an efflux of monovalent cations from the cell. That dissipation of the cytoplasmic membrane potential is the key event in target cell viability loss was recently investigated by Dankert and Esser (18, 18a). Measurement of ΔE_m, either directly by the lipophilic cation tetraphenylphosphonium or indirectly by measuring transport of solutes dependent on ΔE_m, allowed them to establish that complete assembly of C5b-9 complexes on the cell envelope causes immediate and irreversible dissipation of the potential across the cytoplasmic membrane, although transient collapse of ΔE_m also occurred in bacteria treated with C9-deficient, nonlethal serum. Because it has been demonstrated that inhibitors and uncouplers of oxidative phosphorylation, compounds that cause collapse of ΔE_m, can protect against complement attack (33, 77), Dankert and Esser suggested that an energized cytoplasmic membrane is necessary for killing to take place once complement proteins have bound to the bacterial surface. It is likely that the cell attempts to restore ΔE_m as internal pools of ATP are completely utilized during the course of the lethal process (48).

It is clear from the dimensions of the lipid-binding domain on C5b-9 that individual complexes have the capacity to intercalate only into single-lipid bilayers. Since the gram-negative bacterial envelope consists of three essential layers, the outer membrane, the peptidoglycan layer, and the cytoplasmic membrane (50), and since the two membranes are further separated by a periplasmic space of significant volume (73), it is difficult to conceive how the cytoplasmic membrane is damaged if C5b-9 complexes form exclusively on the outer membrane. That lesions do occur on the outer membrane but not on the cytoplasmic membrane following exposure to lysozyme-free serum has recently been established by Taylor and Kroll (79). They separated outer and cytoplasmic membranes from serum-sensitive *E. coli* strains

exposed to lethal doses of complement; covalent binding of C3b to the outer but not to the cytoplasmic membrane was found during the very early stages of the reaction and before the onset of viability loss. Binding of C5b-9 complexes exclusively to the outer membrane was first detected coincident with the onset of viability loss and increased rapidly during the active killing phase of the reaction (Fig. 2). At no time during the reaction could C3 or C5b-9 binding to the cytoplasmic membrane be detected; serum exposure resulted in a dramatic reduction in recoverability of the cytoplasmic membrane that is likely to be due to limited phospholipid degradation. Electron-microscopic studies confirmed that C5b-9 complexes were not deposited on the cytoplasmic membrane of *E. coli* cells undergoing complement-mediated killing; in contrast, large numbers of cylindrical lesions were found in the outer membranes during the active killing phase of the reaction (49).

Insertion of C5b-9 complexes into the outer membranes of rough, serum-susceptible gram-negative bacteria results in disruption of the integrity of this bilayer as evidenced by the release of enzyme markers from the periplasmic space (26, 52, 77). Previous interpretation of these data suggesting enzyme release through the C5b-9 channel is clearly incompatible with biophysical evidence on marker release by complement (79). Furthermore, complement has been shown to release significant amounts of phospholipid from the outer membrane in a dose-dependent manner (37, 87); phospholipid release is accompanied by some degradation. Both release and degradation may be related to activation of the outer membrane-located detergent-resistant phospholipase A as mutants lacking this enzyme release no phospholipid into the reaction mixture when undergoing complement-mediated killing (78).

Monomeric C9 bound to the outer membranes of complement-treated cells could be resolved by immunoblotting techniques into two discrete bands, suggesting proteolytic cleavage of C9 undergoing oligomerization (Fig. 2). This cleavage is probably mediated by the outer

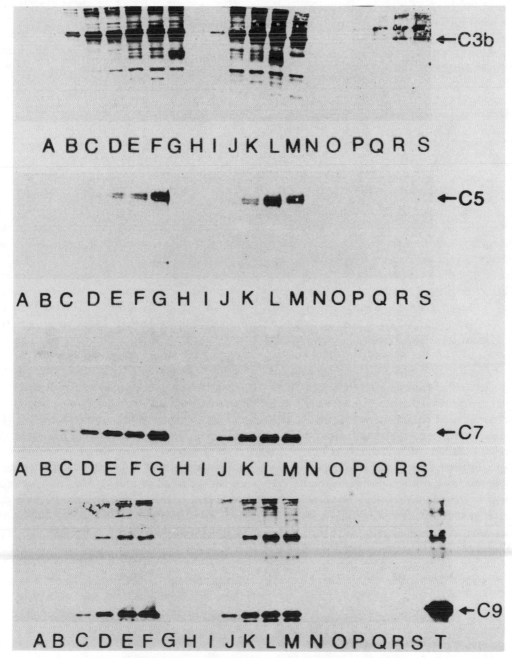

FIGURE 2. Immunoblots of sodium dodecyl sulfate-polyacrylamide gel electrophoresis of outer membranes from two serum-susceptible strains (LP1092 and 17) and one serum-resistant strain (LP1395) of *E. coli* exposed to 20% lysozyme-free human serum for various periods. Blots were developed with polyclonal antisera to complement components C3, C5, C7, and C9. Lanes: A to F, LP1092 for 0, 2.5, 5, 10, 15, and 20 min; G, LP1092 and C8-deficient serum for 20 min; H to M, 17 for 0, 2.5, 5, 10, 15, and 30 min; N to S, LP1395 for 0, 5, 10, 30, 60, and 120 min; T, purified C9.

membrane-associated colicin A protease (*cpr*) described by Cavard et al. (14), since monomeric C9 bound to complement-treated *cpr* mutants appears as a single polypeptide band when visualized by the same technique. However, cleavage of C9 by this enzyme is unlikely to be a necessary step for killing, since *cpr* mutants are as sensitive to the bactericidal action of serum as parent strains are (P. W. Taylor and D. Cavard, unpublished observations). However, the fact that a C9-derived peptide can dissipate ΔE_m of metabolically active cytoplasmic membrane vesicles (18) suggests that C9 fragment-mediated cytoplasmic membrane perturbation is worthy of further investigation. Preliminary experiments with liposome fusion techniques indicate that no serum components other than C5b-9 are necessary for rapid killing of target cells (S. Tomlinson, J. P. Luzio, and P. W. Taylor, *Biochem. Soc. Trans.* 15:646, 1987).

Taken together, these studies lend strong support to the hypothesis that C5b-9 complexes form exclusively on the outer membrane and effect lethal damage from this locus. With certain rough strains possessing an outer-membrane-associated phospholipase A, there is substantial complement-mediated phospholipid removal from the surface of the target cell, which results in the release of the soluble contents of the periplasmic space but is not in itself sufficient to effect killing. Lethal membrane damage, related to dissipation of ΔE_m, may occur when domains at the apolar terminus of the C5b-9 cylinder make contact with the outer surface of the cytoplasmic membrane at zones of transient adhesion between the two bilayers.

ROLE OF THE OUTER MEMBRANE IN DETERMINATION OF COMPLEMENT RESISTANCE

The presence of sialic acid residues at the bacterial surface can restrict activation of the alternative pathway, and so activation of complement on these strains would be expected to proceed by the antibody-dependent classical pathway route. Lack of antibody against relevant surface antigens may therefore enable these strains to escape complement attack through lack of an effective complement-activating mechanism. In practice this seems not to be a common mechanism of circumvention of the complement-mediated bactericidal process, since even heavily sialylated, noncommensular strains such as *Neisseria meningitidis* group B activate complement to a greater or lesser extent (20). However, to date there have been few attempts to systematically address the role of nonactivation of complement as a mechanism for avoidance of complement-mediated killing, particularly with gram-negative bacteria that possess surface antigens that mimic host macromolecules (40).

Many investigators have found that complement-resistant strains activate complement efficiently but escape being killed because the C5b-9 complex fails to insert in an effective way into the bacterial outer membrane. The serum-resistant *E. coli* strain used in the experiment shown in Fig. 2 was opsonized with large amounts of C3b bound covalently to a variety of surface components, and yet no C5, C7, or C9 could be found in stable association with the outer membrane even after long periods of incubation. Similarly, Reynolds et al. (65) found equivalent amounts of C3 deposited on the surfaces of serum-resistant *Salmonella typhimurium* cells and on the same bacteria that had been rendered susceptible to complement by treatment with Tris and EDTA, and Fierer and Finley (27) demonstrated equivalent deposition of C3 by immunofluorescence on a serum-resistant *E. coli* strain before and after conversion of the strain to serum sensitivity with diphenylamine. Joiner et al. (44, 45) have studied the interaction of complement components with a smooth, serum-resistant *Salmonella minnesota* strain and a deep, rough, serum-susceptible mutant derived from it. On the sensitive strain the bulk of the C5b-9 was in stable association with the cell envelope and in all probability was inserted into hydrophobic domains on the outer membrane. In contrast, the resistant parent activated complement efficiently and C5b-9 complexes were formed on the surface of the cell, but they did not insert into the outer membrane bilayer and were subsequently released from the surface. Analogous effects have since been found with a range of *E. coli* and *Salmonella* strains (42).

It is clear that the presence of certain structures at the gram-negative surface is responsible for the failure of C5b-9 complexes to intercalate into the outer membrane, but the process by which this occurs has not been defined with any degree of certainty. Joiner et al. have demonstrated (43) that C3b binds preferentially to long, O-specific side chains of lipopolysaccharide during alternative-pathway activation on the surface of *Salmonella montevideo*. As a consequence, C5 convertase is formed at sites distant from hydrophobic domains on the bacterial surface, and C5b-9 may thus be assembled at a locus where it is unable to insert effectively into the hydrocarbon core of the target membrane; complexes are therefore attached to O side chains by weak ionic interactions and are released spontaneously from the surface. Long and numerous O side chains may also prevent access of C5b-9 to hydrophobic membrane domains by steric hindrance.

Alternatively, determinants known to increase resistance to complement do so by reducing the fluidity of the target membrane. Kato and Bito (47) established that C5b-9 failed to insert into *E. coli* membranes when the experiments were performed at temperatures below the phase transition point and with membrane phospholipids in a state of gel packing with their acyl chains in a restricted and ordered state. Above the transition point, C5b-9-mediated killing occurred at a high rate, since C5b-9 inserted into a target membrane in which phospholipids were in a liquid crystal state and the acyl chains exhibited a high degree of molecular motion. These and other observations suggest that membrane fluidity is obligatory for the formation of functional complement lesions (74), and it would therefore seem to be relevant to determine whether determinants of complement resistance have an effect on membrane fluidity when present as components of the outer bilayer.

Current models consider the outer membrane to be highly asymmetrical with regard to the distribution of component molecules within the bilayer. Lipopolysaccharides are located exclusively on the outer surface, whereas phospholipids occupy mainly the inner leaflet of the outer membrane (50). Macromolecules occupying the outer leaflet are likely to be of critical importance in determining whether C5b-9 assembly and insertion occur, and there is a wide body of evidence implicating the O-specific side chain of lipopolysaccharide as the major determinant of complement resistance in all groups of gram-negative bacteria so far examined. Mutations from smooth to rough colony form, usually but not invariably associated with loss of ability to synthesize O side chains, have long been known to be accompanied by large increases in susceptibility to complement (74). In fact, Dlabac (21) has demonstrated a progressive increase in susceptibility to serum corresponding to sequential loss of sugar residues from the lipopolysaccharide core. Compounds such as diphenylamine (24) and mecillinam (80), which cause a reduction in the length of individual O side chains and probably also a reduction in the degree of substitution of lipopolysaccharide core with O side chains, have been found to markedly increase the susceptibility of enterobacteria to complement. Evidence that increased coverage of lipid A-core with O antigen precludes access of C5b-9 to hydrophobic domains on the cell surface was provided by Goldman et al. (31) in a study of serum-resistant *E. coli* mutants in a serogroup associated with enteric disease. The critical role played by O side chains in determining complement resistance has been demonstrated for many species of gram-negative bacteria, including *Serratia marcescens* (41), *Klebsiella pneumoniae* (83), and *Campylobacter fetus* (59).

It is clear, however, that lipopolysaccharide O side chains are not the only surface structures necessary to determine complete resistance to complement, although they are undoubtedly essential for the expression of resistance. Hfr-mediated transfer of the *rfb* gene cluster, determining biosynthesis of O8-specific O side chains, to an extremely complement-susceptible rough *E. coli* strain yielded recombinants expressing the O8 mannan side chain to high levels; recombinants were not completely resistant to complement, but were killed at a much lower rate than the recipient was (82). Complement resistance could be further increased by inheritance of plasmid-borne genes determining synthesis of outer membrane proteins. Recombinants therefore behaved like many smooth, serum-susceptible, wild-type enterobacteria with respect to kinetics of complement killing. One such wild-type *E. coli* strain, isolated from a patient with a urinary tract infection, was grown in the chemostat under conditions of nutrient limitation at various dilution rates (75); the degree of killing observed was directly related to the ratio of the lipopolysaccharide O-side-chain sugar mannose to the core sugar L-glycero-D-mannoheptose. Such studies emphasize that complete resistance to complement is a multifunctional phenomenon, but that lipopolysaccharide containing a high degree of substitution of core for O-side-chain oligosaccharide is an essential prerequisite for expression of resistance.

The contribution of capsules, most of which are acidic exopolysaccharides, to the resistance of gram-negative bacteria to serum is unclear; recent work has established that low-molecular-weight capsular polymers are anchored to the cell envelope by a lipid moiety linked to the reducing end of the polysaccharide chain (40). The presence of a capsule is not essential for expression of complete resistance to serum, and members of some groups of bacteria, such as salmonellae, are almost always acapsular and predominantly refractory to complement attack when isolated from infected individuals. In general, epidemiological studies do not provide convincing evidence that acidic exopolysaccharides are major determinants of complement resistance in gram-negative bacteria; in fact, at least two groups of strains, *Klebsiella* spp. (28) and *Pseudomonas aeruginosa* isolates from patients with cystic fibrosis (35), which characteristically synthesize and produce copious amounts of extracellular and capsular acidic

polysaccharide, are usually highly susceptible to complement. Similarly, there is genetic evidence that K antigens of *E. coli* do not have a significant role in the determination of resistance to serum (82).

E. coli strains synthesizing the K1 antigen, an (α2-8)-linked *N*-acetylneuraminic acid homopolymer, are frequently responsible for meningitis in neonates; although K1 isolates are frequently susceptible to complement, there is evidence that they confer on some strains the potential to circumvent the lethal effects of serum. Because of the structural identity of the oligo-*N*-acetylneuraminic acid moiety of neuronal cell adhesion molecule, a glycoprotein found in developing neuronal cell membranes (30), with the *E. coli* K1 antigen, it is likely that some K1 strains may not be recognized by the neonatal immune system as foreign cells. Pluschke et al. have provided evidence that the K1 antigen on the surface of complement-resistant strains restricts activation of both the alternative and the antibody-independent classical pathways (60, 61). Therefore, although it is clear that K1, and perhaps other polymers that bear a structural relationship to host cell components, may provide the cell with protection against cellular and humoral defense mechanisms as a consequence of restricted complement activation, there is little or no evidence that the K1 antigen can interfere with the insertion of polymerizing C5b-9 complexes into the outer membrane.

Acquisition by rough *E. coli* strains of some plasmids of the FII incompatibility group has been shown to decrease the rate of killing by serum from humans and from a variety of animal species (29, 64, 76). There has, however, been some controversy over the degree of resistance that plasmids may confer, since the use of widely differing techniques and the use of serum from a variety of sources and at different concentrations make meaningful comparisons between such studies difficult. Effects are manifested only at low serum concentrations when rough strains are used as hosts for plasmids, and tend to be small and difficult to demonstrate. However, much larger effects on complement resistance owing to plasmid acquisition can be achieved if smooth strains with a certain intrinsic lack of resistance are used as hosts (6, 76), again emphasizing the essentially multifactorial, interactive nature of complement resistance. Similarly, curing enterobacterial isolates of antibiotic resistance and bacteriocin determinants led to a small but significant increase in susceptibility to complement (76). A number of groups have cloned the genes encoding determinants responsible for increased survival in serum; Binns et al. (6) found that the *iss* gene on plasmid ColV,I-K94 mapped to a 5.3-kilobase sequence within a *Bam*HI-generated fragment and was closely linked to, although not coincident with, genes for colicin V production. The gene on the IncF plasmid R6-5 that determines increased survival in serum is coincident with the *traT* locus, one of two loci involved in surface exclusion in conjugation (55). Both *iss* and *traT* gene products are proteins located in the outer membrane; the *traT* gene product has been particularly well studied. It has a molecular weight of 25,000 and is exposed on the outer surface of the outer membrane; it is, however, unlikely to play a significant role in determining complement resistance of wild strains and clinical isolates, because careful epidemiological studies have shown that the *traT* gene product is expressed as frequently in complement-susceptible as in complement-resistant populations of *E. coli* (46, 56).

A number of other outer membrane proteins have been shown to contribute to the resistance of gram-negative bacteria to serum. A serum-resistant mutant derived from a smooth, susceptibile urinary isolate of *E. coli* produced more of a 46,000-molecular-weight envelope protein than the parental strain did (81); the amount of this protein was subject to variation as a result of alterations in growth conditions and was well correlated with environmentally induced modification of the response to serum (75). A protein modifying the response of *N. gonorrhoeae* to serum has been identified in strains producing disseminated gonococcal infection (34). The principal virulence factor for *Aero-*

TABLE 1
Serum-resistant gram-negative strains from blood cultures

Strain	No. examined	% Serum resistant	References
Enterobacteria	21	85	67
Enterobacteria	120	90	28
Enterobacteria	76	37	23
E. coli	53	87	84
E. coli	195	64	54
E. coli	20	95	58
S. marcescens	11	100	72
Bacteroides fragilis	5	80	13
N. gonorrhoeae	29	97	22

monas salmonicida, the causative agent of systemic furunculosis in salmonid fishes, is the 49,000-molecular-weight A protein at the surface of the outer membrane (51). It is highly likely that all these proteins function only as determinants of complement resistance when present at the cell surface with a full complement of lipopolysaccharide O side chains.

ROLE OF HUMORAL DEFENSE MECHANISMS AGAINST GRAM-NEGATIVE BACTERIA

Because the host mounts a concerted immune attack against potentially pathogenic gram-negative bacteria, it is difficult to assess the contribution of direct complement-mediared killing to the overall protective process. However, there are a number of infectious states in which the available epidemiological data suggest a key role for complement-mediated killing in the maintenance of an infection-free host. For example, a large number of studies have shown a strong relationship between complement resistance and the ability of a strain to cause bacteremia or septicemia, and some of these studies are listed in Table 1. The position is less clear for other infectious diseases of humans, mainly because so few data are available. In urinary infection with gram-negative bacteria, there is some evidence that strains able to infect renal tissue tend to be more complement resistant than those causing infections confined to the lower urinary tract (32). Susceptibility to complement appears to be a key factor in determining the pathogenesis of infection due to *Neisseria* spp. There is a striking correlation between patients with homozygous deficiencies in the late-acting components of the complement cascade and recurrent infections due to *N. meningitidis* and *N. gonorrhoeae* (68), suggesting that humoral defense is far more important in protecting the host against these pathogens than against other gram-negative bacteria. Complementary to these observations are findings that gonococci isolated from patients with uncomplicated symptomatic local gonococcal infection are serum sensitive, whereas strains from individuals with disseminated gonococcal infection are almost always serum resistant (66, 69). Intriguingly, in patients with homozygous late-acting complement deficiencies, most systemic infections are also due to serum-resistant gonococci and meningococci, indicating that these patients do not acquire neisserial infection with an organism that normal individuals would inevitably ward off owing to their intact complement bactericidal system. Ross and Densen (68) have suggested that this is because sensitive *Neisseria* spp. are phagocytosed readily by neutrophils in both complement-deficient and normal sera, whereas resistant isolates are not efficiently ingested in either deficient or normal serum. Therefore, even in the absence of an intact complement system, complement-susceptible strains would remain inept systemic pathogens because they would be readily eliminated by local phagocytic cells or by the reticuloendothelial system. On the other hand, resistant strains would be expected to be equally pathogenic in patients with or without an intact complement system. Thus, no data now exist to support the concept that normally nonpathogenic serum-sensitive bacteria are etiologic in the absence of the late-acting components of the complement cascade.

Epidemiological studies have also suggested relationships between complement resistance and infections in animals. Carroll and Jasper (12) found the overwhelming majority of enterobacteria causing bovine mastitis to be resistant to serum; the serum bactericidal system is likely to be an important defense against udder infection, because there is evidence that milk neutophils are less active in phagocytic assays than blood neutrophils, even in the presence of opsonic agents (39). However, a higher proportion of serum-susceptible *E. coli* isolates was found by Ward and Sebunya (85) in a study involving the use of fresh bovine serum and isolates from acute coliform mastitis. *Haemophilus somnus* strains isolated from individuals during a variety of clinical diseases, including thromboembolic meningoencephalitis, pneumonia, and reproductive disorders, tended to be more resistant to fresh bovine serum than vaginal and prepuce isolates of the same bacterial species from normal animals (16); the killing of susceptible isolates was almost exclusively via the classical pathway. Ward and Sebunya suggested that although resistant strains from carriers may be pathogenic, susceptible isolates could be used as vaccine strains.

COMPLEMENT AND GRAM-POSITIVE BACTERIA

Gram-positive bacteria are not susceptible to direct killing by C5b-9 complexes, since the peptidoglycan layer, which underlies the outer membrane in gram-negative bacteria, is generally the outermost layer of the gram-positive cell; this thick layer acts as an inpenetrable barrier to the components of the membrane attack pathway of complement and thus protects the cytoplasmic membrane. However, the complement system plays a major role in elimination of gram-positive bacteria by the host owing to its ability to opsonize bacteria as a signal for their ingestion and destruction by phagocytic cells. The interaction of gram-positive microorganisms with complement is the topic of a recent excellent review by Brown (10).

LITERATURE CITED

1. **Agnello, V.** 1978. Complement deficiency states. *Medicine* (Baltimore) 57:1–23.

2. Atkinson, J. P., and M. M. Frank. 1980. Complement, p. 219–271. *In* C. W. Parker (ed.), *Clinical Immunology*. The W. B. Saunders Co., Philadelphia.

3. Ballow, M. 1977. Phylogenetics and ontogenetics of the complement systems, p. 183–204. *In* N. K. Day and R. A. Good (ed.), *Biological Amplification Systems in Immunology*, vol. 2: *Comprehensive Immunology*. Plenum Publishing Corp., New York.

4. Bhakdi, S., and J. Tranum-Jensen. 1978. Molecular nature of the complement lesion. *Proc. Natl. Acad. Sci. USA* 75:5655–5659.

5. Bhakdi, S., and J. Tranum-Jensen. 1983. Membrane damage by complement. *Biochim. Biophys. Acta* 737:343–372.

6. Binns, M. M., D. L. Davis, and K. G. Hardy. 1979. Cloned fragments of the plasmid ColV,I-K94 specifying virulence and serum resistance. *Nature* (London) 279:778–781.

7. Bloch, E. F., M. A. Schmetz, J. Foulds, C. H. Hammer, M. M. Frank, and K. A. Joiner. 1987. Multimeric C9 within C5b-9 is required for inner membrane damage to *Escherichia coli* J5 during complement billing. *J. Immunol.* 138:842–848.

8. Born, J., and S. Bhakdi. 1986. Does complement kill *E. coli* by producing transmural pores? *Immunology* 59:139–145.

9. Boyle, M. D. P., A. P. Gee, and T. Borsos. 1979. Studies on the terminal stages of immune hemolysis. VI. Osmotic blockers of differing Stokes' radii detect complement-induced transmembrane channels of differing size. *J. Immunol.* 123:77–82.

10. Brown, E. J. 1985. Interaction of Gram-positive microorganisms with complement. *Curr. Top. Microbiol. Immunol.* 121:159–187.

11. Buchner, H. 1889. Uber die bakterientotende Wirkung des zellfreien Blutserums. *Zentralbl. Bakteriol. Parasitenkd. Infektionskr. Hyg. Abt. 1 Orig.* 5:817–823.

12. Carroll, E. J., and D. E. Jasper. 1977. Bactericidal activity of standard bovine serum against coliform bacteria isolated from udders and the environment of dairy cows. *Am. J. Vet. Res.* 38:2019–2022.

13. Casciato, D. A., J. E. Rosenblatt, R. Bluestone, L. S. Goldberg, and S. M. Finegold. 1979. Susceptibility of isolates of *Bacteroides* to the bactericidal activity of normal human serum. *J. Infect. Dis.* 140:109–113.

14. Cavard, D., J. M. Pages, and C. J. Lazdunski. 1982. A protease as a possible sensor of environmental conditions in *E. coli* outer membrane. *Mol. Gen. Genet.* 188:508–512.

15. Clas, F., G. Schmidt, and M. Loos. 1985. The role of the classical pathway for the bactericidal effect of normal sera against Gram-negative bacteria. *Curr. Top. Microbiol. Immunol.* 121:19–72.

16. Corbeil, L. B., K. Blau, D. J. Prieur, and A. C. S. Ward. 1985. Serum susceptibility of *Haemophilus somnus* from bovine clinical cases and carriers. *J. Clin. Microbiol.* 22:192–198.

17. Dankert, J. R., and A. F. Esser. 1985. Proteolytic modifications of human complement protein C9: loss of poly-C9 and circular lesion formation without impairment of function. *Proc. Natl. Acad. Sci. USA* 82:2128–2132.

18. Dankert, J. R., and A. F. Esser. 1986. Complement-mediated killing of *Escherichia coli*: dissipation of membrane potential by a C9-derived peptide. *Biochemistry* 25:1094–1100.

18a. Dankert, J. R., and A. F. Esser. 1987. Bacterial killing by complement: C9-mediated killing in the absence of C5b-8. *Biochem. J.* 244:393–399.

19. Davis, S. D., E. S. Boatman, D. Gemsa, A. Iannetta, and R. J. Wedgwood. 1969. Biochemical and fine structural changes induced in *Escherichia coli* by human serum. *Microbios* 1:69–86.

20. Di Ninno, V. L., and V. K. Chenier. 1981. Activation of complement by *Neisseria meningitidis*. *FEMS Microbiol. Lett.* 12:55–60.

21. Dlabac, V. 1968. The sensitivity of smooth and rough mutants of *Salmonella typhimurium* to bactericidal and bacteriolytic action of serum, lysozyme and to phagocytosis. *Folia Microbiol.* 13:439–449.

22. Eisenstein, B. I., T. J. Lee, and P. F. Sparling. 1977. Penicillin sensitivity and serum resistance are independent attributes of strains of *Neisseria gonorrhoeae* causing disseminated gonococcal infection. *Infet. Immun.* 15:834–841.

23. Elgefors, B., and S. Olling. 1978. The significance of serum-sensitive bacilli in Gram-negative bacteraemia. *Scand. J. Infect. Dis.* 10:203–207.

24. Feingold, D. S. 1969. The serum bactericidal reaction. IV. Phenotypic conversion of *Escherichia coli* from serum-resistance to serum-sensitivity by diphenylamine. *J. Infect. Dis.* 120:437–444.

25. Feingold, D. S., J. N. Goldman, and H. M. Kurtiz. 1968. Locus of the action of serum and the role of lysozyme in the serum bactericidal reaction. *J. Bacteriol.* 96:2118–2126.

26. Feingold, D. S., J. N. Goldman, and H. M. Kuritz. 1968. Locus of the lethal event in the serum bactericidal reaction. *J. Bacteriol.* 96:2127–2131.

27. Fierer, J., and F. Finley. 1979. Lethal effect of complement and lysozyme on polymyxin-treated, serum-resistant, Gram-negative bacilli. *J. Infect. Dis.* 140:581–588.

28. Fierer, J., F. Finley, and A. I. Braude. 1972. A plaque assay on agar for detection of Gram-negative bacilli sensitive to complement. *J. Immunol.* 109:1156–1158.

29. Fietta, A., E. Romero, and A. G. Siccardi. 1977. Effect of some R factors on the sensitivity of rough *Enterobacteriaceae* to human serum. *Infect. Immun.* 18:273–282.

30. Finne, J. 1982. Occurrence of unique polysialyl carbohydrate units in glycoprotein of developing brain. *J. Biol. Chem.* 257:11966–11970.

31. Goldman, R. C., K. Joiner, and L. Leive. 1984. Serum-resistant mutants of *Escherichia coli* O111 contain increased lipopolysaccharide, lack an O-antigen-containing capsule, and cover more of their lipid A core with O antigen. *J. Bacteriol.* 159:877–882.

32. Gower, P. E., P. W. Taylor, K. G. Koutsaimanis, and A. P. Roberts. 1972. Serum bactericidal activity in patients with upper and lower urinary tract infections. *Clin. Sci.* 43:13–22.

33. Griffiths, E. 1974. Metabolically controlled killing of *Pasteurella septica* by antibody and complement. *Biochim. Biophys. Acta* 462:598–602.

34. Hildebrandt, J. F., L. W. Mayer, S. P. Wang, and T. M. Buchanan. 1978. *Neisseria gonorrhoeae* acquire a new principal outer membrane protein when transformed to resistance to serum bactericidal activity. *Infect. Immun.* 20:267–273.

35. Høiby, N., and S. Olling. 1977. *Pseudomonas aeruginosa* infection in cystic fibrosis. Bactericidal effect of serum from normal individuals and patients with cystic fibrosis or *P. aeruginosa* strains from patients with cystic fibrosis or other diseases. *Acta Pathol. Microbiol. Scand. Sect. C* 85:107–114.

36. Inoue, K. 1972. Immune bacteriolytic and bactericidal reactions. *Res. Immunochem. Immunobiol.* 1:177–222.

37. Inoue, K., T. Kinoshita, M. Okada, and Y. Akiyama. 1977. Release of phospholipids from complement-mediated lesions on the surface structure of *Escherichia coli*. *J. Immunol.* 119:65–72.

38. Inoue, K., K. Yonemasu, A. Takamizawa, and T. Amano. 1968. Studies on the immune bacteriolysis. XIV. Requirement of all nine components of complement for immune bacteriolysis. *Biken J.* 11:203–206.

39. Jain, N. C., and J. Lasmanis. 1978. Phagocytosis of serum-resistant and serum-sensitive coliform bacteria (Klebsiella) by bovine neutrophils from blood and mastitic milk. *Am. J. Vet. Res.* 39:425–427.

40. Jann, K., and B. Jann. 1985. Cell surface components and virulence: *Escherichia coli* O and K antigens in relation to virulence and pathogenicity, p. 157–175. *In* M. Sussman (ed.), *The Virulence of Escherichia coli*. Academic Press, Inc. (London), Ltd., London.

41. Jessop, H. L., and P. A. Lambert. 1986. The role of surface polysaccharide in determining the resistance of *Serratia marcescens* to serum killing. *J. Gen. Microbiol.* 132:2505–2514.

42. Joiner, K. A. 1985. Studies on the mechanism of bacterial resistance to complement-mediated killing and on the mechanism of action of bactericidal antibody. *Curr. Top. Microbiol. Immunol.* 121:135–158.

43. Joiner, K. A., N. Grossman, M. Schmetz, and L. Leive. 1986. C3 binds preferentially to long chain lipopolysaccharide during alternative pathway activation by *Salmonella montevideo*. *J. Immunol.* 136:710–715.

44. Joiner, K. A., C. H. Hammer, E. J. Brown, R. J. Cole, and M. M. Frank. 1982. Studies on the mechanism of bacterial resistance to complement-mediated killing. I. Terminal complement components are deposited and released from *Salmonella minnesota* S218 without causing bacterial death. *J. Exp. Med.* 155:797–808.

45. Joiner, K. A., C. H. Hammer, E. J. Brown, and M. M. Frank. 1982. Studies on the mechanism of bacterial resistance to complement-mediated killing. II. C8 and C9 release C5b67 from the surface of *Salmonella minnesota* S218 because the terminal complex does not insert into the bacterial outer membrane. *J. Exp. Med.* 155:809–819.

46. Kanukollu, V., S. Bieler, S. Hull, and R. Hull. 1985. Contribution of the *traT* gene to serum resistance among clinical isolates of enterobacteriaceae. *J. Med Microbiol.* 19:61–67.

47. Kato, K., and Y. Bito. 1978. Relationship between bactericidal action of complement and fluidity of cellular membranes. *Infect. Immun.* 19:12–17.

48. Kroll, H.-P., S. Bhakdi, and P. W. Taylor. 1983. Membrane changes induced by exposure of *Escherichia coli* to human serum. *Infect. Immun.* 42:1055–1066.

49. Kroll, H.-P., W.-H. Voigt, and P. W. Taylor. 1984. Stable insertion of C5b-9 complement complexes into the outer membrane of serum treated, susceptible *Escherichia coli* cells as prerequisite for killing. *Zentralbl. Bakteriol. Mikrobiol. Hyg. Abt 1 Orig. Reihe A* 258:316–326.

50. Lugtenberg, B., and L. van Alphen. 1983. Molecular architecture and functioning of the outer membrane of *Escherichia coli* and other Gram-negative bacteria. *Biochim. Biophys. Acta* 737:51–115.

51. Mann, C. B., E. E. Ishiguro, W. W. Kay, and T. J. Trust. 1982. Role of surface components in serum resistance of virulent *Aeromonas salmonicida*. *Infect. Immun.* 36:1069–1075.

52. Martinez, R. J., and S. F. Carroll. 1980. Sequential metabolic expressions of the lethal process in human serum-treated *Escherichia coli*: role of lysozyme. *Infect. Immun.* 28:735–745.

53. Mayer, M. M. 1984. Complement: historical perspectives and some current issues. *Complement* 1:2–26.

54. McCabe, W. R., B. Kaijser, S. Olling, M. Uwaydah, and L. A. Hanson. 1978. *Escherichia coli* in bacteremia: K and O antigens and serum sensitivity of strains from adults and neonates. *J. Infect. Dis.* 138:33–41.

55. Moll, A., P. A. Manning, and K. N. Timmis. 1980. Plasmid-determined resistance to serum bactericidal activity: a major outer membrane protein,

the *traT* gene product, is responsible for plasmid-specified serum resistance in *Escherichia coli*. *Infect. Immun.* 28:359–367.

56. Montenegro, M. A., D. Bitter-Suermann, J. K. Timmis, M. E. Aguero, F. C. Cabello, S. C. Sanyal, and K. N. Timmis. 1987. *traT* gene sequences, serum resistance and pathogenicity-related factors in clinical isolates of *Escherichia coli* and other Gram-negative bacteria. *J. Gen. Microbiol.* 131:1511–1521.

57. Nuttal, G. 1888. Experimente uber die bakterienfeindliche Einflusse des tierischen Korpers. *Z. Hyg. Infektionskr.* 4:353–394.

58. Opferkuch, W. 1984. Die Scrumbaktcrizidie, p. 19–27. *In* C. Krasemann (ed.), *Infektiologisches Kolloquium* no. 2. *Der abwehrgeschwachte Patient.* Walter de Gruyter, Berlin.

59. Perez, G. I. P., and M. J. Blaser. 1985. Lipopolysaccharide characteristics of pathogenic campylobacters. *Infect. Immun.* 47:353–359.

60. Pluschke, G., and M. Achtman. 1984. Degree of antibody-independent activation of the classical complement pathway by K1 *Escherichia coli* differs with O antigen type and correlates with virulence of meningitis in newborns. *Infect. Immun.* 43:684–692.

61. Pluschke, G., J. Mayden, M. Achtman, and R. P. Levine. 1983. Role of the capsule and the O antigen in resistance of O18:K1 *Escherichia coli* to complement-mediated killing. *Infect. Immun.* 42:907–913.

62. Podack, E. R., and J. Tschopp. 1984. Membrane attack by complement. *Mol. Immunol.* 21:589–603.

63. Ramm, L. E., M. B. Whitlow, and M. M. Mayer. 1982. Size of the transmembrane channels produced by complement proteins C5b-8. *J. Immunol.* 129:1143–1146.

64. Reynard, A. M., and M. E. Beck. 1976. Plasmid-mediated resistance to the bactericidal effects of normal rabbit serum. *Infect. Immun.* 14:848–850.

65. Reynolds, B. L., U. A. Rother, and K. O. Rother. 1975. Interaction of complement components with a serum-resistant strain of *Salmonella typhimurium*. *Infect. Immun.* 11:944–948.

66. Rice, P. A., W. M. McCormick, and S. L. Kasper. 1980. Natural serum bactericidal activity against *Neisseria gonorrhoeae* isolates from disseminated, locally invasive and uncomplicated disease. *J. Immunol.* 124:2105–2109.

67. Roantree, R. J., and L. A. Rantz. 1960. A study of the relationship of the normal bactericidal activity of human serum to bacterial infection. *J. Clin. Invest.* 35:82–88.

68. Ross, S. C., and P. Densen. 1984. Complement deficiency states and infection: epidemiology, pathogenesis and consequences of neisserial and other infections in an immune deficiency. *Medicine* (Baltimore) 63:243–273.

69. Schoolnik, G. K., T. M. Buchanan, and K. K. Holmes. 1976. Gonococci causing disseminated gonoccocal infection are resistant to the bactericidal action of normal human sera. *J. Clin. Invest.* 58:1163–1173.

70. Schreiber, R. D., D. C. Morrison, E. R. Podack, and H.-J. Muller-Eberhard. 1979. Bactericidal activity of the alternative complement pathway generated from eleven isolated plasma proteins. *J. Exp. Med.* 149:870–882.

71. Sevag, M. G., and R. E. Miller. 1948. Studies on the effect of immune reactions on the metabolism of bacteria. I. Methods and results with *Eberthella typhosa*. *J. Bacteriol.* 55:381–392.

72. Simberkoff, M. S., I. Ricupero, and J. J. Rahal. 1976. Host resistance to *Serratia marcescens* infection: serum bactericidal activity and phagocytosis by normal blood leukocytes. *J. Lab. Clin. Med.* 87:206–217.

73. Stock, J. B., B. Rauch, and S. Roseman. 1977. Periplasmic space in *Salmonella typhimurium* and *Escherichia coli*. *J. Biol. Chem.* 252:7850–7861.

74. Taylor, P. W. 1983. Bactericidal and bacteriolytic activity of serum against gram-negative bacteria. *Microbiol. Rev.* 47:46–83.

75. Taylor, P. W. 1984. Growth environment effects on pathogenicity of Gram-negative bacteria, p. 10–21. *In* A. C. R. Dean, D. C. Ellwood, and C. G. T. Evans (ed.), *Continuous culture*, vol. 8. *Biotechnology, Medicine and the Environment*. Ellis Horwood, Chichester, England.

76. Taylor, P. W., and C. Hughes. 1978. Plasmid carriage and the serum sensitivity of enterobacteria. *Infect. Immun.* 22:10–17.

77. Taylor, P. W., and H.-P Kroll. 1983. Killing of an encapsulated strain of *Escherichia coli* by human serum. *Infect. Immun.* 39:122–131.

78. Taylor, P. W., and H.-P. Kroll. 1984. Interaction of human complement proteins with serum-sensitive and serum-resistant strains of *Escherichia coli*. *Mol. Immunol.* 21:609–620.

79. Taylor, P. W., and H.-P. Kroll. 1985. Effect of lethal doses of complement on the functional integrity of target enterobacteria. *Curr. Top. Microbiol. Immunol.* 121:135–158.

80. Taylor, P. W., H.-P. Kroll, and S. Tomlinson. 1982. Effect of subinhibitory concentrations of mecillinam on expression of *Escherichia coli* surface components associated with serum resistance. *Drugs Exp. Clin. Res.* 8:625–631.

81. Taylor, P. W., and R. Parton. 1977. A protein factor associated with serum resistance in *Escherichia coli*. *J. Med. Microbiol.* 10:225–232.

82. Taylor, P. W., and M. K. Robinson. 1980. Determinants that increase the serum resistance of *Escherichia coli*. *Infect. Immun.* 29:278–280.

83. Tomas, J. M., V. J. Benedi, B. Ciurana, and J.

Jofre. 1986. Role of capsule and O antigen in resistance of *Klebsiella pneumoniae* to serum bactericidal activity. *Infect. Immun.* 54:85–89.

84. **Vosti, K. L., and E. Randall.** 1970. Sensitivity of serologically classified strains of *E. coli* of human origin to the serum bactericidal systems. *Am. J. Med. Sci.* 259:114–119.

85. **Ward, G. E., and T. K. Sebunya.** 1981. Somatic and capsular factors of coliforms which affect resistance to bovine serum bactericidal activity. *Am. J. Vet. Res.* 42:1937–1940.

86. **Wilson, L. A., and J. K. Spitznagel.** 1968. Molecular and structural damage to *Escherichia coli* produced by antibody, complement, and lysozyme systems. *J. Bacteriol.* 96:1339–1348.

87. **Wilson, L. A., and J. K. Spitznagel.** 1971. Characteristics of complement-dependent release of phospholipid from *Escherichia coli*. *Infect. Immun.* 4:23–28.

88. **Winkelstein, J. A.** 1983. Complement and natural immunity. *Clin. Immunol. Allergy* 3:421–439.

89. **Wright, S. D., and R. P. Levine.** 1981. How complement kills *E. coli*. I. Locus of the lethal lesion. *J. Immunol.* 127:1146–1151.

Chapter 8

High-Affinity Iron Uptake Systems and Bacterial Virulence

E. GRIFFITHS

National Institute for Biological Standards and Control
South Mimms, Potters Bar
Hertfordshire EN6 3QG
England

H. CHART

Division of Enteric Pathogens
Public Health Laboratory Service,
Central Public Health Laboratory
London NW9 5EQ
England

P. STEVENSON

National Institute for Biological Standards and Control
South Mimms, Potters Bar
Hertfordshire EN6 3QG
England

INTRODUCTION

An essential factor in any infection is the ability of the invading pathogen to proliferate successfully in the environment of the host. Some pathogens initiate infection by attaching to cells on mucosal surfaces. Others invade these and other tissue cells and become intracellular. Yet others invade the bloodstream and cause generalized infections. To be successful, all must be able to evade or resist host antibacterial defenses which would otherwise kill or eliminate them. Thus, the abilities to resist the bactericidal action of serum, to resist phagocytosis, and to survive within phagocytic cells are well-known virulence properties, which have been studied in considerable detail (13, 14, 27, 42, 44, 49, 51, 98, 106, 107, 120, 130). However, bacterial pathogens must, in addition to simply evading these host defenses, be able to multiply successfully under conditions found in vivo. Indeed, the actual multiplication of pathogens in the largely undefined and changing environment of host tissues is an essential feature of any infection. Factors that might be expected to influence bacterial multiplication in vivo include temperature, pH, osmotic pressure, oxygen tension, and the availability of essential nutrients. Perhaps the best-understood property of the environment encountered by pathogens in host tissues, and its effect on bacterial growth, is the availability of iron. Our understanding of the way the host normally restricts the availability of iron and the effect of restriction on bacterial metabolism and multiplication has increased enormously in recent years and is the subject of the present paper.

AVAILABILITY OF IRON IN VIVO

Although there is a considerable amount of iron present in the body fluids of humans and animals, it is now known that the amount of free iron, which might be readily available to bacteria, is normally extremely small (57). Most iron in the body is found intracellularly, in ferritin, hemosiderin, and heme, and extracellular iron in body fluids is attached to high-affinity iron-binding glycoproteins, transferrin in serum and lymph, and lactoferrin in external secretions and milk (2, 9, 10, 100). A related protein called ovotransferrin is found in avian egg white (3). These proteins have high association constants for iron (about 10^{36}) and are normally only partly saturated. For example, human serum transferrin is usually only 30 to 40% saturated with iron. Lactoferrin has the additional property of being able to bind iron tightly under the more acidic conditions which often prevail at sites of inflammation (100), whereas transferrin has optimal iron-binding properties at neutral pH. The reasons why iron should be transported in this way in vertebrates relate both to the extreme insolubility of ferric hydroxide complexes at neutral pH and to the toxicity of iron, and they have been discussed by Halliwell and Gutteridge (67) and Griffiths (57). Thus, although there is normally an abundance of iron present in body fluids, the amount of free iron in equilibrium

with the iron-binding proteins is of the order of 10^{-18} M, which is far too low to sustain bacterial growth. In addition, during infection the host reduces even further the amount of iron bound to serum transferrin (28). This decrease is called the hypoferremia of infection. Nevertheless, pathogenic bacteria can multiply successfully under these conditions to establish extracellular infections. They must therefore be able to adapt to this iron-restricted environment and possess mechanisms for assimilating protein-bound iron or for acquiring it from liberated heme. So far, little is known about the availability of iron inside cells such as polymorphs and macrophages (38) or about the characteristics which intracellular pathogens may need to multiply inside these and other tissue cells.

HIGH-AFFINITY IRON UPTAKE SYSTEMS OF BACTERIAL PATHOGENS

Siderophore-Mediated Iron Uptake

The best-understood systems whereby bacterial pathogens assimilate iron from host iron-binding proteins are those which depend on the production of soluble, low-molecular-mass, high-affinity iron-chelating compounds known as siderophores (85,102). Some siderophores are able to remove iron from the iron-binding proteins, and the best understood of these are those used by enteric organisms. Bacteria of the genera *Salmonella, Escherichia,* and *Klebsiella* and some *Shigella* species secrete the phenolate iron chelator enterobactin (also called enterochelin) under conditions of iron restriction in vitro (87, 105, 112, 115, 121, 122). This siderophore is synthesized only during iron-restricted growth, and it efficiently removes iron from the iron-binding proteins and transports it to the bacterial cell; the process is represented diagrammatically in Fig. 1. Enterobactin has also been shown to be produced in vivo during infection (60), and Yancey et al. (148) reported that the loss by mutation of the ability to synthesize this siderophore significantly

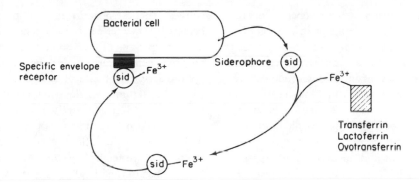

FIGURE 1. Schematic representation of siderophore-mediated iron uptake by bacteria.

reduced the virulence of *Salmonella typhimurium* for mice and prevented the bacteria from multiplying in human serum. More recently, however, Benjamin et al. (8) reported that although they, too, found that enterobactin-negative mutants of *Salmonella typhimurium* failed to multiply in normal mouse serum, the inability to make enterobactin had no effect on the virulence of the organism for several inbred strains of mice. Since *Salmonella typhimurium* is an intracellular pathogen, it has been suggested that the failure of the enterobactin mutation to affect virulence occurs because this siderophore may not be required for growth once the pathogen has entered the cells of the mouse reticuloendothelial system.

Although enterobactin seems to be the main endogenous siderophore made by *Escherichia coli* and *Salmonella* and *Klebsiella* spp. during iron restriction, several enterobacteria also synthesize a hydroxamate type of iron chelator called aerobactin (58). In particular, many strains of *E. coli* that cause generalized extraintestinal infections in humans and animals produce aerobactin (91, 99, 133), the genes for which have been located on a ColV plasmid (40) or in the chromosome (12, 140, 141). Considerable work has been carried out to analyze the aerobactin operon carried by ColV plasmids of *E. coli* (40), and recently both the promoter region and the operator sequences have been identified (43). The invasive pathogen *Shigella flexneri* also produces aerobactin during iron restriction, and here the genes involved

are located in the chromosome (61, 87). Analysis of various *E. coli* K-12–*Shigella* transconjugants has shown that these genes are linked to the *mtl* chromosomal marker of *S. flexneri*, one of three chromosomal segments associated with the virulence of this pathogen (61, 66). Interestingly, it seems that most clinical isolates of *S. flexneri* do not produce enterobactin, although some of the genetic information is present in the cells (109). Enteroinvasive strains of *E. coli*, which produce dysenterylike illnesses, also synthesize aerobactin (61), as do some *Klebsiella* clinical isolates (83, 101; Paul Williams, personal communication). In addition, certain epidemic *Salmonella* strains produce aerobactin as well as enterobactin, the relevant genes being carried on FI*me* plasmids (33). FI*me* plasmids range in size from 100 to 180 kilobase pairs and encode multiple drug resistance genes. Some of the plasmids also encode the aerobactin operon. *Salmonella* strains which harbor these particular plasmids not only are resistant to many antibiotics but also produce disease characterized by a high incidence of septicemia and meningitis (4, 33, 118). The data suggest that plasmids encoding the aerobactin-mediated iron uptake system promote the ability of these pathogens to cause septicemia in much the same way as does the presence of a ColV plasmid encoding the aerobactin system in *E. coli*. However, it should be noted that neither *S. flexneri* nor the enteroinvasive strains of *E. coli* usually cause septicemias, although they, too, produce aerobactin.

The distribution of the aerobactin operon in the bacterial chromosome or in various plasmids suggests that it might be a genetically mobile recombinational unit which can integrate at different sites in various genomes. Recent studies by Waters and Crosa (144) have shown that the genetic information encoding the aerobactin-mediated iron uptake system in plasmids is highly conserved, as is an upstream IS1-like sequence and an overlapping replication region (REPI) (94, 110). In contrast, the downstream flanking region is variable. This includes a downstream copy of IS1 and a corresponding replication region (REPII). Conservation of the upstream REPI sequence appears to be the rule among the IncFI plasmids coding for aerobactin biosynthesis, and Crosa (40) suggested that this may have been instrumental in the preservation and possible extrachromosomal spread of aerobactin genes among ColV and other plasmids of the FI incompatibility group, which includes the *Salmonella* R plasmids. In contrast, the chromosomal aerobactin genes do not seem to have the same pattern of conserved flanking sequences as do those on plasmids, although the aerobactin sequences themselves are highly conserved (40). This suggests that although chromosomal and plasmid aerobactin genes may have evolved from a common ancestral origin, recombination and selective pressures may have resulted in the conservation of different flanking sequences.

Although there is no doubt that the production of aerobactin plays an important part in the virulence of certain pathogens, it is not yet clear how acquiring the ability to make this chelator confers a selective advantage on bacteria that already can make enterobactin. At pH 7.4, enterobactin is by far the most effective siderophore characterized (58, 69). One possible important difference between the modes of action of enterobactin and aerobactin is that the latter seems to be recycled (17). Enterobactin is denatured once the ferric siderophore has been transported into the bacterial cell, and it is clearly an energetically expensive way of assimilating iron (119). In addition, results obtained by Williams and Carbonetti (147)

suggest that aerobactin is able to stimulate bacterial growth at external concentrations much lower than those of enterobactin. Moreover, the effective concentration, and hence the siderophore activity, of enterobactin is significantly reduced in serum since the enterobactin is bound to albumin (82); aerobactin is not affected in this way. Also, the presence of other factors in body fluids could influence the overall effectiveness of different siderophores, and it is known that in the blood stream at least, several factors act to reduce the efficacy of enterobactin-mediated iron uptake, thus favoring aerobactin-mediated iron transport (58). These include the already mentioned effect of albumin, the presence of anti-O-polysaccharide antibodies, which seem to interfere with enterobactin secretion, and the presence of anions, which promote aerobactin-mediated iron uptake (58).

The results of Smith and Huggins (131) suggest that the aerobactin-mediated iron uptake system may be particularly important at a low infective dose of bacterial pathogen. What is not clear at present is whether both enterobactin and aerobactin are required for full virulence. So far no Ent^- Aer^+ strains of *E. coli* have been found among the clinical isolates studied, although most strains of *S. flexneri* seem to produce only aerobactin (109). Interestingly, the few *S. flexneri* strains which did produce both siderophores had an advantage when growing in iron-restricted media in the laboratory (109), although care must be taken when using such data to predict what might be happening in vivo during infection. *Shigella* species are, of course, invasive pathogens and multiply intracellularly (66), and it has been suggested that their ability to remove iron from ferritin might be more important than their ability to utilize iron in transferrin or lactoferrin (58). Enterobactin can remove iron from ferritin, but it is not known whether aerobactin can do so (136). Lawlor et al. (86) believe that aerobactin plays no part in the intracellular multiplication of *Shigella* spp. They found that the ability, or otherwise, to synthesize aerobactin had no effect on the rate of multiplication of *Shigella* spp. within HeLa cells.

However, it should be noted that iron-replete bacteria were used in these experiments, and bacterial growth seems to have been monitored for only 4 h. More work is therefore needed before it can be stated with confidence that siderophore-mediated iron transport is not required for intracellular growth because sufficient iron is available at this location. Furthermore, only model systems have been used to date, and it will be of interest to see whether aerobactin mutants of *Shigella* spp. multiply equally well within other tissue cells, especially colonic epithelial cells.

An integral part of the high-affinity iron uptake systems based on siderophores is the production of outer membrane proteins which act as receptors for ferric siderophores, as well as mechanisms for the release of chelator-bound iron (46, 58, 103, 114). The strict requirement for outer membrane receptor proteins in siderophore-mediated iron uptake is shown by the fact that mutants lacking such proteins are completely devoid of transport activity (40, 53). Although the outer membrane receptors are siderophore specific, inner membrane components, also necessary for siderophore-mediated iron transport, are less specific. Hydroxamate siderophores use common transport functions specified by the *fhuC*, *fhuD*, and *fhuB* genes (18, 19, 48). A functional locus called *tonB* is required for the utilization of all high-affinity iron carriers (18, 103, 117). However, the *tonB* function does not seem to be regulated by iron, nor is it specific for iron transport; it is also involved in the utilization of vitamin B_{12} (68, 103).

The enteric bacteria produce several new outer membrane proteins under iron-restricted growth conditions, but so far only some have been identified as ferric siderophore receptors (56, 58). For example, an 81-kDa protein in *E. coli* functions as the receptor for ferric enterobactin (17, 50, 74, 103), and a ColV plasmid-encoded 74-kDa protein functions as the receptor for aerobactin (11, 53). Until recently, most of the work on the iron-regulated outer membrane proteins of *E. coli* had been carried out with laboratory strains, such as *E.*

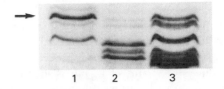

FIGURE 2. Three characteristic sodium dodecyl sulfate-polyacrylamide gel electrophoresis patterns of iron-regulated outer membrane proteins of *E. coli*. Each lane contained about 30 μg of protein, and electrophoresis was carried out for an extended period as described by Griffiths et al. (63). Lanes: 1, *E. coli* O25:H⁻ (an enterotoxigenic strain); 2, *E. coli* O1:K1 (isolated during a human urinary tract infection); 3, *E. coli* O18:K1 (isolated from a neonatal human with meningitis). The arrow indicates the position of the 81-kDa protein.

coli K-12. However, it is now known that pathogenic strains produce similar new proteins when grown in vitro in the presence of iron-binding proteins and in vivo during infection (31, 55, 63).

Results show considerable qualitative and quantitative variation in the expression of iron-regulated outer membrane proteins by different strains of pathogenic *E. coli*, many strains appearing to produce larger amounts of these proteins than *E. coli* K-12 does. Furthermore, some produce iron-regulated proteins not seen in laboratory strains of *E. coli*. Figure 2 shows three different sodium dodecyl sulfate-polyacrylamide gel electrophoresis patterns of iron-regulated outer membrane proteins recently recognized in different isolates of pathogenic *E. coli* which cause diseases in humans (31, 62, 63; unpublished data). Only isolates giving rise to patterns seen in Fig. 2, lanes 2 and 3, seem to be associated with extraintestinal infections of humans. Interestingly, these two patterns have not yet been observed in *E. coli* strains isolated from cases of human enteric diseases or animal septicemia or enteric diseases. All of the 30 or so animal isolates examined to date produced an iron-regulated outer membrane protein profile essentially similar to that shown in Fig. 2, lane 1. Enteroinvasive strains of *E. coli* which synthesize aerobactin and which produce shigellosislike illnesses in humans exhibit an iron-regulated outer membrane protein profile similar to that seen in Fig. 2, lane 1, except that they synthesize an additional iron-regulated 76-kDa protein (61). Indeed, the pattern of the iron-regulated proteins expressed by these enteroinvasive strains of *E. coli* is identical to that seen with laboratory-constructed *E. coli* K-12–*Shigella* hybrids under the same growth conditions. The *S. flexneri* parent strain used in these constructions also produced a 76-kDa protein during iron-restricted growth, and this is thought to be the receptor for aerobactin in these particular organisms. As mentioned previously, in *E. coli* carrying the ColV plasmid-encoded aerobactin system, the siderophore receptor protein is known to have a molecular mass of 74,000 (11, 40, 53, 58). In the laboratory, the iron-regulated proteins discussed above can be induced in pathogens by adding iron-chelating agents such as α, α'-dipyridyl, ethylenediamine-di(*o*-hydroxyphenylacetic acid) (EDDA), or Desferal (CIBA-GEIGY Corp.), instead of an iron-binding protein, to culture media. Although these agents are certainly more convenient and economical to use than an iron-binding protein, the pattern of bacterial iron-regulated proteins obtained is not always identical to that obtained by using a naturally occurring iron-binding protein (29). Caution should therefore be exercised when interpreting data concerning the nature of iron-regulated proteins produced by different strains when the data were obtained with such systems. (29, 58).

Since surface components play such an important part in host-bacterium interactions, alterations induced in the envelopes of invading bacterial pathogens by host iron-binding proteins are clearly of interest, especially now it has been shown that the iron-regulated membrane proteins are synthesized not only by *E. coli* but also by other bacterial pathogens growing in vivo during clinical infection of humans and animals (Table 1). Antibodies which react with some of the iron-regulated proteins of *E. coli* and other pathogens have been detected in human and animal serum samples (58, 127). Whether such antibodies play any part in protecting the host against infection, possibly by interfering with siderophore-mediated iron up-

take, is unclear. As part of an investigation into the protective role of anti-receptor antibodies, Chart and Griffiths (31; unpublished data) examined the antigenic homology of the ferric-enterobactin receptor protein in different strains of *E. coli* by using polyclonal and monoclonal antibodies. Results showed that the molecular weight and at least some of the antigenic properties of the enterobactin receptor were highly conserved. However, antibodies raised to purified and denatured enterobactin receptor protein appeared not to react with the protein in situ on the surface of the *E. coli* strain tested. Not surprisingly, these antibodies had no effect on bacterial multiplication. However, specific antibodies, raised in rabbits, to the 78-kDa FhuA protein of *E. coli,* which is the receptor for ferrichrome, a siderophore produced not by *E. coli* itself but by other microorganisms (102, 103), as well as for bacteriophage T5, were found to partially inhibit ferrichrome-mediated iron transport (34). These antibodies also blocked the adsorption of phage T5 onto the 78-kDa protein. The work suggests that the antibodies bind to epitopes distal to the sites involved in iron uptake via ferrichrome. It must be borne in mind, however, that even if antibodies did recognize the appropriate antigen on the bacterial cell surface, they would not necessarily always be able to interact with the receptor in situ in all strains of *E. coli*. In some cases lipopolysaccharide might interfere with antibody-antigen interaction by masking the membrane proteins (142, 143). Nevertheless, Bolin and Jensen (15) have recently reported that turkeys passively immunized with antibodies against the iron-regulated outer membrane proteins of *E. coli* O78:K80:H9 were protected against experimental colisepticemia.

Although much of our understanding of iron-sequestering systems based on siderophores and outer membrane protein receptors and of their role in bacterial virulence has come from studies on enteric bacteria, there is now an increasing awareness that similar systems play an equally important role in the pathogenicity of other bacteria (40, 58). A particularly in-

TABLE 1
Pathogenic bacteria shown to express iron-regulated proteins in vivo during infection

Organism	Source	Host	References
E. coli	Peritoneal cavity	Guinea pig	62
E. coli	Urine	Human with urinary tract infection	84, 127
Klebsiella pneumoniae	Urine	Human with urinary tract infection	127
Proteus mirabilis	Urine	Human with urinary tract infection	127
P. aeruginosa	Lungs	Human with cystic fibrosis	22
V. cholerae	Intestines	Rabbit	126

teresting case is that of the fish pathogen *Vibrio anguillarum*, which is responsible for a devastating septicemic disease in fish (40). Some highly virulent strains of *V. anguillarum* carry a 65-kilobase plasmid, named pJM1, which encodes an efficient iron uptake system that allows the organism to grow under iron-restricted conditions. On losing the plasmid, *V. anguillarum* loses its ability to grow under such conditions and also loses its virulence (39, 41). In some other virulent strains of *V. anguillarum*, the genes encoding this high-affinity iron transport system are located in the chromosome (40, 137). Analysis has shown that the *V. anguillarum* iron uptake system is based on a phenolic siderophore and an 86-kDa iron-regulated outer membrane protein receptor (40) and that the whole operon, like the aerobactin operon, may be part of a recombinational unit. The discovery of repeated sequences flanking the iron uptake region of plasmid pJM1 is consistent with this idea (40).

The human pathogen *Vibrio cholerae* also produces a siderophore-mediated high-affinity iron uptake system and produces new outer membrane proteins during iron-restricted growth. The structure of the *V. cholerae* siderophore, called vibriobactin, has recently been elucidated (64), and the iron-regulated outer membrane proteins have been found in in vivo-grown vibrios (126). However, Sigel et al. (128) claim that the ferric-vibriobactin iron transport system is not needed for virulence and base their view on experiments which showed that two *V. cholerae* mutants defective in the vibriobactin-mediated iron transport system retained their ability to multiply and to produce disease in

an infant-mouse infection model. It is claimed that both mutants multiplied normally in vivo. Indeed, the number of mutant bacteria recovered from infected animals was similar to the number obtained from the wild-type parent strain. However, high inocula of iron-replete bacteria were used in these experiments, and considerable multiplication of mutant *V. cholerae* would be expected before the organisms became starved of iron and failed to multiply. It is interesting that another *Vibrio* species, *Vibrio vulnificus*, does not seem to possess a high-affinity iron uptake system of its own, although it does have many other virulence determinants (52). This organism becomes highly virulent and produces life-threatening septicemia only when the host iron metabolism has been perturbed to such an extent that iron is freely available in the tissues, such as in individuals suffering from idiopathic hemochromatosis or other iron overload diseases (30, 58, 65).

Pseudomonas aeruginosa is an opportunistic pathogen that produces high-affinity iron uptake systems which sequester iron. Indeed, *Pseudomonas* species produce several siderophores during iron restriction, of which only two, pyochelin and pyoverdin, are considered to be interesting as regards infection (5, 35, 37, 132, 145). *Pseudomonas* species also synthesize new outer membrane proteins during iron restriction in vitro and in vivo during infection (6, 22, 127). However, it seems that these siderophores may not always be produced or be suited for removing iron from transferrin in vivo, and it has been suggested that another product, called pyocyanin, could participate in a reduction mechanism capable of removing iron from transferrin (36). Preliminary studies concerning the uptake of iron by another fish pathogen, *Aeromonas salmonicida,* suggest that this species has at least two means of obtaining iron (32). All the strains examined expressed an iron-regulated outer membrane protein of 83 kDa, and all but one secreted a soluble siderophore. The exception was a strain which required direct contact with the iron-binding protein for iron acquisition. Strains of *Neisseria meningitidis* and *Neisseria gonorrheae* also obtain iron from ferric glycoproteins by direct contact (see below). Little is known about the iron transport systems of gram-positive pathogens, although recent studies have shown that a siderophore-mediated iron transport system does operate for *Corynebacterium diphtheriae* (123–125); the chelator itself has not yet been fully characterized.

Siderophore-Independent Iron Uptake

Quite clearly, the best-understood systems used by pathogenic bacteria to assimilate iron from host iron-binding proteins are those which depend on the production of siderophores. The fact that such systems are the best understood at present does not, of course, mean that they are the most common, nor indeed the most efficient for sequestering iron in vivo. Some pathogens appear to use a mechanism involving the direct interaction between the bacterial cell surface and the iron-binding protein in a manner analogous to the reaction occurring between transferrin and the reticulocyte (38, 76, 138).

There is no doubt that pathogenic *Neisseria* species can remove iron from iron-binding proteins, but the means by which this is accomplished is poorly understood. Although there has been conflicting evidence concerning the role of siderophores in the process, it is now generally accepted that *N. gonorrhoeae* and *N. meningitidis* do not synthesize their own siderophores, and it is virtually certain that iron uptake by these two pathogens involves the direct interaction between an iron-binding protein and

the bacterial cell surface (7, 97, 108, 129, 146, 149). Perhaps one of the most significant features regarding the acquisition of iron from iron-binding proteins by the *Neisseria* species is the highly specific nature of the process. This contrasts sharply with the known siderophore-mediated iron uptake systems which appear to be able to take iron from any one of the three iron-binding proteins: transferrin, lactoferrin, and ovotransferrin. All gonococci and meningococci seem to be able to obtain iron from human transferrin, whereas most commensal *Neisseria* species are unable to do so. The growth of the latter is therefore inhibited by this particular iron-binding protein (96, 129). Similarly, Mickelsen et al. (95) found that all meningococci could obtain iron from human lactoferrin, but only about 50% of the gonococci and 25% of commensal *Neisseria* species could do so. Strains which could not remove iron from lactoferrin were unable to multiply in the presence of the protein; this inhibition was abolished when sufficient iron was added to saturate the iron-binding capacity of the protein. Ovotransferrin was found to be bacteriostatic for all the *Neisseria* species tested, suggesting that it could not act as a source of iron for any of these organisms (7, 96). Since transferrin, lactoferrin, and ovotransferrin are closely related proteins (10, 38), the above observations suggest that the mechanism by which gonococci and meningococci obtain iron from host iron-binding proteins is extremely protein specific. A similar specificity exists for the reticulocyte. For example, rabbit reticulocytes can distinguish among ovotransferrin, transferrin, and lactoferrin and will remove iron only from transferrin (100, 150). The reticulocyte and other mammalian cells remove iron from transferrin by a process involving a direct association between the iron-binding protein and a specific cell surface transferrin receptor (38, 76, 138). For the reticulocyte and other mammalian cells, it is thought that the iron is released from the receptor-bound ferric transferrin by a localized lowering of the pH within internalized vesicles containing the transferrin-receptor protein complex, but the means by which iron

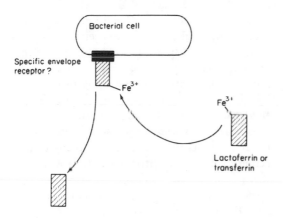

FIGURE 3. Schematic representation of iron uptake by pathogenic bacteria, involving a direct interaction with the host iron-binding glycoprotein.

is removed from iron-binding proteins bound by *Neisseria* spp. is unknown. Indeed, it is not known whether a specific receptor molecule is involved in the bacterial system, which is depicted diagrammatically in Fig. 3. It is known, however, that the uptake of iron from transferrin depends on a functional respiratory chain (129), as is the case with a certain strain of *A. salmonicida* (32). Also, only iron-starved meningococci, in contrast to iron-replete organisms, can remove iron from the transferrin. Like the pathogens which use siderophore-mediated iron uptake systems, *Neisseria* spp. also produce new outer membrane proteins during iron restriction in vitro, although little is known about the relation of these proteins to the process of assimilating iron and to growth in vivo (97, 104, 146).

Clearly, for the gonococci and meningococci, the iron-binding proteins seem to provide specific sources of iron, and Holbein (72) has shown that the level of iron in the circulatory transferrin pool of mice determines the course of experimental *N. meningitidis* infection. In mice, meningococcal infection leads to hypoferremia, and this controls the infection by depriving the pathogen of iron, since it seems that the organism depends on transferrin iron for growth in the host (73, 89, 90). It is not known whether an ability to take iron from lactoferrin plays any part in the pathogenicity

of either gonococci or meningococci. An ability to use the iron in lactoferrin does not seem to be essential for the survival of *Neisseria* spp. on mucosal surfaces, since most commensal species cannot use lactoferrin iron. It has been suggested that since all of these bacteria can use heme as a source of iron, the heme released by dying cells sloughed from the epithelium may be one source of iron on mucosal surfaces (95).

Acquisition of Iron from Heme

In addition to obtaining iron from the iron-binding proteins, a number of pathogens may, under certain circumstances, obtain sufficient iron in vivo from cell-free heme or hemoglobin in serum or from that liberated by hemolysis (58). Generally it seems that this iron is more readily available than that bound to the iron-binding proteins, although little is known about the mechanism whereby pathogens are able to utilize the iron in heme or hemoglobin. Indeed, it is not certain that this should be classed as a high-affinity iron uptake system. Normally there is only a trace of free heme in serum, and this is bound to hemopexin or serum albumin; the very small amounts of hemoglobin present are bound by haptoglobin. Except in very special cases, such as *Yersinia pestis* (25, 111), there is insufficient heme or hemoglobin present to promote infection and it is necessary to liberate hemoglobin from erythrocytes by hemolysis to provide a sufficient iron supply for most pathogens. The effect of hemolysis produced experimentally or by injury or disease on increasing the susceptibility of the host to infection is well documented, and it has been clearly shown that the iron is responsible for stimulating bacterial growth (25, 56, 88). The α-hemolysins produced by certain pathogenic strains of *E. coli* have also been considered to be virulence factors, since they may enable hemolytic strains to obtain the iron needed for growth from lysed erythrocytes in vivo; it must be emphasized, however, that α-hemolysins can also act as cytotoxins (58). In some cases, such as with *E. coli* (45), the administration of haptoglobin protects against experimental infections promoted by free hemoglobin, and this has suggested the use of haptoglobin in the treatment of potentially fatal hemoglobin-mediated bacterial infections (45). However, it is important to note that this may not apply in all cases. *V. vulnificus,* for example, can utilize the hemoglobin in the hemoglobin-haptoglobin complex (70).

IRON AND SUSCEPTIBILITY TO INFECTION

The metabolic changes discussed above, the synthesis and secretion of siderophores, the expression of iron-regulated proteins, and, for *E. coli* and *Salmonella, Klebsiella,* and *Pseudomonas* spp., the changes in the posttranscriptional modification of certain tRNA molecules which take place during iron-restricted growth (56, 58) can all be considered to be features of cellular adaptation to growth under iron-restricted conditions. Clearly, some bacteria have the genetic capability to undergo these sometimes quite substantial alterations in their metabolism required to enable them to sequester essential iron and to multiply in vivo. Another consequence of limiting the availability of iron is that the rate of bacterial multiplication is generally reduced (54). Even a modest reduction in the rate of bacterial growth can make a big difference to the size of a bacterial population over a matter of hours, and this might be crucial in deciding the outcome of an infection. Reducing the rate of bacterial multiplication gives the host an advantage in that it has time to mount other defensive actions which may be able to control the infection. On the other hand, supplying free iron in one form or another bypasses the effect of the iron-binding proteins, and the bacteria grow faster than and are phenotypically different from the iron-restricted organisms. Such an increase in the rate of growth may be sufficient to tip the balance in favor of the invading pathogen, since other host defenses may then be unable to contain the multiplying pathogen and thus control the

infection. It is, of course, well known that increasing the availability of iron, either as heme or as Fe^{3+}, greatly enhances the susceptibility of animals and humans to a variety of bacterial infections (57, 80). However, the mechanism by which excess iron promotes bacterial infections may not be the same in all cases. Although the enhancement of bacterial infections by iron appears in some cases to be due to the action of iron as a nutrient, there is evidence that iron may sometimes also interfere with the activity of some antibacterial systems (25, 55, 81). It has been suggested that a distinction should be made between the role of iron compounds in providing an essential growth factor and their ability to abolish the bactericidal action of certain sera (55). The mechanism whereby iron inhibits the bactericidal action of immune serum is unknown.

CONCLUDING REMARKS

Although iron clearly modulates the interactions between host and pathogen, it must be emphasized that the key to its importance lies in the fact that normally it is not readily available to invading bacteria. Organisms which are unable to obtain iron in vivo are unable to proliferate, and iron-binding proteins can therefore be considered part of the host defense system (59). However, the restricted availability of iron is not sufficient to suppress the growth of all organisms, and, clearly, pathogens multiply sufficiently rapidly in the tissues of normal animals and humans to produce disease. The nature of the disease produced, whether localized or disseminated, extracellular or intracellular, may, however, be influenced by the ability of a pathogen to sequester iron at different body sites. Of course, other virulence determinants play an essential part in pathogenicity, and the factors which decide the outcome of an infection are numerous and complex. Nevertheless, the availability of iron for the essential metabolism of pathogenic organisms and the need of the host to bind and sequester the metal are central issues. The dis-

covery that bacteria undergo specific phenotypic changes both in their metabolism and in
the composition of their outer membrane proteins to enable them to acquire iron and multiply in the iron-restricted environment of host
tissues adds another dimension to the complex
pattern of virulence determinants already found
in iron-replete pathogens. Possible connections
between these, usually cryptic, iron-related
changes and other bacterial properties, such as
resistance to phagocytosis or to the bactericidal
action of serum, must now be explored. It has
already been reported that a large increase in
virulence of N. *meningitidis* occurs after growth
under iron-restricted conditions at low pH (pH
6.6) (21). It is also known that some of the
toxins which play such an important part in
certain diseases are produced by the pathogens
mainly or entirely during iron-restricted growth
(40, 58).

Without a doubt, current developments
are rapidly increasing our understanding of the
critical role of iron in infection and are providing a fresh insight into the capacity of bacteria to multiply in vivo and to cause disease.
This information is leading to new ideas concerning the development and testing of antibacterial agents, including the use of haptoglobin and various iron chelators, and to the
development of new vaccines (15, 23, 24, 45,
71, 78, 79, 93). Much of what is currently
known about the conditions encountered by
bacterial pathogens in host tissues concerns the
extracellular environment, and a great deal of
what we know about the bacterial response to
this environment comes from work with gram-
negative pathogens. Little is known about how
gram-positive organisms acquire iron in vivo or
about the changes they may undergo in these
circumstances. Also, little is known about the
environment encountered by intracellular
pathogens and about the availability of iron inside different tissue cell types. It will be important in future work to compare the ability
of pathogens such as *Shigella* and *Salmonella* spp.
to multiply both extracellularly and intracellularly and to consider the availability of intracellular iron.

Even less is known about the ability of
nonbacterial pathogens to sequester iron in vivo
and about the effects of the iron-restricted environment on the properties of the organisms.
It is known, for example, that the growth of
Candida albicans is inhibited in vitro in the
presence of iron-binding proteins or serum and
that this inhibition can be abolished by adding
iron (47). Abe et al. (1) have shown that excess
iron promotes the proliferation of *Candida* infection in mice, and there is a suggestion that
systemic candidiasis in patients with acute leukemia might be related to the increased satu-
ration of their serum transferrin with iron (26).
However, the mechanism whereby *C. albicans*
normally acquires iron when growing in its human host is not known, although it is known
that a number of fungi, including *C. albicans*,
can secrete siderophores (75, 77). Similarly, little
is known about the way parasites obtain iron,
although again there is a growing interest in
the role of iron in parasitic diseases caused by
organisms such as *Plasmodium falciparum* and
Trypanosoma cruzi (92, 113, 116). The critical
role of iron in the growth of tumor cells and
other rapidly proliferating cells is also now appreciated and is under active investigation (16,
38, 134, 135, 138, 139).

ACKNOWLEDGMENTS.   The research from our
laboratory reported in this paper was supported
in part by grants from the World Health Organization and the Medical Research Council.

LITERATURE CITED

1. Abe, F., M. Tateyama, H. Shibuya, N. Azumi,
   and Y. Ommura. 1985. Experimental candidiasis
   in iron overload. *Mycopathologia* **89**:59–63.
2. Aisen, P. 1980. The transferrins, p. 87–129. *In*
   A. Jacobs and M. Worwood (ed.), *Iron in Biochemistry and Medicine*. vol. 2. Academic Press, Inc.
   (London), Ltd., London.
3. Alderton, G., W. H. Ward, and H. L. Fevold.
   1946. Identification of the bacteria-inhibiting iron-
   binding protein of egg white as conalbumin. *Arch.
   Biochem. Biophys.* **11**:9–13.
4. Anderson, E. S., E. J. Threlfall, J. M. Carr, M.
   M. McConnell, and H. R. Smith. 1977. Clonal

distribution of resistance plasmid-carrying *Salmonella typhimurium* mainly in the Middle East. *J. Hyg.* 79:425–448.

5. Ankenbauer, R., S. Sriyosachati, and C. D. Cox. 1985. Effects of siderophores on the growth of *Pseudomonas aeruginosa* in human serum and transferrin. *Infect. Immun.* 49:132–140.

6. Anwar, H., M. R. W. Brown, A. Day, and P. H. Weller. 1984. Outer membrane antigens of mucoid *Pseudomonas aeruginosa* isolated directly from the sputum of a cystic fibrosis patient. *FEMS Microbiol. Lett.* 24:235–239.

7. Archibald, F. S., and I. W. DeVoe. 1979. Removal of iron from human transferrin by *Neisseria meningitidis*. *FEMS Microbiol. Lett.* 6:159–162.

8. Benjamin, W. H., Jr., C. L. Turnbough, Jr., B. S. Posey, and D. E. Briles. 1985. The ability of *Salmonella typhimurium* to produce the siderophore enterobactin is not a virulence factor in mouse typhoid. *Infect. Immun.* 50:392–397.

9. Bezkorovainy, A. 1980. *Biochemistry of Non-Heme Iron*. Plenum Publishing Corp., New York.

10. Bezkorovainy, A. 1987. Iron proteins, p. 27–67. In J. J. Bullen and E. Griffiths (ed.), *Iron and Infection: Molecular, Physiological and Clinical Aspects*. John Wiley & Sons Ltd., Chichester, England.

11. Bindereif, A., V. Braun, and K. Hantke. 1982. The cloacin receptor of ColV-bearing *Escherichia coli* is part of the Fe^{3+}-aerobactin transport system. *J. Bacteriol.* 150:1472–1475.

12. Bindereif, A., and J. B. Neilands. 1985. Aerobactin genes in clinical isolates of *Escherichia coli*. *J. Bacteriol.* 161:727–735.

13. Binns, M. M., J. Mayden, and R. P. Levine. 1982. Further characterization of complement resistance conferred on *Escherichia coli* by the plasmid genes *traT* of R100 and *iss* of ColV, I-K94. *Infect. Immun.* 35:654–659.

14. Bjorsten, B., and B. Kaijser. 1978. Interaction of human serum and neutrophils with *Escherichia coli* strains: differences between strains isolated from urine of patients with pyelonephritis or asymptomatic bacteruria. *Infect. Immun.* 22:308–311.

15. Bolin, C. A., and A. E. Jensen. 1987. Passive immunization with antibodies against iron-regulated outer membrane proteins protects turkeys from *Escherichia coli* septicemia. *Infect. Immun.* 55:1239–1242.

16. Bowern, N., I. A. Ramshaw, P. Badenoch-Jones, and P. C. Doherty. 1984. Effect of an iron-chelating agent on lymphocyte proliferation. *Aust. J. Exp. Biol. Med. Sci.* 62:743–754.

17. Braun, V., C. Brazel-Faisst, and R. Schneider. 1984. Growth stimulation of *Escherichia coli* in serum by iron (III)-aerobactin: recycling of aerobactin. *FEMS Microbiol. Lett.* 21:99–103.

18. Braun, V., R. Burkhardt, R. Schneider, and L. Zimmermann. 1982. Chromosomal genes for ColV plasmid-determined iron (III)-aerobactin transport in *Escherichia coli*. *J. Bacteriol.* 151:553–559.

19. Braun, V., R. Gross, W. Koster, and L. Zimmermann. 1983. Plasmid and chromosomal mutants in the iron (III)-aerobactin transport system of *Escherichia coli*. Use of streptonigrin for selection. *Mol. Gen. Genet.* 192:131–139.

20. Braun, V., and K. Hantke. 1981. Bacterial cell surface receptors, p. 1–73. In B. K. Ghosh (ed.), *Organization of Prokaryotic Cell Membranes*, vol. 2. CRC Press, Inc. Boca Raton, Fla.

21. Brener, D., I. W. DeVoe, and B. E. Holbein. 1981. Increased virulence of *Neisseria meningitidis* after in vitro iron-limited growth at low pH. *Infect. Immun.* 33:59–66.

22. Brown, M. R. W., H. Anwar, and P. A. Lambert. 1984. Evidence that mucoid *Pseudomonas aeruginosa* in the cystic fibrosis lung grows under iron-restricted conditions. *FEMS Microbiol. Lett.* 21:113–117.

23. Brown, M. R. W., and P. Williams. 1985. Influence of substrate limitation and growth phase on sensitivity to antimicrobial agents. *J. Antimicrob. Chemother.* 15(Suppl. A):7–14.

24. Brown, M. R. W., and P. Williams. 1985. The influence of environment on envelope properties affecting survival of bacteria in infections. *Annu. Rev. Microbiol.* 39:527–556.

25. Bullen, J. J. 1981. The significance of iron in infection. *Rev. Infect. Dis.* 3:1127–1137.

26. Caroline, L., F. Rosner, and P. J. Kozinn. 1969. Elevated serum iron, low unbound transferrin and candidiasis in acute leukaemia. *Blood* 34:441–451.

27. Carrol, M. E. W., P. S. Jackett, V. R. Arber, and D. B. Lowrie. 1979. Phagolysosome formation, cyclic adenosine 3',5'-monophosphate and the fate of *Salmonella typhimurium* within mouse peritoneal macrophages. *J. Gen. Microbiol.* 110:421–429.

28. Cartwright, G. E., A. Lauritsen, S. Humphreys, P. J. Jones, I. M. Merrill, and M. M. Wintrobe. 1946. The anemia of infection. II. The experimental production of hypoferremia and anemia in dogs. *J. Clin. Invest.* 25:81–86.

29. Chart, H., M. Buck, P. Stevenson, and E. Griffiths. 1986. Iron regulated outer membrane proteins of *Escherichia coli*: variations in expression due to the chelator used to restrict the availability of iron. *J. Gen. Microbiol.* 132:1373–1378.

30. Chart, H., and E. Griffiths. 1985. The availability of iron and the growth of *Vibrio vulnificus* in sera from patients with haemochromatosis. *FEMS Microbiol. Lett.* 26:227–231.

31. Chart, H., and E. Griffiths. 1985. Antigenic and molecular homology of the ferric-enterobactin receptor protein of *Escherichia coli*. *J. Gen. Microbiol.* 131:1503–1509.

32. **Chart, H., and T. S. Trust.** 1983. Acquisition of iron by *Aeromonas salmonicida. J. Bacteriol.* 156:758–764.

33. **Colonna, B., M. Nioletti, P. Visca, M. Casalino, P. Valenti, and F. Maimone.** 1985. Composite Is*1* elements encoding hydroxamate-mediated iron uptake in FI*me* plasmids from epidemic *Salmonella* spp. *J. Bacteriol.* 162:307–316.

34. **Coulton, J. W.** 1982. The ferrichrome-iron receptor of *Escherichia coli* K12: antigenicity of the fhuA protein. *Biochim. Biophys. Acta* 717:154–162.

35. **Cox, C. D.** 1982. Effect of pyochelin on the virulence of *Pseudomonas aeruginosa. Infect. Immun.* 36:17–23.

36. **Cox, C. D.** 1986. Role of pyocyanin in the acquisition of iron from transferrin. *Infect. Immun.* 52:263–270.

37. **Cox, C. D., and P. Adams.** 1985. Siderophore activity of pyoverdin for *Pseudomonas aeruginosa. Infect. Immun.* 48:130–138.

38. **Crichton, R. R., and M. Charloteaux-Wauters.** 1987. Iron transport and storage. *Eur. J. Biochem.* 164:485–506.

39. **Crosa, J. H.** 1980. A plasmid associated with virulence in the marine fish pathogen *Vibrio anguillarum* specifies an iron sequestering system. *Nature* (London) 284:556–568.

40. **Crosa, J. H.** 1987. Bacterial iron metabolism, plasmids and other virulence factors, p. 139–170. *In* J. J. Bullen and E. Griffiths (ed.), *Iron and Infection: Molecular, Physiological and Clinical Aspects.* John Wiley & Sons Ltd. Chichester, England.

41. **Crosa, J. H., and L. L. Hodges.** 1981. Outer membrane proteins induced under conditions of iron limitation in the marine fish pathogen *Vibrio anguillarum. Infect. Immun.* 31:223–227.

42. **Cross, A. S., K. S. Kim, O. C. Wright, J. C. Sadoff, and P. Gemski.** 1986. Role of lipopolysaccharide and capsule in the serum resistance of bacteremic strains of *Escherichia coli. J. Infect. Dis.* 154:497–503.

43. **DeLorenzo, V., S. Wee, M. Herrero, and J. B. Neilands.** 1987. Operator sequences of the aerobactin operon of plasmid ColV-K30 binding the ferric uptake regulation (*fur*) repressor. *J. Bacteriol.* 169:2624–2630.

44. **Draper, P.** 1981. Mycobacterial inhibition of intracellular killing, p. 143–157. *In* F. O'Grady and H. Smith (ed.), *Microbial Perturbation of Host Defences.* Academic Press, Inc. (London), Ltd., London.

45. **Eaton, J. W., P. Brandt, J. R. Mahoney, and J. T. Lee.** 1982. Haptoglobin: a natural bacteriostat. *Science* 215:691–693.

46. **Ecker, D. J., B. F. Matzanke, and K. N. Raymond.** 1986. Recognition and transport of ferric enterobactin in *Escherichia coli. J. Bacteriol.* 167:666–673.

47. **Elin, R. J., and S. M. Wolff.** 1973. Effect of pH and iron concentration on growth of *Candida albicans* in human serum. *J. Infect. Dis.* 127:705–708.

48. **Fecker, L., and V. Braun.** 1987. Cloning and expression of the *fhu* genes involved in iron (III)-hydroxamate uptake by *Escherichia coli. J. Bacteriol.* 156:1301–1314.

49. **Fields, P. I., R. V. Swanson, C. G. Haidaris, and F. Heffron.** 1986. Mutants of *Salmonella typhimurium* that cannot survive within the macrophage are avirulent. *Proc. Natl. Acad. Sci. USA* 83:5189–5193.

50. **Fiss, E. H., P. Stanley-Samuelson, and J. B. Neilands.** 1982. Properties and proteolysis of ferric enterobactin outer membrane receptor in *Escherichia coli* K12. *Biochemistry* 21:4517–4522.

51. **Glynn, A. A.** 1972. Bacterial factors inhibiting host defence mechanisms, p. 75–112. *In* H. Smith and J. H. Pearce (ed.), *Microbial Pathogenicity in Man and Animals.* Society for General Microbiology Symposium no. 22. Society for General Microbiology, Reading, England.

52. **Gray, L. D., and A. S. Kreger.** 1987. Mouse skin damage caused by cytolysin from *Vibrio vulnificus* and by *V. vulnificus* infection. *J. Infect. Dis.* 155:236–241.

53. **Grewel, K. K., P. J. Warner, and P. H. Williams.** 1982. An inducible outer membrane protein involved in aerobactin mediated iron transport by ColV strains of *Escherichia coli. FEBS Lett.* 140:27–30.

54. **Griffiths, E.** 1981. Iron and the susceptibility to bacterial infection, p. 463–476. *In* R. F. Beers and E. G. Bassett (ed.), *Nutritional Factors: Modulating Effects on Metabolic Processes.* Raven Press, New York.

55. **Griffiths, E.** 1983. Availability of iron and survival of bacteria in infection, p. 150–177. *In* C. S. F. Easmon, M. Brown, and P. A. Lambert (ed.), *Medical Microbiology,* vol. 3. Academic Press, Inc. (London), Ltd., London.

56. **Griffiths, E.** 1985. Candidate virulence markers, p. 193–226. *In* M. Sussman (ed.), *The Virulence of Escherichia coli.* Society for General Microbiology Special Publication 13. Academic Press, Inc. (London), Ltd., London.

57. **Griffiths, E.** 1987. Iron in biological systems, p. 1–25. *In* J. J. Bullen and E. Griffiths (ed.), *Iron and Infection: Molecular, Physiological and Clinical Aspects.* John Wiley & Sons Ltd., Chichester, England.

58. **Griffiths, E.** 1987. The iron-uptake systems of pathogenic bacteria, p. 69–137. *In* J. J. Bullen and E. Griffiths (ed.), *Iron and Infection: Molecular, Physiological and Clinical Aspects.* John Wiley & Sons Ltd., Chichester, England.

59. **Griffiths, E., and J. J. Bullen.** 1987. Iron-binding proteins and host defence, p. 171–209. *In* J. J. Bullen and E. Griffiths (ed.), *Iron and Infection:*

Molecular, Physiological and Clinical Aspects. John Wiley & Sons Ltd., Chichester, England.

60. Griffiths, E., and J. Humphreys. 1980. Isolation of enterochelin from the peritoneal washings of guinea-pigs lethally infected with *Escherichia coli. Infect. Immun.* 28:286–289.

61. Griffiths, E., P. Stevenson, T. L. Hale, and S. B. Formal. 1985. The synthesis of aerobactin and 76,000-dalton iron-regulated outer membrane protein by *Escherichia coli* K-12–*Shigella* hybrids and by enteroinvasive strains of *Escherichia coli. Infect. Immun.* 49:67–71.

62. Griffiths, E., P. Stevenson, and P. Joyce. 1983. Pathogenic *Escherichia coli* express new outer membrane proteins when growing *in vivo. FEMS Microbiol. Lett.* 16:95–99.

63. Griffiths, E., P. Stevenson, R. Thorpe, and H. Chart. 1985. Naturally occurring antibodies in human sera that react with the iron-regulated outer membrane proteins of *Escherichia coli. Infect. Immun.* 47:808–813.

64. Griffiths, G. L., S. P. Sigel, S. M. Payne, and J. B. Neilands. 1984. Vibriobactin, a siderophore from *Vibrio cholerae. J. Biol. Chem.* 259:383–385.

65. Gutteridge, J. M. C., D. A. Rowley, E. Griffiths, and B. Halliwell. 1985. Low-molecular-weight iron complexes and oxygen radical reactions idiopathic-haemochromatosis. *Clin. Sci.* 68:463–467.

66. Hale, T. L., and S. B. Formal 1986. Genetics of virulence in *Shigella. Microb. Pathogenesis* 1:511–518.

67. Halliwell, B., and J. M. C. Gutteridge. 1985. *Free Radicals in Biology and Medicine.* Oxford University Press, Oxford.

68. Hantke, K. 1981. Regulation of ferric iron transport in *Escherichia coli* K12; isolation of a constitutive mutant. *Mol. Gen. Genet.* 182:288–292.

69. Harris, W. R., C. J. Carrano, S. R. Cooper, S. R. Sofen, A. E. Avdeef, J. V. McArdle, and K. N. Raymond. 1979. Co-ordination chemistry of microbial iron transport compounds. 19. Stability constants and electrochemical behavior of ferric enterobactin and model complexes. *J. Am. Chem. Soc.* 101:6097–6104.

70. Helms, S. D., J. D. Oliver, and J. C. Travis. 1984. Role of heme compounds and haptoglobin in *Vibrio vulnificus* pathogenicity. *Infect. Immun.* 45:345–349.

71. Hoiseth, S. K., and B. A. D. Stocker. 1981. Aromatic dependent *Salmonella typhimurium* are nonvirulent and effective as live vaccines. *Nature (London)* 291:238–239.

72. Holbein, B. E. 1980. Iron-controlled infection with *Neisseria meningitidis* in mice. *Infect. Immun.* 29:886–891.

73. Holbein, B. E. 1981. Enhancement of *Neisseria meningitidis* infection in mice by addition of iron bound to transferrin. *Infect. Immun.* 34:120–125.

74. Hollifield, W. C., Jr., and J. B. Neilands. 1978. Ferric enterobactin transport system in *Escherichia coli* K12: extraction, assay and specificity of the outer membrane receptor. *Biochemistry* 17:1922–1928.

75. Holzberg, M., and W. M. Artis. 1983. Hydroxamate siderophore production by opportunistic and systemic fungal pathogens. *Infect. Immun.* 40:1134–1137.

76. Huebers, H. A., and C. A. Finch. 1987. The physiology of transferrin and transferrin receptors. *Physiol. Rev.* 67:520–587.

77. Ismail, A., G. W. Bedell, and D. M. Lupan. 1985. Siderophore production by the pathogenic yeast *Candida albicans. Biochem. Biophys. Res. Commun.* 130:885–891.

78. Kadurugamuwa, J. L., H. Anwar, M. R. W. Brown, and O. Zak. 1985. Effect of subinhibitory concentrations of cephalosporins on surface properties and siderophore production in iron-depleted *Klebsiella pneumoniae. Antimicrob. Agents Chemother.* 27:220–223.

79. Kadurugamuwa, J. L., H. Anwar, M. R. W. Brown, and O. Zak. 1985. Protein antigens of encapsulated *Klebsiella pneumoniae* surface exposed after growth in the presence of subinhibitory concentrations of cephalosporins. *Antibmicrob. Agents Chemother.* 28:195–199.

80. Kluger, M. J., and J. J. Bullen. 1987. Clinical and physiological aspects, p. 243–282. *In* J. J. Bullen and E. Griffiths (ed.), *Iron and Infection: Molecular, Physiological and Clinical Aspects.* John Wiley & Sons Ltd., Chichester, England.

81. Kochan, I., J. Wasynczuk, and M. A. McCabe. 1978. Effects of injected iron and siderophores on infections in normal and immune mice. *Infect. Immun.* 22:560–567.

82. Konopka, K., and J. B. Neilands. 1984. Effect of serum albumin on siderophore-mediated utilization of transferrin iron. *Biochemistry* 23:2122–2127.

83. Krone, W. J. A., F. Stegehuis, G. Koningstein, C. van Doarn, B. Roosendaal, F. K. de Gray, and B. Oudega. 1985. Characterization of the pColV-K30 encoded cloacin DF13/aerobactin outer membrane receptor protein of *Escherichia coli,* isolation and purification of the protein and analysis of its nucleotide sequence and primary structure. *FEMS Microbiol. Lett.* 26:153–161.

84. Lam, C., F. Turnowsky, E. Schwarzinger, and W. Neruda. 1984. Bacteria recovered without subculture from infected human urines expressed iron-regulated outer membrane proteins. *FEMS Microbiol. Lett.* 24:255–259.

85. Lankford, C. E. 1973. Bacterial assimilation of iron. *Crit. Rev. Microbiol.* 2:273–331.

86. Lawlor, K. M., P. A. Daskaleros, R. E. Robinson, and S. M. Payne. 1987. Virulence of iron transport mutants of *Shigella flexneri* and utilization

of host iron compounds. *Infect. Immun.* 55:594–599.

87. Lawlor, K. M., and S. M. Payne. 1984. Aerobactin genes in *Shigella* spp. *J. Bacteriol.* 160:266 272.

88. Lee, J. T., Jr., D. H. Ahrenhoz, R. D. Nelson, and R. L. Simmons. 1979. Mechanisms of the adjuvant effect of hemoglobin in experimental peritonitis. V. The significance of the co-ordinated iron component. *Surgery* 86:41–48.

89. Letendre, E. D., and B. E. Holbein. 1983. Turnover in the transferrin iron pool during the hypoferremic phase of experimental *Neisseria meningitidis* infection in mice. *Infect. Immun.* 39:50–59.

90. Letendre, E. D., and B. E. Holbein. 1984. Mechanism of impaired iron release by the reticuloendothelial system during the hypoferremic phase of experimental *Neisseria meningitidis* infection in mice. *Infect. Immun.* 44:320–325.

91. Linggood, M. A., M. Roberts, S. Ford, S. H. Parry, and P. H. Williams. 1987. Incidence of the aerobactin iron uptake system among *Escherichia coli* isolates from infections of farm animals. *J. Gen. Microbiol.* 133:835–842.

92. Loo, V. G., and R. G. Lalonde. 1984. Role of iron in intracellular growth of *Trypanosoma cruzi*. *Infect. Immun.* 45:726–730.

93. Mattie, H. 1984. Animal models in antibacterial drug research. *J. Antimicrob. Chemother.* 14:101–104.

94. McDougall, S., and J. B. Neilands. 1984. Plasmid and chromosome-coded aerobactin synthesis in enteric bacteria: insertion sequences flank operon in plasmid-mediated systems. *J. Bacteriol.* 159:300–305.

95. Mickelsen, P. A., E. Blackman, and P. F. Sparling. 1982. Ability of *Neisseria gonorrhoeae*, *Neisseria meningitidis*, and commensal *Neisseria* species to obtain iron from lactoferrin. *Infect. Immun.* 35:915–920.

96. Mickelsen, P. A., and P. F. Sparling. 1981. Ability of *Neisseria gonorrhoeae*, *Neisseria meningitidis*, and commensal *Neisseria* species to obtain iron from transferrin and iron compounds. *Infect. Immun.* 33:555–564.

97. Mietzner, T. A., G. H. Luginbuhl, E. Sandstrom, and S. A. Morse. 1984. Identification of an iron-regulated 37,000-dalton protein in the cell envelope of *Neisseria gonorrhoeae*. *Infect. Immun.* 45:410–416.

98. Moll, A., P. A. Manning, and K. N. Timmis. 1980. Plasmid-determined resistance to serum bactericidal activity: a major outer membrane protein, the *traT* gene product, is responsible for plasmid-specified serum resistance in *Escherichia coli*. *Infect. Immun.* 28:359–367.

99. Montgomerie, J. Z., A. Bindereif, J. B. Neilands, G. M. Kahmanson, and L. B. Guze. 1984. Association of hydroxamate siderophore (aerobatin) with *Escherichia coli* isolated from patients with bacteremia. *Infect. Immun.* 46:835–838.

100. Morgan, E. H. 1981. Transferrin, biochemistry, physiology and clinical significance. *Mol. Aspects. Med.* 4:1–123.

101. Nassif, X., and P. J. Sansonetti. 1986. Correlation of the virulence of *Klebsiella pneumoniae* K1 and K2 with the presence of a plasmid encoding aerobactin. *Infect. Immun.* 54:603–608.

102. Neilands, J. B. 1981. Microbial iron compounds. *Annu. Rev. Biochem.* 50:715–731.

103. Neilands, J. B. 1982. Microbial envelope proteins related to iron. *Annu. Rev. Microbiol.* 36:285–309.

104. Norqvist, A., J. Davies, L. Norlander, and S. Normark. 1978. The effect of iron starvation on the outer membrane protein composition of *Neisseria gonorrhoeae*. *FEMS Microbiol. Lett.* 4:71–75.

105. O'Brien, I. G., and F. Gibson. 1970. The structure of enterochelin and related 2,3-dihydroxy-N-benzoylserine conjugates from *Escherichia coli*. *Biochim. Biophys. Acta* 215:393–402.

106. Ogata, R. T., C. Wintens, and R. P. Levine. 1982. Nucleotide sequence analysis of the complement resistance gene from plasmid R100. *J. Bacteriol.* 151:819–827.

107. Opal, S., A. Cross, and P. Gemski. 1982. K antigen and serum sensitivity of rough *Escherichia coli*. *Infect. Immun.* 37:956–960.

108. Payne, S. M., and R. A. Finkelstein. 1978. The critical role of iron in host-bacterial interactions. *J. Clin. Invest.* 61:1428–1440.

109. Payne, S. M., D. W. Neisel, S. S. Peixotto, and K. M. Lawlor. 1983. Expression of hydroxamate and phenolate siderophores by *Shigella flexneri*. *J. Bacteriol.* 155:949–955.

110. Perez-Casal, J. F., and J. H. Crosa. 1984. Aerobactin iron uptake sequences in plasmid ColV-K30 are flanked by inverted IS1-like elements and replication regions. *J. Bacteriol.* 160:256–265.

111. Perry, R. D., and R. R. Brubaker. 1979. Accumulation of iron by *Yersiniae*. *J. Bacteriol.* 137:1290–1298.

112. Perry, R. D., and C. L. San Clemente. 1979. Siderophore synthesis in *Klebsiella pneumoniae* and *Shigella sonnei* during iron deficiency. *J. Bacteriol.* 140:1129–1132.

113. Peto, T. E. A., and J. L. Thompson. 1986. A reappraisal of the effects of iron and desferrioxamine on the growth of *Plasmodium falciparum* 'in vitro': the unimportance of serum iron. *Br. J. Haematol.* 63:273–280.

114. Plaha, D. S., and H. J. Rogers. 1987. Effect of osmotic shock and shearing forces on ferric enterochelin transport in *Escherichia coli* K12. *J. Gen. Microbiol.* 133:1227–1234.

115. Pollack, J. R., and J. B. Neilands. 1970. Enterobactin, an iron transport compound from *Salmonella typhimurium*. *Biochem. Biophys. Res. Commun.* 38:989–992.

116. Pollack, S., and J. Fleming. 1984. *Plasmodium falciparum* takes up iron from transferrin. *Br. J. Haematol.* 58:289–293.

117. Prody, C. A., and J. B. Neilands. 1984. Genetic and biochemical characterization of the *Escherichia coli* K-12 *fhu* mutation. *J. Bacteriol.* 157:874–880.

118. Rangneker, V. M., D. D. Banker, and H. I. Jhala. 1983. Antimicrobial resistance and incompatibility groups of R plasmids in *Salmonella typhimurium* isolated from human sources in Bombay from 1978 to 1980. *Antimicrob. Agents Chemother.* 23:54–58.

119. Raymond, K. N., and C. J. Carrano. 1979. Coordination chemistry of microbial iron transport. *Acc. Chem. Res.* 12:183–190.

120. Robbins, J. B., R. Schneerson, W. B. Egan, W. Vann, and D. T. Liu. 1980. Virulence properties of bacterial capsular polysaccharide—unanswered questions, p. 115–132. *In* H. Smith, J. J. Skehel, and M. J. Turner (ed.), *The Molecular Basis of Microbial Pathogenicity*. Verlag Chemie GmbH, Weinheim, Federal Republic of Germany.

121. Rogers, H. J. 1973. Iron-binding catechols and virulence in *Escherichia coli*. *Infect. Immun.* 7:445–456.

122. Rogers, H. J., C. Synge, B. Kimber, and P. M. Bayley. 1977. Production of enterochelin by *Escherichia coli* O111. *Biochim. Biophys. Acta* 497:548–557.

123. Russell, L. M., S. J. Cryz, Jr., and R. K. Holmes. 1984. Genetic and biochemical evidence for a siderophore-dependent iron transport system in *Corynebacterium diphtheriae*. *Infect. Immun.* 45:143–149.

124. Russell, L. M., and R. K. Holmes. 1983. Initial characterization of the ferric iron transport system of *Corynebacterium diphtheriae*. *J. Bacteriol.* 155:1439–1442.

125. Russell, L. M., and R. K. Holmes. 1985. Highly toxigenic but avirulent Park-Williams 8 strain of *Corynebacterium diphtheriae* does not produce siderophore. *Infect. Immun.* 47:575–578.

126. Sciortino, C. V., and R. A. Finkelstein. 1983. *Vibrio cholerae* expresses iron-regulated outer membrane proteins *in vivo*. *Infect. Immun.* 42:990–996.

127. Shand, G. H., H. Anwar, J. Kadurugamuwa, M. R. W. Brown, S. H. Silverman, and J. Melling. 1985. *In vivo* evidence that bacteria in urinary tract infection grow under iron-restricted conditions. *Infect. Immun.* 48:35–39.

128. Sigel, S. P., J. A. Stoebner, and S. M. Payne. 1985. Iron-vibriobactin transport system is not required for virulence of *Vibrio cholerae*. *Infect. Immun.* 47:360–362.

129. Simonson, C., D. Brener, and I. W. DeVoe. 1982. Expression of a high-affinity mechanism for acquisition of transferrin iron by *Neisseria meningitidis*. *Infect. Immun.* 36:107–113.

130. Smith, H. 1976. Survival of vegetative bacteria in animals. *Symp. Soc. Gen. Microbiol.* 26:299–326.

131. Smith, H. W., and M. B. Huggins. 1980. The association of the O18 K1 and H7 antigens and the ColV plasmid of a strain of *Escherichia coli* with its virulence and immunogenicity. *J. Gen. Microbiol.* 121:387–400.

132. Sokol, P. A. 1986. Production and utilization of pyochelin by clinical isolates of *Pseudomonas cepacia*. *J. Clin. Microbiol.* 23:560–562.

133. Stuart, S. J., J. K. T. Greenwood, and R. K. J. Luke. 1982. Iron-suppressible production of hydroxamate by *Escherichia coli* isolates. *Infect. Immun.* 36:870–875.

134. Taetle, R., K. Rhyner, J. Castagnola, D. To, and J. Mendelsohn. 1985. Role of transferrin, Fe and transferrin receptors in myeloid leukemia cell growth; studies with an antitransferrin receptor monoclonal antibody. *J. Clin. Invest.* 75:1061–1067.

135. Testa, U. 1985. Transferrin receptors: structure and function. *Curr. Top. Hematol.* 5:127–161.

136. Tidmarsh, G. F., P. E. Klebba, and L. T. Rosenberg. 1983. Rapid release of iron from ferritin by siderophores. *J. Inorg. Biochem.* 18:161–168.

137. Toranzo, A. E., J. L. Barja, S. A. Potter, R. R. Colwell, F. M. Hetrich, and J. H. Crosa. 1983. Molecular factors associated with virulence of marine vibrios isolated from striped bass in Chesapeake Bay. *Infect. Immun.* 39:1220–1227.

138. Trowbridge, I. S., R. A. Newman, D. L. Domingo, and C. Sauvage. 1984. Transferrin receptors: structure and function. *Biochem. Pharmacol.* 33:925–932.

139. Trowbridge, I. S., and M. B. Omary. 1981. Human cell surface glycoprotein related to cell proliferation is the receptor for transferrin. *Proc. Natl. Acad. Sci. USA* 78:3039–3043.

140. Valvano, M. A., and J. H. Crosa. 1984. Aerobactin iron transport genes commonly encoded by certain ColV plasmids occur in the chromosome of a human invasive strain of *Escherichia coli* K1. *Infect. Immun.* 46:159–167.

141. Valvano, M. A., R. P. Silver, and J. H. Crosa. 1986. Occurrence of chromosome- or plasmid-mediated aerobactin iron transport systems and hemolysin production among clonal groups of human invasive strains of *Escherichia coli* K1. *Infect. Immun.* 52:192–199.

142. Van der Ley, P., P. DeGraaff, and J. Tommassen. 1986. Shielding of *Escherichia coli* outer membrane proteins as receptors for bacteriophages and colicins by O-antigenic chains of lipopolysaccharide. *J. Bacteriol.* 168:449–451.

143. Van der Ley, P., O. Knipers, J. Tommassen, and B. Lugtenberg. 1986. O-antigenic chains of lipopolysaccharide prevent binding of antibody molecules to an outer membrane pore protein in *Enter-*

obacteriaceae. Microb. Pathogenesis 1:43–49.

144. Waters, V. L., and J. H. Crosa. 1986. DNA environment of the aerobactin iron uptake system genes in prototype ColV plasmids. *J. Bacteriol.* 167:647–654.

145. Wendenbaum, S., P. Demange, A. Dell, J. M. Meyer, and M. A. Abdallah. 1983. The structure of pyoverdine Pa, the siderophore of *Pseudomonas aeruginosa. Tetrahedron Lett.* 24:4877–4880.

146. West, S. E. H., and P. F. Sparling. 1985. Response of *Neisseria gonorrhoeae* to iron limitation: alteration in expression of membrane proteins without apparent siderophore production. *Infect. Immun.* 47:388–394.

147. Williams, P. H., and N. H. Carbonetti. 1986.

Iron, siderophores, and the pursuit of virulence: independence of the aerobactin and enterochelin iron uptake systems in *Escherichia coli. Infect. Immun.* 51:942–947.

148. Yancey, R. J., S. A. L. Breeding, and C. E. Lankford. 1979. Enterochelin (enterobactin): virulence factor for *Salmonella typhimurium. Infect. Immun.* 24:174–180.

149. Yancey, R. J., and R. A. Finkelstein. 1981. Siderophore production by pathogenic *Neisseria* spp. *Infect. Immun.* 32:600–608.

150. Zapolski, E. J., and J. V. Princiotto. 1976. Failure of rabbit reticulocytes to incorporate conalbumin or lactoferrin iron. *Biochim. Biophys. Acta* 421:80–86.

Section III: Bacterial Resistance to Cellular Defense Mechanisms

Chapter 9

Bacterial Evasion of Cellular Defense Mechanisms: an Overview

Charles J. Czuprynski

Department of Pathobiological Sciences
School of Veterinary Medicine
University of Wisconsin
Madison, Wisconsin 53706

INTRODUCTION

The vigilance of mammalian cellular defense mechanisms is critical for successful resistance against the horde of bacteria that are encountered daily. The complex cellular and molecular interactions that regulate cellular defenses usually provide a decisive advantage to the host. Pathogenic bacteria, however, have developed a wide array of strategies to circumvent the cellular defenses of their intended host. The explosive growth of the literature on cellular defense mechanisms and bacterial evasion of these mechanisms makes a comprehensive review of the subject an almost unachievable goal. Previous authors have provided detailed examinations of various aspects of this subject; these earlier treatises amplify the material presented here (49, 71, 89, 142, 182, 187). My objectives in this review are severalfold. First, I briefly describe the principal events required for successful elimination of invading bacteria by host leukocytes. Second, I consider some of the tactics that have been devised by bacteria to evade this cellular response. Although I view the battle between phagocytic cells and bacteria as central to the process of cellular defense, the influence of pathogenic bacteria on related responses, such as lymphocyte activation, is of obvious relevance and is considered as well. Finally, I briefly discuss recent information about the immunoregulation of phagocyte antibacterial activity. My goal throughout this review is to identify mechanisms of bacterial resistance common to the cellular defenses of humans and domestic animals. I hope that this general approach will provide an overview that might prove useful for subsequent evaluation of specific bacterial pathogens in both human and veterinary medicine.

GENERAL EVENTS IN CELLULAR ANTIBACTERIAL DEFENSE

Resistance to pathogenic microorganisms requires the careful orchestration of a series of molecular and cellular interactions. During the past few years considerable progress has been made in elucidating the mechanistic basis of this response. Broadly speaking, the requisite events for a successful cellular response are as follows: (i) directed migration of resident and blood-borne phagocytes; (ii) attachment and ingestion of bacteria; (iii) stimulation of oxidative burst; (iv) phagosome-lysosome fusion; (v) activation of specific immune response; (vi) phagocyte response to cytokines; and (vii) removal of bacterial and cellular debris. The initial defense is provided by local phagocytic cells (principally mononuclear phagocytes) that normally reside in most, if not all, tissue. If the bacterial inoculum is relatively low in number and virulence, these resident macrophages may be sufficient to contain the threat of bacterial infection. If the bacterial inoculum is of greater magnitude, or if the invading bacteria multiply rapidly at the site of primary inoculation, it is likely that the host will recruit polymorphonuclear and mononuclear phagocytes from the bloodstream to aid in local defense of the infected tissue. The directed migration of phagocytic cells, which may be in response to stimuli of either bacterial (171) or host (184) origin, is therefore an essential early event in antibacterial resistance. Once they have entered the focus of infection, the phagocytes must pursue and attach to the invading bacteria. Although in certain instances binding may occur in the absence of identifiable opsonins on the bacterial surface (203), the presence of serum opsonins (e.g., immunoglobulin G, C3b, and other plasma proteins) usually facilitates this process (89). After binding has occurred, the phagocyte will attempt to internalize the attached bacteria into an invaginated plasma membrane-lined vesicle called a phagosome. Perturbation of the phagocyte plasma membrane during this process triggers an intracellular cascade that results in activation and mobilization of cytochrome oxidase to the inner surface of the phagosome and transportation of lysosomes to the phagosome, with which they fuse and extrude their granule contents into the resulting phagolysosome (49, 71). Concomitant with this process is a progressive decrease in the pH of the phagosome and a marked increase in both oxygen uptake and glucose utilization via the hexose-monophosphate pathway. The last two events provide energy and reducing power for the stepwise reduction of oxygen to water, resulting in production of a number of highly reactive oxygen intermediates (e.g., hydroxyl radical, superoxide anion, and hydrogen peroxide) (71). The sum of these events creates an intravacuolar environment that is extremely hostile to many bacteria because of the reduced pH (90), the presence of microbicidal oxygen intermediates (14), and the lytic and degradative capabilities of the peptides and hydrolases that are released into the phagolysosome during granule fusion (188). These events occur quite rapidly and may cause irreversible bacterial injury within minutes. In these cases there may be no need for intervention by the immune system. In instances when the invading bacteria succeed in avoiding or surviving ingestion, however, the host must initiate an appropriate immune response to augment the defense mechanisms that the bacteria have eluded. The final task facing a vertebrate host in its struggle with pathogenic bacteria is to degrade and eliminate the resulting bacterial and cellular debris so that normal tissue architecture can be maintained or restored.

The above is, of course, a very simplistic outline of the actual process of cellular defense. Failure to accomplish any one of the steps involved in this process, however, may allow continued multiplication of the invading bacteria and result in either local or systemic tissue damage. There are ample examples of pathogenic bacteria that circumvent one or more of the events outlined above. In some instances the bacteria use guile to sidestep cellular defenses in a fashion that may be nearly imperceptible. Under other circumstances, the bacteria become the aggressors and unleash an attack against host leukocytes that compromises the function of the leukocytes or even causes their demise. In the remainder of this paper, I discuss examples of tactics that have been developed by bacteria to avoid destruction by host cells. Although I do not claim that this examination is all-inclusive, I hope to give sufficient specific examples to illustrate the common strategies used by pathogenic bacteria of humans and domestic animals.

EFFECTS OF BACTERIA ON LEUKOCYTE LOCOMOTION

There is substantial in vitro evidence for the directed migration of leukocytes toward bacteria or bacterial products. This response may be stimulated by a component of the bacterium itself, such as the N-formylated tripeptides (68), or it may require the presence of serum for the cotaxigenic generation of chemoattractants such as C5a (184). Similar responses in vivo are presumed to be critical for mobilization of leukocytes to sites of infection. In contrast to the stimulatory effects of bacteria on leukocyte locomotion, there is considerable evidence that toxins produced by a diverse group of bacteria (e.g., streptolysin O, perfringolysin, staphylococcal alpha toxin and leucocidin, cholera toxin, and pertussis toxin) can impede the directed migration of leukocytes toward various chemoattractants. This subject has received careful reviews (6, 218), which provide additional information regarding the cell biology of these effects. These principally in vitro studies are supported by reported alterations in neutrophil chemotactic activity during bacterial infection. In separate studies, active bacterial infection was reported to enhance (87, 157) and decrease (134) locomotion by neutrophils. Differences in donor age, type and severity of infection, and prior antibiotic therapy may account for the discrepancies among these reports. Perhaps neutrophil migration may be either enhanced or depressed, depending on the time at which activity is assessed, during a single episode of infection. Temporal evaluation of alterations in neutrophil migratory activity during bacterial infection is required to address this point. Defective neutrophil chemotaxis during lepromatous leprosy has been reported (208) and confirmed (207). In both studies, preincubation of neutrophils from healthy controls, with serum or plasma from lepromatous patients, reduced neutrophil chemotaxis in vitro. It is not clear whether these effects were mediated directly by circulating products of *Mycobacterium leprae* or whether they required the production of humoral factors by the host that impaired neutrophil chemotaxis.

AVOIDANCE OF PHAGOCYTOSIS

Capsular Polysaccharide

Once the host leukocytes have detected and migrated toward a site of bacterial invasion, they must first attach to and then internalize the offending microorganisms. Bacteria have adapted various strategies for circumventing this process. One crude but effective mechanism of eluding phagocytosis may be simply to grow as aggregates or filaments that are sufficiently large to discourage easy ingestion by phagocytes. This strategy may explain in part the chronic, progressive lesions formed by members of the *Actinomycetales* such as *Actinomyces viscosus* (167) and *Dermatophilus congolensis* (2). In addition, some of the *Actinomycetales* produce surface components that under normal conditions stimulate release of inflammatory mediators by neutrophils (167) and induce lymphocyte proliferation (54). The net result provides the bacteria with an extracellular nidus from which they can provoke the intense and prolonged inflammatory response that characterizes mycetoma and other types of actinomycotic infections.

The most familiar strategy of bacterial avoidance of phagocytosis is the production of antiphagocytic surface components, either polysaccharide or protein in nature, that prevent the phagocytes from successfully internalizing their prey. The mechanisms by which encapsulated bacteria resist phagocytosis may include decreased binding of serum opsonins (205), inaccessibility of ligands (e.g., immunoglobulin G and C3b) required for phagocyte binding (153, 217), and decreased hydrophobicity of the bacterial surface (203); detailed discussions are given in previous reviews of this subject (49, 89, 184, 187). A classic example of the role of an antiphagocytic polysaccharide capsule in the pathogenesis of bacterial infection is provided by pneumococci (129). Numerous other examples in human and veterinary microbiology have been recorded, including *Escherichia coli* (79, 86, 92, 190), *Staphylococcus aureus* (4, 153, 217), *Bacteroides fragilis* (179),

Pasteurella haemolytica (1, 43), *Pasteurella multocida* (130), *Corynebacterium equi* (219), *Streptococcus equi* (219), *Haemophilus influenzae* (98), *Klebsiella pneumoniae* (183), and *Neisseria meningitidis* (160).

Protein Antiphagocytic Determinants

Other bacteria produce peptide antiphagocytic structures that may form a capsule-like outer layer (as on *Bacillus anthracis* [106]) or projections such as the M protein of group A streptococci (60) and the fimbriae of group E streptococci (46). In certain instances the presence of some of these structures might actually be detrimental to the bacteria. Pili on *Pseudomonas aeruginosa* (186), oral *Actinomyces* spp. (167), and *E. coli* (13, 131), which facilitate adherence to epithelial cells, also promote attachment and ingestion of the bacteria by phagocytes. Apparently these bacteria gain more from pilus-mediated enhanced adherence to their favored niche (mucosal epithelium) than they lose by being at increased risk of destruction by phagocytes.

Inconspicuous Adherence

Some bacteria readily attach to phagocytic cells but manage to avoid subsequent internalization. They then proliferate on the leukocyte surface in defiance of the antimicrobial arsenal of their adjacent neighbor. This mode of pathogenesis is perhaps best demonstrated by the mycoplasmas. These small procaryotes, which lack even the physical barrier of a peptidoglycan outer layer, may quietly persist on the cell surface for long periods without announcing their presence (as has been woefully noted by many investigators working with lymphocytes or other cells in culture). The effects of this symbiotic relationship may be benign or even inapparent, depending on the mycoplasmal species involved, the cell surface being used as a residence, and the extracellular milieu. Mycoplasmas are not invincible, as has been demonstrated by the ability of specific antibodies to promote ingestion and killing of mycoplasmas by neutrophils and macrophages

(193). Under certain conditions, however, some mycoplasmas compromise the ability of phagocytes to ingest and kill a second bacterial target (93). This may be one mechanism by which mycoplasmas contribute to respiratory disease in humans and domestic animals. Mycoplasmas also can have particularly striking effects on the activity of T and B lymphocytes. When mycoplasmas bind to lymphocytes, they induce capping on the lymphocyte surface, which stimulates lymphocyte proliferation much as do mitogenic lectins (194). This inappropriate stimulation of lymphocytes, which has been mistaken for lymphokine activity in some experimental systems (163), has been proposed to contribute to autoimmune phenomena such as rheumatoid arthritis (189).

Besides mycoplasmas, gonococci also may persist, and perhaps even thrive, in intimate association with leukocytes (24, 50). Some strains of gonococci adhere to neutrophils via pili, but appear to be resistant to internalization (114, 115). There is controversy in the literature regarding the susceptibility of gonococci to neutrophil antimicrobial activity (48, 195). These discrepancies may result from differences in the target strain and assay conditions used in the various studies. There seems to be general agreement that even when internalized, a percentage of gonococci are resistant to killing and are able to survive for extended periods (31, 204). It has been proposed that part of the oxidative burst that can be detected by various means during the interaction of neutrophils and gonococci may actually represent increased respiration by the gonococci (23). Unpublished data suggest that lactate released by the neutrophils may be the component that stimulates gonococcal oxidative activity (M. Cohen, unpublished data).

PARASITIZATION OF NONPROFESSIONAL PHAGOCYTES

One mechanism by which bacteria can minimize their interaction with the cellular defenses of the host is to enter and multiply within nonprofessional phagocytes. Although this mode of pathogenesis is well recognized for the preferential infection of endothelial and epithelial cells by rickettsiae and chlamydiae, respectively, it receives infrequent consideration in regard to the pathogenesis of other bacteria that have demonstrated the ability to enter and grow within various cell types (at least in vitro). *Shigella* spp. and invasive *E. coli* both use this strategy when they invade intestinal epithelial cells (80, 168). Evidence, both direct and indirect, has also been provided for invasion of nonphagocytic cells by *Listeria monocytogenes* (9, 85, 223) and *Brucella abortus* (76). The significance of these observations to the natural pathogenesis of the infections caused by these agents requires further investigation. An intracellular site, however, may not provide the bacteria with the privileged niche they seek. Recent evidence suggests that cloned cytotoxic T cells can recognize and lyse, in a class I antigen-restricted fashion, macrophages infected with *L. monocytogenes* (47) or *M. leprae* (38). These data raise the possibility that infection of nonphagocytic cells, which universally express class I antigens, also results in assault by cytotoxic T cells, much as has been described for virus-infected cells.

Two families of bacteria (related to the rickettsiae) that are unique to veterinary medicine deserve mention at this time. These are the *Haemobartonellaceae* and the *Anaplasmataceae*. These organisms parasitize the erythrocytes of dogs and cats (*Haemobartonella* spp.) and ruminants (*Anaplasma* spp.), respectively. These tick-borne agents cause anemia that can vary in severity from mild to life-threatening. *Haemobartonella* spp. are epicellular pathogens that reside within invaginations on the erythrocyte membrane (82), whereas *Anaplasma* spp. can be visualized as inclusion bodies within Giemsa-stained erythrocytes (99). In most instances haemobartonellosis and anaplasmosis result in chronic infections, suggesting that the association of these microorganisms with erythrocytes promotes evasion of host defense mechanisms. Although bacterial pathogens of human erythrocytes have been reported periodically,

they are not routinely perceived as a significant health problem (159).

SURVIVAL AND GROWTH WITHIN PROFESSIONAL PHAGOCYTES

A number of bacteria have solved the problem of dealing with cellular defense mechanisms by adapting to life within phagocytes. Because neutrophils are relatively short-lived cells that probably do not allow prolonged intracellular multiplication of bacteria, most of the attention in this area has focused on parasitization of mononuclear phagocytes (e.g., macrophages). A partial list of these important facultative intracellular pathogens of humans and animals includes *Mycobacterium tuberculosis* (127), *Mycobacterium paratuberculosis* (224), *Legionella pneumophila* (91), *Yersinia pestis* (191, 192), *B. abortus* (59), *L. monocytogenes* (128), *Nocardia asteroides* (21), *Salmonella typhimurium* (56), *Francisella tularensis* (61), *Haemophilus somnus* (116), and *Rhodococcus equi* (53). For some of these organisms there is considerable evidence for the role of virulence determinants that allow the bacteria to thwart the antibacterial action of the phagocyte (25, 36, 201, 202), whereas for other species there is little information available at present. It is likely that genetic factors of both the host and the microorganism influence the success of intracellular parasitism for any given pathogen (17, 121, 154, 211).

In addition to the facultative intracellular pathogens listed above, we must also consider the obligate intracellular pathogens *Rickettsia* and *Chlamydia* spp. The latter are discussed in detail in Chapter 10 of this volume. Both *Rickettsia* and *Chlamydia* spp. are specialized intracellular pathogens that can multiply within mononuclear phagocytes, although that cell type is not necessarily the preferred host cell. An exception to this statement is provided by the rickettsial agent *Ehrlichia canis,* which preferentially and persistently infects mononuclear phagocytes in dogs (77). Some of the mechanisms used by the obligate and facultative intracellular bacterial pathogens to avoid intracellular destruction are discussed separately below.

Perturbations of the Phagolysosome

After a bacterium has been internalized, the normal progression results in the fusion of lysosomes with the membrane-bound bacterium to form a phagolysosome. *Rickettsia tsutsugamushi* (158), *M. leprae* (141), and *M. tuberculosis* (143) have been reported to escape from disrupted phagosomes or phagolysosomes and obtain refuge in the more hospitable environment of the cytoplasm.

Other intracellular bacteria have devised a somewhat different strategy. Although these bacteria remain within an intact phagosome, lysosomal fusion with the bacteria-containing phagosome is blocked. This protects the ingested bacteria from the peptides and lysosomal enzymes present in the lysosomal granules. This observation was first made by Armstrong and Hart (8), who noted that fusion of ferritin-labeled secondary lysosomes did not occur, as evaluated by electron microscopy, with phagosomes that contained viable virulent *M. tuberculosis*. Phagosome-lysosome fusion was not impaired when nonviable or opsonized viable bacilli were used. Similar observations have been made with *Mycobacterium avium* (63) and with *Mycobacterium microti* and *Mycobacterium lepraemurium,* although for the last two species fusion was inhibited in macrophages (125) but not in neutrophils (181). Inhibition of phagosome-lysosome fusion also has been documented for *B. abortus*-infected (64) and *Chlamydia*-infected (196) macrophages. A series of reports by Goren and co-workers suggested that inhibition of fusion by *M. tuberculosis* was mediated by sulfatides: a finding that was subsequently extended to other polyanionic agents (73). This conclusion has recently been reevaluated in the same laboratory (74, 75); a detailed discussion of this analysis is contained in Chapter 11 of this volume. These recent observations bring into question the extent to which inhibition of

phagosome-lysosome fusion occurs and the validity of various methodologies that have been used to determine its occurrence. Nonetheless, it is likely that inhibition of fusion contributes to the intracellular survival of at least some intracellular pathogens.

Avoidance of Oxygen-Dependent Killing Mechanisms

Phagocytes are thought to rely heavily on a potent array of reactive oxygen intermediates, formed during the oxidative burst that accompanies phagocytosis, for killing ingested bacteria (14). It is therefore not surprising that bacteria have developed various tactics for evading the oxidative attack of phagocytes. Some bacteria fail to stimulate an oxidative burst when they are ingested, or they elicit an oxidative burst that is weak and short-lived. This strategy has been adopted by *Yersinia enterocolitica* (120), *Salmonella typhi* (111, 136), *H. somnus* (44), *Mycobacterium intracellulare* (67), *M. leprae* (88), *Actinobacillus actinomycetemcomitans* (137), and *M. paratuberculosis* (B. Zurbrick, D. Follett, and C. Czuprynski, submitted for publication). The effects of *Y. enterocolitica* were shown to be dependent on plasmid-mediated expression of outer membrane proteins (120). The weak oxidative response elicited from bovine neutrophils by *H. somnus* may be related to the presence of high-molecular-weight cell wall components (94) and low-molecular-weight nucleotides of *H. somnus* (37) that are reported to inhibit neutrophil function. The resistance of *B. abortus* to phagocyte-mediated killing has been correlated with a reduced oxidative response attributed to the presence of a smooth lipopolysaccharide (LPS) (112) or the putative release of nucleotides that compromise neutrophil function (18, 29, 30). The effects of *B. abortus* may be related to the conditions used: some investigators have reported limited killing of *B. abortus* (222) and elicitation of a respectable oxidative response upon ingestion of opsonized *B. abortus* organisms by neutrophils (J. R. Taylor, M.S. thesis, Auburn University, Auburn, Ala., 1981).

Rather than diminishing the oxidative response of the phagocyte, other bacteria survive the oxidative onslaught by virtue of their resistance to the various oxygen radicals that are produced. Superoxide dismutase has been suggested to protect *N. asteroides* (57, 58) and *L. monocytogenes* (215) against killing by phagocytes, although evidence discounting the importance of oxidative killing of *L. monocytogenes* has also been reported (70, 83). Catalase activity appears to be associated with the resistance of *S. aureus* (133) and *Neisseria gonorrheae* (7) to killing by human neutrophils. Other investigators have noted examples of substantial resistance to oxidative attack that were not obviously related to levels of either superoxide dismutase or catalase (95).

Resistance to Oxygen-Independent Killing

Besides the oxygen-dependent mechanisms described above, phagocytes also exert a number of oxygen-independent killing mechanisms against intracellular bacteria (117, 132, 188, 214). These include acidification of the phagosome and release of various peptides and degradative enzymes into the phagolysosome during degranulation. *L. pneumophila* (90) inhibited phagosome acidification of monocytes obtained from a single donor. This effect, which required viable *L. pneumophila* cells, may be biologically relevant in light of the pH sensitivity of *L. pneumophila* for growth on artificial media. Workers in several laboratories have described the presence of highly microbicidal cationic peptides in neutrophils and macrophages (117, 188, 214). Bovine neutrophils are reported to be a particularly rich source of these peptides (170). Although the described molecular nature of these peptides varies somewhat among laboratories, as does the list of susceptible bacterial targets, it is likely that these antimicrobial components are similar in their modes of action and exert their effects principally via damage to bacterial membranes (117, 188, 214). Resistance of gram-negative bacteria to these agents is greater for smooth- than rough-LPS strains (138, 173). The antibacter-

ial activity of these peptides is enhanced at the reduced pH that would occur within the phagolysosome (174). Anaerobiosis reduces, but does not eliminate, the antibacterial activity of these peptides (31).

Role of Iron

The promotion of bacterial virulence by iron and iron-containing compounds is a well-recognized phenomenon. A detailed review of the list of bacteria so affected is given elsewhere (210). Iron is likely to be especially important for bacteria that establish long-term residence within macrophages. This situation becomes particularly critical for certain organisms, such as *M. paratuberculosis,* that are exquisitely dependent on an adequate extracellular source of iron for their growth (12). Recent evidence suggests that macrophages accumulating in the granulomatous lesions that develop in the intestinal mucosa during bovine paratuberculosis contain ferritin, lactoferrin, and transferrin (140). This observation suggests that the redistribution of iron in the granulomatous lesions of chronic infections may provide intracellular bacteria with a source of iron that could be utilized for intracellular growth (152).

INFLUENCE OF BACTERIAL PRODUCTS ON LEUKOCYTE FUNCTION

Effects of LPS

The pluripotential biological effects of bacterial LPS have been the subject of numerous investigations. Thorough discussion of these effects and their implications for host defense have been reviewed in great detail (155); I will therefore touch only briefly on this subject. It would seem that the spectrum of biological effects mediated by LPS is limited chiefly by the imagination and persistence of the investigator. Nonetheless, there appears to be general agreement on certain effects of LPS that are pertinent to host defense. Bacterial LPS is probably the most frequently described second signal for activation of macrophage cytotoxic activity. The importance of this biological response has been clearly demonstrated for macrophage-mediated killing of tumor and protozoal targets. Although it is inferred that a similar process is critical for antibacterial resistance, elucidation of the molecular basis for immunoregulation of macrophage antibacterial activity requires additional investigation. Neutrophils appear to be readily influenced by LPS. Purified rough LPS or lipid A, but not smooth LPS, induces neutrophil chemiluminescence (102). Conversely, pretreatment with high doses of LPS was shown to inhibit human neutrophil bactericidal activity and depress the oxidative burst (156). More recent evidence suggests that LPS, and other bacterial products such as muramyl dipeptide, can prime neutrophils for an enhanced oxidative response to various stimuli (78) and induce cytoskeletal alterations that may be related to locomotive activity (84). These in vitro observations are consistent with the hypothesis that promiscuous activation of neutrophils by LPS in vivo, as a sequela to traumatic injury or infection, may contribute to the neutrophil-mediated tissue damage that can be observed in diseases such as adult respiratory distress syndrome (220). In addition to its effects on neutrophils, LPS performs a defensive function by protecting enterobacteria against the antimicrobial activity of neutrophil-derived cationic peptides (138, 173).

Exotoxins of Gram-Negative Bacteria

Besides the plethora of effects mediated by LPS, various species of gram-negative bacteria release exotoxins that are potent modulators of leukocyte activity. In some instances these toxins have been purified, and their molecular mode of action is well described. For others, little progress has been made in purification, and evaluation of the biological effects of the toxin has been inferred from rather crude preparations that may contain significant LPS contamination.

Considerable attention has been paid to the various components elaborated by *Bordetella*

pertussis (212). In particular, a number of elegant studies have defined the effects of pertussis toxin on leukocytes. Pertussis toxin ADP ribosylates GTP regulatory proteins (Ni) on the cell surface that mediate receptor-induced activation of leukocytes. The effects of pertussis toxin appear to be dose dependent (212). Pertussis toxin inhibits chemotaxis by neutrophils and lymphocytes (15, 135, 185) and degranulation by neutrophils (15). Besides the implications for its role in host defense against *Bordetella* spp. (41), studies of pertussis toxin have provided cell biologists with a powerful tool for dissociating receptor-mediated events from those that result from direct stimulation of calcium influx or protein kinase C activity (15). The mechanism by which nucleotides and nucleotide receptors regulate leukocyte functions requires further clarification. The information gathered from studies of pertussis toxin, however, is bolstered by other approaches, which clearly indicate the influence of nucleosides and nucleic acids on leukocytes. Several provocative reports have demonstrated that nucleotide fractions of *B. abortus* (18, 29, 30) and *H. somnus* (37) markedly inhibit bovine neutrophil function. Although it is suggested that this effect may contribute to the resistance of these bacteria to killing by neutrophils and macrophages, the mechanism by which these bacteria might selectively release these nucleotides and compromise neutrophil function remains to be explained. The influence of nucleotides on intracellular bacterial survival is not restricted to gram-negative bacteria; *M. microti* and other mycobacteria are reported to release cyclic AMP, which prevents phagosome-lysosome fusion and promotes intracellular survival of the bacilli (126).

Other species of gram-negative bacteria are reported to produce toxins that compromise leukocyte activity. *L. pneumophila* releases an extracellular toxin that impairs neutrophil bactericidal activity and release of superoxide anion in response to some stimuli (123). Other investigators have reported a cell-associated acid phosphatase on *L. pneumophila* that inhibits superoxide production in response to fMet-Leu-

Phe (165). Perhaps one or both of these factors contributes to the intraphagocytic survival of *L. pneumophila*. The slime (113) and extracellular alkaline protease and elastase (107) of *P. aeurginosa* are reported to inhibit chemotaxis by human neutrophils and to influence endocytic (113) and oxidative (107) activity. *Fusobacterium necrophorum* produces a leukotoxin that may be related to the pathogenesis of foot rot (55).

Certain strains of *E. coli* contain a plasmid-encoded hemolysin (alpha-hemolysin) which has been shown to be associated with virulence in a rat peritonitis model (216). This hemolysin has potent effects on various functions of human leukocytes. Low doses of hemolysin stimulate human neutrophil chemiluminescence (33), neutrophil release of lysosomal enzymes and leukotrienes (110), and mast cell release of histamine (110). Larger doses of hemolysin, or of intact hemolytic *E. coli,* decrease neutrophil phagocytic and chemotactic activities and eventually lead to cell death (65). Alpha-hemolysin is known to be a high-molecular-weight polypeptide (M_r, 107,000) that inserts itself into target cell membranes, where it forms pores that upset the ionic balance of the cell (19). A detailed analysis of the biochemical characteristics and biological activity of alpha-hemolysin is presented elsewhere (32). Taken as a whole, the data present a persuasive argument for the role of this component in the pathogenesis of extraintestinal *E. coli* infections.

Many species in the family *Pasteurellaceae* possess components that inhibit various leukocyte functions. These include human species such as the oral pathogen *A. actinomycetemcomitans* (198) and important veterinary pathogens such as *P. multocida* (164), *P. haemolytica* (11, 176), and *Haemophilus pleuropneumoniae* (16). The taxonomy of this family is currently under reevaluation, and probably some species will be shifted from one genus to another; therefore, it is not surprising that a number of these bacteria produce leukotoxins with similar biological characteristics. In particular, considerable attention has focused on the leukotoxin of *P. haemolytica,* an important agent in bovine and ovine respiratory disease. This toxin was first noted by investigators who observed that large numbers of log-phase bacteria of certain strains of *P. haemolytica,* or their culture filtrates, were cytotoxic to bovine leukocytes (11, 176). This cytotoxic activity requires viable bacteria, is rapidly released into the culture filtrate during log-phase growth, and is somewhat specific in its cytotoxicity for bovine leukocytes versus those obtained from other mammalian species (176). Purification of this cytotoxin has proven to be problematic; the available information on the biological activity of *P. haemolytica* leukotoxin therefore is based largely on studies involving the use of crude or partially purified toxin preparations. It has been suggested that this toxin may be a neutral protease specific for sialoglycopeptides (149). Although most studies have focused on the cytotoxic effects of large numbers of *P. haemolytica* organisms or relatively large amounts of cytotoxin (11, 176), recent evidence has demonstrated that relatively small amounts of toxin can markedly reduce the chemiluminescence response of ruminant, but not nonruminant, leukocytes (34, 35). The *P. haemolytica* leukotoxin gene has been cloned into *E. coli* K-12 (122). Recent unpublished evidence from that laboratory suggests that *P. haemolytica* leukotoxin is very similar to that of *E. coli* alpha-hemolysin (122a). This very exciting observation is supported by numerous reported similarities between the two toxins (production only during log-phase growth, extracellular release, molecular weight greater than 100,000, stimulatory effects of iron-binding proteins on toxin production, requirement of calcium for cytotoxic activity, etc.). These observations suggest that the leukocyte-modulating effects of *P. haemolytica* may be very relevant to the pathogenesis of pulmonary pasteurellosis. This hypothesis is supported by the report of Slocombe et al. (180), who showed that neutrophil depletion reduced pulmonary damage during the early stages (up to 6 h after challenge) of acute pulmonary pasteurellosis. Perhaps the initial interaction of neutrophils with the small amounts of leukotoxin present in the lungs activates neutrophils to release oxygen radicals and granule constituents that contribute to subsequent pulmonary damage.

Components of Gram-Positive Bacteria

A number of toxins and cell wall constituents of gram-positive bacteria are reported to impair cellular defense mechanisms. The combined presence of *B. anthracis* protective antigen and edema factor markedly enhances intracellular cyclic AMP levels (119), thus inhibiting phagocytosis and chemiluminescence by human neutrophils (145) and preventing priming of oxidative activity by LPS (221). Low doses of the alpha toxin of *S. aureus,* which by itself does not stimulate neutrophil chemiluminescence, enhance the chemiluminescence response of neutrophils that are ingesting staphylococci (68). At doses greater than 20 U/ml, however, it suppresses chemiluminescence, and at still higher doses it is cytotoxic (172). A number of gram-positive bacteria release thiol-activated hemolysins that bind to cholesterol in eucaryotic cell membranes. Streptolysin O, one such hemolysin, directly stimulated canine lymphocytes to proliferate (22) and human neutrophils to chemiluminesce (3). At higher doses, loss of neutrophil viability was observed (124). Similar effects have been noted for pneumolysin, a related thiol-activated hemolysin. Release of myeloperoxidase by degranulating neutrophils inactivates pneumolysin (40), suggesting an extracellular toxin-neutralizing role for myeloperoxidase. Genetic studies of the thiol-activated hemolysin of *L. monocytogenes* indicate that possession of hemolytic activity is associated with virulence for mice (66, 103). Thus, secretion of these hemolysins, which were first noted for their ability to lyse erythrocytes, may be an important virulence determinant for a number of pathogenic gram-positive bacteria.

Various cell-wall components of gram-positive bacteria have been reported to influence leukocyte function in vitro and antibacterial resistance in vivo. In most instances, these effects do not require the presence of viable bacteria. Certain species (e.g., *Propionibacterium*

acnes and *Lactobacillus casei*) are potent macrophage activators in vivo and in vitro (39, 104). The lipid components of the outer layer of nocardiae and mycobacteria elicit a variety of biological responses in vitro and in vivo (72, 100). Surface lipids of *Corynebacterium pseudotuberculosis* are lethal for mice and cause cytopathic effects in mouse, but not rabbit or guinea pig, macrophages (81). Intraperitoneal injection of purified *L. monocytogenes* cell wall material markedly reduced resistance to *L. monocytogenes* and *S. typhimurium* in the absence of any obvious defect in phagocyte activity (10). Peptidoglycan-polysaccharide of group A streptococci inhibited human neutrophil phagocytic and bactericidal activity (118). This finding may be significant in light of the described long-term ability of streptococcal cell walls to resist intracellular degradation (69).

CIRCUMVENTION OF IMMUNE-MEDIATED RESISTANCE

I have concentrated above on innate cellular defense mechanisms that would operate during a primary bacterial infection. It is also important to consider how the properties of pathogenic bacteria might influence the execution of immunologically regulated cellular defense. Although this is an extremely broad topic, I will address only situations in which some property of the bacteria, or the host response to it, plays a pivotal role in the pathogenesis of the infection.

Bacterial Antigenic Shift

One mechanism by which bacteria might elude host defense would be to change their antigenic composition, much as has been described for trypanosomes and influenza virus. There are several examples of pathogenic bacteria that elude the host in this fashion. Antigenic variation by *Campylobacter fetus* was repeatedly observed during infection of the bovine genital tract (42). Phase changes associated with virulence of *B. pertussis* have also been de-

scribed (151, 213). It is likely that other examples will become apparent as genetic evaluation of the molecular basis of bacterial
virulence extends to additional pathogenic species.

Immunosuppression

Although, strictly speaking, this might
not be regarded as a virulence mechanism,
chronic infection with certain organisms, particularly mycobacteria, results in a paradoxical
suppression of lymphocyte activity in vitro (45,
62, 148). Although it has been suggested that
this effect is mediated by induction of suppressor T cells (62, 209), recent evidence suggests that macrophages activated by the chronic
infection release prostaglandin E_2, and perhaps
other suppressive factors, that impair lymphocyte proliferation in vitro (52, 206). A similar
effect may occur in lepromatous leprosy (166,
169, 175). Removal of macrophages, addition
of indomethacin, and addition of interleukin-
2 all have been reported to abrogate this apparent suppression in vitro (52, 139, 147, 148,
200). In contrast, a recent report indicates that
the lipoarabinomannan of *M. leprae* suppresses
in vitro proliferation of lymphocytes from both
leprosy patients and healthy controls (101). This
suggests that *M. leprae* lipoarabinomannan may
contribute to the immunological anergy that
characterizes lepromatous leprosy. Whether such
suppressive factors are produced by other mycobacteria remains to be seen.

Immunotherapy of Intracellular Bacterial Pathogens

A brief consideration of the literature on
the immunoregulation of macrophage antibacterial activity is appropriate. Considerable evidence indicates that gamma interferon is a potent, and perhaps the foremost, activating agent
for macrophage-mediated killing of tumor and
protozoal targets (197). It generally has been
assumed that gamma interferon activation of
macrophage antibacterial activity is a similarly
important component in host defense. There is
substantial evidence for the ability of gamma

interferon to activate macrophages to restrict
the growth of and kill obligate intracellular
pathogens such as *Chlamydia* spp. (27, 162) and
Rickettsia spp. (97, 199). Critical examination
of the literature regarding other bacterial targets, however, reveals considerable controversy
(28, 146). Exogenous and endogenous gamma
interferon significantly influences resistance to
the facultative intracellular pathogen *L. monocytogenes* (26, 109). Although the authors of those
studies implied that this response was mediated by activation of macrophage listericidal
activity, the supporting data were not com-
pelling (26). Other investigators have provided
data suggesting that gamma interferon may induce some anti-*Listeria* activity in mouse macrophages (109) and human monocytes (105,
150). Paradoxical data have been obtained when
mycobacteria are used as the target organism.
Douvas et al. (51) reported that gamma interferon pretreatment of human monocytes enhanced intracellular growth of *M. tuberculosis*
under conditions that activated tumoricidal and
leishmanicidal activity. Rook et al. (161) observed that gamma interferon inhibited the
growth of *M. tuberculosis* in mouse macrophages, but had no effect or slightly enhanced
growth in human monocytes. A separate study
indicated that gamma interferon treatment of
mouse macrophages induced a bacteriostatic effect against *M. microti* (108). One group of investigators reported that *M. leprae*-infected
mouse macrophages were refractory to activation by gamma interferon (177, 178). In contrast, other investigators observed that intradermal injection of human leprosy patients with
recombinant gamma interferon enhanced production of hydrogen peroxide by monocytes
(144). Intracellular growth of *M. paratuberculosis* in bovine monocytes was inhibited by recombinant alpha interferon and enhanced by a
pH 2-labile factor in crude lymphokine supernatants; recombinant gamma interferon alone
did not have growth-enhancing activity (Zur
brick et al., submitted). Pretreatment of human alveolar macrophages (96) and monocytes
(20) with gamma interferon inhibited the intracellular growth of *L. pneumophila*. Because of

the variable results and controversy surrounding the effects of gamma interferon on macrophage antibacterial activity, it may be prudent to examine carefully the effects of gamma interferon on mononuclear phagocyte interaction with each specific bacterial pathogen rather than issue a sweeping statement regarding its general efficacy in antibacterial resistance. The present explosion of information about cytokines other than gamma interferon, some of which have macrophage-activating activity (5), will probably further complicate evaluation of this matter.

ACKNOWLEDGMENTS.   Work performed in my laboratory was supported by funds from the U.S. Public Health Service, U.S. Department of Agriculture, Wisconsin Agriculture Experiment Station, National Foundation for Ileitis and Colitis, Office of Naval Research, and the University of Wisconsin Graduate School.

I acknowledge the contributions of Jim Brown, Beth Noel, Brenda Zurbrick, Holly Hamilton, Denise Follett, and Jim Lederer to these projects. The extraordinary assistance of Barbara Polce and Janelle Manning in the preparation of this manuscript is greatly appreciated.

LITERATURE CITED

1. Adlam, C., M. Knights, A. Mugridge, J. C. Lindon, P. R. W. Baker, J. E. Beesley, B. Spacey, G. R. Craig, and L. K. Nagy. 1984. Purification, characterization, and immunological properties of the serotype-specific capsular polysaccharide of *Pasteurella haemolytica* (serotype A-1) organisms. *J. Gen. Microbiol.* 130:2415–2426.

2. Amakiri, S. F., and K. J. Nwufoh. 1981. Changes in cutaneous blood vessels in bovine dermatophilosis. *J. Comp. Pathol.* 91:439–442.

3. Anderson, B. R., and J. L. Duncan. 1980. Activation of human neutrophil metabolism by streptolysin O. *J. Infect. Dis.* 141:680–685.

4. Anderson, J. C., and M. R. Williams. 1985. The contribution of a capsule to survival of staphylococci within bovine neutrophils. *J. Med. Microbiol.* 20:317–323.

5. Andrew, P. W., A. D. M. Rees, A. Scoging, N. Dobson, R. Mathews, J. T. Whittall, A. R.

M. Coates, and D. B. Lowrie. 1984. Secretion of a macrophage activing factor distinct from interferon-γ by human T-cell clones. *Eur. J. Immunol.* 14:962–964.

6. Arbuthnott, J. P. Membrane-damaging toxins in relation to interference with host defence mechanisms, p. 97–120. *In* J. E. Alouf (ed.), *Bacterial Protein Toxins.* Elsevier Publishing Co., New York.

7. Archibald, F. S., and M. N. Duong. 1986. Superoxide dismutase and oxygen toxicity defenses in the genus *Neisseria. Infect. Immun.* 51:631–641.

8. Armstrong, J. A., and P. D. Hart. 1975. Phagosome-lysosome interactions in cultured macrophages infected with virulent tubercle bacilli. *J. Exp. Med.* 142:1–16.

9. Asahi, O. T., T. Hosoda, and Y. Akiyama. 1957. Studies on the mechanism of infection of the brain with *Listeria monocytogenes. Am. J. Vet. Res.* 18:147–157.

10. Baker, L. A., and P. A. Campbell. 1978. *Listeria monocytogenes* cell walls induce decreased resistance to infection. *Infect. Immun.* 20:99–107.

11. Baluyut, C. S., R. R. Simondson, W. J. Bemrick, and S. K. Maheswaran. 1981. Interaction of *Pasteurella haemolytica* with bovine neutrophils: identification and partial characterization of a cytotoxin. *Am. J. Vet. Res.* 42:1920–1926.

12. Barclay, R., and C. Ratledge. 1983. Iron-binding compounds of *Mycobacterium avium, M. intracellulare, M. scrofulaceum,* and mycobactin-dependent *M. paratuberculosis* and *M. avium. J. Bacteriol.* 153:1138–1146.

13. Bar-Shavit, Z., I. Ofek, R. Goldman, D. Mirelman, and N. Shanon. 1977. Mannose residues on phagocytes as receptors for the attachment of *Escherichia coli* and *Salmonella typhi. Biochem. Biophys. Res. Commun.* 78:455–460.

14. Beaman, L. V., and B. L. Beaman. 1984. The role of oxygen and its derivatives in microbial pathogenesis and host defense. *Annu. Rev. Microbiol.* 38:27–48.

15. Becker, E. L., J. C. Kermode, P. H. Naccache, R. Yassin, M. L. Marsh, J. J. Munoz, and R. I. Sha'afi. 1985. The inhibition of neutrophil granule enzyme secretion and chemotaxis by pertussis toxin. *J. Cell Biol.* 100:1641–1646.

16. Bendixen, P. H., P. E. Shewen, S. Rosendal, and B. N. Wilkie. 1981. Toxicity of *Haemophilus pleuropneumoniae* for porcine lung macrophages, peripheral blood monocytes, and testicular cells. *Infect. Immun.* 33:673–676.

17. Benjamin, W. H., Jr., C. L. Turnbogh, Jr., D. S. Posey, and D. E. Briles. 1986. *Salmonella typhimurium* virulence genes necessary to exploit the Ity genotype of the mouse. *Infect. Immun.* 51:872–878.

18. Bertram, T. A., P. C. Canning, and J. A. Roth.

1986. Preferential inhibition of primary granule release from bovine neutrophils by a *Brucella abortus* extract. *Infect. Immun.* 52:285–292.

19. Bhakdi, S., N. Mackman, J. M. Nicaud, and I. B. Holland. 1986. *Escherichia coli* hemolysin may damage target cell membranes by generating transmembrane pores. *Infect. Immun.* 52:63–69.

20. Bhardwaj, N., T. W. Nash, and M. A. Horwitz. 1986. Interferon γ activated human monocytes inhibit the intracellular multiplication of *Legionella pneumophila*. *J. Immunol.* 137:2662–2669.

21. Black, C. M., B. L. Beaman, R. M. Donovan, and E. Goldstein. 1985. Intracellular acid phosphatase content and ability of different macrophage populations to kill *Nocardia asteroides*. *Infect. Immun.* 47:375–383.

22. Bloch, E. F., and R. D. Schultz. 1985. The canine lymphocyte: effect of streptolysin O on the proliferative response of canine lymphocytes. *Vet. Immunol. Immunopathol.* 8:125–135.

23. Britigan, B. E., and M. S. Cohen. 1986. Effects of human serum on bacterial competition with neutrophils for molecular oxygen. *Infect. Immun.* 52:657–663.

24. Britigan, B. E., M. S. Cohen, and P. F. Sparling. 1985. Gonococcal infection: a model of molecular pathogenesis. *N. Engl. J. Med.* 312:1683–1694.

25. Brubaker, R. R. 1984. Molecular biology of the dread black death. *ASM News* 50:240–245.

26. Buchmeir, N. A., and R. D. Schreiber. 1985. Requirement of endogenous interferon-γ production for resolution of *Listeria monocytogenes* infection. *Proc. Natl. Acad. Sci. USA* 82:7404–7408.

27. Byrne, G. I., and C. L. Faubion. 1982. Lymphokine-mediated microbiostatic mechanisms restrict *Chlamydia psittaci* growth in macrophages. *J. Immunol.* 128:469–474.

28. Campbell, P. A. 1986. Are inflammatory phagocytes responsible for resistance against facultative intracellular bacteria? *Immunol. Today* 7:70–72.

29. Canning, P. C., J. A. Roth, and B. L. Deyoe. 1986. Release of 5'-guanosine monophosphate and adenine by *Brucella abortus* and their role in the intracellular survival of the bacteria. *J. Infect. Dis.* 154:464–470.

30. Canning, P. C., J. A. Roth, L. B. Tabatabai, and B. L. Deyoe. 1985. Isolation of components of *Brucella abortus* responsible for inhibition of function in bovine neutrophils. *J. Infect. Dis.* 152:913–921.

31. Casey, S. G., W. M. Shafer, and J. K. Spitznagel. 1986. *Neisseria gonorrhoeae* survive intraleukocytic oxygen-independent antimicrobial capacities of anaerobic and aerobic granulocytes in the presence of pyocin lethal for extracellular gonococci. *Infect. Immun.* 52:384–389.

32. Cavalieri, S. J., G. A. Bohach, and I. S. Snyder. 1984. *Escherichia coli* α-hemolysin: characteristics and probable role in pathogenicity. *Microbiol. Rev.* 48:326–343.

33. Cavalieri, S. J., and I. S. Snyder. 1982. Effect of *Escherichia coli* α-hemolysin on human peripheral leukocyte function in vitro. *Infect. Immun.* 37:966–974.

34. Chang, Y. F., H. W. Renshaw, and J. L. Augustine. 1985. Bovine pneumonic pasteurellosis: chemiluminescent response of bovine peripheral blood leukocytes to living and killed *Pasteurella haemolytica, Pasteurella multocida*, and *Escherichia coli. Am. J. Vet. Res.* 26:2266–2271.

35. Chang, Y. F., H. W. Renshaw, and A. B. Richards. 1986. *Pasteurella haemolytica* leukotoxin: physicochemical characteristics and susceptibility of leukotoxin to enzymatic treatment. *Am. J. Vet. Res.* 47:716–723.

36. Charnetzky, W. T., and W. W. Shuford. 1985. Survival and growth of *Yersinia pestis* within macrophages and an effect of the loss of the 47-megadalton plasmid on growth in macrophages. *Infect. Immun.* 47:234–241.

37. Chiang, Y. W., M. L. Kaeberle, and J. A. Roth. 1986. Identification of suppressive components in *Haemophilus somnus* fractions which inhibit bovine polymorphonuclear leukocyte function. *Infect. Immun.* 52:792–797.

38. Chiplunkar, S., G. De Libero, and S. H. E. Kaufman. 1986. *Mycobacterium leprae*-specific Lyt2⁺ T lymphocytes with cytolytic activity. *Infect. Immun.* 54:793–797.

39. Christie, G. H., and R. Bomford. 1975. Mechanisms of macrophage activation by *Corynebacterium parvum* I: in vitro experiments. *Cell. Immunol.* 171:141–149.

40. Clark, R. A. 1986. Oxidative inactivation of pneumolysin by the myeloperoxidase system and stimulated human neutrophils. *J. Immunol.* 136:4617–4622.

41. Confer, D. L., and J. W. Eaton. 1982. Phagocyte impotence caused by an invasive bacterial adenylate cylase. *Science* 217:948–950.

42. Corbeil, L. B., G. G. D. Schurig, P. J. Bier, and A. J. Winter. 1975. Bovine venereal vibriosis: antigenic variation of the bacterium during infection. *Infect. Immun.* 11:240–244.

43. Corstvet, R. E., M. J. Gentry, P. R. Newmann, J. A. Rummage, and A. W. Confer. 1982. Demonstration of age-dependent capsular material on *Pasteurella haemolytica* serotype 1. *J. Clin. Microbiol.* 16:1123–1126.

44. Czuprynski, C. J., and H. L. Hamilton. 1985. Bovine neutrophils ingest but do not kill *Haemophilus somnus* in vitro. *Infect. Immun.* 50:431–436.

45. Davies, D. H., L. Corbeil, D. Ward, and J. R.

Duncan. 1974. A humoral suppressor of in vitro lymphocyte transformation responses in cattle with Johne's disease. *Proc. Soc. Exp. Biol. Med.* 145:1372–1377.

46. Daynes, R. A., and C. H. Armstrong. 1973. An antiphagocytic factor associated with group E streptococcus. *Infect. Immun.* 7:298–304.

47. De Libero, G., and S. H. E. Kaufmann. 1986. Antigen-specific Lyt2$^+$ cytolytic T lymphocytes from mice infected with the intracellular bacterium *Listeria monocytogenes*. *J. Immunol.* 137:2688–2694.

48. Densen, P., and G. L. Mandell. 1978. Gonococcal interactions with polymorphonuclear neutrophils: importance of the phagosome for bacteriocidal activity. *J. Clin. Invest.* 62:1161–1171.

49. Densen, P., and G. L. Mandell. 1980. Phagocyte strategy vs. microbial tactics. *Rev. Infect. Dis.* 2:817–838.

50. Devoe, I. W. 1982. The meningococcus and mechanisms of pathogenicity. *Microbiol. Rev.* 46:162–190.

51. Douvas, G. S., D. L. Looker, A. E. Vatter, and A. J. Crowle. 1985. Gamma interferon activates human macrophages to become tumoricidal and leishmanicidal but enhances replication of macrophage-associated mycobacteria. *Infect. Immun.* 50:1–8.

52. Edwards, C. K., III, H. B. Hedegaard, A. Zlotnik, P. R. Gangadharam, R. B. Johnston, Jr., and M. J. Pabst. 1986. Chronic infection due to *Mycobacterium intracellularae* in mice: association with macrophage release of prostaglandin E_2 and reversal by injection of indomethacin, muramyl dipeptide or interferon-γ. *J. Immunol.* 136:1820–1827.

53. Ellenberger, M. A., M. L. Kaeberle, and J. A. Roth. 1984. Effect of *Rhodococcus equi* on equine polymorphonuclear leukocyte function. *Vet. Immunol. Immunpathol.* 7:315–324.

54. Engel, D., D. Van Epps, and J. Claggett. 1976. In vivo and in vitro studies on possible pathogenic mechanisms of *Actinomyces viscosus*. *Infect. Immun.* 14:548–554.

55. Fales, W. H., J. F. Warner, and G. W. Tleresa. 1977. Effects of *Fusobacterium necrophorum* leukotoxin on rabbit peritoneal macrophages in vitro. *Am. J. Vet. Res.* 38:491–495.

56. Fields, P. I., R. V. Swanson, C. J. Haidaris, and F. Heffron. 1986. Mutants of *Salmonella typhimurium* that cannot survive within the macrophage are avirulent. *Proc. Natl. Acad. Sci. USA* 83:5189–5193.

57. Filice, G. A. 1983. Resistance of *Nocardia asteroides* to oxygen dependent killing by neutrophils. *J. Infect. Dis.* 148:861–867.

58. Filice, G. A., B. L. Beaman, J. A. Krick, and J. S. Remington. 1980. Effects of human neutrophils and monocytes on *Nocardia asteroides*: failure of killing despite occurrence of the oxidative metabolic burst. *J. Infect. Dis.* 142:432–438.

59. Fitzgeorge, R. B., M. Solotorovsky, and H. Smith. 1967. The behavior of *Brucella abortus* within macrophages separated from the blood of normal and immune cattle by adherence to glass. *Br. J. Exp. Pathol.* 48:522–528.

60. Foley, M. J., and W. B. Wood, Jr. 1959. Studies on the pathogenicity of group A streptococci. II. The antiphagocytic effects of the M protein and the capsular gel. *J. Exp. Med.* 110:617–628.

61. Foshay, L. 1950. Tularemia. *Annu. Rev. Microbiol.* 4:313–330.

62. Fossum, C., R. Bergman, and B. Morein. 1985. Suppressor activity of bovine FCγ cells during a persistent infection with *Mycobacterium avium*. *Res. Vet. Sci.* 38:270–274.

63. Frehel, C., C. De Chastellier, T. Lang, and N. Rastogi. 1986. Evidence for inhibition of fusion of lysosomal and prelysosomal compartments with phagosomes in macrophages infected with pathogenic *Mycobacterium avium*. *Infect. Immun.* 52:252–262.

64. Frenchick, P. J., R. J. F. Markham, and A. H. Cochran. 1985. Inhibition of phagosome-lysosome fusion in macrophages by soluble extracts of virulent *Brucella abortus*. *Am. J. Vet. Res.* 46:332–335.

65. Gadeberg, O. V., and I. Ørskov. 1984. In vitro cytotoxic effect of α-hemolytic *Escherichia coli* on human blood granulocytes. *Infect. Immun.* 45:255–260.

66. Gaillard, J. L., P. Berche, and P. Sansonetti. 1986. Transposon mutagenesis as a tool to study the role of hemolysins in the virulence of *Listeria monocytogenes*. *Infect. Immun.* 52:50–55.

67. Gangadharam, P. R. J., and P. F. Pratt. 1984. Susceptibility of *Mycobacterium intracellulare* to hydrogen peroxide. *Am. Rev. Respir. Dis.* 130:309–311.

68. Gemmell, C. G., P. K. Peterson, L. Landstrom, and P.G. Quie. 1983. Stimulation of particle-induced chemiluminescence in human polymorphonuclear leukocytes by staphylococcal α toxin. *J. Infect. Dis.* 147:729–732.

69. Ginsburg, I. 1972. Mechanisms of cell and tissue injury induced by group A streptococci: relation to post-streptococcal sequelae. *J. Infect. Dis.* 126:294–340.

70. Godfrey, R. W., and M. S. Wilder. 1984. Relationships between oxidative metabolism, macrophage activation, and antilisterial activity. *J. Leukocyte Biol.* 36:533–543.

71. Goren, M. B. 1977. Phagocyte lysosomes: interactions with infectious agents, phagosomes, and experimental perturbations in function. *Annu. Rev.*

Microbiol. 31:507–533.

72. Goren, M. B. 1982. Immunoreactive substances of mycobacteria. *Am. Rev. Respir. Dis.* 125:50–69.

73. Goren, M. B., P. D'Arcy Hart, M. R. Young, and J. A. Armstrong. 1976. Prevention of phagosome-lysosome fusion in cultured macrophages by sulfatides of *Mycobacterium tuberculosis. Proc. Natl. Acad. Sci. USA* 73:2510–2514.

74. Goren, M. B., A. E. Vatter, and J. Fiscus. 1987. Polyanionic agents as inhibitors of phagosome lysosome fusion in cultured macrophages: evolution of an alternative interpretation. *J. Leukocyte Biol.* 41:111–121.

75. Goren, M. B., A. E. Vatter, and J. Fiscus. 1987. Polyanionic agents do not inhibit phagosome-lysosome fusion in cultured macrophages. *J. Leukocyte Biol.* 41:122–129.

76. Greene, C. E., and L. W. George. 1984. Canine brucellosis, p. 646–662. *In* C. E. Greene (ed.), *Clinical Microbiology and Infectious Diseases of the Dog and Cat.* The W. B. Saunders Co., Philadelphia.

77. Greene, C. E., and J. W. Harvey. 1984. Canine ehrlichiosis, p. 545–561. *In* C. E. Greene (ed.), *Clinical Microbiology and Infectious Diseases of the Dog and Cat.* The W. B. Saunders Co., Philadelphia.

78. Guthrie, L. A., L. C. McPhail, P. M. Henson, and R. B. Johnston, Jr. 1984. Priming of neutrophils for enhanced release of oxygen metabolites by bacterial lipopolysaccharide. *J. Exp. Med.* 160:1656–1671.

79. Hadad, J. J., and C. L. Gyles. 1982. Scanning and transmission electron microscopic study of the small intestine of colostrum-fed calves infected with selected strains of *Escherichia coli. Am. J. Vet. Res.* 43:41–49.

80. Hale, T. L., P. J. Sansonetti, P. A. Schad, S. Austin, and S. B. Formal. 1983. Characterization of virulence plasmids and plasmid-associated outer membrane proteins in *Shigella flexneri, Shigella sonnei,* and *Escherichia coli. Infect. Immun.* 40:340–350.

81. Hard, G. C. 1975. Comparative toxic effect of the surface lipid of *Corynebacterium ovis* on peritoneal macrophages. *Infect. Immun.* 12:1439–1449.

82. Harvey, J. W. 1984. Haemobartonellosis, p. 576–587. *In* C. E. Greene (ed.), *Clinical Microbiology and Infectious Diseases of the Dog and Cat.* The W. B. Saunders Co., Philadelphia.

83. Hashimoto, S., K. Nomoto, and T. Yokokura. 1986. The role of superoxide anion and lysosomal enzymes in antilisterial activity of elicited peritoneal macrophages. *Scand. J. Immunol.* 24:429–436.

84. Haslett, C., L. A. Guthrie, M. M. Kopaniak, R. B. Johnston, Jr., and P. M. Henson. 1985. Modulation of multiple neutrophil functions by preparative methods or trace concentrations of bacterial lipopolysaccharide. *Am. J. Pathol.* 119:101–110.

85. Havell, E. A. 1986. Synthesis and secretion of interferon by murine fibroblasts in response to intracellular *Listeria monocytogenes. Infect. Immun.* 54:787–792.

86. Hill, A. W., D. J. S. Heneghan, and M. R. Williams. 1983. The opsonic activity of bovine milk whey for the phagocytosis and killing by neutrophils of encapsulated and non-encapsulated *Escherichia coli. Vet. Microbiol.* 8:293–300.

87. Hill, H. R., J. M. Gerrard, N. A. Hogan, and P. G. Quie. 1974. Hyperactivity of neutrophil leukotactic responses during active bacterial infection. *J. Clin. Invest.* 53:996–1002.

88. Holzer, T. J., K. E. Nelson, V. Schauf, R. G. Crispen, and B. R. Anderson. 1986. *Mycobacterium leprae* fails to stimulate phagocytic cell superoxide anion generation. *Infect. Immun.* 51:514–520.

89. Horwitz, M. A. 1982. Phagocytosis of microorganisms. *Rev. Infect. Dis.* 4:104–123.

90. Hørwitz, M. A., and F. R. Maxfield. 1984. *Legionella pneumophila* inhibits acidification of its phagosome in human monocytes. *J. Cell Biol.* 99:1936–1943.

91. Horwitz, M. A., and S. C. Silverstein. 1980. Legionnaire's disease bacterium (*Legionella pneumophila*) multiplies intracellularly in human monocytes. *J. Clin. Invest.* 66:441–450.

92. Howard, C. J., and A. A. Glynn. 1971. The virulence for mice of strains of *Escherichia coli* related to the effects of K antigens on their resistance to phagocytosis and killing by complement. *Immunology* 20:767–777.

93. Howard, C. J., G. Taylor, J. Collins, and R. N. Gourlay. 1976. Interaction of *Mycoplasma dispar* and *Mycoplasma agalactiae* subsp. *bovis* with bovine alveolar macrophages and bovine lacteal polymorphonuclear leukocytes. *Infect Immun.* 14:11–17.

94. Hubbard, R. D., M. L. Kaeberle, J. A. Roth, and Y. W. Chiang. 1986. *Haemophilus somnus*-induced interference with bovine neutrophil functions. *Vet. Microbiol.* 12:77–85.

95. Jackett, P. S., V. R. Aber, and D. B. Lowrie. 1978. Virulence and resistance to superoxide, low pH and hydrogen peroxide among strains of *Mycobacterium tuberculosis. J. Gen. Microbiol.* 104:37–45.

96. Jensen, W. A., R. M. Rose, A. S. Wasserman, T. H. Kalb, K. Anton, and H. G. Remold. 1987. In vitro activation of the antibacterial activity of human pulmonary macrophages by recombinant γ interferon. *J. Infect. Dis.* 3:574–577.

97. Jerells, T. R., J. Turco, H. H. Winkler, and G. L. Spitalny. 1986. Neutralization of lymphokine-mediated antirickettsial activity of fibroblasts and macrophages with monoclonal antibody specific for murine interferon gamma. *Infect. Immun.* 51:355–359.

98. Johnson, R. B., Jr., P. Anderson, F. S. Rosen, and D. H. Smith. 1973. Characterization of human antibody to polyribosephosphate, the capsular antigen of *Haemophilus influenzae,* type B. *Clin. Immunol. Immunopathol.* 1:234–240.

99. Jones, T. C., and R. D. Hunt. 1983. *Veterinary Pathology,* p. 538–547. Lea & Febiger, Philadelphia.

100. Kaneda, K., Y. Sumi, F. Kurano, Y. Kato, and I. Kato. 1986. Granuloma formation and hemopoiesis induced by C_{36-48} mycolic acid-containing glycolipids from *Nocardia rubra. Infect. Immun.* 540:869–875.

101. Kaplan, G., R. R. Ghandi, D. E. Weinstein, W. R. Levis, M. E. Patarroyo, P. J. Brennan, and Z. A. Cohn. 1987. *Mycobacterium leprae* antigen-induced suppression of T cell proliferation in vitro. *J. Immunol.* 138:3028–3034.

102. Kapp, A., M. Freudenberg, and C. Galanos. 1987. Induction of human granulocyte chemiluminescence by bacterial lipopolysaccharides. *Infect. Immun.* 55:758–761.

103. Kathariou, S., P. Metz, H. Hof, and W. Goebel. 1987. Tn916-induced mutations in the hemolysin determinant affecting virulence of *Listeria monocytogenes. J. Bacteriol.* 169:1291–1297.

104. Kato, I., T. Yokokura, and M. Mutai. 1983. Macrophage activation by *Lactobacillus casei* in mice. *Microbiol. Immunol.* 27:611–618.

105. Kemmerich, B., G. J. Small, and J. E. Pennington. 1986. Relation of cytosolic calcium to the microbicidal activation of blood monocytes by recombinant γ interferon. *J. Infect. Dis.* 154:770–777.

106. Keppie, J., P. W. Harris-Smith, and H. Smith. 1963. The chemical basis of the virulence of *Bacillus anthracis.* IX. Its aggressins and their mode of action. *Br. J. Exp. Pathol.* 44:446–453.

107. Kharazmi, A., G. Doring, N. Høiby, and N. H. Valerius. 1984. Interaction of *Pseudomonas aeruginosa* alkaline protease and elastase with human polymorphonuclear leukocytes in vitro. *Infect. Immun.* 43:161–165.

108. Khor, M., D. B. Lowrie, and D. A. Mitchison. 1986. Effects of recombinant interferon-γ and chemotherapy with isoniazid and rifampicin on infections of mouse peritoneal macrophages with *Listeria monocytogenes* and *Mycobacterium microti* in vitro. *Br. J. Exp. Pathol.* 67:707–717.

109. Kiderlen, A. F., S. H. E. Kaufman, and M. L. Lohmann-Matthes. 1984. Protection of mice against the intracellular bacterium *Listeria monocytogenes* by recombinant immune interferon. *Eur. J. Immunol.* 14:964–967.

110. König, B., W. König, J. Scheffer, J. Hacker, and W. Goebel. 1986. Role of *Escherichia coli* alpha-hemolysin and bacterial adherence in infection:

requirement for release of inflammatory mediators from granulocytes and mast cells. *Infect. Immun.* 54:886–892.

111. Kossack, R. E., R. L. Guerrant, P. Densen, J. Schadelin, and G. L. Mandell. 1981. Diminished neutrophil oxidative metabolism after phagocytosis of virulent *Salmonella typhi. Infect. Immun.* 31:74–678.

112. Kreutzer, D. L., L. A. Dreyfus, and D. C. Robertson. 1979. Interaction of polymorphonuclear leukocytes with smooth and rough strains of *Brucella abortus. Infect. Immun.* 23:737–742.

113. Laharrague, P. F., J. X. Corberand, G. Fillola, B. G. Gleizes, A. M. Fontanilles, and E. Gyrard. 1984. In vitro effect of the slime of *Pseudomonas aeruginosa* on the function of human polymorphonuclear neutrophils. *Infect. Immun.* 44:760–762.

114. Lambden, P. R., J. E. Heckles, H. McBride, and P. J. Watt. 1981. The identification and isolation of novel pilus types produced by variants of *N. gonorrhoeae* P9 following selection in vivo. *FEMS Microbiol. Lett.* 10:339–341.

115. Lambden, P. R., J. N. Robertson, and P. J. Watt. 1980. Biological properties of two distinct pilus types produced by isogenic variants of *Neisseria gonorrhoeae* P9. *J. Bacteriol.* 141:393–396.

116. Lederer, J. A., J. F. Brown, and C. J. Czuprynski. 1987. "*Haemophilus somnus*": a facultative intracellular pathogen of bovine mononuclear phagocytes. *Infect. Immun.* 55:381–387.

117. Lehrer, R. I., M. E. Selsted, D. Szklarek, and J. Fleischmann. 1983. Antibacterial activity of microbicidal cationic proteins 1 and 2, natural peptide antibiotics of rabbit lung macrophages. *Infect. Immun.* 42:10–14.

118. Leong, P. A., and M. S. Cohen. 1984. Group A streptococcal peptoglycan-polysaccharide inhibits phagocytic activity of human polymorphonuclear leukocytes. *Infect. Immun.* 45:378–383.

119. Leppla, S. H. 1982. Anthrax toxin edema factor: a bacterial adenylate cylase that increases cAMP concentrations in eukaryotic cells. *Proc. Natl. Acad. Sci. USA* 79:3162–3166.

120. Lian, C. J., and C. H. Pai. 1985. Inhibition of human neutrophil chemiluminescence by plasmid-mediated outer membrane proteins of *Yersinia enterocolitica. Infect. Immun.* 49:145–151.

121. Lissner, C. R., D. L. Weinstein, and A. D. O'Brien. 1985. Mouse chromosome 1 Ity locus regulates microbicidal activity of isolated peritoneal macrophages against a diverse group of intracellular and extracellular bacteria. *J. Immunol.* 135:544–547.

122. Lo, R. Y. C., P. E. Shewen, C. A. Strathdee, and C. N. Greer. 1985. Cloning and expression of the leukotoxin gene of *Pasteurella haemolytica* A1

in *Escherichia coli* K12. *Infect. Immun.* 50:667–671.

122a. Lo, R. Y. C., C. A. Strathdee, and P. E. Shewen. 1987. Nucleotide sequence of the leukotoxin genes of *Pasteurella haemolytica* A1. *Infect. Immun.* 55:1987–1996.

123. Lochner, J. E., R. H. Bigley, and B. H. Iglewski. 1985. Defective triggering of polymorphonuclear leukocyte oxidative metabolism by *Legionella pneumophila* toxin. *J. Infect. Dis.* 151:42–46.

124. Loeffler, D. A., K. A. Schat, and N. L. Norcross. 1986. Use of ^{51}Cr release to measure the cytotoxic effects of staphylococcal leukocidin and toxin neutralization on bovine leukocytes. *J. Clin. Microbiol.* 23:416–420.

125. Lowrie, D. B., V. R. Aber, and P. S. Jackett. 1979. Phagosome-lysosome fusion and cyclic adenosine 3':5'-monophosphate in macrophages infected with *Mycobacterium microti*, *Mycobacterium bovis* BCG, or *Mycobacterium lepraemurium*. *J. Gen. Microbiol.* 110:431–441.

126. Lowrie, D. B., P. S. Jackett, and N. A. Ratcliffe. 1975. *Mycobacterium microti* may protect itself from intracellular destruction by releasing cyclic AMP into phagosomes. *Nature* (London) 254:600–602.

127. Lurie, M. B. 1942. The fate of tubercle bacilli ingested by phagocytes from normal and immunized animals. *J. Exp. Med.* 75:247–267.

128. Mackaness, G. B. 1964. The immunological basis of acquired cellular resistance. *J. Exp. Med.* 120:105–120.

129. Macleod, C. M., and M. R. Krauss. 1950. Relation of virulence of pneumococcal strains for mice to the quantity of capsular polysaccharide formed in vitro. *J. Exp. Med.* 92:1–9.

130. Maheswaran, S. K., and E. S. Thies. 1979. Influence of encapsulation on phagocytosis of *Pasteurella multocida* by bovine neutrophils. *Infect. Immun.* 26:76–81.

131. Managan, D. F., and I. S. Snyder. 1979. Mannose-sensitive interaction of *Escherichia coli* with human peripheral leukocytes in vitro. *Infect. Immun.* 26:526–527.

132. Mandell, G. L. 1974. Bactericidal activity of aerobic and anaerobic polymorphonuclear neutrophils. *Infect. Immun.* 9:337–341.

133. Mandell, G. L. 1975. Catalase, superoxide dismutase, and virulence of *Staphylococcus aureus*. In vitro and in vivo studies with emphasis on staphylococcal-leukocyte interaction. *J. Clin. Invest.* 55:561–566.

134. McCall, C. E., D. A. Bass, L. R. DeChatelet, A. S. Link, Jr., and M. Mann. 1979. In vitro responses of human neutrophils to N-formyl-methionyl-leucyl-phenylalanine: correlation with the effects of acute bacterial infection. *J. Infect. Dis.* 140:277–286.

135. Meade, B. D., P. D. Kind, and C. R. Manclark. 1984. Lymphocytosis-promoting factor of *Bordetella pertussis* alters mononuclear phagocyte circulation and response to inflammation. *Infect. Immun.* 46:733–739.

136. Miller, R. M., J. Carbus, and R. B. Hornick. 1972. Lack of enhanced oxygen consumption by polymorphonuclear leukocytes on phagocytosis of virulent *Salmonella typhi*. *Infect. Immun.* 31:674–678.

137. Miyasaki, K. T., M. E. Wilson, H. S. Reynolds, and R. J. Genco. 1984. Resistance of *Actinobacillus actinomycetemcomitans* and differential susceptibility of oral *Haemophilus* species to the bactericidal effects of hydrogen peroxide. *Infect. Immun.* 46:644–648.

138. Modrzakowski, M. C., and J. K. Spitznagel. 1979. Bactericidal activity of fractionated granule contents from human polymorphonuclear leukocytes: antagonism of granule cationic proteins by lipopolysaccharide. *Infect. Immun.* 25:597–602.

139. Mohagheghpour, N., R. H. Gelber, J. W. Larrick, D. T. Sasaki, P. J. Brennan, and E. G. Engelman. 1985. Defective cell-mediated immunity in leprosy: failure of T cells from lepromatous leprosy patients to respond to *Mycobacterium leprae* is associated with defective expression of interleukin-2 receptors and is not reconstituted by interleukin-2. *J. Immunol.* 135:1443–1449.

140. Momotani, E., K. Furugouri, Y. Obara, Y. Miyata, Y. Ishikawa, and T. Yoshino. 1986. Immunohistochemical distribution of ferritin, lactoferrin, and transferrin in granulomas of bovine paratuberculosis. *Infect. Immun.* 52:623–627.

141. Mor, N. 1983. Intracellular location of *Mycobacterium leprae* in macrophages of normal and immune-deficient mice and effect of rifampin. *Infect. Immun.* 42:802–811.

142. Moulder, J. W. 1985. Comparative biology of intracellular parasitism. *Microbiol. Rev.* 49:298–337.

143. Myrvik, Q. N., E. S. Leake, and M. J. Wright. 1984. Disruption of phagosomal membranes of normal alveolar macrophages by the H37Rv strain of *Mycobacterium tuberculosis*. *Am. Rev. Respir. Dis.* 129:322–328.

144. Nathan, C. F., G. Koplan, W. R. Levis, A. Nusrat, M. O. Witner, S. A. Sherwin, C. K. Job, C. R. Horawitz, R. M. Steinman, and Z. A. Cohn. 1986. Local and systemic effects of intradermal recombinant interferon-γ in patients with lepromatous leprosy. *N. Engl. J. Med.* 315:6–15.

145. O'Brien, J., A. Friedlander, T. Dreier, J. Ezzell, and S. Leppla. 1985. Effects of anthrax toxin components on human neutrophils. *Infect. Immun.* 47:306–310.

146. Orme, I. M., and F. M. Collins. 1983. Resistance of various strains of mycobacteria to killing by activated macrophages in vivo. *J. Immunol.* 131:1452–1454.

147. Orme, I. M., and F. M. Collins. 1984. Immune response to atypical mycobacteria: immunocompetence of heavily infected mice measured in vivo fails to substantiate immunosuppression data obtained in vitro. *Infect. Immun.* 43:32–37.

148. Orme, I. M., M. J. H. Ratcliffe, and F. M. Collins. 1984. Acquired immunity to heavy infection with *Mycobacterium bovis* bacillus Calmette-Guerin and its relationship to the development of nonspecific unresponsiveness in vitro. *Cell. Immunol.* 88:285–296.

149. Otulakowski, G. L., P. E. Shewen, A. E. Udoh, A. Mellors, and B. N. Wilkie. 1983. Proteolysis of sialoglycoprotein by *Pasteurella haemolytica* cytotoxic culture supernatant. *Infect. Immun.* 42:64–70.

150. Peck, R. 1985. A one-plate assay for macrophage bactericidal activity. *J. Immunol. Methods* 82:131–140.

151. Peppler, M. S., and M. E. Schrumpf. 1984. Phenotypic variation and modulation in *Bordetella bronchiseptica*. *Infect. Immun.* 44:681–687.

152. Perry, R. D., and R. R. Brubaker. 1979. Accumulation of iron by yersiniae. *J. Bacteriol.* 137:1290–1295.

153. Peterson, P. K., Y. Kim, B. J. Wilkinson, D. Schmeling, A. F. Michael, and P. G. Quie. 1978. Dichotomy between opsonization and serum complement activation by encapsulated staphylococci. *Infect. Immun.* 20:770–775.

154. Pollack, C., S. C. Straley, and M. S. Klempner. 1986. Probing the phagolysosomal environment of human macrophages with a Ca^{2+} responsive operon fusion in *Yersinia pestis*. *Nature* (London) 322:834–836.

155. Proctor, R. A. (ed.). 1986. *Handbook of Endotoxin*, vol. 4: *Clinical Aspects of Endotoxin Shock*. Elsevier Publishing Co., New York.

156. Proctor, R. A. 1979. Endotoxin in vitro interactions with human neutrophils: depression of chemiluminescence, oxygen consumption, superoxide production, and killing. *Infect. Immun.* 25:912–921.

157. Repine, J. E., C. C. Clauson, and F. C. Goetz. 1980. Bactericidal function of neutrophils from patients with acute bacterial infections and from diabetics. *J. Infect. Dis.* 142:869–875.

158. Rikihisa, Y., and S. Ito. 1982. Entry of *Rickettsia tsutsugamushi* into polymorphonuclear leukocytes. *Infect. Immun.* 38:343–350.

159. Ristic, M., and J. P. Kreier. 1979. Hemotrophic bacteria. *N. Engl. J. Med.* 301:937–939.

160. Roberta, R. B. 1970. The relationship between group A and group C meningococcal polysaccharide and serum opsonins in man. *J. Exp. Med.* 131:499–513.

161. Rook, G. A. W., J. Steele, M. Ainsworth, and

B. R. Champion. 1986. Activation of macrophages to inhibit proliferation of *Mycobacterium tuberculosis:* comparison of the effects of recombinant γ interferon on human monocytes and murine peritoneal macrophages. *Immunology* 59:333–338.

162. Rothermel, C. D., B. Y. Rubin, and H. W. Murray. 1983. γ Interferon is the factor in lymphokine that activates human macrophages to inhibit intracellular *Chlamydia psittaci* replication. *J. Immunol.* 131:2542–2544.

163. Ruuth, E., M. Ranby, B. Friedrich, H. Persson, A. Goustin, T. Leanderson, A. Coutinho, and E. Lundgren. 1985. Mycoplasma mimicry of lumphokine activity in T-cell lines. *Scand. J. Immunol.* 21:593–600.

164. Ryu, H., M. L. Kaeberle, J. A. Roth, and R. W. Griffith. 1984. Effect of type A *Pasteurella multocida* fractions on bovine polymorphonuclear leukocyte functions. *Infect. Immun.* 43:66–71.

165. Saha, A. K., J. N. Dowling, K. L. LaMarco, S. Das, A. T. Remaley, N. Olomu, M. T. Pope, and R. H. Glew. 1985. Properties of acid phosphatase from *Legionella micdadei* which blocks superoxide anion production by human neutrophils. *Arch. Biochem. Biophys.* 243:150–160.

166. Salgame, P. R., P. R. Mahadevan, and N. H. Antia. 1983. Mechanism of immunosuppression in leprosy: presence of suppressor factor(s) from macrophages of lepromatous patients. *Infect. Immun.* 40:1119–1126.

167. Sandberg, A. L., L. L. Mudrick, J. O. Cisar, M. J. Brennan, S. E. Mergenhagen, and A. E. Vatter. 1986. Type 2 fimbrial lectin-mediated phagocytosis of oral *Actinomyces* spp. by polymorphonuclear leukocytes. *Infect. Immun.* 54:472–476.

168. Sansonetti, P. J., A. Ryter, P. Clerc, A. T. Maurelli, and J. Mounier. 1986. Multiplication of *Shigella flexneri* within HeLa cells: lysis of the phagocytic vacuole and plasmid-mediated contact hemolysis. *Infect. Immun.* 51:461–469.

169. Sathish, M., L. K. Bhutani, A. K. Sharma, and I. Nath. 1983. Monocyte-derived soluble suppressor factor(s) in patients with lepromatous leprosy. *Infect. Immun.* 42:890–899.

170. Savoigni, A., R. Marzari, L. Dolzani, D. Serrano, G. Graziosi, R. Gennaro, and D. Romeo. 1984. Wide-spectrum antibiotic activity of bovine granulocyte polypeptides. *Antimicrob. Agents Chemother.* 26:405–407.

171. Schiffmann, E., B. A. Corcoran, and S. A. Wahl. 1975. N-formyl methionyl peptides as chemoattractants for leukocytes. *Proc. Natl. Acad. Sci. USA* 72:1059–1062.

172. Schmeling, D. J., C. G. Gemmell, P. R. Craddock, P. G. Quie, and P. K. Peterson. 1981. Effect of staphylococcal alpha toxin on neutrophil migration and adhesiveness. *Inflammation* 5:313–322.

173. Shafer, W. M., S. G. Casey, and J. K. Spitznagel. 1984. Lipid A and resistance of *Salmonella typhimurium* to antimicrobial granule proteins of human neutrophil granulocytes. *Infect. Immun.* 43:834–838.

174. Shafer, W. M., L. E. Martin, and J. K. Spitznagel. 1986. Late intraphagosomal hydrogen ion concentration favors the in vitro antimicrobial capacity of a 37-kilodalton cationic protein of human neutrophil granulocytes. *Infect. Immun.* 53:651–655.

175. Shankar, P., F. Agis, D. Wallach, B. Flageul, F. Cottenot, J. Augier, and M. A. Bach. 1986. *M. leprae* and PPD-triggered T cell lines in tuberculoid and lepromatous leprosy. *J. Immunol.* 136:4255–4263.

176. Shewen, P. E., and B. N. Wilkie. 1982. Cytotoxin of *Pasteurella haemolytica* acting on bovine leukocytes. *Infect. Immun.* 35:91–94.

177. Sibley, L. D., S. G. Franzblau, and J. L. Krahenbuhl. 1987. Intracellular fate of *Mycobacterium leprae* in normal and activated mouse macrophages. *Infect. Immun.* 55:680–685.

178. Sibley, L. D., and J. L. Krahenbuhl. 1987. *Mycobacterium leprae*-burdened macrophages are refractory to activation by gamma interferon. *Infect. Immun.* 55:446–450.

179. Simon, G. L., M. S. Klempner, D. L. Kasper, and S. L. Gorbach. 1982. Alterations in opsonophagocytic killing by neutrophils of *Bacteroides fragilis* associated with animal and laboratory passage: effect of capsular polysaccharide. *J. Infect. Dis.* 145:72–77.

180. Slocombe, R. F., J. Malark, R. Ingersoll, F. J. Derksen, and N. E. Robinson. 1985. Importance of neutrophils in the pathogenesis of acute pneumonic pasteurellosis in calves. *Am. J. Vet. Res.* 46:2253–2258.

181. Smith, C. C., R. M. Barr, and J. Alexander. 1979. Studies on the interaction of *Mycobacterium microti* and *Mycobacterium lepraemurium* with mouse polymorphonuclear leukocytes. *J. Gen. Microbiol.* 112:185–189.

182. Smith, H. 1977. Microbial surfaces in relation to pathogenicity. *Bacteriol. Rev.* 41:475–500.

183. Smith, M. R., and W. B. Wood, Jr. 1947. Studies on the mechanism of recovery in pneumonia due to Friedlander's bacillus. III. The role of "surface phagocytosis" in the destruction of the microorganisms in the lung. *J. Exp. Med.* 86:257–265.

184. Snyderman, R., H. S. Shin, J. K. Phillips, H. Gewurz, and S. E. Mergenhagen. 1969. A neutrophil chemotactic factor derived from C5 upon interaction of guinea pig serum with endotoxin. *J. Immunol.* 103:413–422.

185. Spangrude, G. J., F. Sacchi, H. R. Hill, D. E. Van Epps, and R. A. Daynes. 1985. Inhibition

of lymphocyte and neutrophil chemotaxis by pertussis toxin. *J. Immunol.* 135:4135–4143.

186. Speert, D. P., B. A. Loh, D. A. Cabral, and I. E. Salit. 1986. Nonopsonic phagocytosis of nonmucoid *Pseudomonas aeruginosa* by human neutrophils and monocyte-derived macrophages is correlated with bacterial piliation and hydrophobicity. *Infect. Immun.* 53:207–212.

187. Spitznagel, J. K. 1983. Microbial interactions with neutrophils. *Rev. Infect. Dis.* 5:S806–S822.

188. Spitznagel, J. K., and W. M. Shafer. 1985. Neutrophil killing of bacteria by oxygen-independent mechanisms: a historical summary. *Rev. Infect. Dis.* 7:398–403.

189. Standbridge, E. J. 1982. Mycoplasma-lymphocyte interactions and their possible role in immunopathologic manifestations of mycoplasmal disease. *Rev. Infect. Dis.* 4:S219–S226.

190. Stevens, P., S. Huancy, W. D. Welch, and L. S. Young. 1978. Restricted complement activation by *Escherichia coli* with the K-1 capsular serotype: a possible role in pathogenicity. *J. Immunol.* 121:2174–2180.

191. Straley, S. C., and P. A. Harmon. 1984. Growth in mouse peritoneal macrophages of *Yersinia pestis* lacking established virulence determinants. *Infect. Immun.* 45:649–654.

192. Straley, S. C., and P. A. Harmon. 1984. *Yersinia pestis* grows within phagolysosomes in mouse peritoneal macrophages. *Infect. Immun.* 45:655–659.

193. Taylor, G., and C. J. Howard. 1980. Interaction of *Mycoplasma pulmonis* with mouse peritoneal macrophages and polymorphonuclear leukocytes. *J. Med. Microbiol.* 13:19–30.

194. Thomsen, A. C., and I. Heron. 1979. Effect of mycoplasmas on phagocytosis and immunocompetence in rats. *Acta Pathol. Microbiol. Scand. Sect. C* 87:67–71.

195. Thongthai, C., and W. D. Sawyer. 1973. Studies on the virulence of *Neisseria gonorrhoeae*. I. Relation of colonial morphology and resistance to phagocytosis by polymorphonuclear leukocytes. *Infect. Immun.* 7:373–379.

196. Todd, W. J., and J. Storz. Ultrastructural cytochemical evidence for the activation of lysosomes in the cytocidal effect of *Chlamydia psittaci*. *Infect. Immun.* 12:638–646.

197. Trinchieri, G., and B. Perussia. 1985. Immune interferon: a pleiotropic lymphokine with multiple effects. *Immunol. Today* 6:131–136.

198. Tsai, C. C., B. J. Shenker, J. M. DiRienzo, D. Malamud, and N. S. Taichman. 1984. Extraction and isolation of a leukotoxin from *Actinobacillus actinomycetemcomitans* with polymyxin B. *Infect. Immun.* 43:700–705.

199. Turco, J., and H. H. Winkler. 1983. Comparison of the properties of antirickettsial activity and

interferon in mouse lymphokines. *Infect. Immun.* 42:27–32.

200. Turcotte, R., and D. Legault. 1986. Mechanisms underlying the depressed production of interleukin-2 in spleen and lymph node cell cultures of mice infected with *Mycobacterium bovis* BCG. *Infect. Immun.* 51:826–831.

201. Une, T., and R. R. Brubaker. 1984. Roles of V antigen in promoting virulence and immunity in yersiniae. *J. Immunol.* 133:2226–2230.

202. Une, T., and R. R. Brubaker. 1984. In vivo comparison of a virulent VWA⁻ and PGM⁻ or PST^r phenotypes of yersiniae. *Infect. Immun.* 43:895–900.

203. Van Oss, C. J. 1978. Phagocytosis as a surface phenomenon. *Annu. Rev. Microbiol.* 32:19–39.

204. Veale, D. R., M. Goldner, C. W. Penn, J. Ward, and H. Smith. 1979. The intracellular survival and growth of gonococci in human phagocytes. *J. Gen. Microbiol.* 113:383–393.

205. Verbrugh, H. A., W. C. van Dijk, M. E. van Erne, R. Peters, P. K. Peterson, and J. Verhoef. 1979. Quantitation of the third component of human complement attached to the surface of opsonized bacteria: opsonin-deficient sera and phagocytosis-resistant strains. *Infect. Immun.* 26:808–814.

206. Wadee, A. A., and A. R. Rabson. 1981. Production of a suppressor factor by adherent cells from *Mycobacterium tuberculosis* infected guinea pigs. *Clin. Exp. Immunol.* 45:427–432.

207. Wahba, A., H. Cohen, and J. Sheskin. 1980. Neutrophil chemotactic responses in lepromatous leprosy: an in vitro study of 52 patients. *Clin. Immunol. Immunopathol.* 17:556–561.

208. Ward, P. A., S. Goralnick, and W. E. Bullock. 1976. Defective leukotaxis in patients with lepromatous leprosy. *J. Lab. Clin. Med.* 87:1025–1032.

209. Watson, S. R., and F. M. Collins. 1980. Development of suppressor T cells in mice heavily infected with mycobacteria. *Immunology* 39:367–373.

210. Weinberg, E. D. 1978. Iron and infection. *Microbiol. Rev.* 42:45–66.

211. Weinstein, D. L., M. Carsiotis, C. R. Lissner, and A. D. O'Brien. 1984. Flagella help *Salmonella typhimurium* survive within murine macrophages. *Infect. Immun.* 46:819–825.

212. Weiss, A. A., and E. L. Hewlett. 1986. Virulence factors of *Bordetella pertussis*. *Annu. Rev. Microbiol.* 40:661–686.

213. Weiss, A. A., and S. Falkow. 1984. Genetic analysis of phase change in *Bordetella pertussis*. *Infect. Immun.* 43:263–269.

214. Weiss, J., M. Victor, O. Stendahl, and P. Elsbach. 1982. Killing of gram-negative bacteria by polymorphonuclear leukocytes. Role of an O_2-independent bactericidal system. *J. Clin. Invest.* 69:959–970.

215. Welch, D. F., C. P. Sword, S. Brehm, and D. Dusanic. 1979. Relationship between superoxide dismutase and pathogenic mechanisms of *Listeria monocytogenes*. *Infect. Immun.* 23:863–872.

216. Welch, R. A., and S. Falkow. 1984. Characterization of *Escherichia coli* hemolysins conferring quantitative differences in virulence. *Infect. Immun.* 43:156–160.

217. Wilkinson, B. J., S. P. Sisson, Y. Kim, and P. K. Peterson. 1979. Localization of the third component of complement on the cell wall of encapsulated *Staphylococcus aureus* M: implications for the mechanism of resistance to phagocytosis. *Infect. Immun.* 26:1159–1163.

218. Wilkinson, P. C. 1980. Leukocyte locomotion and chemotaxis: effects of bacteria and viruses. *Rev. Infect. Dis.* 2:293–318.

219. Woolcock, J. B., and M. D. Mutimer. 1978. The capsules of *Corynebacterium equi* and *Streptococcus equi*. *J. Gen. Microbiol.* 109:127–130.

220. Worthen, G. S., C. Haslett, L. A. Smedly, A. J. Rees, R. S. Gumbay, J. E. Henson, and P. M. Henson. 1986. Lung vascular injury induced by chemotactic factors: enhancement by bacterial endotoxins. *Fed. Proc.* 45:7–12.

221. Wright, G. G., and G. L. Mandell. 1986. Anthrax toxin blocks priming of neutrophils by lipopolysaccharide and by muramyl dipeptide. *J. Exp. Med.* 164:1700–1709.

222. Young, E. J., M. Borchert, F. L. Kreotzer, and D. M. Musher. 1985. Phagocytosis and killing of *Brucella* by human polymorphonuclear leukocytes. *J. Infect. Dis.* 151:682–690.

223. Zimianski, M. C., C. R. Dawson, and B. Togni. 1974. Epithelial cell phagocytosis of *Listeria monocytogenes* in the conjunctiva. *Invest. Ophthalmol.* 13:623–626.

224. Zurbrick, B. G., and C. J. Czuprynski. 1987. Ingestion and intracellular growth of *Mycobacterium paratuberculosis* within bovine blood monocytes and monocyte-derived macrophages. *Infect. Immun.* 55:1588–1593.

Chapter 10

Chlamydial Infection: Breach of Host Cellular Barriers

J. STORZ, W. J. TODD, AND K. L. SCHNORR

Department of Veterinary Microbiology and Parasitology
School of Veterinary Medicine
Louisiana State University
Baton Rouge, Louisiana 70803

INTRODUCTION

Chlamydial agents are now recognized as pathogenic microorganisms that depend absolutely on the intracellular environment of animal cells for multiplication. Specifically, the following conditions for chlamydial survival and perpetuation are required by these obligate intracellular parasites. Chlamydiae must enter a suitable host cell, avoid destruction by the host, multiply therein without destroying host cellular functions essential for the parasite multiplication, and, finally, find a way to be released from the host cell and survive during passage to new hosts (50, 51).

Chlamydiae are of medical interest because of the diverse diseases they cause in humans and in animals (64, 73, 74). They are of research interest because of their interaction with eucaryotic host cells and their specialized life cycle with its unique features of parasitism. Currently, the two species *Chlamydia trachomatis* and *Chlamydia psittaci* compose the genus *Chlamydia*. Humans are the primary and perhaps the only natural hosts for *C. trachomatis*, which is associated with diseases such as tra-

choma, inclusion conjunctivitis, pneumonia, lymphogranuloma venereum, and genital tract infections (21, 55, 64). Animals susceptible to infections with *C. psittaci* are widely distributed in the animal kingdom and range from wild and domesticated birds to mammals, including humans. These infections have been recognized to lead to a variety of different disease conditions such as pneumonia, enteritis, encephalitis, conjunctivitis, polyarthritis, abortions and other reproductive disorders, and, significantly, clinically inapparent, persistent infections (73, 74).

The relationship that chlamydiae establish with host cells is an intimate association that has evolved between two very different forms of life. The invasion of host cells by chlamydiae represents the incursion of one genetic system by another genetic system. Chlamydiae have evolved mechanisms to exploit cellular functions (27, 28, 50, 51), including mechanisms for penetrating into different cellular compartments. Once inside the host cell, they do little damage initially and may even go unnoticed as chlamydial multiplication advances within the cell. They change their intracellular form of existence and finally exert a cytocidal effect on the infected host cell. Under other conditions, chlamydiae may persist for extended periods within the surviving host cell (55, 58, 78).

The mechanisms by which chlamydiae invade the host cells and control their fate and functions are important topics of investigation. This review concentrates on the different host cellular barriers that chlamydiae have to overcome and the functions of the host cell that are pirated by this intracellular pathogen. Information on these phenomena was obtained frequently by using inhibitors or compounds that modulate particular cell barriers. The actual mechanisms by which chlamydial developmental forms hurdle cellular barriers and harness cellular functions are not fully understood. Characterizing the hurdles that are overcome in the invasion of the host cellular genetic spheres revealed much about these uniquely efficient and diverse parasites.

FUNCTIONS OF CHLAMYDIAL FORMS IN THE DEVELOPMENTAL CYCLE

The developmental cycle of chlamydiae, which is synonymous with the infectious cycle, proceeds through a series of functional and morphological changes during intracellular multiplication (50, 63, 75). Chlamydiae are structurally and functionally reorganized during multiplication. The developmental cycle may be divided into the following stages: (i) adsorption of infectious elementary bodies (EBs) to cellular membranes; (ii) uptake of EBs and translocation into cytoplasmic sites; (iii) primary reorganization of the infecting EB into a larger dispersing form with further differentiation into a reticulate body (RB) ready to divide, during which time the EB envelope changes and the genome unfolds for expression; (iv) growth and multiplication by binary division of the noninfectious but metabolically active RBs; (v) secondary reorganization of the RBs into infectious EBs through a transition stage called condensing forms; and (vi) release

of infectious EBs from host cells.

Chlamydiae thus have several morphologies, depending on the stage of multiplication and the function the form plays in the chlamydial developmental cycle (50, 75). Chlamydial forms can be differentiated according to their morphology, chronological appearance during multiplication, and function. The following forms are distinguishable: EBs, dispersing forms, RBs, dividing RBs, and condensing forms. The different forms will be analyzed for features that facilitate interaction with host cells.

Chlamydial infectivity declines after adsorption and uptake, passes through a period without infectivity, lasting for about 20 to 48 h depending on species and biotype, and then rises rapidly along with the number of extracellular EBs. The rise in extracellular infectivity of *C. psittaci* correlates with a decline in host viability, as measured by trypan blue exclusion; and cells are extensively lysed after 40 h of infection. Reorganization of the EB into the dispersing form is comparable to the lag phase and lasts for about 6 to 8 h, which is much longer than the lag period of the typical bacterial growth curve (51). Multiplication and division of the noninfectious RBs correspond to the exponential growth phase. The estimated mean generation time of *C. psittaci* growing exponentially in L cells is about 2 h. The exponential growth phase lasts from 8 to 20 h, and then the organisms enter the retardation and stationary growth phases. Beginning with the appearance of condensing forms (about 20 h after infection) and continuing until the host cell dies, secondary reorganization of RBs into EBs occurs and is asynchronous. Emergence of infectivity coincides with the formation of EBs. The duration of the developmental cycle differs among chlamydial strains and host cell systems (75).

During reorganization of the EB into dispersing form, the following characteristic changes occur. The disulfide bonds that crosslink the protein moieties of outer membrane proteins of EBs are reduced, making the membrane more fluid (9, 29, 31, 57). The infecting

EB enlarges to a diameter of 400 to 500 nm. The dense nucleoid of the EB disperses into less electron-dense, filamentous material and becomes mixed with scattered, granular, ribosomelike particles. Division signals the completed change from the dispersing form into the RB. Infectious chlamydial EBs entering a host cell must contain and be able to express the genetic information governing their growth and development as well as their control of some host cell functions. The biochemical changes in the early chlamydial inclusions are difficult to distinguish from the metabolic activity of host cells. Parasite metabolic functions cannot be measured accurately at this developmental stage (51, 75). The mechanism of interaction of the dispersing form with the host cell is most critical in understanding early control mechanisms, yet this phase is poorly understood because it is so difficult to dissect experimentally.

The RBs range in size from 500 to 1,000 nm, are characteristically plastic and pleomorphic, and predominate throughout most of the development cycle. After numerous divisions the RBs become smaller and more circular, and reorganization into condensing forms occurs. This event is marked by condensation of fibrillar material in the centers of the smaller RBs. The condensing forms develop into the mature, infectious EBs by polarization of the electron-dense nucleoid to an eccentric location and by further decrease in size. Disulfide cross-linked proteins are formed during this phase (30). Secondary reorganization and formation of EBs occur while many dividing RBs are still present in chlamydial inclusions, producing additional progeny for maturation.

EBs, the extracellular infectious forms, have diameters of 200 to 280 nm. The internal organization of EBs as viewed in thin sections of chlamydial inclusions and purified particles is identical, sometimes having the appearance of a closely packed tuft of fibrils. The remaining semilunar area contains closely packed, round ribosomelike structures approximately 20 nm in diameter. EBs have smooth, limiting, trilaminar membranes 9 to 10 nm thick that are rigid and provide high resistance in the extra-

cellular environment. A second, narrower and less distinct, trilaminar plasma membrane is frequently detected beneath the outer cell membrane. Peptidoglycan is not found between the two layers, in contrast to other gram-negative bacteria. The EB envelope contains disulfide cross-linked protein complexes, because reducing agents are required for solubilization in sodium dodecyl sulfate. The major outer membrane protein has a molecular mass of about 40 kilodaltons (10, 31, 57). Other disulfide cross linked complexes in the envelopes of EBs of *C. psittaci* are three minor cysteine-rich proteins of 12, 59, and 62 kilodaltons (9, 11, 29–31, 57). Disulfide cross-linkage is postulated to determine the rigidity of the EB envelope. The eccentrically located electron-dense nucleoid is in contact with the plasma membrane.

Using scanning electron microscopy, Matsumoto (47) observed projections on the outside surfaces of EBs of *C. psittaci* and button structures on the inside surface after freeze-fracture. The projections were arranged hexagonally. Stokes demonstrated by high-voltage electron microscopy that these projections were distributed over about half the chlamydial surface and often were located opposite the concave side of the electron-dense, crescent-shaped chlamydial nucleoid (72). Patches of regular arrays of hemispheric projections were observed on EBs of *C. psittaci* and *C. trachomatis*. Louis et al. (45) studied the structure and modification of the envelope of *C. psittaci* during the chlamydial growth cycle by freeze-fracture and complementary replicas obtained in ultrahigh vacuum at very low temperature. They observed progressive differentiation of craterlike structures on the chlamydial membranes similar to the button structures described above. The localized patches of surface projections opposite the nucleoid confer a polarity on the chlamydial EB. Theoretically, these structures could function as transmembrane pores in the transfer of molecules from cellular to chlamydial sites during the developmental cycle. The significance of the projections is not known, but they may be related to projection-associated binding sites important for attachment to the host cells. The interaction with the host cell of all developmental forms of chlamydiae, except the EBs, is mediated through the inclusion membrane.

The reorganization from infectious EBs to noninfectious RBs proceeds through the dispersing forms. They are seen as single forms in thin sections of cells during the early stage of infection. These forms are round or ovoid and have diameters of 400 to 500 nm. They contain a granular matrix that is less electron dense than the nucleoid of the EBs but denser than the RBs. They are surrounded by an outer trilaminar membrane and an inner, less pronounced plasma membrane. The disulfide-linked membrane complexes are probably reduced during this transition (30). A fine fibrillar network is distributed throughout this form and contains round, ribosomelike structures. Interactions with the host cell are mediated through the endosomal membrane. Control of lysosomes and avoidance of their fusion with the chlamydia-containing endosome remain essential functions (75, 80).

The RBs arise from the dispersing forms as divided large and intermediate-sized pleomorphic, noninfectious chlamydial forms that may reach a size of 500 to 1,000 nm. They are surrounded by an outer membrane, which contains major outer membrane protein monomers that are not disulfide cross-linked, and an inner, ill-defined plasma membrane (31, 57). Fine reticulated fibrils are interspersed with numerous ribosomes as their internal structure. They remain within the confines formed by the inclusion membrane.

The smaller RBs are transformed, through the condensing forms, into the infectious EBs. Each 300- to 500-nm-diameter condensing form has a centrally located, electron-dense nucleoid. The central nucleoid mass is surrounded by an electron-lucent fibrillar zone connected through fibrils with an outer, electron-dense, granulofibrillar matrix of ribosomelike material and fibrils. These forms also have a trilaminar cell membrane and an inner, less prominent plasma membrane (50, 75).

ENTRY INTO THE HOST CELLULAR METABOLIC SPHERES

The failure to detect mechanisms by which host-free chlamydiae might generate useful energy led Moulder to propose the concept that they are energy parasites (50, 51). Recent findings revealed that chlamydiae directly utilize some host cellular energy intermediates. This concept implies that the successful chlamydial parasite sequesters the products of host energy-yielding reactions for its own use. The increase in glucose uptake by chlamydia-infected cells compared with uptake by control cells was significant, and increased utilization coincided with chlamydial multiplication (18). Addition of antimycin, an inhibitor of aerobic respiration at the cytochrome level, or other inhibitors of cellular respiration, decreased chlamydial yields (18).

The first demonstration of the use of an energy-rich product of cell metabolism by multiplying chlamydiae was done by Hatch (28). The direct utilization of host cell nucleoside triphosphates by multiplying chlamydiae became evident from analysis of equilibrium labeling of nucleotides in infected cells and from incorporation of labels into 16S chlamydial RNA. The kinetics of CMP:UMP and GMP:AMP labeling of chlamydial 16S RNA indicated that the chlamydial parasite utilized preformed host nucleoside triphosphate pools. Exogenous thymidine was incorporated at a minimal level into chlamydial DNA. Hatch (28) suggested that the failure of chlamydiae to utilize host thymidine pools efficiently may be due to the concentration of the TTP pools in the nucleus and to the more successful competition of the host for this substrate.

The strong evidence that chlamydiae depend on and utilize energy intermediates such as host cellular nucleosides implies that the membranes of multiplying chlamydiae and their inclusions must have unusual properties. The cytoplasmic chlamydial inclusions are bounded by a membrane initially derived from the host plasmalemma and are subsequently modified and enlarged. In addition, chlamydial forms have cell walls and plasma membranes. Chlamydiae must have evolved mechanisms for the transport of nucleoside triphosphates across these three membranes, perhaps via the specialized surface structures found on EBs or RBs. The interaction of chlamydiae with cellular membranes and the intracellular environment provides factors that induce changes in the envelopes of the EBs and the inclusion membrane (75).

Isoleucine was identified by Hatch (27) as a limiting factor in chlamydial multiplication. Insufficient levels of this essential amino acid prevented the L-cell hosts from dividing. Chlamydial multiplication did not proceed when isoleucine levels were too low to permit L-cell growth. An overall reduction in the rate of protein synthesis by both host and parasite resulted from the deficiency of isoleucine. Under these conditions, C. psittaci persisted in a noninfectious latent state within the host cell. The host cell and the chlamydial parasite competed for the same limiting factor, isoleucine. Addition of isoleucine to starved cells containing chlamydiae in a latent state activated the parasite to complete the developmental cycle. Addition of cycloheximide induced a similar effect, whereby the infection was activated because cycloheximide prevented host protein synthesis and made host isoleucine available for chlamydial protein synthesis and multiplication.

Another interesting aspect of host cell dependence of chlamydiae was identified by Fan and Jenkin (16) in studies of lipid biosynthesis in chlamydia-infected cells. Host cell lipid synthesis appeared to be inhibited in cells infected with the LGV strain of C. trachomatis. This observation suggested that chlamydial agents also exploit the host cell capacity for lipid synthesis. Since chlamydiae were found to lack aldolases for glucose utilization, they must derive the three-carbon compounds required for the glycerol moiety of lipids from the host cells. Phosphatidic acid, glycerol phosphate, and dihydroxyacetone were considered sufficient to satisfy the requirements for three-carbon units. By reducing the formation of host cellular diglycerides, which are important in lipid bio-

synthesis in mammalian cells, chlamydiae could divert phosphatidic acid for the synthesis of cytidine diphosphate diglyceride, leading to the formation of chlamydial phosphatidyl ethanolamine.

Another level of host cell dependence is observed with strains of C. psittaci. These strains utilize cellular folic acid or its precursors for chlamydial biosynthetic processes (21, 54).

EVIDENCE FOR CHLAMYDIAL LIGANDS AND CELLULAR RECEPTORS

The nature of the EB surface ligand that recognizes and interacts with the host cell surface was explored (13, 22, 23, 84). The previous finding that EB cell walls attach to and are taken up by host cells nearly as efficiently as are intact EBs assigns the functions of adsorption to cell wall components. The ligand molecules involved appear to be proteins, because heating of EBs inhibited adsorption (7, 17).

Electroblotting procedures were developed to demonstrate the association of radiolabeled host cell components with chlamydial proteins. EB preparations were solubilized and separated by polyacrylamide gel electrophoresis. The resolved chlamydial antigens were then electrophoretically transferred to nitrocellulose. Labeled and solubilized plasma membrane proteins from cell lines grown in culture were then exposed to the nitrocellulose-bound chlamydial proteins to detect chlamydial ligand proteins. The two proteins binding labeled membrane components of host cells had molecular masses of approximately 18 and 31 kilodaltons and were present on EBs of C. trachomatis serovars. They were not detected in RBs (84). Hackstadt (22) found that two strains of C. psittaci had ligand proteins of 18 and 32 kilodaltons, but failed to detect the larger protein in the presence of 2-mercaptoethanol. He detected serologic activity of these proteins in antisera which had been raised against Formalin-killed EBs (22). These sera did not neutralize infectivity, nor did they recognize the 18- or 32-kilodalton protein by immunoprecipitation. Wenman and Meuser (84) produced antisera, monospecific by Western blotting, for either the 18- or 31-kilodalton protein antigen, which blocked binding of eucaryotic cell membranes to the chlamydial proteins and also neutralized infectivity.

Treatment of cells with trypsin reduced adsorption of EBs, and recovery of this refractive cellular state was prevented by adding cycloheximide (7, 8). Dextran sulfate, fetuin, ovomucoid, N-acetylneuraminic acid, and neuraminidase pretreatment of monolayers decreased the susceptibility of HeLa cells for trachoma stains (39). It was proposed that sialic acids may function as possible receptors for chlamydial ligands (38). Infectivity of LGV strains was not affected by these treatments; however, treatment of cells with wheat germ agglutinin inhibited their infectivity (44). Because of the complementarity of this agglutinin for N-acetylglucosamine, a receptor with this specificity was postulated. Unfortunately, nonspecific high-affinity association of wheat germ agglutinin with N-acetylneuraminic acid also occurs, leaving the specificity somewhat in doubt (1, 82). Other LGV strains were not affected, indicating the existence of additional cellular binding sites.

Other recent experimental evidence minimizes the significance of specific chemical moieties of cellular receptors. Many saccharides tested had no inhibitory effect on the association of trachoma strains with cells, but N-acetylneuraminic acid, galactosamine, and mannosamine caused significant inhibition, and this effect was mediated by their amino groups (1). Furthermore, insect cells or mutant BHK Ric R14 cells depleted or deficient in N-acetylglucosamine were susceptible to infection with an oculogenital chlamydial strain. Allan and Pearce (1) explained these results in terms of electrostatic repulsion rather than blocking of receptor-ligand interaction. Increased electrostatic repulsion caused by addition of N-acetylneuraminic acid to the negatively charged host and EB surfaces, and reduced electrostatic forces for

N-acetylneuraminic acid-depleted cells, could explain these phenomena. These authors (1) proposed the important new idea that the initial attachment of chlamydiae to host cells may be more complex than that mediated by a simple mono- or oligosaccharide. Chlamydiae might be capable of more than one specific ligand-receptor interaction. Furthermore, the inhibitory effects of glucosamine and mannosamine may depend on induced depletion of host cell receptors through inhibition of receptor recycling (25, 82).

EARLY EB-HOST CELL INTERACTION

Interaction between chlamydial EBs and host cells has been studied by using radiolabeled EBs and analysis of whole-cell populations (7, 17) and by ultrastructural evaluation of cells infected during early stages of the cycle (15, 17, 32, 78, 82, 86, 87). Fluorescent-antibody techniques or cytological examination was used for qualitative assessment of inclusion formation after infection. These methods were not sensitive enough to monitor quantitatively the behavior of EBs and individual cells or subpopulations of cells. The combination of flow cytometry and fluorescence-microscopic observations has the promise for precise quantitative analysis of EB-host cell interactions (43, 81).

The following pattern emerges on the basis of interpretations of experimental evidence and some speculation. Adsorption of EBs to the plasmalemma occurs by specific but yet undefined binding between chlamydial ligands and receptors on the host cell. Through this specific interaction, the host cell is committed to take up the EB, a process that can explain the observation of facilitated uptake whereby chlamydiae preferentially enter host cells (7, 17). The process of entry most probably occurs by receptor-mediated endocytosis via coated pits (32, 82, 87). EBs within the endocytic vacuole are then transported to the area of the Golgi apparatus in harmony with primary reorganization (15). The development of the inclusion at the site of the Golgi apparatus is consistent with the coated-pit concept of entry, because this endocytic pathway usually cycles through the Golgi apparatus rather than through lysosomes. The energy required for the uptake of EBs comes from the host cell, because the uptake by either L cells or macrophages is interfered with by glycolytic or oxidative inhibitors (17, 18).

It is agreed that chlamydiae are relatively efficient in inducing different types of cells as well as professional phagocytic cells to take them up. Chlamydiae are taken up by nonprofessional phagocytes at a rate approximately 10 to 100 times faster than that of latex beads or *Escherichia coli* cells. The term parasite-specified phagocytosis was coined to stress the influence of the organism on this enhanced rate of uptake (7, 8). Classical phagocytosis is characterized ultrastructurally by particle uptake through pseudopodial enclosure. This process of phagocytosis is inhibited by microfilament inhibitors such as cytochalasin B (7). Uptake of chlamydiae is unaffected by cytochalasin B, but methylamine and monodansylcadaverine, inhibitors of receptor-mediated endocytosis, block EB uptake (34, 82).

Chlamydial EBs are seen principally along the tips and sides of microvilli in the early stages of adsorption (15, 32, 66, 79). The binding of EBs to cellular microvilli might help to bridge electronegative barriers between EBs and host cells by increasing the chances of contact and adherence. With time the EBs are associated with depressions in the cell membranes at the base of the microvilli, which are known sites of clathrin-coated pits. If gold-labeled α2 macroglobulin is mixed with EBs, both can be seen in the same coated pits or alone in separate coated pits (32). Parasitism of this entry process offers an attractive explanation for the escape from fusion with lysosomes.

Interpretation of experimental evidence obtained with other chlamydial strains appears to contradict the scheme of uptake described above (82). The use of various inhibitors to pinpoint cellular functions has shortcomings. High multiplicities of EBs per host cell in investigations of the early events in chlamydial infections make it impossible to determine which configuration will lead to productive infection.

Flow-cytometric analysis of the chlamydial infectious process may bring new insight. Previous experimental investigations of EB-host cell interactions differentiated neither the number of cells interacting with EB nor the relative number of EBs interacting with cells. Levitt et al. (43) devised an experimental design which furnishes this accuracy. Fewer than 50% of cells internalized 25% of the bound EB following pronase treatment in the L_2 McCoy fibroblast system. There was a relatively rapid inactivation of L_2 EBs prior to detection of chlamydial inclusion formation. Uptake was complete by 4 h, and 90% of the cells took up almost 70% of the EBs that were initially bound. Although 45% of McCoy cells developed inclusions after exposure to one 50% infective dose of L_2, another 35% of the cells internalized EBs that did not proliferate. It was assumed previously that EB entering a permissive host cell initiated an infectious cycle. Evidently all EBs may not have the same infectious potential, yet defective properties have not been explored. Flow cytometry should permit more conclusive assessment of the effects of various sugars, lectins, polycations, or polyanions on the chlamydial infectious process and the susceptibility of host cells (43, 81).

EFFECT OF CYTOACTIVE AGENTS ON CELLULAR SUSCEPTIBILITY TO CHLAMYDIAL INFECTIONS

Methods used to enhance the infectivity of chlamydiae for cultured cells resulted in important observations on the host-parasite relationship. Irradiation was one of several methods used to prepare nondividing cells for chlamydial culture (19). Irradiated cells no longer divided, but over several days they became large, flattened, and multinucleated. An advantage of this system is that the large cytoplasm of irradiated cells allows the development of extensive, easily recognized inclusions. Other methods which have been used to produce nondividing cells are treatment with cytochalasin B or 5-iodo-2'-deoxyuridine. These treatments were equivalent to X irradiation for increasing the susceptibility of cells to chlamydial infection (12).

Additional approaches to enhancing chlamydial uptake and infectivity are pretreatment of the cells with the polycation DEAE-dextran (DEAE-D) or centrifugation of the cells along with the inoculum (20, 26, 68, 69). A solution containing 20 to 30 µg of DEAE-D (molecular weight, 2×10^6) per ml was used to wash the monolayer prior to infection. Treatment with DEAE-D enhanced the infectivity of some strains of C. psittaci and C. trachomatis. The infectivity of LGV strains was not enhanced. Weiss and Dressler (83) were the first to show that centrifugation could enhance the infectivity of obligate intracellular parasites for cultured cells. A 1,200-fold increase in infectivity of C. psittaci was reported when chlamydiae were centrifuged in the presence of L-cell monolayers. Maximum infectivity resulted from centrifugation for 1 h at 2,000 $\times$ g. It was also shown that lower centrifugal forces are satisfactory for enhancing the infectivity of chlamydiae. Although centrifuge-enhanced infectivity did increase when the centrifugal force was increased, infectivity did not increase after 10 min of centrifugation. Observations are not compatible with sedimentation onto cells as the mechanism for centrifuge-enhanced infectivity, and it is theorized that centrifugation may expose cellular receptors.

Chlamydiae have a net negative surface charge (pI 4 to 5) at neutral pH (1, 12). Cells also have a net negative surface charge. The low spontaneous infectivity of chlamydiae for cultured cells may well be due to their mutually repulsive surface charges. Treatment of cells with the polycation DEAE-D enhances the infectivity of C. trachomatis or C. psittaci for cells, presumably by neutralizing mutually repulsive electrostatic forces. The DEAE-D effect varies quantitatively with both the cell type used and the chlamydial strain. Although centrifugation

is much more efficient than DEAE-D treatment of cells in enhancing infectivity, the effects of centrifugation and DEAE-D are not additive at high centrifugal forces. Centrifuge-enhanced adsorption occurs rapidly, within 10 min or less, and is not dependent on additional time of stationary adsorption.

Cycloheximide consistently enhances chlamydial inclusion formation in treated cells (27). Treatment of L cells with cycloheximide at 2 µg/ml enhanced inclusion formation 1.75-fold for C. psittaci LW-613 and 2.50-fold for C. psittaci B-577 (12, 68, 69). It is believed that cycloheximide enhances infectivity by increasing the soluble pool of amino acids and by allowing the parasite to compete better for the host cellular pool of nutrients. Consequently, it does not affect adsorption or uptake.

Cytochalasin B has no effect on chlamydial infectivity for either phagocytic or nonphagocytic cells treated with this drug (7). The absence of an inhibitory effect is alone quite important. Cytochalasin B inhibits polymerization of actin and formation of microfilaments. At the levels used (1 µg/ml), cytochalasin B inhibits energy-requiring microfilament activity, including cellular motility and cytoplasmic streaming. Chlamydial uptake requires energy. Cytochalasin B does not inhibit energy-independent micropinocytosis, which functions during uptake of soluble nutrients. Accordingly, the mechanism of chlamydial uptake must differ from any of these three mechanisms.

Enhanced infectivity of C. trachomatis for HeLa cells treated with cyclic GMP or drugs that enhance intracellular levels of cGMP, namely carbachol and prostaglandins FS2 and E_2, was reported (12). Treatment of L cells with similar doses of carbachol or cGMP had little, if any, enhancing effect on C. psittaci inclusion formation (33). The lack of inhibitory action alone is important in understanding chlamydia-host cell interactions. Although the exact effect of cGMP on phagocytosis is largely unknown, it is generally believed that increased levels of cGMP enhance lysosomal mobilization by stimulating microtubules and phagolysosome formation.

Stewart (70) reported an increase in infectivity of *C. psittaci* for L cells treated with hydrocortisone at levels up to 100 μg/ml. Although no effect on infectivity of *C. trachomatis* in hydrocortisone-treated mouse macrophages was found, increased infectivity of *C. trachomatis* in hydrocortisone-treated McCoy cells was observed by others. Bushell and Hobson (6) reported a twofold increase in infectivity at doses of 0.1 to 10.0 μg/ml. Our findings of enhanced inclusion formation in hydrocortisone-treated L cells confirm the previous observations. At a hydrocortisone dose of 10.0 μg/ml, *C. psittaci* inclusion formation increased 1.40-fold for strain LW-613 and 2.25-fold for strain B-577. Enhanced chlamydial infectivity in hydrocortisone-treated cells is difficult to explain (12). Hydrocortisone is most effective in enhancing chlamydial inclusion formation when given before infection. This drug is known to have a stabilizing effect on plasma and lysosomal membranes and is also known to reduce host cellular RNA and DNA synthesis. In analogy with the theory on cycloheximide-enhanced chlamydial infectivity, Bushell and Hobson (6) suggested that reduced host-parasite competition for nutrients allowed chlamydiae to prosper.

When cells were treated to depolymerize microtubules, equal enhancement of *C. psittaci* infectivity for L cells was seen when colchicine (1 μg/ml) was used to treat cells 2 h before, during, or 2 h after centrifuge-enhanced adsorption (12). The results of this experiment are not compatible with the theory that depolymerization of microtubules alters adsorption or uptake. The enhancing effect of colchicine was rapid and appeared to be irreversible. The early events in chlamydial multiplication after uptake proceeded faster in colchicine-treated cells, so that the inclusions were larger at 48 h after infection. Evidently, cells with depolymerized microtubules provide favorable conditions for the early phases of chlamydial multiplication (12).

Infectivity of chlamydiae for colchicine-treated L cells showed a 1.50-fold (for strain B-577) to 1.83-fold (for strain LW-613) increase over that for untreated cells. The increase in infectivity was found at doses of 0.1 to 10.0 μg/ml. The best understood of the many effects of colchicine on cells is that it binds to tubulin, inhibiting the formation of microtubules and depolymerizing those already formed in cells. Microtubules are essential in maintaining cytoskeletal integrity and in phagolysosome formation. Lumicolchicine and vinblastine were also used to treat L cells before they were infected with *C. psittaci*. Lumicolchicine is a photoinactivated product of colchicine. Lumicolchicine and colchicine have identical effects on cells, except that lumicolchicine does not bind to tubulin. Vinblastine is similar to colchicine in that it binds to tubulin and inhibits microtubule formation and function. Results of these experiments are not conclusive, and the mechanism of colchicine-enhanced infectivity remains elusive (12). It is possible that uptake of chlamydiae is the same in colchicine- and lumicolchicine-treated cells. Events in chlamydial multiplication after uptake are enhanced in colchicine-treated cells and seem to be reduced in cells in which tubulin functions to maintain the cytoskeleton.

DEFECTIVE DEVELOPMENT UNDER ENHANCING CONDITIONS

The polycation DEAE-D is thought to cause increased uptake of some types of chlamydiae by host cells, which results in the development of more inclusions in DEAE-D-treated cells. DEAE-D treatment caused little change in either the number of inclusion-containing cells or the yield of infectious progeny produced by a serotype 1 strain of mammalian *C. psittaci* (67–69). In contrast, a serotype 2 strain infected nine times the number of cells in a DEAE-D treated monolayer, but the yield per infected cell was much lower than from untreated cells. This indicates that although more of the serotype 2 EBs began the developmental cycle, many of the resulting inclusions did not mature normally in the treated cells.

Strain LW-613 exhibited a different pattern of inclusion formation in untreated cells from that of strain B-577. Instead of forming an inclusion with an entire margin, the RBs of the serotype 2 strain often indented individually into the surrounding host cell cytoplasm, giving the inclusion a highly irregular shape, yet retaining the inclusion membrane.

In cycloheximide-treated cells, many chlamydial forms of strain LW-613 were highly pyknotic. The chlamydial forms stained darkly, and numerous miniature RBs appeared within the cell walls of the altered RBs. The RBs had amorphous areas and areas packed with dark-staining granules the size of ribosomes. Segregated lighter patches containing filamentous material were seen in some aberrant RBs. The rough endoplasmic reticulum of the host cell was dilated within a cytoplasm more electron dense than that of neighboring uninfected cells. The mitochondria had condensed matrices, and the membranes of the cristae were irregular and indistinct. When inclusions were small and contained only RBs, fewer abnormalities were observed.

The serotype 2 strain exhibited several additional changes in DEAE-D-treated cells. The RBs were often enlarged and more electron lucent than normal. The chlamydial forms were abnormally pleomorphic, with less-distinct boundaries between RBs. Amorphous areas of intermediate electron density appeared within chlamydial forms. The cytoplasm of some chlamydial forms appeared degenerated and consisted of membranes and cell walls that enclosed a few strands of the previous reticulum. Similar abnormal chlamydial forms were observed in colchicine-treated L cells (12, 67).

The decreased yields of infectious progeny from *C. psittaci* serotype 2 grown in cells treated with DEAE-D, cycloheximide, or colchicine can be explained by the aberrant chlamydial forms observed. The pyknotic forms in cycloheximide-treated monolayers were not caused by a specific effect of the cycloheximide, because these aberrant forms were also seen in colchicine or DEAE-D-treated cells. The configuration of the

mitochondria in host cells that contained pyknotic chlamydial forms suggested that the eucaryotic cells had received an injury and perhaps were no longer able to supply the parasite with the energy it required. The chlamydial infection probably contributed to the injury of the host cells, since mock-infected control cell monolayers did not show the same changes, even though some degenerating cells were present (67). Although chlamydiae multiply in balance with a normal host cell, the serotype 2 strains may overtax a stessed host, because this serotype appears to require more host-specific synthesis than serotype 1.

CYTOPATHIC FUNCTIONS AND RELEASE OF CHLAMYDIAE FROM HOST CELLS

Intracellular bacteria are released by a variety of mechanisms that are dependent upon the host cell and the particular genus, species, and biotype of the pathogen. Although it is well established that different intracellular bacteria are released from infected cells by different mechanisms, it is also true that the same pathogen may exit from different cell types by entirely different mechanisms.

Members of the genus *Chlamydia* are responsible for a diverse spectrum of clinical diseases in animals and humans. Consequently, we can expect an equal variety of interactions with host cells, especially with respect to the cell type infected, duration of infection, persistence, and mechanisms of release. Experimental analysis has documented the two mechanisms that may be possible extremes: release associated with lysis of the infected host cell and release by a process of exocytosis without concomitant host cell death (78, 80).

Host cell lysis is the most commonly documented mechanism of chlamydial release in nature (35, 80). The process of chlamydia-induced cell lysis was studied by using the highly pathogenic bovine chlamydial strain designated LW-613. To gain insight into the cytolytic events potentially important to this invasive pathogenic strain, the mechanisms of chlamydial release and host cell lysis were studied in detail under defined laboratory conditions by using cultured bovine fetal spleen cells analyzed by enzyme reactions, cell fractionation methods, and ultrastructural cytochemical techniques. All methods of analysis led to the conclusion that extensive release of lysosomal enzymes from host cells occurs during later stages of the chlamydial developmental cycle. These enzymes digest most of the host cell constituents, resulting in concomitant lysis of the host cell and release of the infectious EBs. The involvement of lysosomal enzymes in the lytic events of chlamydial release may be a common characteristic of highly invasive strains of C. psittaci (80) and may by itself account for some of the pathologic changes in vivo.

Persistent infections with chlamydiae are common and important. Which release mechanisms function in persistent or noncytocidal infections? Chlamydiae classified as C. trachomatis are surprisingly distinct from members of the species C. psittaci. Although both species share a similar developmental cycle and several key antigens, such as the genus-specific antigen, there is little genetic or antigenic relatedness between them (54, 63, 64). Although they may have had a common ancestor, the two species clearly have evolved along different evolutionary paths. C. trachomatis is specifically a human pathogen, whereas C. psittaci is an animal pathogen that occasionally infects humans. Only one strain of C. psittaci, the TWAR agent, appears to infect humans as its primary host (37).

C. trachomatis strains can be divided into two biological variants: biovar I and biovar II. Biovar I comprises the LGV strains, which, like C. psittaci, commonly produce invasive infections (64). In cell culture they induce plaques and thus exit cells by lysis of the infected cells, presumably by in situ release of host lysosomal enzymes as exemplified by lytic release of C. psittaci in cell culture. In contrast, the C. trachomatis isolates classified as biovar II possess

decidedly different biological and pathogenic properties. These isolates are normally not invasive in vivo. Infections are limited largely to mucosal epithelial cells of the conjunctiva and the genital tract, causing primarily hyperendemic trachoma and sexually transmitted urogenital tract infections (64).

Perhaps the most curious puzzle concerning chlamydial release and disease is the clinical observation of the carrier state for the sexually transmitted biovar II chlamydiae in human subjects. Many carriers produce and release large numbers of EBs without showing any clinical signs of disease (64). The interactions of these chlamydiae with host cells are therefore likely to be much more diverse than the cell lysis that commonly occurs with C. psittaci and biovar I of C. trachomatis. Some insight into this apparent paradox of multiplication and release of large numbers of chlamydiae, without any overt cytopathic changes, was gained through the investigations of Todd and Caldwell (78), who furnished evidence for the release of EBs without concomitant death of the host cells in culture. This observation is likely to be essential to understanding the mechanisms of pathogenesis produced by biovar II in vivo and may have some bearing on the in vivo mechanisms of persistent infections with C. psittaci.

Although many aspects of and all of the molecular mechanisms responsible for noncytocidal release remain unknown, the following relevant information emerged: the earliest step in this mechanism of release is the disruption of the inclusion membrane, which occurs after the formation of EBs commences. This observation was unexpected, considering the previous evidence of cell lysis by C. psittaci, which indicated that the inclusion membrane is one of the last structures to be destroyed. The next step in noncytolytic release is the dislocation of host cell cytoplasm from the apical portion of the inclusion and the plasmalemma. The inclusion is now separated from the extracellular environment only by the plasmalemma of the host cell. The events that follow are less well documented. The plasmalemma over the area of the inclusion rup-

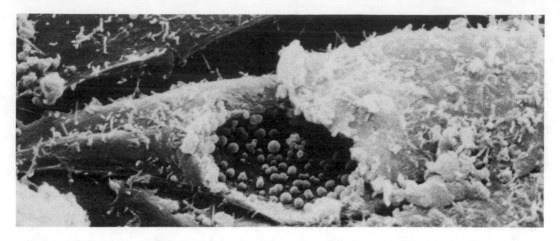

FIGURE 1. Release of *C. trachomatis* serotype D from infected HeLa cells by rupture of the host cell at the site of the inclusion. This scanning electron micrograph shows chlamydial particles attached to the inner surface of the opened chlamydial inclusion at 72 h postinfection. Despite such openings, the host cells remain viable as determined by vital stains and will eventually repair the lesions (78).

tures, and the contents of the inclusion reach the extracellular environment. This became evident through scanning electron microscopy (Fig. 1) and was confirmed by fluorescent-antibody studies on unfixed cells (78).

While the inclusions are opened and chlamydial EBs escape, the infected host cell remains viable, as determined by vital staining with trypan blue. To protect the osmotic integrity of the host cell, a new portion of plasmalemma appears to be formed underneath the protruding inclusion. This process begins with the accumulation of a microfilamentlike network just below the basal portion of the inclusion membrane, which seems to wall off the inclusion from the main body of the host cell. A new portion of plasmalemma is then formed, effectively separating the area of the inclusion from the rest of the host cell. One plausible interpretation is that during the latter stages of infection, after loss of the inclusion membrane, the host cell can recognize the presence of the inclusion, effectively wall off that portion of the cell, and expel its contents of EBs. Thus, the infectious EBs are released without concomitant death of the host cell. The infected monolayers remain intact throughout the cycle of infection.

Moulder et al. (53) analyzed the toxic effect of EBs at the cellular level by studying the reactions of L cells on exposure to high multiplicities of different chlamydial strains. When L cells were exposed to 500 to 1,000 50% infective doses of chlamydiae, they began to die 8 h after exposure and were dead long before the chlamydial developmental cycle was completed. This phenomenon is called immediate toxicity. Chlamydial EBs inactivated by UV irradiation retained their ability to injure cells, but heat inactivation destroyed this activity. Cells exposed in suspension to high multiplicities did not attach to the surfaces of culture vessels and failed to spread out. Their phagocytic and protein-synthesizing activities were reduced. For induction of immediate toxicity, chlamydial EBs had to be ingested in large numbers by the host cells. Chlamydiae did not need to synthesize macromolecules or to reproduce to cause the immediate toxic effect. Evidence for release of lysosomal enzymes was not found, nor could depression of cellular metabolism explain the rapid injury and death of the host cells. The immediate toxicity was thought to derive from injuries to the plasma membrane of the host cell by the high rate of chlamydial uptake through endocytosis (53, 87).

THE PLASMALEMMA DURING CHLAMYDIAL INFECTION

The most obvious role of the plasmalemma in chlamydial infections occurs during the initial stages of infection, adsorption, and uptake of the infectious EBs. Other functions of the plasmalemma during the course of the chlamydial infectious cycle may be significant. The plasmalemma may function to protect intracellular chlamydiae from immune surveillance. During the terminal stages of cellular infection, it must be either lysed during cytolytic mechanisms of chlamydial release or repaired during exocytotic mechanisms of chlamydial release (16, 71, 78, 79).

Between the early and late stages of infection, the plasmalemma may also play a direct role in chlamydial infection. Reportedly, chlamydiae modify the surfaces of the infected cells by inserting chlamydia-specific antigens. This observation is important because of possible immune clearance of infected cells. The first experimental protocol to detect chlamydial antigens on the surfaces of infected cells by polyclonal fluorescent-antibody assay involved air drying, which could by itself disrupt and translocate chlamydial antigens (61). Recently, Wilde et al. (85) reported transient presence of chlamydial proteins on the host cell surface and long-term presence of chlamydia-specific lipopolysaccharide (LPS). These observations were made with monoclonal antibodies on unfixed infected cells without air drying. The accumulation of LPS was associated with a decrease in the fluidity of the plasmalemma. These data suggest a dynamic interaction between antigens of chlamydiae and the plasmalemma.

PROPERTIES AND FUNCTIONS OF THE INCLUSION MEMBRANE

Chlamydial EBs are taken up by cells through a process of endocytosis. Importantly, they continue to reside in the cytoplasmic inclusion vacuole, which is bounded by a plasmalemma-derived unit membrane. This cytoplasmic inclusion membrane enlarges as chlamydiae grow and multiply. Consequently, the inclusion membrane becomes expanded and possibly modified. It continues to have important containment and transport functions throughout chlamydial development (17, 50, 65, 75, 76).

Matsumoto (47, 48) defined some properties of inclusions of L cells infected with the meningopneumonitis-causing strain of *C. psittaci*. The membrane can be considered part of the inclusion. The inclusion membranes were less stable in 0.25 M sucrose solution than the plasmalemma was. Addition of bovine serum albumin or fetal bovine serum stabilized the membranes. Isolated inclusions were relatively stable in 10 mM Tris buffer with 5% bovine serum albumin. Chlamydial inclusions behaved similarly whether they were isolated from mouse macrophages or L cells in discontinuous dextran or sucrose gradients, and they exibited similar sensitivities to detergent (88). Macrophage inclusion membranes had at least nine proteins with equal mobilities in sodium dodecyl sulfate-polyacrylamide gel electrophoresis. Only two of these proteins had mobilities equal to those of plasmalemma proteins.

Ultrastructurally it was observed that RBs also have surface projections and that RBs are connected directly with the host cytoplasm through the canals of the projections. It may be possible that RBs within an inclusion communicate and interchange directly with the host cell cytoplasm in this manner (47, 48). Importantly, it was not resolved whether mitochondria form direct contacts with the inclusion membranes.

The morphology of the inclusion membrane as revealed by freeze-replica techniques appears to differ from that of the plasmalemma (48). Since the inclusion membrane is derived from the plasmalemma, it follows that the P and E faces are reversed. The convex surface of the inclusion membrane corresponds to the E face, and the P face represents the concave surface. Membrane particles were not found on the convex surface, but many are present on the concave surface. Biochemical studies by Stokes

(71) also indicate that the inclusion membrane may be modified by chlamydia-directed glycosylation.

CONTROL OF LYSOSOMES

Lysosomes are an important hurdle for chlamydiae to clear in becoming successful intracellular parasites. Bacteria that have adapted successfully to the intracellular habitat have evolved a variety of ways to deal with lysosomes. The typical function of lysosomes is fusion with the endosomes that are formed as the plasmalemma engulfs extracellular particles, including bacteria. Within these fused endosome-lysosome vacuoles, or secondary lysosomes or phagolysosomes, the engulfed particles are digested by acid hydrolases (35, 80).

Some obligate intracellular bacteria such as *Rickettsia* spp. avoid this hydrolytic fate by digesting their way out of the endosome before lysosomal fusion can occur. These bacteria multiply freely within the cytoplasm of the host cell. They do not seem to be recognized by the intracellular constituents and appear to be treated as a host cell organelle. Other bacteria such as *Coxiella* spp. have evolved mechanisms to resist digestion by lysosomal enzymes and, in fact, require the acid environment of lysosomes to activate their metabolite transport mechanisms to begin growth and multiplication (24).

A third group of bacteria, including the members of the genus *Chlamydia*, remain within the endosome, but prevent that endosome from fusing with lysosomes (17, 32, 80). If fusion occurs, chlamydiae are digested by the lysosomal enzymes. In fact, endosomes containing chlamydiae that were coated with specific antibodies or that were heated at 90°C for 30 min fuse with lysosomes and are digested. How is fusion between lysosomes and endosomes that contain viable chlamydial EBs prevented? There are two hypotheses. The first hypothesis is that chlamydiae modify the endosomal membrane by insertion of a chlamydial component (32,

71, 75). Chlamydia-specified protein synthesis is not required to prevent endosome-lysosome fusion, which implies that the putative component must be preformed, perhaps as a surface constituent of the infectious EB. Solid data to demonstrate such a component are presently lacking, even though intact inclusions have been isolated. The second and more intriguing hypothesis is that chlamydiae can recognize and exploit specific receptor sites on the plasmalemma that trigger formation of a type of endosome that normally does not fuse with lysosomes (32, 34). Evidence in support of this hypothesis can be derived from the observation that chlamydiae enter host cells by the coated-pit pathway of entry, which is not programmed for lysosomal fusion. The specific chlamydial ligands and host cell receptors involved have not been elucidated.

EFFECTS ON OTHER HOST CELL ORGANELLES

Although some effects of chlamydial infection on the host cell lysosomes and the plasmalemma have been studied by immunochemical, biochemical, and cytochemical techniques, the data generated for interactions between chlamydiae and other host cell organelles are limited primarily to ultrastructural observations and interpretations. With respect to chlamydial infections that result in lytic release of EBs, the host cell organelles within infected cells retain their typical ultrastructural morphology until late in the chlamydial developmental cycle (79). Then, all of the host cell organelles, including lysosomes, the nucleus, smooth and rough endoplasmic reticula, Golgi apparatus, mitochondria, and ribosomes, appear to lose their fine ultrastructural features and disintegrate. This destruction of host cell organelles is coincident with the release of lysosomal enzymes (80). The molecular basis for this release is not documented. Consequently, it is not certain whether the breakdown in lysosomes is merely a consequence of, or is itself the cause of, this destruction of cell organelles (35, 80). Once lysosomal enzyme release occurs, it can by itself explain the chlamydial cytopathic effect on infected cells.

As the inclusion develops in the central portion of the cell, it gradually forces the organelles of the host to peripheral positions (80). The lysosomes become dislocated to peripheral sites near the plasmalemma (Fig. 2). In contrast, mitochondria frequently are detected in close association with the inclusion membrane, and they remain well preserved during chlamydial development until the stage of cell lysis, as one would expect, because the functioning of mitochondria is important for meeting energy requirements of chlamydial multiplication (18, 51, 75). At the terminal stages of the lytic infection, mitochondria became affected: they swell and round up, and their cristae become distorted and fragmented. Eventually they disintegrate along with the other host cell organelles, including smooth and rough endoplasmic reticula, ribosomes, cytoskeletal network, nucleus, and plasmalemma. The inclusion membrane remains intact, while most of the host cell organelles disintegrate, until the last event of actual release of chlamydiae occurs in cell lysis (80).

All organelles remain ultrastructurally intact in nonlytic, exocytotic mechanisms of

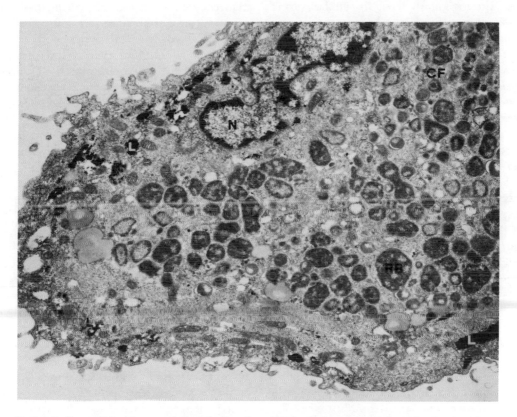

FIGURE 2. Transmission electron micrograph of a cultured bovine fetal spleen cell infected by *C. psittaci* LW-613. To monitor the fate of lysosomes, we processed the infected cells cytochemically for the lysosomal enzyme acid phosphatase. The lysosomes are marked by the electron-dense reaction products of this enzyme. Toward the latter stages of infection, the lysosomes are located exclusively near the peripheral areas of infected cells. The mechanism of host cell lysis includes the release of lysosomal enzymes into the cytoplasm of infected cells (80).

chlamydial release. The exceptions are the inclusion membrane, which is removed during the late stages of the developmental cycle, and the portion of the plasmalemma, which opens during release and later appears as a smooth surface (78).

MODELS FOR PERSISTENCE OF CHLAMYDIAL INFECTIONS

An important state of the host-parasite interaction in some of these chlamydial infections is the persistent, clinically inapparent infection, which plays a significant role in spreading the organism within animal populations. Very little is known about the mechanisms of persistence at the cellular level in the infected animals. A few cell culture models of *C. psittaci* persistence have been described. The cultures were deprived of important metabolites for chlamydial multiplication, and the persistent state was lost after correction of the nutrient deficiency (26, 52, 55, 58).

Persistent infections were established in vitro with the psittacine 6BC strain of *C. psittaci* (55) and the abortigenic serotype 1 strain B-577, but not with the arthropathogenic serotype 2 strain LW-613 (58). This observation may be relevant from the point of view of chlamydia-host interactions in naturally occuring infections of animals. The B-577 persistent state is characterized by cycles of low cytopathic expression and cycles of high cytopathic expression. These cycles seem to be determined, at least in part, by temporary changes in the susceptibility of L cells to chlamydial infection and by the selection of a chlamydial mutant better adapted to the cultural conditions.

Immunofluorescence studies, together with centrifugation and cycloheximide treatments, revealed that the persistently infected cultures go through periods of resistence in which infectious EBs may adsorb but productive infection does not occur. These changes in susceptibility are not absolute but relative, and they can be abolished by cycloheximide treatment,

a situation similar to that described for L cells treated with alpha interferon and infected with *C. trachomatis*. Efforts to detect an antiviral activity indicative of alpha interferon in supernatants collected from persistently infected L-cell cultures were unsuccessful. Consequently, the factors responsible for changing the susceptibility of persistently infected cultures remain unknown (58).

In the model of the avian 6BC strain of *C. psittaci*, the behavior of the persistently infected L-cell population was explained by assuming that every cell is cryptically infected and that the cryptic infection makes the cultures completely resistant to superinfection with exogenous chlamydiae (52, 55). Morphological evidence for the presence of a chlamydial cryptic body was not obtained in the B-577 study (58). Chlamydial agents are procaryotic organisms which maintain their cellular entity throughout the infectious process. Theoretically, the presence of a cryptic body should be revealed by a specific and sensitive fluorescent-antibody test. Penicillin-sensitive chlamydial infectivity was required for maintenance of the persistent state of B-577. Persistently infected cultures could be cured from the chlamydial infection by repeated subculture of the cells at very low cell densities, indicating that not every cell in the population was infected.

HOST CELL RANGE OF CHLAMYDIAL INFECTIONS

Although the infectivity of *C. trachomatis* for cultured cells is relatively low, it can be enhanced significantly by treatment of cells with cytoactive agents. The lymphogranuloma biotypes of *C. trachomatis* and most strains of *C. psittaci* infect cultured cells efficiently. The cell types include fibroblasts, kidney and conjunctival epithelial cells, synovial cells, L cells, McCoy cells, HeLa cells, astrocytes, macrophages, liver cells of lizards, a cell line from fat head minnows, and mosquito cells (42, 64, 73, 86).

The cell types subject to in vivo infections with *C. trachomatis* are principally epithelial cells. The cells include conjunctival cells, respiratory epithelial cells, columnar and transitional endocervical epithelial cells, and urethral epithelial cells. The infections with non-LGV strains remain localized in mucous membranes and are not invasive (49, 64, 76), while the invasive LGV strains also infect macrophages and other cells of the lymphatic system.

In addition to epithelial cells, a wide range of other cell types were found ultrastructurally to be productively or nonproductively infected with strains of C. psittaci (14, 15, 65, 79). These cell types were studied in greatest detail for immunotype 2 infections of the intestinal mucosa of calves and in the inclusion conjunctivitis infection of the conjunctival and genital mucous membranes of guinea pigs. Ultrastructural examination of sections from the terminal ileum revealed productive chlamydial infections of the absorptive epithelial cells of tips and intervillous zones, undifferentiated epithelial cells of the crypts, enterochromaffin cells, follicle-associated epithelial or M cells of Peyer's patches, fibroblasts, endothelial cells, macrophages, and synovial cells. Strains of C. psittaci also infect ciliated epithelial cells and pneumocytes of the respiratory tract of many animal species. Furthermore, C. psittaci strains of immunotype 1, involved in placental and fetal infections, cytolytically parasitize endometrial cells and trophoblastic epithelial cells of the placenta (73, 74). Epithelial cells of the endocervix are the main target cells in the genital infection of guinea pigs (65, 66). Liver cells are parasitized extensively in chlamydial infections of frogs (56).

The following cells were observed to be invaded by chlamydiae in vivo, but the developmental cycle appeared always interrupted or arrested before dense-centered EBs were formed: plasma cells, goblet cells, monocytes, and neutrophilic leukocytes (14, 15). The chlamydial forms present in these cell types from in vivo infections had morphological features of degeneration. Leukocytes were attracted to chlamydia-infected cells and often pavemented infected mucous membranes. Degenerating chlamydial forms were found in macrophages and fibroblasts under certain conditions.

INTERACTIONS OF CHLAMYDIAE WITH CELLS OF THE IMMUNE SYSTEM

The interactions between chlamydial EBs and cells of the immune system are complex and varied (2, 4, 43, 60, 62, 86, 87, 89). Consideration of the nature of this interaction between chlamydiae and any of the cell types of the immune system is confounded owing to the dual nature of the cells. They may be viewed as chlamydial host cells and/or as cells with specific roles in defense mechanisms in the body. Is a confrontation between infectious EBs and phagocytes an infection of the cells, a clearance of the organisms, or a combination of both? Uptake of infectious EBs by macrophages has been reported to be cytochalasin B insensitive and therefore indicative of receptor-mediated endocytosis (7), yet ultrastructural evidence also supports a role for phagocytosis in these cells. The uptake of heat-activated EBs is cytochalasin B sensitive. Receptosomes containing EBs and lysosomes fuse in monocytes, and this often leads to EB digestion, yet with age, monocyte-derived macrophages lose their ability to kill ingested chlamydiae.

Investigation of the capability of cultured lymphocyte lines to support the growth of chlamydiae in vitro revealed the potential for the transport and dissemination of chlamydiae by normal lymphocytes in vivo. Different human cell lines were tested for their ability to bind, ingest, and support multiplication of C. trachomatis (L_2 serovar). The 12 different lymphocytic cell lines studied could be divided into four categories with various levels of chlamydial interaction: (i) minimal EB binding, uptake, and multiplication; (ii) EB binding without uptake or multiplication; (iii) high EB binding, moderate uptake, and low multiplication; and (iv) high EB binding, uptake, and multiplication. Factors governing these processes in each of these cell lines were not defined (3). EB interactions with these lymphocytic cell lines probably depend on properties inherent to each cell line. Additionally, each cell in each of these lines functions as an individual entity that is affected by factors such as cell maturity, cell cycle stage, and stimuli of the local environment.

Peripheral blood leukocytes were also examined for their ability to take up and support the replication of chlamydiae. EBs bound to B cells, neutrophils, and monocytes at the exclusion of T lymphocytes (3, 4, 41). Adsorption was differentiated as a step distinct from uptake or intracellular multiplication. Fifty percent of B cells bound EBs, but none of them ingested EBs. In contrast, both monocytes and granulocytes bound and ingested chlamydial EBs. The killing functions of neutrophils for EBs proceeded in the absence of opsonization.

Infants with chlamydial pneumonitis were found to have elevated levels of circulatory immunoglobulins, B lymphocytes, and plasma cells (4, 41, 43). The direct stimulatory effect of chlamydiae on B lymphocytes in vitro was investigated. Exposure to chlamydial antigen induced large relative and absolute numbers of B lymphoblasts in 3- to 6-day-old cultures (41). Increased levels of immunoglobulins in the media of these cultures were also observed.

Enterobacterial LPS stimulates B cells to undergo division to increase immunoglobulin synthesis. Efforts were made to determine whether chlamydial LPS had a similar effect on B cells. Polymyxin B, an inhibitor of LPS-induced stimulation of B cells, failed to inhibit B-cell stimulation by intact EBs. Additionally, EBs were able to stimulate B cells in LPS-resistant mice as well as in LPS-sensitive mice. Other chlamydial surface components were suggested to exert this function, because the results are so different from the results with LPS from other bacteria. An explanation for the apparent failure of chlamydial LPS to stimulate B cells may derive from the inaccessible location of some portions of the molecule beneath the EB surface. Immunoelectron-microscopic probing with LPS-specific monoclonal antibodies indicated that portions of the LPS are unreactive in the intact EB.

Interactions between EBs and monocytes at ratios of 5:1 or less are generally nonproductive (77). This varies with the chlamydial species and type. Human and murine monocytes exposed to *C. trachomatis* generally develop inclusions in 0.5 to 4% of the cells exposed. A total of 20 to 30% of cultured human monocytes inoculated with the 6BC strain of *C. psittaci* developed inclusions, whereas the same cell population prevented multiplication of *C. trachomatis* (L_2 serovar). Cultured monocyte-derived macrophages developed inclusion bodies in 40 to 50% of the cells following exposure to *C. trachomatis* or *C. psittaci* (46). The increasing susceptibility of monocytes to chlamydial infection as a function of their time in culture is well known and has been linked, in part, to loss of respiratory burst capability.

EB uptake by monocytes or macrophages appears to occur via two pathways. Infectious EBs enter via parasite-specified endocytosis (8), which is receptor mediated, whereas heat-inactivated EBs are taken up by a host-specified route typical of phagocytosis. Two different forms of vacuoles have been observed ultrastructurally in macrophages which had been exposed to chlamydiae (40). These may provide partial insight into the uptake and intracellular disposition of chlamydiae (46). At low EB-to-monocyte ratios, single EBs are seen intracellularly after 1 h of incubation. Most EBs are tightly surrounded by inclusion membranes, while other vacuoles contain a single EB with loosely associated membranes. Tight vacuoles were the only type observed in BHK-21 cells, a nonphagocytic cell line. An inference could therefore be made that tight vacuoles are derived from receptor-mediated uptake, while vacuoles with loosely apposed membranes are formed during phagocytosis.

Two different types of endosomes have also been isolated from macrophages exposed to infectious or heat-killed EB preparations of the 6BC strain. The principal difference between the endosomes was the presence of a 70-kilodalton protein in the membranes of vacuoles taken from macrophages exposed to infectious EBs. Membranes from endosomes with heat-inactivated EBs contained a 25-kilodalton protein (88). The effect of these proteins on the avoidance of fusion of receptosomes with lysosomes would be of interest because heat-inactivated EBs are digested by lysosomal enzymes, in contrast to infectious EBs.

Within 1 h of exposure of monocytes to EBs at multiplicities greater than 10, a large number become swollen and no longer exclude dyes. The number of monocytes demonstrating such cytotoxic changes and the number of infectious units per cell are directly related (36). This resembled the immediate toxicity observed in L cells (53). Heat-killed EBs retained their toxic effect, although at a lower level than infectious organisms did. The toxicity was associated with EBs, because equal numbers of RBs were not found to be toxic. Toxicity of affected monocytes for surrounding monocytes and epithelial cells was observed. The toxicity was found to be due to the release of lysosomal enzymes into the extracellular environment. Four of nine mice intravenously inoculated with sonically disrupted, EB-laden macrophages died within 1 h. In contrast, mice survived after receiving an equal number of EBs alone or disrupted macrophages alone (40).

The toxicity of EBs in vivo was established by Rake and Jones (59). The nature of the toxin responsible for this damage is somewhat unclear. Rake and Jones (59) originally suspected an endotoxin, primarily because the toxic factor copurified with EBs. Gross lesions found in mice intravenously inoculated with the chlamydial EBs were similar to lesions found in mice given LPS from other gram-negative bacteria. However, the chlamydial toxin described is heat labile and is inactivated by 0.1% Formalin, characteristics which are not common to other bacterial LPS. In addition, antisera protecting mice against homologous toxin failed to protect mice against heterologous toxin challenge. Currently there are three known antigenic sites on the chlamydial LPS molecule. One is uniquely chlamydial, and the other two are shared with other host-independent gram-negative bacteria (5). Consequently, this should confer cross-protection.

PERSPECTIVES AND VISTAS

Chlamydial agents emerge as very successful and diverse procaryotic parasites of eucaryotic host cells. They have evolved unique modes of interaction with the host cell that include not only mechanisms designed to overcome cellular barriers or evade cellular defenses, but also effective control of different host cellular functions.

The early interaction of chlamydiae with animal cells emerges as a fascinating phenomenon that appears to be more complex than initially expected when evidence for possible specific receptors emerged. The EB surface structures functioning as ligands must be explored further. Different modes of uptake appear to function and may explain the diversity of chlamydial interaction with cells and intact hosts. There are host cell-specified factors and EB-specified factors that determine chlamydial uptake, including the coated-pit theory of entry into host cells. The mode of uptake significantly influences the modes of lysosomal control. The inclusion membrane appears to play a cardinal role in governing the interplay between chlamydiae developing within the inclusion and the diverse cellular constituents in the cytoplasm. The persistence of the inclusion membrane is a feature that distinguishes chlamydiae from other host cell-dependent bacteria.

Factors that influence the release of chlamydiae also are of biological and medical importance. Again, this process appears to be diverse, involving mechanisms that destroy the host cells and other mechanisms that are noncytocidal and permit persistence with coexistence of host cell and parasite. Both have pathogenetic potential and epidemiological implications.

The host cell range in vivo can be narrow or broad, depending on the chlamydial strain involved. The wide host cell range of *C. psittaci* points toward high potential for invasive infections, while the narrower range of *C. trachomatis* confines it to local infections involving mucous membranes. Simultaneously, the cytocidal effects on infected host cells seem to play a role. The interaction of chlamydiae with cells of the immune system emerges as an important phase in the modulation of the immune-mediated host defense systems. The interaction with leukocytes may be unique because they ingest and kill EBs. The adsorption of EBs to lymphocytes emerges as a function that must be investigated to define specific mechanisms in the immune response.

From a medical perspective, the overriding concerns are (i) prevention and (ii) clearance of chlamydial infections. These objectives have focused the attention of investigators on the early events of chlamydia-host cell interaction such as attachment, entry, and mechanisms to avoid destruction by lysosomes. These early events provide the best opportunities to abort the infection. The experimental designs for analysis of interactions between two complex biological systems such as chlamydiae and host cells usually harbor too many variables to yield unequivocal data for precise interpretations. Eventually more definitive answers may be obtained by using flow cytometry and by investigating the products of cloned chlamydial genes. For example, expression of cloned gene products to permit facilitated uptake, entry into eucaryotes by the coated-pit route, or prevention of endosome fusion with lysosomes would be the most direct method to elucidate these critical early functions in chlamydial infection.

ACKNOWLEDGMENTS. Our research was supported by research grants from the Science and Education Administration of the Department of Agriculture, by Public Health Service research grants from the National Institute of Allergy and Infectious Diseases, and by intramural programs through the Rocky Mountain Laboratories, Hamilton, Mont.

We thank Rhonda C. Aydell and Cecilia H. Boudreaux for excellent secretarial help in preparing this manuscript.

LITERATURE CITED

1. Allan, I., and J. H. Pearce. 1987. Association of *Chlamydia trachomatis* with mammalian and cultured insect cells lacking chlamydial receptors. *Microb. Pathogenesis* 2:63–70.

2. Bard, J., and D. Levitt. 1984. *Chlamydia trachomatis* stimulates human peripheral blood B lymphocytes to proliferate and secrete polyclonal immunoglobulins in vitro. *Infect. Immun.* 43:84–92.

3. Bard, J., and D. Levitt. 1985. Binding, ingestion, and multiplication of *Chlamydia trachomatis* (L$_2$ serovar) in human leukocyte cell lines. *Infect. Immun.* 50:935–937.

4. Bard, J., and D. Levitt. 1986. *Chlamydia trachomatis* (L$_2$ serovar) binds to distinct subpopulations of human peripheral blood leukocytes. *Clin. Immunol. Immunopathol.* 38:150–160.

5. Brade, L., F. E. Nano, S. Schlecht, S. Schramek, and H. Brade. 1987. Antigenic and immunogenic properties of recombinants from *Salmonella typhimurium* and *Salmonella minnesota* rough mutants expressing in their lipopolysaccharide a genus-specific chlamydial epitope. *Infect. Immun.* 55:482–486.

6. Bushell, A. C., and D. Hobson. 1978. Effect of cortisol on the growth of *Chlamydia trachomatis* in McCoy cells. *Infect. Immun.* 21:946–953.

7. Byrne, G. I. 1976. Requirements for ingestion of *Chlamydia psittaci* by mouse fibroblasts (L cells). *Infect. Immun.* 14:645–651.

8. Byrne, G. I., and J. W. Moulder. 1978. Parasite-specified phagocytosis of *Chlamydia psittaci* and *Chlamydia trachomatis* by L and HeLa cells. *Infect. Immun.* 19:598–606.

9. Caldwell, H. D., J. Kromhout, and J. Schachter. 1981. Purification and partial characterization of the major outer membrane protein of *Chlamydia trachomatis*. *Infect Immun.* 31:1161–1176.

10. Caldwell, H. D., and L. J. Perry. 1982. Neutralization of *Chlamydia trachomatis* infectivity with antibodies to the major outer membrane protein. *Infect. Immun.* 38:745–754.

11. Caldwell, H. D., and J. Schachter. 1982. Antigenic analysis of the major outer membrane protein of *Chlamydia* spp. *Infect. Immun.* 35:1024–1031.

12. Dennis, M. W., and J. Storz. 1982. Infectivity enhancement of *Chlamydia psittaci* of bovine and ovine origin for cultured cells. *Am. J. Vet. Res.* 43:1897–1901.

13. Dhir, S. P., S. Hakomori, G. E. Kenny, and J. T. Grayston. 1972. Immunochemical studies on chlamydial group antigen (presence of a 2-keto-3-deoxycarbohydrate as immunodominant group). *J. Immunol.* 109:116–122.

14. Doughri, A. M., K. P. Altera, and J. Storz. 1973. Host cell range of chlamydial infection in the neonatal bovine gut. *J. Comp. Pathol.* 83:107–114.

15. Doughri, A. M., J. Storz, and K. P. Altera. 1972. Mode of entry and release of chlamydiae in infections of intestinal epithelial cells. *J. Infect. Dis.* 126:652–657.

16. Fan, V. S. C., and H. M. Jenkin. 1975. Biosynthesis of phospholipids and neutral lipids of monkey kidney cells (LLC-MK-2) infected with *Chlamydia trachomatis* strain lymphogranuloma venereum. *Proc. Soc. Exp. Biol. Med.* 148:351–357.

17. Friis, R. R. 1972. Interaction of L cells and *Chlamydia psittaci:* entry of the parasite and host responses to its development. *J. Bacteriol.* 110:706–721.

18. Gill, S. D., and R. B. Stewart. 1970. Effect of metabolic inhibitors on the production of *Chlamydia psittaci* by infected L cells. *Can. J. Microbiol.* 16:1076–1085.

19. Gordon, F. B., H. R. Dressler, A. L. Quan, W. T. McQuilkin, and J. I. Thomas. 1972. Effect of ionizing irradiation on susceptibility of McCoy cell cultures to *Chlamydia trachomatis. Appl. Microbiol.* 23:123–129.

20. Gordon, F. B., I. A. Harper, A. L. Quan, J. D. Treharne, R. S. C. Dwyer, and J. A. Garland. 1969. Detection of chlamydia (bedsonia) in certain infections of man. I. Laboratory procedures: comparison of yolk sac and cell culture for detection and isolation. *J. Infect. Dis.* 120:451–462.

21. Gordon, F. B., and A. L. Quan. 1965. Occurrence of glycogen in inclusions of the psittacosis lymphogranuloma venereum-trachoma agents. *J. Infect. Dis.* 115:186–196.

22. Hackstadt, T. 1986. Identification and properties of chlamydial polypeptides that bind eucaryotic surface components. *J. Bacteriol.* 165:13–20.

23. Hackstadt, T., and H. D. Caldwell. 1985. Effect of proteolytic cleavage of surface-exposed proteins on infectivity of *Chlamydia trachomatis. Infect. Immun.* 48:546–551.

24. Hackstadt, T., and J. C. Williams. 1981. Biochemical stratagem for obligate parasitism of eukaryotic cells by *Coxiella burnetti. Proc. Natl. Acad. Sci. USA* 78:3240–3244.

25. Harding, C., J. Heuser, and P. Stahl. 1983. Receptor-mediated endocytosis of transferrin and recycling of the transferrin receptor in rat reticulocytes. *J. Cell Biol.* 97:329–339.

26. Harrison, M. J. 1970. Enhancing effect of DEAE-dextran on inclusion counts of an ovine chlamydia (Bedsonia) in cell culture. *Aust. J. Exp. Biol. Med. Sci.* 48:207–213.

27. Hatch, T. P. 1975. Competition between *Chlamydia psittaci* and L cells for host isoleucine pools: a limiting factor in chlamydial multiplication. *Infect. Immun.* 12:211–220.

28. Hatch, T. P. 1975. Utilization of L cell nucleoside triphosphates by *Chlamydia psittaci* for ribonucleic acid synthesis. *J. Bacteriol.* 122:393–400.

29. Hatch, T. P., I. Allan, and J. H. Pearce. 1984. Structural and polypeptide differences between envelopes of infective and reproductive life cycle forms of *Chlamydia* spp. *J. Bacteriol.* 157:13–20.

30. Hatch, T. P., M. Miceli, and J. E. Sublett. 1986. Synthesis of disulfide-bonded outer membrane proteins during the developmental cycle of *Chlamydia psittaci* and *Chlamydia trachomatis. J. Bacteriol.* 165:379–385.

31. Hatch, T. P., D. W. Vance, Jr., and E. Al-Hossainy. 1981. Identification of a major envelope protein in *Chlamydia* spp. *J. Bacteriol.* 146:426–429.

32. Hodinka, R. L., and P. B. Wyrick. 1986. Ultrastructural study of mode of entry of *Chlamydia psittaci* into L-929 cells. *Infect. Immun.* 54:855–863.

33. Kaul, R., and W. M. Wenman. 1986. Cyclic AMP inhibits developmental regulation of *Chlamydia trachomatis. J. Bacteriol.* 168:722–727.

34. Kihlstrom, E., and G. Soderlund. 1986. Early phases in the interaction between *Chlamydia trachomatis* and eukaryotic cells, p. 82–85. *In* L. Leive (ed.), *Microbiology–1986.* American Society for Microbiology, Washington, D.C.

35. Kordova, N., J. C. Wilt, and M. Sadig. 1971. Lysosomes in L cells infected with *Chlamydia psittaci* 6BC strain. *Can. J. Microbiol.* 17:955–959.

36. Kuo, C.-C. 1978. Immediate mouse cytotoxicity of *Chlamydia trachomatis* for mouse peritoneal macrophages. *Infect. Immun.* 20:613–618.

37. Kuo, C.-C., H.-H. Chen, S.-P. Wang, and J. T. Grayston. 1986. Identification of a new group of *Chlamydia psittaci* strains called TWAR. *J. Clin. Microbiol.* 24:1034–1037.

38. Kuo, C.-C., and E. Y. Chi. 1987. Ultrastructural study of *Chlamydia trachomatis* surface antigens by immunogold staining with monoclonal antibodies. *Infect. Immun.* 55:1324–1328.

39. Kuo, C.-C., S.-P. Wang, and J. T. Grayston. 1973. Effect of polycations, polyanions, and neuraminidase on the infectivity of trachoma-inclusion conjunctivitis and lymphogranuloma venereum organisms in HeLa cells: sialic acid residues as possible receptors for trachoma-inclusion conjunctivitis. *Infect. Immun.* 8:74–79.

40. Lawn, A. M., W. A. Blyth, and J. Taverne. 1973. Interactions of TRIC agents with macrophages and BHK-21 cells observed by electron microscopy. *J. Hyg.* 71:515–528.

41. Levitt, D., R. Danen, and J. Bard. 1986. Both species of chlamydia and two biovars of *Chlamydia trachomatis* stimulate mouse B lymphocytes. *J. Immunol.* 136:4249–4254.

42. Levitt, D., R. Danen, and P. Levitt. 1986. Selective infection of astrocytes by *Chlamydia trachomatis* in primary mixed neuron-glial cell cultures. *Infect. Immun.* 54:913–916.

43. Levitt, D., B. Zable, and J. Bard. 1986. Binding, ingestion, and growth of *Chlamydia trachomatis* (L_2 serovar) analyzed by flow cytometry. *Cytometry* 7:378–383.

44. Levy, N. J. 1979. Wheat germ agglutinin blockage

of chlamydial attachment sites: antagonism by *N*-ace-tyl-D-glucosamine. *Infect. Immun.* 25:946–953.

45. Louis, C., G. Nicolas, F. Eb, J. Lefebvre, and J. Orfila. 1980. Modifications of the envelope of *Chlamydia psittaci* during its developmental cycle: freeze-fracture study of complementary replicas. *J. Bacteriol.* 141:868–875.

46. Manor, E., and I. Sarov. 1986. Fate of *Chlamydia trachomatis* in human monocytes and monocyte-derived macrophages. *Infect. Immun.* 54:90–95.

47. Matsumoto, A. 1973. Fine structures of cell envelopes of *Chlamydia* organisms as revealed by freeze-etching and negative staining techniques. *J. Bacteriol.* 116:1355–1363.

48. Matsumoto, A. 1981. Isolation and electron microscopic observations of intracytoplasmic inclusions containing *Chlamydia psittaci. J. Bacteriol.* 145:605–612.

49. Moorman, D. R., J. W. Sixbey, and P. B. Wyrick. 1986. Interaction of *Chlamydia trachomatis* with human genital epithelium in culture. *J. Gen. Microbiol.* 132:1055–1067.

50. Moulder, J. W. 1969. A model for studying the biology of parasitism: *Chlamydia psittaci* and mouse fibroblasts (L cells). *BioScience* 19:875–881.

51. Moulder, J. W. 1971. The contribution of model systems to the understanding of infectious diseases. *Perspect. Biol. Med.* 14:486–502.

52. Moulder, J. W. 1983. Inhibition of onset of overt multiplication of *Chlamydia psittaci* in persistently infected mouse fibroblasts (L cells). *Infect. Immun.* 39:898–907.

53. Moulder, J. W., T. P. Hatch, G. I. Byrne, and K. R. Kellogg. 1976. Immediate toxicity of high multiplicities of *Chlamydia psittaci* for mouse fibroblasts (L cells). *Infect. Immun.* 14:277–289.

54. Moulder, J. W., T. P. Hatch, C.-C. Kuo, J. Schachter, and J. Storz. 1984. Genus 1. *Chlamydia Jones, Rake and Stearns* 1945 p. 729–739. *In* N. R. Krieg and J. G. Holt (ed.), *Bergey's Manual of Systematic Bacteriology,* vol. 1. The Williams & Wilkins Co., Baltimore.

55. Moulder, J. W., N. J. Levy, and L. P. Schulman. 1980. Persistent infection of mouse fibroblasts (L cells) with *Chlamydia psittaci:* evidence for a cryptic chlamydial form. *Infect. Immun.* 30:874–883.

56. Newcomer, C. E., M. R. Anver, J. L. Simmons, B. W. Wilcke, Jr., and G. W. Nace. 1982. Spontaneous and experimental infections of *Xenopus laevis* with *Chlamydia psittaci. Lab. Anim. Sci.* 32:680–686.

57. Newhall, W. J., and R. B. Jones. 1983. Disulfide-linked oligomers of the major outer membrane protein of chlamydiae. *J. Bacteriol.* 154:998–1001.

58. Perez-Martinez, J. A., and J. Storz. 1985. Persistent infection of L cells with an ovine abortion strain of *Chlamydia psittaci. Infect. Immun.* 50:453–458.

59. Rake, G., and H. P. Jones. 1944. Studies on lym-phogranuloma venereum. II. The association of specific toxins with agents of the lymphogranuloma-psittacosis group. *J. Exp. Med.* 79:463–485.

60. Register, K. B., P. A. Morgan, and P. B. Wyrick. 1986. Interaction between *Chlamydia* spp. and human polymorphonuclear leukocytes in vitro. *Infect. Immun.* 52:664–670.

61. Richmond, S. J., and P. Stirling. 1981. Localization of chlamydial group antigen in McCoy cell monolayers infected with *Chlamydia trachomatis* or *Chlamydia psittaci. Infect. Immun.* 34:561–570.

62. Rothermel, C. D., B. Y. Rubin, E. A. Jaffe, and H. W. Murray. 1986. Oxygen independent inhibition of intracellular *Chlamydia psittaci* growth by human monocytes and interferon-α activated macrophages. *J. Immun.* 137:689–692.

63. Schachter, J., and H. D. Caldwell. 1980. Chlamydiae. *Annu. Rev. Microbiol.* 34:285–309.

64. Schachter, J., and C. R. Dawson. 1978. *Human Chlamydial Infections.* PSG Publishing Co., Littleton, Mass.

65. Soloff, B. L., R. G. Rank, and A. L. Barron. 1982. Ultrastructural studies of chlamydial infection in guinea-pig urogenital tract. *J. Comp. Pathol.* 92:547–558.

66. Soloff, B. L., R. G. Rank, and A. L. Barron. 1985. Electron microscopic observations concerning the in vivo uptake and release of the agent of guinea-pig inclusion conjunctivitis *(Chlamydia psittaci)* in guinea-pig exocervix. *J. Comp. Pathol.* 95:335–344.

67. Spears, P., and J. Storz. 1979. Changes in the ultrastructure of *Chlamydia psittaci* produced by treatment of the host cell with DEAE-dextran and cycloheximide. *J. Ultrastruct. Res.* 67:152–160.

68. Spears, P., and J. Storz. 1979. Biotyping of *Chlamydia psittaci* based on inclusion morphology and response to DEAE-dextran and cycloheximide. *Infect. Immun.* 24:224–232.

69. Spears, P., and J. Storz. 1979. *Chlamdia psittaci:* growth characteristics and enumeration of serotypes 1 and 2 in cultured cells. *J. Infect. Dis.* 140:959–967.

70. Stewart, R. B. 1960. Effect of cortisone on the growth of psittacosis virus in cultures of L cells. *J. Bacteriol.* 80:25–29.

71. Stokes, G. V. 1974. Cycloheximide-resistant glycosylation in L cells infected with *Chlamydia psittaci. Infect. Immun.* 9:497–499.

72. Stokes, G. V. 1978. Surface projections and internal structure of *Chlamydia psittaci. J. Bacteriol.* 133:1514–1516.

73. Storz, J. 1971. *Chlamydia and Chlamydia Induced Diseases.* Charles C Thomas, Publisher, Springfield, Ill.

74. Storz, J., and H. Krauss. 1985. Chlamydial infections and diseases of animals, p. 447–531. *In* H. Blobel and T. Schliesser (ed.), *Handbook on Bacterial*

Infections in Animals, vol. V. Fischer Verlag, Jena, German Democratic Republic.

75. Storz, J., and P. Spears. 1977. Chlamydiales: properties, developmental cycle and effect on eukaryotic host cells. *Curr. Top. Microbiol. Immunol.* 76:165–212.

76. Swanson, J., D. A. Eschenbach, E. R. Alexander, and K. K. Holmes. 1975. Light and electron microscopic study of *Chlamydia trachomatis* infection of the uterine cervix. *J. Infect. Dis.* 131:678–687.

77. Taverne, J., W. A. Blyth, and R. C. Ballard. 1974. Interactions of TRIC agents with macrophages: effects on lysosomal enzymes of the cell. *J. Hyg.* 72:297–309.

78. Todd, W. J., and H. D. Caldwell. 1985. The interaction of *Chlamydia trachomatis* with host cells: ultrastructural studies of the mechanism of release of a biovar II strain from HeLa 229 cells. *J. Infect. Dis.* 151:1037–1044.

79. Todd, W. J., A. M. Doughri, and J. Storz. 1976. Ultrastructural changes in host cellular organelles in the course of the chlaymdial developmental cycle. *Zentralbl. Bakteriol. Microbiol. Hyg. Abt. 1 Orig. Reihe A* 236:359–373.

80. Todd, W. J., and J. Storz. 1975. Ultrastructural cytochemical evidence for activation of lysosomes in the cytocidal effect of *Chlamydia psittaci. Infect. Immun.* 12:638–646.

81. Waldman, F. M., W. K. Hadley, M. J. Fulwyler, and J. Schachter. 1987. Flow cytometric analysis of *Chlamydia trachomatis* interaction with L. cells. *Cytometry* 8:55–59.

82. Ward, M. E., and A Murray. 1984. Control mechanisms governing the infectivity of *Chlamydia trachomatis* for HeLa cells: mechanisms of endocytosis. *J. Gen. Microbiol.* 130:1765–1780.

83. Weiss, E., and H. Dressler. 1960. Centrifugation of rickettsiae and viruses onto cells and its effect on infection. *Proc. Soc. Exp. Biol. Med.* 103:691–695.

84. Wenman, W. M., and R. U. Meuser. 1986. *Chlamydia trachomatis* elementary bodies possess proteins which bind to eucaryotic cell membranes. *J. Bacteriol.* 165:602–607.

85. Wilde, C. E., III, T. McBride, and S. Karimi. 1987. Dynamics of chlamydial antigen exposure on infected cells. *J. Cell. Biochem. Suppl.* 11B:130.

86. Wyrick, P. B., and E. A. Brownridge. 1978. Growth of *Chlamydia psittaci* in macrophages. *Infect. Immun.* 19:1054–1060.

87. Wyrick, P. B., E. A. Brownridge, and B. E. Ivins. 1978. Interaction of *Chlamydia psittaci* with mouse peritoneal macrophages. *Infect. Immun.* 19:1061–1067.

88. Zeichner, S. L. 1983. Isolation and characterization of macrophage phagosomes containing infectious and heat-inactivated *Chlamydia psittaci.* Two phagosomes with different intracellular behaviors. *Infect. Immun.* 40:956–966.

89. Zvillich, M., and I. Sarov. 1985. Interaction between human polymorphonuclear leucocytes and *Chlamydia trachomatis* elementary bodies: electron microscopy and chemiluminescent response. *J. Gen. Microbiol.* 131:2627–2635.

Chapter 11

Recent Developments in Studies on Phagosome-Lysosome Fusion in Cultured Macrophages

MAYER B. GOREN

Department of Molecular and Cellular Biology
National Jewish Center for Immunology and Respiratory Medicine
Denver, Colorado 80206
and
Department of Microbiology and Immunology
University of Colorado Health Sciences Center
Denver, Colorado 80262

NATAN MOR

Department of Molecular and Cellular Biology
National Jewish Center for Immunology and Respiratory Medicine
Denver, Colorado 80206

INTRODUCTION

This review is devoted principally to recent developments in methodology for studying phagosome-lysosome fusion (P-LF) in cultured murine peritoneal macrophages (MΦ) and to newly recognized phenomena governing the delivery of lysosomal constituents to phagosomes. However, the widespread but less than critical adoption of the esthetically pleasing acridine orange (AO) technique for studying P-LF in living cells has confronted us with serious dilemmas respecting valid interpretation of the observations. Indeed, we addressed this problem in earlier publications (8, 11, 12), but now find that the guidelines previously set forth already require further revisions. Accordingly, in this paper we first review the current status of AO as a lysosomal label for studying P-LF, paying particular attention to operational pitfalls. The concept of differential delivery of lysosomal contents during P-LF is introduced. We then describe the behavior in P-LF of MΦ exposed to polyanionic agents such as dextran sulfate and analyze how such cells might be studied with more confidence. This is followed by a discussion of the properties and uses of highly ionized, and therefore membrane nonpermeating, fluorochromes, which may be used in specific instances as alternatives to AO for labeling lysosomes. Finally we describe how the simultaneous sequestration of polymeric hydrosols, of electron-opaque colloidal markers, and of mobile low-molecular-weight fluorochromes in lysosomes led to the recognition that lysosomal contents can be delivered piecemeal instead of simultaneously to phagosomes during P-LF events.

LABELING OF LYSOSOMES TO MONITOR P-LF

Electron-Opaque Markers

When the macrophage culture medium contains certain electron-opaque colloidal substances such as Thorotrast (a hydrated thorium oxide), ferritin, or some colloidal gold preparations, the cells take up the markers by pinocytosis. The markers are delivered to secondary lysosomes and sequester there because they are largely undegradable. Lysosomes labeled with Thorotrast are prominent in the electron micrograph of *Candida albicans* in Fig. 1. The labeled cells then phagocytose viable *C. albicans* cells, and within about 1.5 h, abundant electron-opaque marker is transferred to the phagosomes (24). It is difficult to account for the delivery of this marker by other than a P-LF process. Indeed, this appearance is widely accepted as valid evidence for P-LF.

AO Technique

Mobility and Accumulation in Lysosomes

The appropriate weakly basic properties of AO (Fig. 2) endow it with the ability to penetrate almost unhindered across biomembranes. Within a living cell, therefore, it can distribute to all domains bounded by the plasma membrane. However, it can then redistribute within the cell as well as to extracellular locations. The affinity of AO for various domains and possible domains both within and external to a macrophage, as we have discerned from many studies, is as follows (in decreasing order of affinity): Dowex-50 and other cation exchangers; polyanionic substances in lysosomes; sulfatides of *Mycobacterium tuberculosis;* bacteria

with acidic surfaces; normal lysosomes and cell nuclei; and killed and digesting microorganisms. In the presence of limited AO, only the domains of highest affinity will acquire the dye, so that ultimately the fluorochrome will concentrate in locations where it is most efficiently trapped or complexed. With sufficient AO available, all domains within a closed system may acquire the dye according to their capacities.

Only the free-base form of the acridine derivative permeates membranes freely. Therefore, protonation of the dye, as in lysosomes, traps and concentrates AO in these organelles because of their acidity (pH ca. 4.5) and through augmentation by a membrane ATPase that behaves as a proton pump (5, 25). Therefore, secondary lysosomes can be labeled by the dye through this mechanism and can be easily recognized (1, 15). Primary lysosomes are very probably also labeled: they can be clearly recognized in neutrophils, although they are not ordinarily discernible in macrophages because of size.

Delivery to Phagosomes

Like Thorotrast and the other markers, lysosomally sequestered AO can be delivered along with other lysosomal contents to phagosomes by a P-LF event and ought thereby to reveal the fusion process (15; see also reference 10). Viable bakers' yeast was a fortuitous choice of target for monitoring this behavior (15). Usually within 30 to 45 min of uptake, a variety of vivid fusion figures can be seen (Fig. 3). However, for reasons that have previously been obscure (but which may now be confidently inferred), a presumably "normal" macrophage monolayer may show only insignificant delivery of AO to yeast-containing phagosomes and thus might be judged to be inhibited in P-LF (Fig. 4). As a specific example, the Thorotrast-labeled cells shown in Fig. 1 were simultaneously labeled with AO to allow comparison of fusion by vital fluorescence microscopy on one hand and by electron microscopy (EM) on the other. Although almost universal transfer

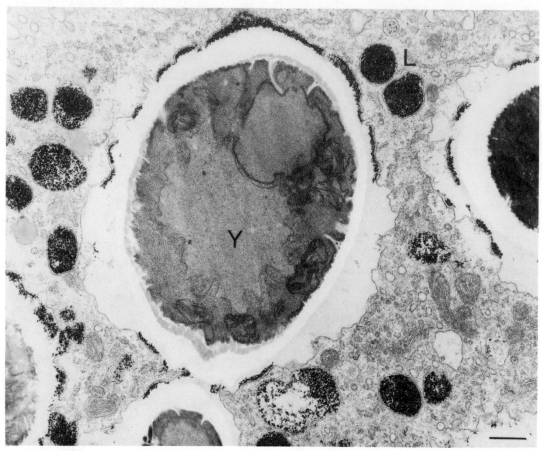

FIGURE 1. Macrophage lysosomes (L) labeled with electron-opaque Thorotrast. After phagocytosis of viable *C. albicans* cells, P-LF has occurred and delivered the marker into the phagosomes. The yeasts (Y) resist killing and digestion. Bar, 500 nm.

of the Thorotrast marker to phagosomes was documented, AO delivery was limited to only about 10% of phagosomes scored (Fig. 4) (24). The dilemma was resolved by the finding that fewer than 20% of the *C. albicans* cells had been rendered nonviable (killed or severely injured) during phagocytosis by the macrophages. PL-F

FIGURE 2. Structure of AO, a lysosomotropic weak base.

was almost universal as revealed by EM, but only the killed or damaged *C. albicans* cells digesting under the influence of the lysosomal hydrolases were evidently rendered sufficiently permeable to allow recognizable staining by the acridine dye. Viable *Candida* spp. and *Saccharomyces cerevisiae* are essentially indifferent to even 50 to 100 µg of AO per ml, becoming stained only a dull green. A similar behavior toward acridine dyes has been described for other microorganisms as well (6, 26, 27). However, those with acidic surfaces, such as tubercle bacilli, are exceptional and acquire the dyes even in the absence of P-LF (see below). Therefore, on the infrequent occasions when normal mac-

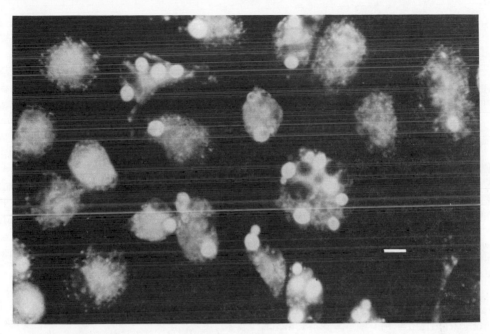

FIGURE 3. Fusion figures in normal macrophages prelabeled with 5 μg of AO per ml and allowed to ingest viable bakers' yeast. Bar, 10 μm.

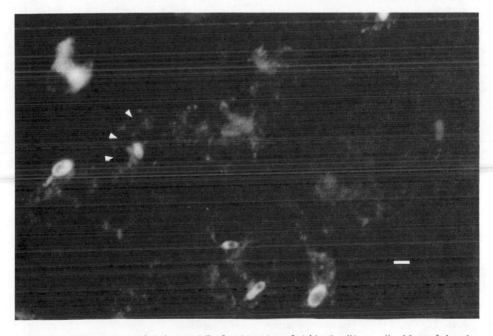

FIGURE 4. Macrophages prelabeled with AO after ingestion of viable *C. albicans* cells. Most of the phagosomes appear to be devoid of dye (not fused, arrowheads), but P-LF was judged to be widespread on the basis of Thorotrast delivery (Fig. 1). Bar, 10 μm. Taken from reference 24.

rophages show presumed inhibition of fusion following ingestion of *S. cerevisiae* cells (11), it seems plausible that the particular macrophage culture may not have killed this ordinarily very susceptible yeast. Fusion is probably abundant, but remains cryptic with AO as the label.

Trapping by Polyanionic Agents

Because AO is a weak base, it is avidly complexed and trapped by acidic substances, especially by polyanionic agents. The domains mentioned above are mostly polyanionic or acidic in character. Coupled with the free movement of the dye, the distribution or redistribution of AO within a cell system from one site to others in which it is more avidly trapped may be readily understood. Figure 5 illustrates the diffusion of AO (free-base form) from the medium into a macrophage, where it is trapped in lysosomes by protonation (an acidic domain). However, Fig. 5 also shows the facile loss of this lyso-somal AO to a potent anionic second domain with higher affinity for the dye. This second domain may be intracellular (a particular pha-gosome, for example), extracellular and free, or located within other cells; the AO reaches the domain by permeation through membranes and may thus be competitively irreversibly trapped.

This domain may be given its character by such agents as Dowex 50 cation exchange beads (9, 11, 12), droplets of free sulfatides from *M. tu-berculosis,* viable or killed *M. tuberculosis* organ-isms because of their surface acidic lipids, and, of particular importance, lysosomes in which certain polyanionic agents have been concen-trated: dextran sulfate, poly-D-glutamic acid, or certain acidic polysaccharides (7, 9, 10, 16, 20). Thus, as an example of trapping by an intracellular domain, although viable virulent *M. tuberculosis* has been shown to inhibit P-LF from within the entrapping phagosomes (in MΦ) (2), these bacteria nevertheless rapidly become fluorescent when phagocytosed by MΦ prela-beled with AO (12), probably not by a P-LF process, but rather because the AO can reach the tubercle bacilli in the phagosomes by per-meation. It is then trapped by the strongly acidic surface lipids. Extracellular bacilli resting on the cover slip are likewise equally fluorescent (12). AO is therefore not suitable for judging P-LF if the viable microorganism itself strongly adsorbs the dye.

In this staining behavior, tubercle bacilli behave with AO-labeled macrophages like par-ticles of cation-exchange resins (Dowex 50, for

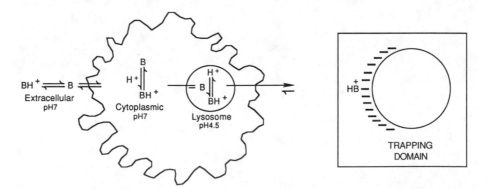

FIGURE 5. Interactions of the permeant AO with a macrophage, with lysosomes, and with a domain that behaves as a powerful trap for the dye. The free base becomes trapped and concentrated in lysosomes by protonation, but it can be drained to even an extracellular potently anionic domain. Because the equilibrium concentration of free base is always finite, even if very small in some cir-cumstances, it can be robbed from lysosomes by powerful trapping agents, such as cation exchange resins, polyanion-containing lysosomes, etc. (9, 11).

example), which have a powerful affinity for AO (21; see also references 9, 11, and 12). Because extracellular ion-exchange resin particles become as vividly colored as their phagocytosed counterparts, it is impossible to judge on the basis of the staining by AO alone how the intracellular particles acquired the dye. Experiments with Thorotrast-labeled cells and ion-exchange resin beads prove, however, that P-LF is not inhibited (14).

P-LF IN POLYANION-CONTAINING CELLS

Over a decade or longer, various investigators have described inhibition of P-LF in MΦ that have lysosomally sequestered a sufficiency of polyanionic substances: suramin (15), *M. tuberculosis* sulfatides (10), dextran sulfate (10, 20), D-polyglutamic acid (16, 17), and oxidized (carboxylated) amylose (7), etc. Thus, when Thorotrast-labeled cells accumulate enough of these polyanionic substances (usually different amounts in each case), delivery of the electron-opaque marker to newly formed yeast-containing phagosomes is severely inhibited. Moreover, if these polyanion-containing cells are labeled in the usually practiced manner, i.e., by exposure for about 15 min to 5 µg of AO per ml before yeast phagocytosis, delivery of the fluorescent marker to the yeasts is highly suppressed, supporting the conclusion of fusion inhibition that was independently derived from the parallel EM studies (7, 10, 15, 16, 20). We have noted earlier (see Fig. 6A) that in polyanion cells labeled in this way the nuclei are invariably dark and have not acquired the dye. In these cells, phagocytosed yeasts are also dark. We described previously, however (11, 12), that if the polyanion macrophages are labeled by exposure to about 20 to 30 µg of AO per ml (instead of 5 µg of AO per ml), the nuclei become green with dye (Fig. 6B), as they are in control cells, and as in control cells, abundant delivery of AO to yeast phagosomes also occurs. These yeasts must therefore be at least

severely injured and be undergoing digestion. However, the polyanion lysosomes still retain much dye, and in counterpart cells also labeled with Thorotrast, the block to transfer of the electron-opaque marker is still maintained (14; for documentation of these phenomena in color plates see especially M. B. Goren, *Curr. Top. Membr. Transp.*, in press.)

In our analyses of these and other curious results (11, 13, 14), we suggested the following. (i) Accumulation of polyanionic agents in secondary lysosomes does not inhibit P-LF, but only antagonizes transfer of the lysosomal markers. (ii) At the inhibitory concentrations, the polyanions are probably present in lysosomes as hydrosols, i.e., viscous, sluggishly moving, gelatinous masses that do not transfer to the phagosome fusion partners. (iii) Particulate colloidal EM markers become physically trapped in the polyanionic hydrosol. (iv) The basic AO becomes ionically trapped in this mass, which behaves like a gelatinous bolus of cation-exchange material. (v) Exposure of these cells to 5 µg of AO per ml for 15 min usually provides insufficient dye to satisfy the demand of the lysosomal polyanionic jelly; the cell nuclei, which have considerable affinity for AO, are invariably devoid of dye in the polyanion cells labeled as described, and this betrays the persisting drain for AO (Fig. 6A). As a corollary, if AO is to be used in studying P-LF or its inhibition in MΦ, the cells should be exposed to sufficient dye to render the nuclei visibly (bright) green. (vi) Labeling with 20 to 30 µg/ml evidently saturates the capacity of the gelatinous lysosomal polyanionic, provides additional unbound dye to the lysosomes and to the nuclei (now green), and allows the P-LF to be visualized (Fig. 6B). The lysosomal polyanion jelly, with its ionically trapped AO (and/or physically trapped Thorotrast), is still not delivered to the phagosomes.

This behavior is powerful evidence that fusion of these secondary lysosomes with phagosomes can result in a differential delivery of lysosomal constituents to the fusion partners: AO and lysosomal hydrolases must be trans-

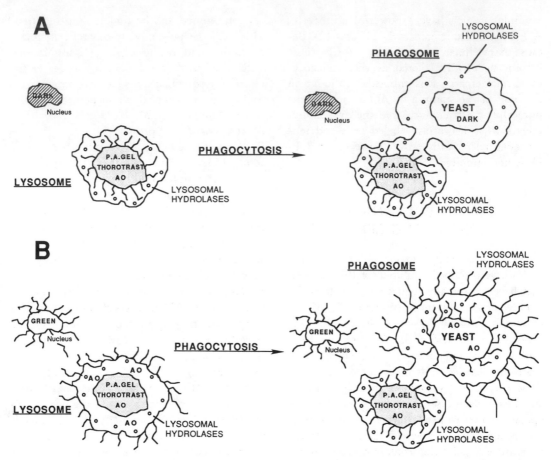

FIGURE 6. (A) Polyanion-containing cell labeled with Thorotrast and with 5 μg of AO per ml, which is insufficient to satisfy the demand of the lysosomes. The nucleus is dark. The polyanion jelly traps Thorotrast and all of the AO. Following phagocytosis and P-LF, only lysosomal enzymes are delivered to the yeast phagosome. (B) Cells as in Fig. 6A, but labeled with an excess of AO (20 μg/ml). The nuclei are bright green; the polyanion gel is saturated with AO, and free AO is present in the lysosome. After phagocytosis of yeast cells and P-LF, free AO is delivered to the phagosome, along with lysosomal hydrolases, but complexed AO and Thorotrast remain trapped in the polyanion jelly.

ferred, while the gelatinous polyanion with its entrapped Thorotrast and the saturating moiety of dye are not. Therefore, the evidence from inhibition of both AO and EM marker transfer is a dual deception stemming from the capacity of the gelatinous polyanionic agent to trap both Thorotrast and the basic AO. It would be expected, however, that a neutral or anionic lysosomal fluorescent marker should not be trapped by the gelatinous polyanionic substance and therefore should transfer to phagosomes, even though the Thorotrast marker colocalized in the same lysosomes is immobilized.

SULFONATED LYSOSOMOTROPIC FLUORESCENT MARKERS

The structures of lissamine rhodamine B (LR), lucifer yellow CH (LY), and sulforhodamine 101 (SR) shown in Fig. 7 allow the deduction that these fluorescent probes of moderate molecular weight should accumulate and concentrate in macrophage secondary lysosomes by a pinocytic process, similar to that for the electron-opaque colloidal markers. Because of their highly ionic nature, they should be membrane impermeant, in contrast to AO,

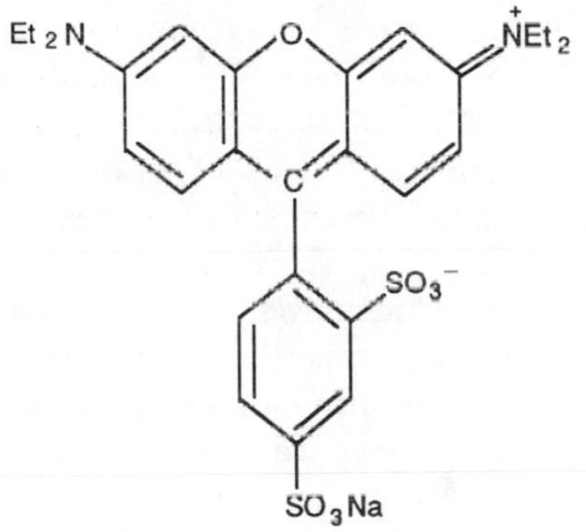

Lissamine Rhodamine

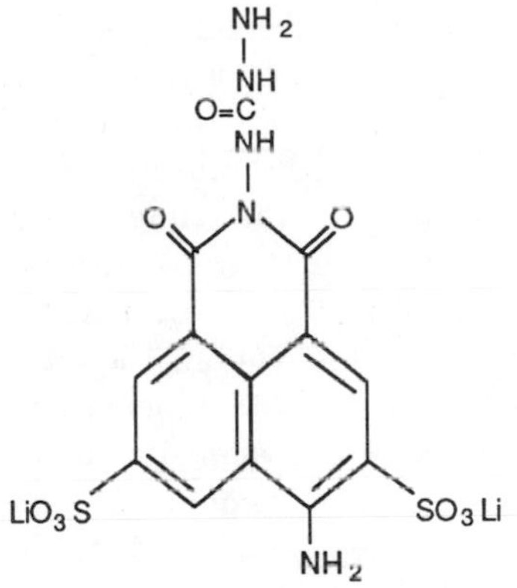

Lucifer Yellow

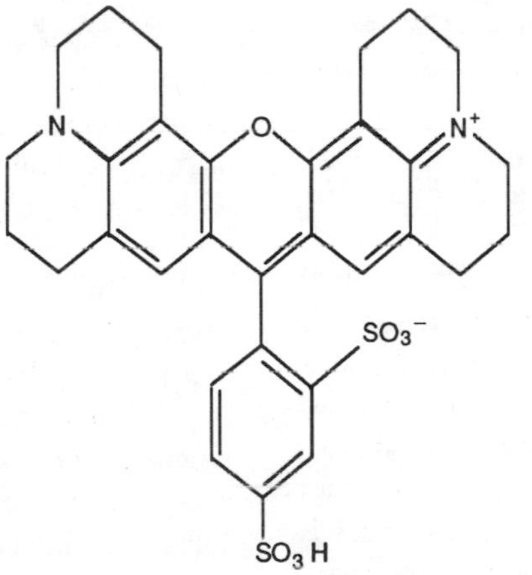

Sulforhodamine

FIGURE 7. Structures of several highly ionized sulfonated fluorescent lysosomal probes. They are not trapped by either nonionic or polyanionic hydrocolloids. Because they are impermeant molecules, they must be delivered to phagosomes by a fusion process.

and therefore should not be free to redistribute easily once sequestered in lysosomes. They should also not be trapped ionically by gelatinous polyanions. On fusion of these labeled lysosomes with yeast phagosomes, it would be expected that the dyes would be delivered to the phagosomes, and if polyanionic agents do not in fact inhibit P-LF, these fluorescent markers should still be delivered to the fusion partners even in the face of immobilization of

EM colloidal marker or AO.

Indeed, the behavior of these dyes was largely as anticipated. We and others (23, 28, 29) have unequivocally demonstrated that they are sequestered in lysosomes; that they are impermeant and, unlike AO, do not redistribute to sites of trapping; and that they undoubtedly are delivered to phagosomes by a P-LF process. However, they are not as mobile as AO, and so they do not permeate yeast-containing phagosomes with the same facility as the acridine dye does. Their behavior as probes for studying lysosomal functions is consistent with these properties and indeed diminishes their utility, but not, we suggest, the validity of results obtained through their use. (i) Although exposure of macrophages to AO at 5 μg/ml for 15 min is adequate for lysosomal labeling, labeling with any one of the impermeant dyes requires concentrations from 150 μg/ml to as much as 2 mg/ml of medium and exposure for up to 2 to 3 days (9, 13, 29). (ii) Viable *S. cerevisiae* cells are poor targets for fusion studies, since extensive lysosomal digestion after killing is needed to render them sufficiently permeable for penetration. Up to 6 h of postphagocytosis incubation is required. (iii) Heat-killed yeasts are satisfactory targets. Within 1 h of a phagocytosis pulse, abundant dye transfer to phagosomes can be seen in control (unmanipulated) macrophages. If the cells contain previously sequestered polyanionic hydrosols, transfer of probe to the phagosomes is delayed, so that about 3 to 4 h of incubation is required (13). Figure 8A and B illustrate the transfer of lysosomal SR to heat-killed and then fluoresceinated yeasts (9, 13) in MΦ that sequestered sufficient dextran sulfate to essentially abolish transfer of Thorotrast from the same lysosomes as discerned from parallel EM studies. This is a second example of differential transfer of lysosomal markers.

The fluoresceinated yeasts (9) are excellent targets for studying P-LF in cells labeled with one of the red fluorochromes LR and SR. Illumination for rhodamine (about 560-nm excitation and 590-nm barrier filter) selects the phagosomes that have accumulated various levels of the red probe (Fig. 8A). With the same field, fluorescein excitation (BG38/BG12 exciter and 530-nm barrier) reveals the total number of yeast cells in the field (Fig. 8B). The shades of color that are elicited, almost pure green (arrows; no fusion) to very bright orange (heavy fusion), contribute a vivid panorama of the spectrum of activities that should be expected for the varied behavior of a biological system. P-LF is not an all black-or-white

phenomenon. There are also all shades of gray.

We have not yet examined the utility of the impermeant probes for studying P-LF with much smaller microorganisms, e.g., *Escherichia coli,* various bacilli (*Bacillus megaterium* and *Bacillus subtilis,* for example), or mycobacteria. The optical limitations may severely restrict exploitation of these dyes. However, if such microscopic targets can be fluoresceinated with retention of viability, then the spectrum of colors that might be revealed under excitation for fluorescein emission (as above) may yield significant information on P-LF or its inhibition for small targets. Collaborative studies with N. Düzgünes are being undertaken to test this ploy.

Nonionic Hydrosols

The gelatinous quality that we envisage for polyanionic agents such as dextran sulfate within lysosomes can also be mimicked with neutral, nonionic hydrosoluble polymers of high molecular weight, e.g., dextran, polyvinylpyrrolidone, polyethylene oxide, and polyacrylamide. These accumulate in lysosomes. At sufficiently high concentrations they probably exist as viscous hydrosols in the organelles, for they trap colloidal markers such as Thorotrast (13). However, because they are nonionic they trap none of the fluorescent probes, including AO. Thus, in the face of Thorotrast immobilization, all of these dyes transfer with relative facility from such jelly-containing lysosomes to yeast phagosomes.

DIFFERENTIAL TRANSFER OF LYSOSOMAL CONSTITUENTS TO PHAGOSOMES

In the preceding sections we described P-LF examples in which apparently mobile components within macrophage lysosomes were delivered to the phagosome fusion partner with concomitant retention in the lysosomes of less-mobile (or possibly even immobilized) constituents. We have assumed that the mobile components invariably include the lysosomal hydrolases, for even in the so-called polyanion-

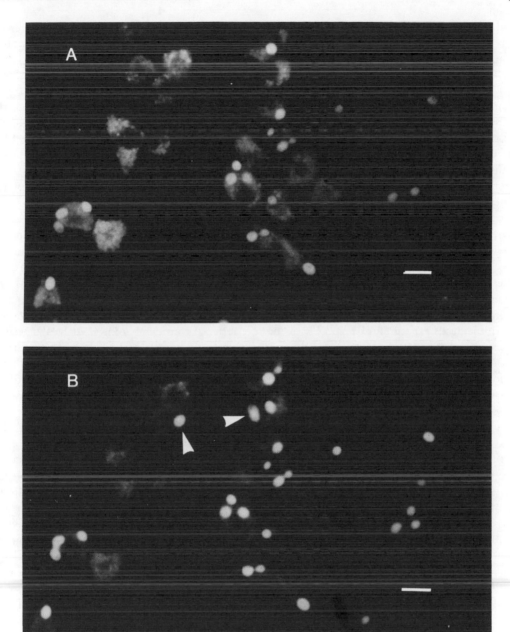

Figure 8. Fusion of lysosomes with phagosomes in cells exposed to sufficient dextran sulfate to immobilize the lysosomal Thorotrast marker. The targets are heat-killed (and then fluoresceinated) bakers' yeast cells. The fluorescent marker is SR. (a) Rhodamine excitation (560 nm) with 590-nm barrier. Yeast phagosomes with delivered SR are visualized. (b) Excitation for fluorescein reveals the total number of yeast cells in the field. Three yeast cells (arrowheads), not visible in panel A, are a pure green. Bar, 10 μm.

inhibited cells, digestion of the phagocytosed targets proceeds apace (9, 14). In the present review we described delivery of AO from polyanion-containing lysosomes when sufficient dye is available even though polymer and Thorotrast were immobilized; we also described delivery of the impermeant ionic dyes from polyanion-containing lysosomes and delivery of any of the fluorescent markers, including AO, from lysosomes sequestering the nonionic hydrosoluble polymers, notably dextran. Exploitation of fluorescein and rhodamine derivatives of dextran and of fluorochromes of low molecular weight in various combinations provided us with the tools for dissection and actual visualization of both concomitant and differential deliveries of lysosomal probes.

As described by Wang and Goren (29), macrophages were lysosomally doubly labeled by simultaneous exposure to LY and LR, or by exposure to SR and to fluoresceinated dextran (molecular weight, 40,000 [FD-40]). After a prolonged period of chase, the markers in each case were proved to be colocalized in the same (lysosomal) vesicles, as recognized from examinations for the two probes by specific fluorescence microscopy. When LY and LR (both labels of low molecular weight) were present together, after phagocytosis of heat-killed yeasts the yellow and the red markers were delivered simultaneously to phagosomes in 1 to 2 h. Fluoresceinated dextran of low molecular weight (4,000) also transferred quite readily to phagosomes. However, the picture was remarkably different when the cells were labeled with the combination of SR (low molecular weight) and FD-40 (29). For 2 to 3 h after a phagocytic pulse, almost universal delivery of the mobile red SR, but essentially no transfer of the polymeric green dye, was documented. Indeed, with some cells, the delivery of red SR to phagosomes was of such magnitude as to essentially deplete the lysosomal compartment of the red dye. At this point, however, the phagosomes contained no detectable FD-40, whereas the lysosomes were a uniform green, i.e., uncontaminated by recognizable SR color. This impressive example of differential delivery of lysosomal

probes was then followed by equally impressive evidence of a sequential transfer process. Not surprisingly, the (green) hydrophilic polymer of modest molecular weight transferred slowly to the yeast phagosomes over a period prolonged for more than 24 h, during which the fraction of phagosomes containing FD-40 increased from about 6% at 3 h to about 85% at 24 h. The FD-40 was found mostly in the same phagosomes that contained the earlier-delivered SR, so that after 1 day, most of the phagosomes contained both probes.

A cautionary note should be added about pitfalls: derivatized dextrans of higher molecular weight (40×10^3 to 70×10^3) should be extensively dialyzed if they are toxic to the cells. Moreover, it was our experience (29; M. B. Goren and Y. Wang, unpublished data) that after dialysis, some preparations still contained species of considerably lower molecular weight that could transfer relatively early to phagosomes. These must be separated from the high-molecular-weight polymer by careful gel filtration. Another serious pitfall is that in some fluorescent dextrans the dye molecule is conjugated to the polymer backbone via amide linkages. These cleave in the lysosomal environment and release the free low-molecular-weight fluor, which of course transfers quickly to phagosomes (Goren and Wang, unpublished data). Such derivatized dextrans are therefore not suitable for studying differential delivery.

The differential and sequential transfer process described above was taken as evidence for a multiple-fusion delivery mechanism, i.e., a nibbling process in which mobile lysosomal components are delivered much more rapidly (but probably not exclusively) to the fusion partners than are substances of relatively low mobility. A nibbling process seems much more in accord with our findings than the alternatives that we have considered. It is highly unlikely that phagosome-lysosome junctions are maintained uninterrupted for the long periods we described, since EM profiles that show such junctions, although encountered, are not abundant. For the same reason, it is unlikely that the junctions are maintained until most of the mobile components have transferred and are then broken and again reestablished for transferring the less mobile components. Indeed, violent saltatory motions of lysosomes, numerous apparent collisions with phagosomes, and ricochets are easily documented by time-lapse video recording (29; Wang and Goren, unpublished data). With some reservations, this behavior seems to be in accord with the mechanisms that we have proposed.

Immobilization of Colloidal Gold

Colloidal gold has been used in the past as an electron-opaque pinosomal and lysosomal label (4, 22). However, currently available commercial materials seem to be too dilute for practical use in P-LF studies. Gold sols of satisfactory concentration can be prepared by reducing $HAuCl_4$ in the presence of hydrocolloidal stabilizing agents such as gelatin, polyvinylpyrrolidone, or polyacrylamide (13). These products gave excellent labeling of macrophage lysosomes, but we observed essentially no transfer of the gold to yeast phagosomes in either polyanion-containing or control cells (13, 14). Therefore, the stabilizing agents apparently form a gelatinous matrix in which the gold is trapped and thus resemble the polyanion-Thorotrast lysosomal mixtures in immobilizing the EM marker.

A specially prepared gold sol (Amersham Corp.), kindly given to us by D. B. Lowrie, contains about 5 mg of Au per ml and is stabilized with 20 mg of gelatin per ml. It is essentially totally immobilized within lysosomes and thus provided us with an additional opportunity to study the differential transfer process. Cells were doubly labeled with the gold and either AO or SR. The AO-labeled cells were given opsonized zymosan prepared by the method of Kielian and Cohn (19), an excellent target which has only low affinity for the dye. The SR cells received opsonized, fluoresceinated, heat-killed yeasts. With SR, an abundance of fusions was observed within 1.5 h of phagocytosis. They were as brilliant as those obtained with dextran sulfate cells after 4 h (Fig.

8). On the other hand, Fig. 9 documents the universal delivery of AO to phagosomes in the counterpart cells labeled with the basic dye. In contrast, EM showed almost no delivery of the gold marker to yeast phagosomes: of 100 profiles scored, only 11 phagosomes contained even a single grain of gold. The immobilization of the colloid in the putative gelatinous matrix is documented in the micrograph shown in Fig. 10. Here, unequivocal fusion of a phagosome with Au-labeled lysosomes has occurred: continuity between phagosomal and lysosomal membranes is clearly evident, and yet no marker has been transferred. Instead, two or three boli of gelatin-entrained colloid are caught, seemingly motionless, on the periphery of the yeast cell, whose appearance reveals the ravages inflicted by the digestive enzymes that have been delivered to the vacuole. A substantially identical section was previously recognized in dextran sulfate-inhibited cells (13; Fig. 5).

CONCLUSIONS

In this paper we have reviewed and further expanded upon the limitations of the AO vital fluorescence techniques for studying P-LF and have also defined certain requirements for improving its reliability.

The macrophages, whether control or polyanion type, should be exposed to sufficient AO for an adequate time to label the nuclei a visible and fairly bright green. Because AO is a permeant marker, the labeling is achieved rapidly (10 to 20 min). It seems likely that for many organisms, killing by the macrophages, or at least severe injury accompanied by digestion, is required to render the targets permeable for penetration of the dye. In the absence of dye delivery, a judgment of P-LF inhibition is unwarranted without supportive evidence from EM. For control cells labeled with, e.g., Thorotrast, retention of the marker is convincing evidence of inhibition. However, with polyanion-containing cells, EM observations may not be reliable, because polyanionic agents can physically trap the lysosomal marker. Provid-

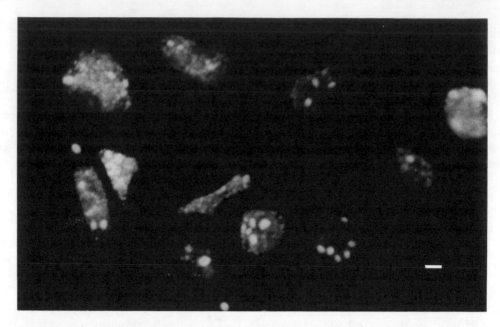

FIGURE 9. Cells labeled with a gelatin-stabilized gold and with AO (5 μg/ml), before phagocytosis of opsonized zymosan, examined by vital fluorescence microscopy. All phagosomes are brilliant. Bar, 10 μm.

ing the cells with a sufficiency of lysosomal AO may yield the most reliable evidence. Furthermore, the dye is not trapped by nonionic hydrosols.

The weakly basic acridine dyes cannot be used to assess P-LF for microorganisms that have significant affinity for the dye (*M. tuberculosis,* for example), since AO can reach the targets by diffusion even when fusion is evidently inhibited (2, 12). As a corollary, this restriction also applies even to inert substances such as particles of cation-exchange resins, since they exhibit very strong affinity for the dye.

The impermeant, highly ionic, lysosomotropic fluorochromes LR, LY, and SR do not suffer from trapping by either anionic or nonionic hydrocolloids. Because of its brilliance, SR is for us the probe of choice. Uptake of these dyes in lysosomes is slow, and they are retarded (compared with AO) in penetrating the phagocytosed targets. These limitations might be alleviated by exposure of the cells for shorter times to very high concentrations of dye or, for very small microorganisms, by surface conjugation of the target with fluorescein.

Exploitation of the impermeant, yet sufficiently mobile LR, LY, or SR in conjunction with electron-opaque colloids as markers for polyanion-containing lysosomes revealed the surprising process of a selective differential delivery of lysosomal constituents to phagosomes. The phenomenon had previously been cautiously inferred from the behavior of polyanion-containing cells in which digestion of endocytosed substrates was entirely unaltered in the face of almost total abolition of Thorotrast delivery (9, 14). The inference became conviction when the EM data could be reinforced with visible evidence from fluorescence microscopy. It was then augmented by the experiments involving double labeling with fluorochromes of considerably different mobility (29).

To explain the differential and sequential transfer of the lysosomal markers, the mechanics of delivery should account for the selective depletion of SR from essentially all of the lysosomes in a given cell, for leaving a large residual population of lysosomes still charged with FD-40 at a time when nearly all of the SR has

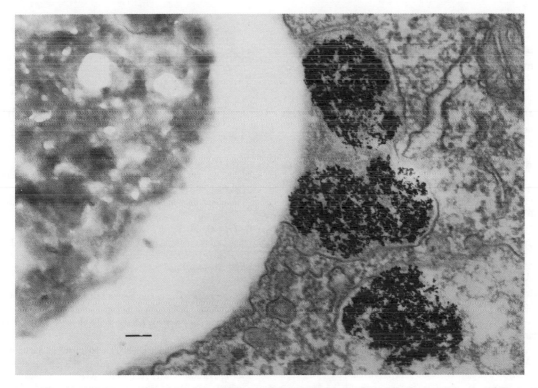

FIGURE 10. EM of cells as in Fig. 9 but with heat-killed yeasts as targets. P-LF is clearly evident in the continuity of lysosomal and phagosomal membranes and from digestion of the yeast, but gold has not been delivered (see text). Bar, 100 nm.

been transferred, and for a continuation of the process which then delivers FD-40. These requirements cannot be accommodated by the conventionally accepted P-LF process with its implicit total delivery of lysosomal contents: this feature was clearly denied by our evidence. Instead we proposed that individual secondary lysosomes might fuse transiently and perhaps repeatedly with phagosomes. During each fusion a partial transfer of the more mobile components (e.g., SR) might occur until depletion. However, only insignificant amounts of FD-40 are transferred at the same time because of its hindered mobility, an interpretation that is supported by the high fluorescence polarization documented for FD-40 within lysosomes (8). Afterward, sluggish delivery of the polymer becomes more evident.

The overall demonstrated behavior is therefore quite different from the temporally briefly separated progression of fusion events documented for the intracellular activities of polymorphonuclear leukocytes. In these it was established that fusion of specific granules with the phagocytic vacuole precedes by several minutes the delivery of azurophilic granule contents (3). Our concept also departs from that conveyed by the well-known classical cinematographic demonstration of leukocytes engulfing bacteria in which Hirsch and colleagues captured the explosive disappearance of cytoplasmic granules during fusion with the developing phagosomes (described in reference 18). Implicit in this behavior was an abrupt total delivery of lysosomal contents with each explosive event. Indeed, this may be the true state of affairs for these kinds of cells with their virgin lysosomes. In contrast, EM profiles have sometimes captured the flaccid appearance of macrophage secondary lysosomes heavily labeled with electron-dense markers, hanging saclike and attached to a phagosomal membrane. This is an aspect that could well accommodate the multiple delivery–pinching-off sequences that we have considered. Evidence for such pinching-off events might be sought by and recognized in EM studies dedicated to this task.

ACKNOWLEDGMENTS. Original investigations reported here were supported in part by grant AI-08401 from the U.S.-Japan Cooperative Medical Science Program, administered by the National Institute of Allergy and Infectious Diseases, and in part by Public Health Service grant AI-17509 from the National Institute of Allergy and Infectious Disease. M.B.G. is the Margaret Regan Investigator in Chemical Pathology, National Jewish Center for Immunology and Respiratory Medicine.

We thank Barry Silverstein for assistance with the illustrations and Shirley Downs for careful preparation of the manuscript.

LITERATURE CITED

1. **Allison, A. C., and M. R. Young.** 1969. Vital staining and fluorescence microscopy of lysosomes, p. 600–628. *In* J. T. Dingle and H. B. Fell (ed.), *Lysosomes in Biology and Pathology,* vol. 2. Elsevier/North Holland Biomedical Press, Amsterdam.

2. **Armstrong, J. A., and P. D. Hart.** 1971. Response of cultured macrophages to *Mycobacterium tuberculosis,* with observations on fusion of lysosomes with phagosomes. *J. Exp. Med.* 134:713–740.

3. **Bainton, D. F.** 1973. Sequential degranulation of the two types of polymorphonuclear leukocyte granules during phagocytosis of microorganisms. *J. Cell Biol.* 58:249–264.

4. **Cohn, Z. A., M. E. Fedorko, and J. G. Hirsch.** 1966. The *in vitro* differentiation of mononuclear phagocytes. V. The formation of macrophage lysosomes. *J. Exp. Med.* 123:757–766.

5. **de Duve, C., T. de Barsy, B. Poole, A. Trouet, P. Tulkens, and F. Vanhoof.** 1974. Lysosomotropic agents. *Biochem. Pharmacol.* 23:2495–2531.

6. **Freidlin, I. S., T. N. Khavkin, N. K. Artemenko, and I. Y. Sakharova.** 1977. Vital fluorescence microscopy of lysosomes in cultured mouse peritoneal macrophages during their interactions with microorganisms and active substances. II. Interac-

tions of macrophages with a non-pathogenic strain of *Escherichia coli. Acta Microbiol. Acad. Sci. Hung.* 24:293–302.

7. **Geisow, M. J., G. H. Beaven, P. D. Hart, and M. R. Young.** 1980. Site of action of a polyanion inhibitor of phagosome-lysosome fusion in cultured macrophages. *Exp. Cell Res.* 126:159–165.

8. **Geisow, M. J., P. D. Hart, and M. R. Young.** 1981. Temporal changes of lysosome and phagosome pH during phagolysosome formation in macrophages: studies by fluorescence spectroscopy. *J. Cell Biol.* 89:645–652.

9. **Goren, M. B.** 1983. Some paradoxes of macrophage functions, p. 31–50. *In* T. K. Eisenstein, P. Actor, and H. Friedman (ed.), *Host Defenses to Intracellular Pathogens.* Plenum Publishing Corp., New York.

10. **Goren, M. B., P. D. Hart, M. R. Young, and J. A. Armstrong.** 1976. Prevention of phagosome-lysosome fusion in cultured macrophages by sulfatides of *Mycobacterium tuberculosis.* Proc. Natl. Acad. Sci. USA 73:2510–2514.

11. **Goren, M. B., C. L. Swendsen, J. Fiscus, and C. Miranti.** 1984. Fluorescent markers for studying phagosome-lysosome fusion. *J. Leukocyte Biol.* 36:273–292.

12. **Goren, M. B., C. L. Swendsen, and J. Henson.** 1980. Factors modifying the fusion of phagosomes and lysosomes: art, fact, and artefact, p. 999–1038. *In* R. van Furth (ed.), *Mononuclear Phagocytes: Functional Aspects,* part II. Martinus Nijhoff, The Hague, The Netherlands.

13. **Goren, M. B., A. E. Vatter, and J. Fiscus.** 1987. Polyanionic agents as inhibitors of phagosome-lysosome fusion in cultured macrophages: evolution of an alternative interpretation. *J. Leukocyte Biol.* 41:111–121.

14. **Goren, M. B., A. E. Vatter, and J. Fiscus.** 1987. Polyanionic agents do not inhibit phagosome-lysosome fusion in cultured macrophages. *J. Leukocyte Biol.* 41:122–129.

15. **Hart, P. D., and M. R. Young.** 1975. Interference with normal phagosome-lysosome fusion in macrophages using ingested yeast cells and suramin. *Nature* (London) 256:47–49.

16. **Hart, P. D., and M. R. Young.** 1978. Manipulations of the phagosome-lysosome fusion response in cultured macrophages. Enhancement of fusion by chloroquine and other amines. *Exp. Cell Res.* 114:486–490.

17. **Hart, P. D., and M. R. Young.** 1980. Manipulation of phagosome-lysosome fusion in cultured macrophages: potentialities and limitations, p. 1039–1055. *In* R. van Furth (ed.), *Mononuclear Phagocytes: Functional Aspects,* part II. Martinus Nijhoff, The Hague, The Netherlands.

18. **Hirsch, J. G.** 1962. Cinemicrophotographic observations on granule lysis in polymorphonuclear leu-

cocytes during phagocytosis. *J. Exp. Med.* 116:827–834.

19. Kielian, M. C., and Z. A. Cohn. 1980. Phagosome-lysosome fusion. Characterization of intracellular membrane fusion in mouse macrophages. *J. Cell Biol.* 85:754–765.

20. Kielian, M. C., R. M. Steinman, and Z. A. Cohn. 1982. Intralysosomal accumulation of polyanions. I. Fusion of pinocytic and phagocytic vacuoles with secondary lysosomes. *J. Cell Biol.* 93:866–874.

21. Lerman, L. S. 1961. Structural considerations in the interaction of DNA and acridines. *J. Mol. Biol.* 3:18–30.

22. Lowrie, D. B., P. S. Jackett, V. R. Aber, and M. E. W. Carol. 1980. Cyclic nucleotides and phagosome-lysosome fusion in mouse peritoneal macrophages, p. 1057–1075. *In* R. van Furth (ed.), *Mononuclear Phagocytes: Functional Aspects*, part II. Martinus Nijoff, The Hague, The Netherlands.

23. Miller, D. K., E. Griffiths, J. Lenard, and R. A. Firestone. 1983. Cell killing by lysosomotropic detergents. *J. Cell Biol.* 97:1841–1851.

24. Mor, N., and M. B. Goren. 1987. Discrepancy in assessment of phagosome-lysosome fusion with two lysosomal markers in murine macrophages infected with *Candida albicans*. *Infect. Immun.* 55:1663–1667.

25. Ohkuma, S., and B. Poole. 1978. Fluorescence probe measurement of the intralysosomal pH in living cells and the perturbation of pH by various agents. *Proc. Natl. Acad. Sci. USA* 75:3327–3331.

26. Pantazis, C. G., and W. T. Kniker. 1979. Assessment of blood leukocyte microbial killing by using a new fluorochrome microassay. *RES J. Reticuloendothel. Soc.* 26:155–170.

27. Strugger, V. S. 1947. Die Vitalfluorochromierung des Protoplasmas. *Naturwissenschaften* 34:267–273.

28. Swanson, J. A., B. D. Yirinec, and S. C. Silverstein. 1985. Phorbol esters and horseradish peroxidase stimulate pinocytosis and redirect the flow of pinocytosed fluid in macrophages. *J. Cell Biol.* 100:851–859.

29. Wang, Y.-l., and M. B. Goren. 1987. Differential and sequential delivery of fluorescent lysosomal probes into phagosomes in mouse peritoneal macrophages. *J. Cell Biol.* 104:1749–1754.

Chapter 12

Acquired Cellular Immunity to Facultative Intracellular Bacterial Parasites

FRANK M. COLLINS

Trudeau Institute, Inc.
Saranac Lake, New York 12983

KELTON P. HEPPER

Marion Laboratories, Inc.
Kansas City, Missouri 64134

INTRODUCTION

The ability of normal, healthy adults to resist a second attack of many childhood diseases was widely recognized long before the infectious nature of these diseases was generally appreciated. On the basis of the pioneering protection studies of Pasteur, von Behring, Koch, Wright, and others, the concept of a protective humoral immunity (antitoxic and opsonic antibodies) was established, and the pivotal role of specific immunoglobulins in the expression of acquired resistance had become generally accepted by the turn of this century (8). On a largely empiric basis, effective vaccines were quickly developed against such diseases as tetanus, diphtheria, fowl cholera, anthrax, and bubonic plague. Enhanced resistance was usually developed after the administration of two or three doses of a suitably inactivated whole bacterial vaccine, although in establishing resistance to some diseases, soluble toxoids were also effective (33).

Despite these early successes, other important bacterial diseases, such as tuberculosis, dysentery, erysipelas, and gonorrhea, were not prevented even by repeated injections of killed vaccine, although some protection against some of these infections, such as cholera, typhoid fever, and bacterial meningitis, was achieved in suitably challenged animals (9). For this reason, attempts were made to develop live attenuated vaccines, with considerable success in several cases (smallpox, yellow fever, tuberculosis, and brucellosis). Such vaccines tend to develop cellular rather than humoral responses on the part of the host defenses, and this can usually be transferred to naive recipients by an infusion of specifically sensitized T lymphocytes harvested from the infected spleen, lymph node, or even peripheral blood (4). On coming into contact with the triggering antigen(s), these T cells release lymphokines, which can bring about the immunologic activation of monocytes entering the infected lesion from the bloodstream. Such cells are drawn into the developing lesion (tubercle) in large numbers from the bloodstream, owing to the release of chemotactic factors within the damaged tissue. Resident macrophages present within the lung, in the peritoneal cavity, or in the nasopharyngeal and intestinal submucosae can phagocytose and kill most environmental or commensal microorganisms that accidentally gain entry to the normal tissues. These bacteria are digested very rapidly, and their antigens are released into the draining lymph node, where they induce a predominantly humoral response, which may play an important protective role for the host defenses by limiting the entry of these organisms (and their cross-reactive relatives) across the gut and nasopharyngeal mucosal membranes (4). These secretory (immunoglobulin A) antibodies can play a major protective role in preventing the commensal flora from entering the tissues, probably by blocking attachment receptors on the bacterial cell walls or flagellae and thus preventing the opportunistic pathogens from reaching the target tissue. Circulating antibodies are less effective in preventing the entry of virulent gut or respiratory pathogens into the submucosa, thereby allowing them to establish a foothold within the host tissues. The opsonized bacilli may continue to multiply within the normal macrophages at the site of infection, where they may be protected against the bactericidal action of normally effective doses of antibiotic (8). The more virulent strains multiply rapidly within the tissue macrophages and are killed only by specifically activated macrophages as they enter the infected lesion later in the infection. Immunization of the host with live *Mycobacterium bovis* BCG produces large numbers of specifically stimulated macrophages; this limits the growth of the challenge inoculum within the lungs and prevents the spread of virulent mycobacteria to uninvolved organs and tissues (5). This depends upon a complex series of cellular interactions which occur within the draining lymph nodes and the lungs and which forms the basis of the present discussion.

HUMORAL AND CELLULAR IMMUNITY DEVELOPED WITHIN THE INFECTED TISSUE

Most infections due to facultative intracellular pathogens induce a response which involves an interplay between specific antibodies, complement, and macrophages within the infected tissue (4). However, some infections (such as tuberculosis, listeriosis, and syphilis) primarily involve the cell-mediated arm of the immune response, with specific antibodies playing little or no direct role in passively protected animals (8, 9). Infusion of specifically sensitized T lymphocytes harvested from the lymph nodes or spleens of convalescent donors can fully protect naive syngeneic recipients against a subsequent virulent challenge (29). This response shows a clear dose-response protection and occurs even in the complete absence of hyperimmune serum. The convalescent host possesses a population of specific memory T cells which activate the mononuclear cell defenses in such a way that they can then express an enhanced nonspecific resistance against a number of other intracellular pathogens (22). Mackaness (22) coined the phrase "angry macrophages" to describe these immunologically activated cells, which are produced by exposure of blood-derived monocytes to a number of lymphokines (including macrophage activation factor) released when sensitized T cells are exposed to the specific sensitin either in vivo or in vitro (40). The activated macrophages are larger and metabolically more active, as well as more phagocytic, and are able to take up and kill more pathogens at an enhanced rate compared with that seen for normal unstimulated phagocytes (26). Despite this activation, most macrophages have difficulty inactivating highly virulent tubercle bacilli, especially in vitro (38). More attenuated strains of mycobacteria may be killed (or at least prevented from multiplying) by the lymphokine-activated macrophages (21). However, virulent atypical mycobacteria do not seem to be killed under optimum experimental conditions (R. W. Stokes and F. M. Collins, submitted for publication), although BCG-vaccinated mice can demonstrate an accelerated bacteriostatic response both in the donor mice and in recipients of specific memory T cells harvested from the vaccinated donors (32). Such mice may also show a substantial level of cross-protection against both aerogenic and intravenous *Mycobacterium avium* challenges, although in most cases, the specific antituberculous immunity (against *Mycobacterium tuberculosis*) seems to be quantitatively more effective. However, the level of protection achieved in these experiments varies considerably with the experimental conditions (the test organism, the dose and route of vaccination and challenge, the time interval between vaccination and challenge, and the genetic susceptibility of the host species). For this reason the experimental conditions must be standardized very carefully to minimize the effect of differences in growth or inhibition of the challenge infection which might be ascribed to the experimental test system itself (7). For instance, growth of a highly virulent strain of tubercle bacillus continues within the lungs long after the emerging cell-mediated immune response has been able to limit the growth of the same organism within the liver and spleen (5). T cells harvested from the spleen during this period will transfer both tuberculin hypersensitivity and acquired antituberculous resistance to syngeneic, T-cell-depleted recipients (30), but the mere presence of sensitized T cells within the donor spleen does not guarantee that the lung counts will decline with time, and eventually the donor animals may die (5). The infusion of immune T cells limits the growth of a secondary challenge infection within the lungs, and eventually the secondary bacterial counts decline slowly and may even reach clinically insignificant levels. However, other virulent mycobacteria (*M. avium*, *Mycobacterium kansasii*, and *Mycobacterium ulcerans*) can give rise to persistent systemic infections with little or no indication of any cell-mediated immune response of the type normally associated with BCG- and *M. tuberculosis*-infected mice (Fig. 1). Previous studies carried out with mice heavily infected with virulent *M. avium* 724

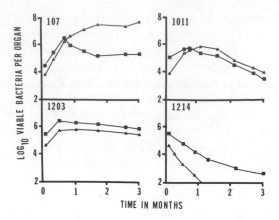

FIGURE 1. Growth of *M. tuberculosis* Erdman (TMC 107), *M. bovis* BCG Pasteur (TMC 1011), *M. kansasii* TMC 1203, and *M. kansasii* TMC 1214 in intravenously infected B6D2 mice. Symbols: ■, spleen; ▲, lungs.

had suggested that this unresponsiveness was due to a population of suppressor T cells which appear in heavily infected spleens (41). However, such in vitro suppression data do not seem to be reflected by a corresponding in vivo depression in T-cell reactivity to other test antigens in the intact animal (15, 31). Therefore, it is not clear how much of the in vitro unresponsiveness can be validly extrapolated to the in vivo situation.

Persister strains of *M. kansasii* (TMC 1201 and TMC 1203) multiply within the spleens of intravenously challenged immunocompetent mice for about 10 days, after which the rate of bacterial growth in vivo falls sharply and the growth curve passes into a prolonged plateau phase. This growth restriction phase coincides with a sharp rise in cellular proliferation, peaking around day 7 (Fig. 2). This was also associated with a marked increase in the number of mononuclear cells present in the spleen, which was responsible for a substantial degree of splenomegaly seen in these animals at that time (Table 1). Mice infected with smaller numbers (10^6 CFU) of *M. kansasii* TMC 1203 showed a delay in the proliferation response (15), which coincided with a later peak in both antilisterial and antituberculous resistance by these mice. Adoptive transfer studies involving the use of T-cell-depleted recipients indicated that im-

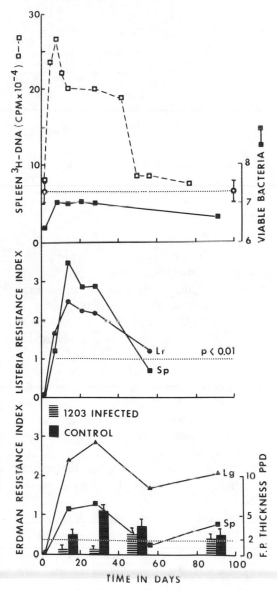

FIGURE 2. Effect of 10^8 CFU of *M. kansasii* TMC 1203 on the proliferation of spleen cells. Top: Growth of *M. kansasii* in spleen (■) compared with tritiated thymidine uptake (□). Middle: Antilisteria activity within the liver (●) or spleen (■). Bottom: Antituberculous resistance to an Erdman challenge, measured as a resistance index for the lungs (Lg) or spleen (Sp), or the level of tuberculin hypersensitivity (2.5 μg of PPD in 30 μl of saline), measured 24 h after footpad injection in *M. kansasii*-infected mice or normal controls. In each panel, the dotted lines represent the limit of significance at the 1% level.

mune T cells did not appear within the spleens of these mice until at least 60 days into the primary infection (16). On the other hand, mice infected with the nonvirulent *M. kansasii* TMC 1214 (Fig. 3) showed proliferative activity within the spleen similar to that seen with mice receiving heat-killed *M. kansasii*, with little or no antilisterial or antituberculous reactivity observed in either group of animals (Table 1).

SUPPRESSION OF T-CELL RESPONSES IN *M. KANSASII*-INFECTED MICE

The normal host response to a virulent mycobacterial challenge is an influx of mononuclear cells into the developing lesion (27). By 14 days, both splenic and peritoneal macrophages show an enhanced rate of killing of an intravenous inoculum of *Listeria monocytogenes* (39). This effect usually reaches its peak between 2 and 3 weeks, regardless of the overall virulence of the primary infecting organism (compare Fig. 2 and 3). On the other hand, heat-killed mycobacteria induce little or no antilisterial activity unless incorporated into a Freund-type adjuvant (3, 10). Antituberculous resistance was measured as the difference ($\log_{10}$) in viable acriflavine-resistant *M. tuberculosis* AR in the lungs compared with that in the normal controls (15). Peak antituberculous responses in the lungs were seen 30 days after the *M. kansasii* infection (Fig. 2), compared with 14 days for the *Listeria* challenge. The splenic response was substantially lower than that in the lungs, but was still significant ($P < 0.01$). The *M. kansasii* infection resulted in a persistent footpad anergy to purified protein derivative (PPD), which was reflected in a substantial suppression in PPD reactivity in the Erdman-challenged mice compared with the controls (Fig. 2).

When mice were infected with 10^0 CFU of *M. kansasii* TMC 1214, the viable counts declined immediately and represented only 0.01% of the initial inoculum after 90 days (Fig. 3). The mice exhibited some antilisterial

TABLE 1

Proliferation following stimulation with 10^7 CFU of viable or 10^8 CFU of heat-killed *M. kansasii* by intravenous inoculation

Time (days)	10^7 CFU of viable cells			10^8 CFU of heat-killed cells		
	Spleen wt (mg)	[^{3}H]TdR[a] uptake (10^3 cpm)	Total cells (10^6 ± SEM)	Spleen wt (mg)	[^{3}H]TdR uptake (10^3 cpm)	Total cells (10^6 ± SEM)
0	85	42 ± 0.2	70 ± 7			
1	88	50 ± 0.5	81 ± 7	75	83 ± 0.7	72 ± 4
5	125	108 ± 1.8	110 ± 7			
10	145	310 ± 3.9 (7.4)[b]	283 ± 2	113	165 ± 3.1	110 ± 10
20	140	178 ± 0.9	357 ± 9	122	184 ± 3.7 (4.0)[b]	135 ± 11
30	147 (173%)	115 ± 2.3	319 ± 16	114 (134%)	151 ± 1.6	115 ± 9

[a] TdR, Thymidine.
[b] Maximum proliferation index.

activity, which peaked on day 14 (coincident with the peak proliferative response). However, there was no significant increase in antituberculous immunity (data not shown).

Normal mice infected with 10^8 CFU of *M. kansasii* TMC 1203 produced specifically sensitized T cells only after a prolonged period of infection. This was determined by infusing increasing numbers of T cells from the *M. kansasii*-infected donor into sublethally irradiated syngeneic recipients which had been challenged intravenously with acriflavine-resistant *M. kansasii* AR. Paradoxically, mice which had been infected with smaller numbers (10^6 CFU) of viable *M. kansasii* TMC 1203 developed detectable numbers of immune T cells more rapidly than animals receiving 100 times that number of vaccinating organisms did (16). This was interpreted to mean that the T-cell response within the heavily infected host was inhibited by the activated macrophages responsible for nonspecifically limiting the further growth of the larger challenge inoculum during the early stages of the infection.

SUPPRESSION OF T-CELL RESPONSES DETECTED DURING CELL MIXING EXPERIMENTS

Increasing the number of cells harvested from heavily infected mouse spleen cocultured with indicator T cells resulted in up to 90% reductions in the level of blastogenic responsiveness (Fig. 4). This peaked 10 days after the *M. kansasii* TMC 1203 infection had been initiated. Treatment of the infected spleen cells with anti-Thy 1.2 antibody plus complement reduced the level of suppression somewhat but did not completely ablate it (Table 2). On the other hand, purified T cells taken from heavily infected donors showed an additive effect which was largely ablated by anti-Thy 1.2 serum and complement treatment. Strong inhibition was mediated by the adherent cell population present in the *M. kansasii*-infected spleen. However, initial attempts to dislodge the adherent cells from the nylon wool column by using EDTA- (35) or lidocaine-enriched buffer (17) failed to yield a sufficient number of viable cells for cell mixing experiments. The problem was overcome by allowing the infected spleen cells to adhere directly to the microtiter well floor by incubating the cell suspension in RPMI 1640 medium plus 5% fetal calf serum in 5% CO_2 in air for 1 h at 37°C. Nonadherent and weakly adherent cells were removed by vigorous washing, and the indicator T cells and mitogen were then added to the well. Tritiated thymidine uptake was reduced in a dose-responsive manner by these cells (Table 2). However, adherent cells harvested from uninfected mice or those stimulated with heat-killed *M. kansasii* did not inhibit mitogenic responsiveness, being, if anything, stimulatory in nature.

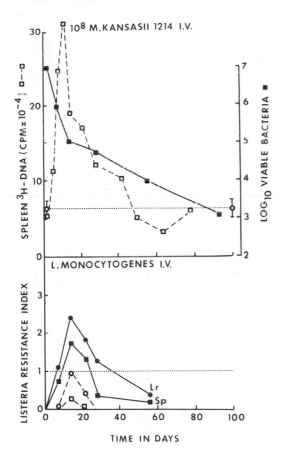

FIGURE 3. Effect of 10^8 CFU of *M. kansasii* TMC 1214 on cell proliferation (top) and antilisterial reistance (bottom). The broken lines and open symbols in the lower graph represent the antilisterial activity in mice injected with 10^8 CFU of heat-killed *M. kansasii*. In each panel, the dotted lines represent the limit of significance at the 1% level.

HUMORAL VERSUS CELL-MEDIATED RESPONSES BY *M. KANSASII*-INFECTED SPLEENS

Infected mice were tested for their responsiveness to a number of unrelated antigenic stimuli in vivo. At increasing time intervals after receiving 10^8 CFU of live or heat-killed *M. kansasii* TMC 1203, groups of mice were sensitized with 5×10^8 sheep erythrocytes, and their spleens were removed 5 days later (12). Plaque-forming cell counts were car-

ried out by the standard procedure of Cunningham and Szenberg (11). The sheep erythrocyte inoculum resulted in a substantial delayed-type hypersensitivity as well as a humoral (plaque-forming cell) response (19). However, prior infection with mycobacteria affected the kinetics of this response, resulting in a substantial and persistent ablation of the delayed footpad response, with little or no change in humoral reactivity. The humoral response seen in the *M. kansasii*-infected mice increased with time, reaching a peak around day 20 of the bacterial infection (Table 3). Heat-killed *M. kansasii* cells also induced a small rise in plaque-forming cell counts, but this was not significant when expressed per 10^6 spleen cells.

Virulent mycobacterial infections induce a substantial degree of splenomegaly and an increasing number of granulomas (tubercles) with time. Both responses result in an increased number of activated macrophages within the tissues, and previous investigators had shown these to be responsible for an increased level of suppression of T-cell activity in vivo (1, 2). The present study also suggests that these activated macrophages are responsible for the early bacteriostatic effect seen in these mycobacterial infections. However, in the absence of specifically sensitized T cells, these cells are unable to do more than reduce the rate of growth by this inoculum in vivo, giving rise to the characteristic plateau seen in the growth curve (Fig. 4). Throughout this time, adoptive transfer studies indicate a virtual absence of specifically immune T cells in the heavily infected spleen (16). Eventually, such cells do appear (day 60), coinciding with the decline in the number of activated macrophages within the spleen (Fig. 2). This raises the possibility that the macrophages somehow block this T-cell response, just as cell mixing experiments with BCG-stimulated macrophages suggest that activated macrophages are responsible for the suppression of blastogenic responsiveness shown by indicator T cells in vitro (13). Live *M. kansasii* TMC 1203 induces the early production of large numbers of suppressor macrophages, whereas heat-killed organisms do not, with the result

TABLE 2
Cell mixing experiment with spleen cells from *M. kansasii*-infected donors and normal T cells

Donor host	Cell no. (10³)	[³H]TdR[a] incorporation (cpm ± SEM) in:			
		Whole spleen	T cells	B cells	Adherent cells
Control			90,026 ± 1,730		
10⁷ viable *M. kansasii*	100	89,690 ± 9,964	194,161 ± 6,230	118,016 ± 4,484	207,053 ± 5,543
10⁷ viable *M. kansasii*	200	28,064 ± 4,552[b]	229,622 ± 2,745	140,038 ± 5,399	4,467 ± 1,025[c]
10⁷ viable *M. kansasii*	400	6,170 ± 1,250[c]	150,773 ± 2,793	115,532 ± 3,133	579 ± 47[c]
10⁷ viable *M. kansasii* + α-Thy 1.2 + C	200	42,894 ± 12,123	91,742 ± 1,430		
10⁸ heat-killed *M. kansasii*	200	155,928 ± 5,284	160,904 ± 3,776	119,016 ± 1,820	216,739 ± 4,040
Uninfected	200	167,249 ± 13,808	253,647 ± 5,788	119,016 ± 1,820	253,960 ± 3,009

[a]TdR, Thymidine.
[b]$P < 0.01$ versus control.
[c]$P < 0.001$ versus control.

that no suppression is seen (Table 2) although such mice develop a substantial splenomegaly (Table 1), indicating that the suppressor effect is not simply due to the presence of large numbers of mononuclear phagocytes within the spleen. Attempts to demonstrate a suppressive role for these activated macrophages by means of direct transfer into normal syngeneic recipients have proven to be unsuccessful so far, presumably because the transferred cells rapidly

TABLE 3
Immune responses to sheep erythrocytes injected into mice stimulated with 10⁸ CFU of live or heat-killed *M. kansasii*

Time (days)	CFU of TMC 1203	No. of PFC[a] in spleen ± SEM	No. of PFC/10⁶ spleen cells ± SEM	Delayed-type hypersensitivity[b] ± SEM
0	None	64,500 ± 12,000	800 ± 140	12.2 ± 0.7
10	None	59,600 ± 9,200	780 ± 120	11.0 ± 0.8
	10⁸ viable	59,000 ± 15,500	926 ± 170	1.8 ± 0.2
	10⁸ heat killed	64,400 ± 12,500	585 ± 130	14.2 ± 1.2
20	None	65,800 ± 5,200	700 ± 150	12.6 ± 0.7
	10⁸ viable	259,000 ± 6,600[c]	725 ± 190	1.8 ± 0.2
	10⁸ heat killed	107,000 ± 11,300	796 ± 150	4.6 ± 1.0
30	None	98,000 ± 12,100	754 ± 130	13.8 ± 0.5
	10⁸ viable	224,750 ± 6,300[c]	1,196 ± 235	2.0 ± 0.3
	10⁸ heat killed	88,100 ± 8,900	766 ± 200	10.8 ± 0.7
60	None	42,320 ± 3,777	555 ± 131	14.6 ± 0.7
	10⁸ viable	117,600 ± 13,700[c]	818 ± 301	5.0 ± 0.9

[a]PFC, Plaque-forming cells.
[b]10 Schnelltäster units = 1 mm.
[c]$P < 0.01$ versus controls.

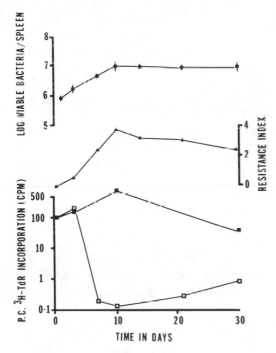

FIGURE 4. Growth of *M. kansasii* TMC 1203 in the spleens of B6D2 mice (top) compared with the listeria resistance indices and blastogenic responses by whole spleen cells (□) and T-cell-enriched suspensions (■) when exposed to concanavalin A in vitro.

lose their activated state once introduced into a normal recipient.

The coincidence of the sharp peak in monocyte numbers within the spleen, the raised antilisterial activity, and the ablated blastogenic responsiveness in vitro (Fig. 4) strongly suggest some sort of causal relationship between these phenomena. Evidence presented by other investigators suggests that activated macrophages (or their soluble factors) are important mediators of the antigenic unresponsiveness seen in lepromatous leprosy patients (18) and may also be responsible for the initiation of the immunosuppressive changes characteristic of this important human disease (34). It is therefore tempting to speculate that the same population of activated macrophages is responsible for the early limitation of the growth of the mycobacterial population as is responsible for the modulation of the immune T-cell re-

sponse which must eventually control the resulting infection.

CONCLUSIONS

Acquired resistance to facultative intracellular parasites is primarily a cell-mediated immune response, with humoral factors usually playing a more minor protective role (23). However, virulent *Salmonella, Brucella, Yersinia,* and *Francisella* infections invoke a substantial humoral response on the part of the host defenses, and these antibodies may play an important protective role against these pathogens. The specific opsonins interact with the smooth somatic and capsular antigens of the pathogen, antagonizing their ability to inhibit phagocytosis (9). When present on a mucosal surface, specific secretory (immunoglobulin A) antibodies play an important protective role against many oral and respiratory opportunistic pathogens by blocking their attachment receptors to nasopharyngeal or intestinal mucosal cells (8). Despite this, highly virulent pathogens may still invade the normal mucosa and establish a temporary foothold within the tissues. Elimination of the resulting systemic infection requires the induction of a specific T-cell-mediated immune response (4). Intervention of this defense involves the interaction of infected mononuclear phagocytes with immunocompetent T cells present in the draining lymph node and spleen (9). For nonpathogens which accidentally gain entry to the tissues, the macrophages normally resident in the tissues can eliminate the infection without requiring this immunological activation. Some opportunistic pathogens may be able to survive this initial period of inactivation and begin to multiply slowly within the tissues, at the same time draining into the local lymph node. Overt pathogens continue this spread to infect uninvolved tissues and organs (14). This systemic spread can be contained only if immune T cells enter the primary lesion in large numbers and immunologically activate the blood monocytes also entering the developing granuloma (27). Eventually, these cells eliminate most of the organisms from the lymphoreticular organs, although it is not unusual for a few viable bacilli to persist within fibrosed or caseated lesions within the lungs, giving rise to the so-called carrier state. The persistence of a few virulent tubercle bacilli within the apparently cured patient, even after prolonged and aggressive chemotherapy, is a double-edged sword. The patient remains resistant to external (exogenous) reinfection as a result of the continued presence of memory T cells within the spleen, but the same residual organisms constitute an important public health threat, since endogenous reactivation of this infection by corticosteroid therapy or age-related immunodepletion can lead to life-threatening disease (37).

Most (95 to 98%) of the immunocompetent individuals exposed to a modest tuberculous infection develop sufficient cell-mediated immunity to limit the spread of the infection to the draining lymph node (23). This local immune response involves the presentation of mycobacterial antigens by the infected macrophages to the T cells which bear specific recognition markers for the sensitin-major histocompatibility complex (36). These stimulated T cells undergo extensive blast transformation (replication) which expands the reactive clone enormously: a response seen as an aggregation of pyroninophilic cells within the developing tubercle and its draining lymph node, beginning 10 to 14 days into the primary infection (27, 39). As a result of this T-cell response, the host can acquire both antimicrobial immunity and tuberculin hypersensitivity (6). These responses can be transferred to naive recipients by means of splenic T cells harvested from the immunized host, although it seems that different T-cell subsets are involved in the two processes (30). Depletion of the T-cell population from the host ablates its ability to mount both of these responses equally (25). Live BCG vaccine induces a specific T-cell response, which peaks at about the time the bacterial population within the spleen undergoes a sharp decline in its growth rate (7). Once the infec-

tion has been brought under control, the production of these T cells will be down-regulated, and the number of expressor T cells present in the tissues declines sharply with time (28). Although the number of expressor T cells declines (20), the convalescent host can still mount an effective immune response to rechallenge owing to the presence of long-lived memory T cells within the spleen (8). These T cells are relatively radiation and cyclophosphamide resistant (32) and may persist within the tissues even in the apparent absence of a stimulating infection (20). However, latent tuberculous infections are notoriously difficult to detect, with small numbers of viable bacilli still present years after combined chemotherapy has apparently cured the patient completely (24). The presence of such a minimal infectious stimulus may maintain the production of memory T cells indefinitely, providing the means for reexpanding the population of expressor T cells needed to control the growth of the original (or even cross-reactive) pathogen whenever the host comes in contact with it again (32). Because of this, the continued debate over the relative efficacy of different BCG preparations (19) may have little validity, since the tuberculous challenge normally serves to reactivate the memory T-cell defenses, regardless of the level of antituberculous protection initially induced in the vaccinated host (7). Recent studies showed that regardless of the immunogenicity of the BCG substrain used to sensitize the mice, growth of the aerogenic challenge was controlled effectively by the memory T cells left by the vaccinating infection (32). The accelerated recall of T-cell-mediated immunity limited the growth of the virulent challenge before the infection could reach clinically significant proportions. Thus, the primary function of any BCG vaccine must be the induction of a sufficient number of long-lived memory T cells to allow the host to prevent the hematogenous spread of any secondary infection (14). We still know surprisingly little about the nature of these memory T cells or the manner by which they can recall an effective immune response in the reinfected host.

However, there is no question that these cells constitute one of the major factors in protecting the host against infections caused by these important human and veterinary pathogens.

ACKNOWLEDGMENTS. This work was supported by Public Health Service grants AI-14067 and HL-19774 from the National Institutes of Health and by a grant from the World Health Organization (Immunology of Tuberculosis).

LITERATURE CITED

1. Bennett, J. A., and J. C. Marsh. 1981. Relationship of bacillus Calmette-Guerin-induced suppressor cells to hematopoietic precursor cells. *Cancer Res.* 40:80–85.

2. Bennett, J. A., V. S. Rao, and M. S. Mitchell. 1978. Systemic bacillus Calmette-Guerin (BCG) activates natural suppressor cells. *Proc. Natl. Acad. Sci. USA* 75:5142–5144.

3. Collins, F. M. 1973. The relative immunogenicity of virulent and attenuated strains of tubercle bacilli. *Am. Rev. Respir. Dis.* 107:1030–1040.

4. Collins, F. M. 1979. Cellular antimicrobial immunity. *Crit. Rev. Microbiol.* 7:27–91.

5. Collins, F. M. 1982. Immunology of tuberculosis. *Am. Rev. Respir. Dis.* 125:S42–S49.

6. Collins, F. M. 1983. Kinetics of the delayed-type hypersensitivity response in tuberculous guinea pigs and mice tested with several mycobacterial antigens. *Am. Rev. Respir. Dis.* 127:599–604.

7. Collins, F. M. 1984. Protection against mycobacterial disease by means of live vaccines tested in experimental animals, p. 787–839. *In* G. P. Kubica and L. G. Wayne (ed.), *The Mycobacteria. A Sourcebook.* Marcel Dekker, Inc., New York.

8. Collins, F. M. 1987. Immunological responses to microbial antigens by the infected host, p. 105–150. *In* C. Wicher (ed.), *Microbial Antigenodiagnosis.* CRC Press, Inc., Boca Raton, Fla.

9. Collins, F. M., and S. G. Campbell. 1982. Immunity to intracellular bacteria. *Vet. Immunol. Immunopathol.* 3:5–66.

10. Collins, F. M., and G. B. Mackaness. 1970. The relationship of delayed hypersensitivity to acquired antituberculous resistance. II. Effect of adjuvant on the allergenicity and immunogenicity of heat killed tubercle bacilli. *Cell. Immunol.* 1:266–275.

11. Cunningham, A. M., and A. Szenberg. 1968. Further improvement in the plaque technique for detecting single antibody-forming cells. *Immunology* 14:599–600.

12. Cunningham, D. S., and F. M. Collins. 1981. Suppressor and helper T-cell populations in *M. kansasii*-infected spleens. *Immunology* 44:473–480.

13. Druker, B. J., and H. T. Wepsic. 1983. BCG-induced macrophages as suppressor cells. *Cancer Invest.* 1:151–161.

14. Fok, J. S., R. S. Ho, P. K. Arora, G. E. Harding, and D. W. Smith. 1976. Host-parasite relationships in experimental airborne tuberculosis. V. Lack of hematogenous dissemination of *M. tuberculosis* to the lungs in animals vaccinated with bacillus Calmette-Guerin. *J. Infect. Dis.* 133:137–144.

15. Hepper, K. P., and F. M. Collins. 1984. Immune responsiveness in mice heavily infected with *M. kansasii. Immunology* 53:357–364.

16. Hepper, K. P., and F. M. Collins. 1984. Adoptive transfer of acquired resistance to *M. kansasii* by T-cells harvested from chronically infected mice. *Immunology* 53:819–825.

17. Holt, P. G. 1979. Alveolar macrophages. 1. A simple technique for the preparation of high numbers of viable alveolar macrophages from small animals. *J. Immunol. Methods* 27:189–198.

18. Kaplan, G., D. E. Weinstein, R. M. Steinman, W. R. Levis, and Z. A. Cohn. 1985. An analysis of *in vitro* T-cell responsiveness in lepromatous leprosy. *J. Exp. Med.* 162:917–929.

19. Lagrange, P. H., T. E. Miller, and G. B. Mackaness. 1976. Parameters conditioning the potentiating effect of BCG in the immune response, p. 23–36. *In* G. Lamoureux, R. Turcotte, and V. Portelance (ed.), *BCG in Cancer Immunotherapy.* Grune and Stratton, New York.

20. Lefford, M. J., and D. D. McGregor. 1974. Immunological memory in tuberculosis. 1. Influence of persisting viable organisms. *Cell. Immunol.* 14:417–428.

21. Lourie, D. B., P. S. Jackett, and P. W. Andrew. 1985. Activation of macrophages for antimycobacterial activity. *Immunol. Lett.* 11:195–203.

22. Mackaness, G. B. 1970. The monocyte in cellular immunity. *Semin. Hematol.* 7:172–184.

23. Mackaness, G. B. 1971. The induction and expression of cell-mediated hypersensitivity in the lung. *Am. Rev. Respir. Dis.* 104:813–828.

24. McCune, R. M., F. M. Feldman, and W. McDermott. 1966. Microbial persistence. II. Characteristics of the sterile state of tubercle bacilli. *J. Exp. Med.* 123:469–486.

25. Morrison, N. E., and F. M. Collins. 1975. Immunogenicity of an aerogenic BCG vaccine in T-cell-depleted and normal mice. *Infect. Immun.* 11:1110–1121.

26. North, R. J. 1978. The concept of the activated macrophage. *J. Immunol.* 121:806–808.

27. North, R. J., G. B. Mackaness, and R. V. Elliott. 1972. The histogenesis of immunologically commit-

ted lymphocytes. *Cell. Immunol.* 3:680–694.

28. North, R. J., and G. S. Spitalny. 1974. Inflammatory lymphocyte in cell-mediated antibacterial immunity: factors governing the accumulation of mediator T cells in peritoneal exduates. *Infect. Immun.* 10:489–498.

29. Orme, I. M., and F. M. Collins. 1983. Protection against *M. tuberculosis* infection by adoptive immunotherapy. *J. Exp. Med.* 158:74–83.

30. Orme, I. M., and F. M. Collins. 1984. Adoptive protection of the *M. tuberculosis* infected lung. Dissociation between cells that passively transfer protective immunity and those that transfer delayed hypersensitivity to tuberculin. *Cell. Immunol.* 84:113–120.

31. Orme, I. M., and F. M. Collins. 1984. The immune response to atypical mycobacteria: immunocompetence of heavily infected mice measured in vivo fails to substantiate immunosuppression data obtained in vitro. *Infect. Immun.* 43:32–37.

32. Orme, I. M., and F. M. Collins. 1986. Cross-protection against nontuberculous mycobacterial infections by *M. tuberculosis*-memory immune T lymphocytes. *J. Exp. Med.* 163:203–208.

33. Robbins, J. B. 1978. Vaccines for the prevention of encapsulated bacterial diseases: current status, problems and prospects for the future. *Immunochemistry* 15:839–854.

34. Salgame, P., D. E. Maladevan, and N. Antia. 1983. Mechanisms of immunosuppression in leprosy: presence of suppressor factors from macrophages of lepromatous patients. *Infect. Immun.* 40:1119–1126.

35. Shon-Hegrad, M. A., and P. G. Holt. 1981. Improved method for the isolation of purified mouse peritoneal macrophages. *J. Immunol. Methods* 43:169–173.

36. Sprent, J., R. Korngold, and K. Molnar-Kimber. 1980. T-cell recognition of antigen *in vivo:* role of the H-2 complex. *Springer Semin. Immunopathol.* 3:213–246.

37. Stead, W. W., J. P. Lofgren, E. Warren, and C. Thomas. 1985. Tuberculosis as an endemic and nosocomial infection among the elderly in nursing homes. *N. Engl. J. Med.* 312:1483–1487.

38. Stokes, R. W., I. M. Orme, and F. M. Collins. 1986. The role of phagocytes in the expression of resistance and susceptibility to *Mycobacterium avium* in mice. *Infect. Immun.* 54:811–819.

39. Truitt, G. L., and G. B. Mackaness. 1971. Cell-mediated resistance to aerogenic infection of the lung. *Am. Rev. Respir. Dis.* 104:829–843.

40. Watson, J. D. 1981. Lymphokines and the induction of the immune response. *Transplantation* 31:313–317.

41. Watson, S. R., and F. M. Collins. 1980. Suppressor T-cell production in heavily infected mice. *Immunology* 39:367–373.

Section IV: Bacterial Toxins in Disease Production

Chapter 13

Bacterial Toxins as Virulence Determinants of Veterinary Pathogens: an Overview

J. M. RUTTER

Agricultural and Food Research Council
Institute for Animal Disease Research
Compton Laboratory
Compton, Berkshire RG16 0NN
England

INTRODUCTION

The ability of any bacterial species to colonize the tissues of an animal depends on a number of interrelated properties. These include whether the bacteria can (i) gain access to one of the body surfaces of the host, (ii) overcome the nonspecific defense mechanisms and establish itself on that surface or in an appropriate ecological niche, and (iii) obtain suitable nutrients from the microenvironment to multiply in the host. Most bacteria gain access to the surfaces of the body such as the skin and conjunctiva or to the mucous membranes of the respiratory tract or gut, but some penetrate the deeper tissues of the body as a result of wounds and abrasions. In most cases the outcome of a primary bacterial challenge is either clearance of the bacteria from the body or a symbiotic relationship with the host, but with pathogenic bacteria the outcome may be clinical signs of disease and sometimes death.

The mechanisms of bacterial pathogenicity have been studied for just over a century, and the earliest and most spectacular investigations were of infections with bacterial pathogens that produced toxins. The concept of harmful poisons being formed as a result of infectious disease was foreseen as early as the 18th century, but it was not until the last three decades of the 19th century that the observations of Klebs, Koch, Loeffler, Roux, and Yersin laid the foundations for the role of bacterial toxins as virulence determinants in disease.

One of the most significant features of these early studies was that laboratory animals that died after experimental infection with, e.g., diphtheria bacillus had widespread lesions in their internal organs, but the organism was localized at the site of inoculation, clearly indicating that "a poison produced at the seat of inoculation must have circulated in the blood." This was confirmed by the demonstration that bacterium-free filtrates of *Corynebacterium diphtheriae* were lethal following injection into animals, which encouraged Roux, in his Croonian Lecture of 1889, to propose that the harmful effects of all pathogenic bacteria were due to poisons and that by administering gradually increasing doses of the toxin it would be possible to render animals refractory to the effects of the poison. The toxins of *Clostridium tetani* and *Clostridium botulinum* were demonstrated soon afterwards, and this was followed by a period when many bacterial products were injected into many animals. These studies led to major advances in veterinary medicine when the major clostridial diseases of sheep were shown to be caused by toxins and prevented by cheap, safe, and effective toxoid vaccines. The introduction of antibiotics has played a major role in the control of bacterial diseases in animal production during the last four decades and has probably reduced the search for bacterial virulence determinants except in diseases in which control measures were inadequate. Nevertheless, a large number of bacterial products from animal and human pathogens have been shown to be toxic, i.e., they are capable of killing laboratory animals when injected by various routes or of affecting mammalian cells in laboratory tests, and in some cases the role of these toxins has been rigorously examined to determine what part they play in the pathogenesis of disease in the target species.

The criteria for judging whether a toxin is responsible for the clinical signs of disease were summarized by van Heyningen (58) as follows: (i) the organism is known to produce a toxin; (ii) virulent variants produce the toxin, and avirulent ones do not; (iii) injection of the toxin separately from the bacteria produces symptoms that mimic the disease; (iv) the infecting organism produces the disease without multiplying profusely or spreading extensively, and organs at a distance from the seat of infection are affected, and (v) the disease can be prevented by immunization against the toxin. There are many problems with these criteria, which are difficult to apply to more than a few examples of toxigenic bacteria. Many bacterial products have been shown to be lethal when injected into laboratory animals by various routes (20) and have therefore been called toxins; in most cases, however, the production and significance of such toxins in natural disease have not been established, although studies of the toxins have frequently provided fundamental new insights into cell structure, metabolism, and immunology. It is more realistic, therefore, to assume that a wide spectrum of disease, from subacute to chronic, is associated with the various products of bacterial metabolism in vivo. These substances may assist colonization of the microniche, enhance invasion of deeper tissues, perturb the normal integrity and physiology of the host cells, or, in some cases, reproduce the clinical signs of disease in the host. Many of these products are toxic for laboratory animals or cultured cells in vitro, but only when they contribute to an essential step in the pathogenetic mechanism of the natural disease should they be termed virulence toxins.

In this overview of bacterial toxins as virulence determinants of veterinary pathogens, I shall briefly review the general concepts of bacterial toxigenicity that have emerged, with particular reference to those of veterinary importance and to mechanisms of pathogenicity in vivo. Each area is itself the subject of a large amount of literature. The intention here is not to cover the whole topic in depth, but rather to provide a framework for the contributions that follow.

MECHANISMS OF BACTERIAL TOXIGENICITY

One of the earliest and most useful distinctions in the classification of bacterial toxins was the differentiation between endotoxins and exotoxins. Endotoxins were considered to be structural components released from the walls of dead gram-negative bacteria after autolysis, whereas exotoxins were soluble products actively released by growing cells. With increasing knowledge, however, it became clear that too rigid a definition was unsatisfactory; endotoxins may be released from intact cells without obvious structural changes to the cell wall, exotoxins can be produced and liberated from within dead bacteria by cell lysis, and several gram-negative species produce exotoxins as well as endotoxins. Nevertheless, the terms endotoxin and soluble bacterial proteins (or exotoxins) are a convenient basis for classification.

Endotoxins

Endotoxins are heat-stable toxic components that elicit a wide range of pathophysiological and pharmacological effects in susceptible hosts. Endotoxin was first recognized by Pfeiffer (41) in late-log-phase cultures of *Vibrio cholerae*. It was called endotoxin to differentiate it from the exotoxin produced by actively growing cultures of this organism, and it eventually became clear that virtually all species of gram-negative bacteria produced endotoxins as part of their cell walls. The classical studies to characterize endotoxin (8, 62, 63) led to our current understanding of endotoxic lipopolysaccharide (LPS), which consists of lipid A, core oligosaccharide, and, on the cell surface, O-specific polysaccharide termed the O antigen. LPS plays an important role in stabilization of the gram-negative cell wall, serves as a receptor for bacteriophages and some bacteriocins, and is the major surface antigen for many gram-negative bacterial species, forming the basis of a serological classification which is a vital aid in the diagnosis of infection. Purification and hydrolysis of LPS indicated that lipid A was the active principle; this was confirmed by the demonstration that preparations from mutant *Salmonella* strains that lacked the ability to synthesize polysaccharide were just as toxic as LPS from the parent strain (61), and studies of the lipid A structure of LPS isolated from a variety of gram-negative species indicated that a $\beta 1$-6 diglucosamine linkage has been essentially conserved (24). Although these observations help to explain the ubiquitous toxicity of endotoxin from pathogenic as well as nonpathogenic bacteria, the polysaccharide component clearly plays an important role in virulence in vivo, because smooth isolates with the repeat polysaccharide side chains are more virulent than rough or semirough variants that lack the O antigen. This may be because surface components assist bacterial penetration of the gut wall or help the bacteria to resist phagocytosis.

No other biological material has such a wide variety of effects as endotoxin after injection into animals. Depending on the species and strain of animal as well as bacterial cell, these effects include fever or pyrogenicity, leukopenia followed by leukocytosis, hyperglycemia, shock, prostration, diarrhea, and death; they also include local generalized Schwartzman reaction, hemorrhagic necrosis of tumors, nonspecific resistance to intraperitoneal injection of gram-negative bacteria, and adjuvant activity. Lipid A appears to be responsible for most of these effects. It has been suggested that the classical endotoxic properties of pyrogenicity and lethal toxicity are due to accumulation of NADH and ADP, leading to enhanced glucolytic metabolism and lactate formation resulting in accumulation of superoxide radicals and H_2O_2 (9).

The role of endotoxins in disease is probably less significant than the above results might suggest. Clearly there are large numbers of gram-negative bacteria in the guts of all animals, and some LPS gains access to the body because antibodies are detectable against O antigen in most normal animals. However, it is likely that endotoxin exhibits a significant pathogenic effect only in the later stages of gram-negative bacteremia and septicemia. This may be purely a dose effect, since it is not until bacteremia occurs that sufficient endotoxin is produced within the body tissues to exert a toxic effect.

A variety of actions of endotoxin on the immune system have attracted considerable interest (37). LPS is a T-independent mitogen that produces polyclonal B-cell activation and a predominantly immunoglobulin M response. It activates complement via the classical and alternative pathways and stimulates macrophages or monocytes associated with increased monokine production. Both core polysaccharide and O-polysaccharide are good antigens, and their antibodies have been associated with protection against the toxic manifestations of LPS and bacteremia. However, the toxicity of lipid A remains a problem in such studies.

In summary, bacterial LPS or endotoxin is a major bacterial toxin of gram-negative species and mediates a wide range of pathophysiological effects in animals. It is produced in vivo, is probably responsible for the characteristic signs of disease and death in gram-negative septicemias, and is a potential contributor to clinical signs of disease in infections with gram-negative bacteria. More importantly, it exerts specific and nonspecific effects on certain components of the immune system, which may play an important role in the symbiotic relation of an animal with its gram-negative bacterial flora.

Bacterial Protein Toxins

Soluble proteins produced extracellularly during active growth or toward the end of the growth cycle of bacteria are the substances most frequently thought of in any consideration of bacterial toxins. These products differ in a number of ways from endotoxin; the classical exotoxins are considerably more toxic than endotoxin (20), they are heat-labile proteins, they can be converted to toxoid with substances such as Formalin, and they stimulate the production of antitoxic antibodies that can neutralize the effects of the toxin before and frequently after it is administered to animals. In addition to the classical toxins such as tetanus, botulinum, and diphtheria toxins and the more recently discovered cholera toxin, *Escherichia coli* heat-labile toxin (LT), and of *Pasteurella multocida* toxin, all of which can reproduce the clinical signs of the disease with which they are associated, many other bacterial products have been described which are toxic for animal cells in vivo or in vitro without reproducing disease. Some unifying concepts have emerged from studies of these bacterial toxins, and it is convenient to divide them into three groups: (i) cytolytic toxins; (ii) toxins with intracellular activity; and (iii) other toxins whose mechanisms of action are less well defined.

Cytolytic Toxins

Bacterial cytolytic toxins were first detected by their ability to cause hemolysis around bacterial cultures on blood agar plates. Although hemolytic activity is still a useful criterion for differentiating bacterial cultures, there is little evidence for its association with mech-anisms of pathogenicity in vivo, apart, perhaps, from bovine bacillary hemoglobinuria caused by *Clostridium novyi* type D. It was soon realized that cells other than erythrocytes could be affected by these products, and the term cytolytic toxin or cytolysin was introduced by Bernheimer (5) to describe bacterial toxins which have the ability to damage cell membranes to such a degree that leakage of intracellular constituents can result in lysis and death of the cell. Cytolysins are produced by a wide range of gram-positive and gram-negative bacteria, and some bacterial species, e.g., *Clostridium perfringens* and *Staphylococcus aureus,* produce a number of different cytolysins. Many cytolytic toxins cause death when injected in sufficient amounts into laboratory animals (20), but some are capable of causing permeability changes in biological membranes without necessarily causing lysis of cells (56), and sublethal amounts of others may impair the chemotactic responses of leukocytes (64). The additive effects of such toxins may contribute to death or to the clinical signs of disease, but their precise role in the pathogenesis of disease in the target species is by no means clear. Information about the mode of action of some of these products has been described by Arbuthnott (1), and in the present review they are divided into phospholipases, thiol-activated cytolysins, and cytotoxins that affect leukocytes.

Phospholipases. The major components of the bilayer structure of plasma membranes of mammalian cells are phospholipids and cholesterol. Many pathogenic and nonpathogenic bacterial species produce a variety of phospholipases, designated A to D, that hydrolyze glycerophospholipids and sphingolipids, which are the two major classes of phospholipids in cell membranes (36). These enzymes are probably required by the bacteria for the metabolism of phospholipids, but attention was focused on them as virulence determinants by the demonstration that the lethal, necrotizing, and hemolytic α-toxin of *C. perfringens* was a phospholipase C (32). The α-toxin is the major toxin of type A strains that cause gas gangrene in humans and animals, as well as being gut commensals. This was the first demonstration that the activity of a bacterial toxin was attributable to an enzyme. Early work provided good evidence that of all the antitoxins present in *C. perfringens* antisera, α-antitoxin was the one required for the protection of guinea pigs, but the essential lesion in both naturally occurring and experimental gas gangrene caused by type A strains of *C. perfringens* is a massive destruction of tissue accompanied by severe toxemia and shock (10). Fatal shock in these infections is associated with changes in vascular permeability in the venules of the mesentery, diaphragm, and peritoneum, leading to loss of plasma protein and severe hemoconcentration, but the central role of α-toxin in these changes has still to be clearly established (10). A number of other enzymes such as collagenase and hyaluronidase are also produced by these strains and may assist the breakdown of tissues and spread of infection in vivo. The other types of *C. perfringens* (B, C, D, and E) that cause disease in sheep, goats, lambs, and piglets produce smaller amounts of the phospholipase C α-toxin, but it is not the major toxin produced by these types.

In addition to *C. perfringens*, *C. novyi* types A, B, and D produce phospholipase C (38). These are termed γ- (type A) and β- (types B and D) toxins and are used for typing purposes. The severe toxemia that occurs during gas gangrene caused by type A strains of *C. novyi* in humans and animals and during black disease caused by type B strains of *C. novyi* in sheep is most likely to be associated with the production of a powerful lethal toxin (α-toxin) which has not been characterized but which is cytopathic for chicken embryo fibroblasts (45). However, type D strains of this organism (formerly called *Clostridium haemolyticum*) produce very large amounts of the phospholipase C termed β-toxin in culture and cause bacillary hemoglobinuria in cattle. This is a rapidly fatal infectious disease characterized by a high fever, hemoglobinuria, and infarcts in the liver (59) and is frequently termed red-water disease. The clinical signs of bacillary hemoglobinuria are consistent with a severe intravascular hemolysis

of erythrocytes that is produced by a hemolytic phospholipase C, and this disease might be the only good example in which hemolytic activity in vitro is reflected by comparable signs in vivo.

An unusual phospholipase D has been identified as the lethal and dermonecrotic toxin of *Corynebacterium pseudotuberculosis*, the cause of suppurative infections mainly in sheep, goats, and horses. The toxin is a basic glycoprotein with a molecular weight of about 14,500 (39), but in natural infections there is no clinical evidence of acute or chronic poisoning. The toxin has no hemolytic activity and does not affect the permeability of cell membranes in culture, so that strictly speaking it is not a cytotoxin (36). However, it may cause platelet aggregation and release vasoactive substances which contribute to the spread of the causative bacteria.

S. aureus produces a wide range of extracellular products, including exfoliative toxin, α-toxin, β-toxin, Δ-toxin, γ-toxin, and leucocidin (44). Many of these extracellular products have the ability to damage tissues, but apart from exfoliative toxins in skin infections in humans, their roles in pathogenicity are not clearly established. The α-toxin has always been considered to be the most significant in the pathogenesis of staphylococcal infections, but its precise role has not been defined. The β-toxin is a phospholipase (a magnesium-dependent sphingomyelinase C) and is a so-called hot-cold lysin for sheep erythrocytes, which means that its potent hemolytic activity is greatly enhanced if the erythrocytes are chilled after being incubated at 37°C. It was thought to be lethal for mice, but this may have been due to contaminating amounts of α-toxin. *S. aureus* also produces a phospholipase C specific for phosphatidylinositol, but this enzyme does not lyse intact erythrocytes, and its biological role is unclear (36). *S. aureus* is an important cause of mastitis in dairy cows, but the role of these toxins in the pathogenesis of the severe clinical signs that occur in staphylococcal infections has not yet been clarified.

Phospholipids constitute the fluid matrix of all biological membranes, and phospholipases produced by bacteria in vivo might be expected to exert an effect on these substrates. Only a small degradation of certain phospholipids in the cytoplasmic membrane of key sensitive cells might have a profound effect on the pathophysiology of the host, but clearly this depends on the location of the bacteria, whether it is producing the enzyme in vivo, and the accessibility of the substrate.

Thiol-activated cytolysins. A large group of thiol- or sulfhydryl-activated cytolysins, otherwise known as oxygen-labile hemolysins, bind and sequester cholesterol in membranes, which leads to cell lysis. They are produced by a wide range of gram-positive bacteria and include the θ-toxin of type B, C, D, and E *C. perfringens*, δ-toxin of *Clostridium chauvoei, Clostridium septicum,* and type A *C. novyi*, and the tetanolysin of *C. tetani* (52). These toxins are lethal and cardiotoxic for laboratory animals, 13 to 16 μg of *C. perfringens* θ-toxin per kg being lethal for mice and 5 to 8 μg/kg being lethal for rabbits by the intravenous route (20). One of the best known thiol-activated cytolysins is streptolysin O, produced by β-hemolytic streptococci (*Streptococcus pyogenes*) isolated from humans, and determination of antibodies against this toxin is one of the basic tests in the diagnosis of streptococcal infection.

Thiol-activated cytolysins are active in picogram amounts in hemolytic tests and are among the most potent cytolytic toxins known. They are inactivated by small amounts of cholesterol and certain other steroids and appear to be antigenically related in that they are cross-neutralized by hyperimmune sera. Striking ultrastructural changes have been seen in cell membranes treated with high concentrations of these toxins, and it has been proposed that the toxin molecules interact with cholesterol at the cell surface, leading to disruption and fragmentation of the membrane. Whether these toxins play a significant role in the pathogenesis of disease has not been established. *C. perfringens* θ-toxin has been shown to impair the chemotaxis of human neutrophils in vitro (64), and subtle alteration in leukocyte membranes could play a role in bacterial pathogenesis.

In addition to a thiol-activated cytolysin (streptolysin O), group A, C, and G streptococci produce an oxygen-stable hemolysin designated streptolysin S. Although there is no evidence that streptolysin S is produced during natural infection in humans, in vivo studies have suggested that it suppresses T-cell-dependent antibody responses and helper T cells (60).

Cytotoxins that affect leukocytes. *Pasteurella haemolytica* is an important cause of pneumonia in cattle and sheep in many countries and is responsible for serious economic losses in livestock production. Current methods for control of this infection must be improved, and an effective biological method would be welcomed, because whole-cell bacterins have given disappointing results. *Pasteurella* infections appear to be ubiquitous in the target species, but successful attempts to reproduce the disease have generally required intratracheal or intrabronchial inoculation or combined infections with either viruses (e.g., parainfluenza virus type 3) or mycoplasmas (e.g., *Mycoplasma bovis*). These results indicate that the mechanisms of pathogenicity in vivo are complex, since they involve concurrent infections with viruses or mycoplasmas that reduce host resistance, and the development of a multicomponent vaccine that protects calves against the respiratory disease complex is an important step in better protection (57).

Once *P. haemolytica* has begun to multiply in vivo, toxic products can be elaborated, and a cytotoxin for bovine pulmonary alveolar macrophages and leukocytes has been found in supernatant fluids obtained during the early-logarithmic growth phase of *P. haemolytica* (3, 4, 27, 33). The cytotoxin is an immunogenic protein, but it has not been purified free of contaminating activities without loss of toxicity (2, 25). The activity of crude toxin can be neutralized by hyperimmune rabbit sera, adult bovine sera, nasal secretions, and lung washings (14, 49). Calves either previously infected with *P. haemolytica* or given a live vaccine of *P. haemolytica* were better protected against experimental challenge than unexposed controls or calves given a killed bacterin, and the protected animals had higher cytotoxin neutralization titers (19). These results suggest that cytotoxin and perhaps other other antigens in vivo during the early stages of infection are associated with protection, and promising areas for better control of this important infection have become apparent. The elevated temperature, dyspnea, and shock that occur prior to death in affected animals may be related to endotoxin release from the large numbers of *P. haemolytica* cells multiplying in the lung tissue, but this must be further investigated.

Another interesting and well-studied leucocidin is that produced by *S. aureus*; it affects polymorphonuclear leukocytes and macrophages from rabbits and humans (43). This leucocidin causes a pronounced granulocytopenia followed by a marked granulocytosis and increased lysozyme levels in serum, but the significance of these changes in human staphylococcal disease has not been determined. Elevated levels of leucocidin antitoxin occur in patients with staphylococcal disease, and its production is greatly enhanced in vivo (22), which may enhance invasiveness by allowing the organism to resist phagocytosis (42). Leucocidin consists of two components with molecular weights of 32,000 and 38,000; it is thermolabile, and its complex action on the cell membrane leads to altered permeability with loss of potassium ions (65). In rabbit leukocytes the toxin stimulated adenylate cyclase activity, which was found to be mainly associated with the plasma membrane (66).

Toxins with Intracellular Activity

A large and well-studied group of toxins, reviewed recently by Eidels et al. (17) and Middlebrook and Dorland (35), affect metabolic activity following binding to receptors on the plasma membranes of target cells and transport across the cell membranes. The main examples are (i) *E. coli* LT, cholera toxin, and pertussis toxin, which activate intracellular adenylate cyclase; and (ii) diphtheria toxin, *Pseudomonas* exotoxin A, and *Shigella* toxin, which inhibit protein synthesis inside the cell.

Many of these toxins have common features. They are polypeptides either synthesized as a single polypeptide chain and cleaved by proteolytic enzymes to a two-chain structure linked by disulfide bonding (e.g., diphtheria toxin and *Pseudomonas* exotoxin A) or synthesized separately and then associated to form a two-chain or subunit structure (e.g., cholera toxin, *E. coli* LT, and pertussis toxin). The B chain is the larger of the two and binds the toxin molecule to receptors on the target cell, which enables the molecule to enter the cell by receptor-mediated endocytosis. The A chain or subunits of it have enzymatic activities that affect intracellular target sites, and for those that have been characterized, usually in in vitro systems, this occurs by modification of either protein synthesis or plasma membrane enzymes. The enzymatic activity is usually not associated with the intact toxin, but requires activation by release of the A chain or a fragment of it, either by limited proteolysis or by reduction. The enzymatic activity can be demonstrated in cell-free preparations with free A chains, but these are not toxic for animal cells, apparently because the B chain is required to transport the active moiety into the cell. An interesting feature of some of these bacterial toxins is their similarity to polypeptide hormones such as luteinizing hormone, chorionic gonadotrophin, and thyroid-stimulating hormone (17). These hormones also have an A-B structure: the β-subunit recognizes receptors on the target cells, and the α-subunit increases intracellular cyclic AMP (cAMP) levels. Thus, bacterial products with toxic activities may represent cell-regulatory substances that have evolutionary significance.

Activators of adenylate cyclase. One of the major advances in veterinary medicine during the last two decades has been the identification of adhesins and toxins as major virulence determinants of *E. coli*. Enterotoxins were first recognized as plasmid-transmitted virulence determinants in isolates of *E. coli* that caused neonatal diarrhea in pigs (51). They were differentiated on the basis of heat lability or stability, and both forms have been intensively studied, purified, and characterized (17). There are structural and immunological variations between enterotoxins produced by human and animal strains, but there are also similarities between the B subunit from either source, between the heat-stable toxin (ST) from either source, and between LT and cholera toxin, with which LT has considerable homology. Most information has been obtained about LT from *E. coli* isolated from humans; this LT has a molecular weight of about 91,000, with an A subunit of molecular weight 25,000 to 29,000 and a B subunit of molecular weight 59,000. The B subunit is nontoxic and consists of five identical polypeptide chains (21); it binds to receptors on cell membranes including the ganglioside GM1, which is the major receptor for cholera toxin, although GM1 is probably not the only receptor for LT. The A subunit is nicked by trypsin to form a smaller polypeptide chain that is enzymatically active. It is transported into the enterocyte by a receptor-mediated endocyte pathway, where it catalyzes NAD-dependent activation of adenylate cyclase. This results in an increase in cAMP, leading to fluid loss into the gut, watery diarrhea, dehydration, and sometimes death.

Intracellular cAMP plays a major role as a regulator in animal cells, and high levels of it may be toxic in a number of ways: it may result in the breakdown and release of cellular energy stores, and it has been shown to inhibit several processes associated with phagocyte activity in polymorphonuclear neutrophils (34). LT is a good antigen, and vaccines that contain LT to stimulate sows to produce antitoxin, which is passively transferred via colostrum and milk to the small intestines of her piglets, are available commercially, usually in combination with the adhesin antigen K88.

Recently a second type of LT produced by *E. coli* and designated LT-II has been purified and characterized (26). Its role in the pathogenesis of diarrheal disease has not yet been established, but it also activates adenylate cyclase; it is serologically distinct from LT-I, and the structural genes responsible for its production are located on the bacterial chromosome and not a plasmid (23).

The other well-characterized bacterial toxin that activates adenylate cyclase is pertussis toxin. This protein is produced by strains of *Bordetella pertussis* and is thought to be involved in the pathogenesis of whooping cough in children. It is the histamine-sensitizing factor, lymphocytosis- or leukocytosis-promoting factor, and islet-activating protein of *B. pertussis* and has a molecular weight of 117,000. It is a hexameric protein and consists of an A protomer and a B oligomer which associate to form the active toxin (55). The toxin affects adenylate cyclase activity in vivo, causing enhanced insulin secretion and accumulation of cAMP in pancreatic islets in rats, but the effect is believed to be on a regulatory inhibitor subunit of adenylate cyclase compared with that of cholera toxin, which is thought to affect a stimulator subunit of the cyclase. *Bordetella bronchiseptica* is related to *B. pertussis* and produces a cytotoxin that causes turbinate atrophy in pigs (see below), but whether this toxin activates adenylate cyclase has not been determined.

Inhibitors of protein synthesis. The toxin of *Corynebacterium diphtheriae*, the cause of diphtheria in children, was one of the first toxins to be recognized and has been well characterized (17, 35). It has many similarities with *Pseudomonas* exotoxin A (17, 67); they have similar molecular weights (62,000 and 66,000), and both appear to conform to the A-B structure in which the B fragment carries a binding domain for the cell receptor and the A subunit acts intracellularly to uncouple protein synthesis by an NAD-dependent ADP ribosylation of elongation factor 2. They are secreted as single polypeptide chains which are converted by proteolysis into the active subunits, and their production is enhanced by depletion of iron in the culture medium, although *Pseudomonas* mutants that produce toxin A in medium containing high levels of iron have also been isolated (67). However, the toxins have different receptors, because cells from mice and rats are resistant to diphtheria toxin but sensitive to *Pseudomonas* toxin.

Shigella (Shiga) toxin, produced by strains

of *Shigella dysenteriae* that cause shigellosis in humans, also inhibits protein synthesis in vitro (11, 17). Shiga toxin causes a number of effects, including cytotoxic activity for HeLa cells in culture, enterotoxic activity resulting in fluid accumulation in ligated ileal loops, and neurotoxic activity resulting in the death of mice, rabbits, and monkeys. There appears to be no increase in intracellular cAMP levels associated with enterotoxic activity (16), so that its activity is different from that of cholera toxins and *E. coli* LT. Shiga toxin is identical to the verotoxin (VT) produced by *E. coli* associated with the hemolytic uremic syndrome and hemorrhagic colitis in humans (11). However, at least two Shiga-like VTs have now been identified in these strains of *E. coli* (53), and a third VT in other strains infecting humans and perhaps a fourth in isolates that cause edema disease in pigs may exist (40). Edema disease occurs in weaned pigs and is associated with infection by certain serotypes of *E. coli*. The clinical signs include edema of the stomach and large intestine, ataxia, and death. A disease that resembled edema disease clinically and pathologically was reproduced in pigs following intravenous inoculation of cell extracts from a K-12 strain of *E. coli* into which the VT genes of a strain of *E. coli* infecting pigs had been transferred (50). However, the activity of this porcine VT has not been characterized.

Dysentery in calves has recently been shown to be caused by an isolate of *E. coli* that has subsequently been shown to produce VT (12). This strain is comparable in many ways to the VT-positive enteropathogenic *E. coli* strains that cause disease in humans. They attach to enterocytes and cause effacement of microvilli in the large intestine, but in gnotobiotic pigs a VT-negative strain caused similar but milder lesions (G. A. Hall, personal communication), indicating that this lesion is not pathognomic for VT production.

Other toxins. There are several other important toxins whose structures have been well characterized but whose activities are less well defined. These include tetanus and botulinum toxins and *E. coli* ST.

Although the neurotoxin of *C. tetani* is one of the classical exotoxins and its structure has been well characterized (6), there is still no in vitro assay for the toxin, which must be titrated in mice. The spores of *C. tetani* are widely distributed in the environment, and after gaining access to the body, usually via an infected wound such as during castration of lambs, the organism multiplies locally with little power of invasion and produces the powerful neurotoxin which causes the spastic paralysis and death associated with tetanus. The toxin has been purified, and its physical and chemical properties have been characterized. Most of the toxin is released at the end of the active phase of growth as a single polypeptide chain with a molecular weight of about 160,000. The toxin can be nicked by mild proteolysis to form an α chain (molecular weight 55,000) and a β chain (molecular weight 105,000) held together by a disulfide bond and noncovalent bonds. The β-chain possesses the domain binding to the ganglioside receptors on target cell membranes. The main mechanism of pathogenesis is interference with the release of an inhibitory neurotransmitter at nerve synapses, but the precise action of the toxin is unknown. There is no evidence that enzymatic activity occurs or that the toxin has to enter neurons to exert its effect.

Several studies have suggested that tetanus toxin might use the receptor system of thyroid-stimulating hormone (17), but the relevance of these observations to its in vivo activity is not clear. The various serotypes of *C. tetani* differ in their ability to produce toxin, but all are antigenically and pharmacologically similar. Tetanus can be prevented by immunization with toxoid, although toxoid therapy is unsuccessful once the clinical signs have appeared. Nevertheless, tetanus vaccines have been widely used in sheep production and have been very successful.

The neurotoxin of *C. botulinum* is one of the most powerful toxins known, 0.4 to 2.5 ng/kg being lethal for mice by the intravenous or intraperitoneal route (20). It is a large protein, of molecular weight ca. 150,000, which can be nicked by proteolysis to give an α chain of molecular weight ca. 50,000 and a β chain of molecular weight ca. 100,000 (17, 54). The toxin binds to ganglioside receptors, blocking the release of acetylcholine from cholinergic nerve endings and transmission of impulses, which causes flaccid paralysis and impairment of respiratory function, leading to death. Eight types of immunologically distinct toxin have been recognized, but they all produce a similar pharmacological effect.

The ST of *E. coli*, STa, is different from the other toxins described above in that it is a small molecule with a molecular weight of between 2,000 and 10,000. However, a common active element consisting of only 18 or 19 amino acids, which has been synthesized chemically, is crucial (17). STa is antigenically different from LT and cholera toxin, is methanol soluble, and is heat and protease stable. It causes diarrhea in neonatal but not weaned piglets and humans and acts by stimulating fluid secretion which is preceded by an increase in cGMP owing to activation of guanylate cyclase. It is not clear whether STa must be transported into the cell to be active or whether it has enzymatic activity (36). The human and porcine toxins are immunologically related, and there is a high degree of amino acid sequence homology between them. The binding component on rat intestinal brush borders may be a protein with a molecular weight of about 100,000 (28). Synthetic preparations of ST have been linked to the B subunits of LT and have more potent immunological properties than those of the synthetic preparation alone (28). A different, methanol-insoluble ST, STb, is active in weaned pigs but inactive in infant mice. It is immunologically and genetically distinct from STa, but comparatively little is known about it.

Toxins with Uncharacterized Biochemical Activities

There is another group of veterinary pathogens that produce toxins, often with good evidence that they are the major determinants in the pathogenesis of disease, but little is known of their biochemical activities or whether

they conform to the A-B structure. They include anthrax toxin, the β- and ε-toxins of *C. perfringens*, and the toxins of *B. bronchiseptica* and *P. multocida* that cause turbinate atrophy in pigs.

Anthrax toxin. Toxic activities in broth cultures of *Bacillus anthracis*, the cause of anthrax in animals and humans, can be readily demonstrated (31). Three components, termed protective antigen, edema factor, and lethal factor, have been recognized; they are proteins and may conform to an A-B structure, with the protective antigen acting as the B chain and either lethal or edema factor serving as the active A chain (36). The combination of edema factor and protective antigen caused elevated cellular cAMP levels (30), and edema factor itself appeared to be acting directly as an adenylate cyclase. However, a massive septicemia is a prominent feature of the terminal stages of anthrax, and the significance of toxemia in the pathogenesis of anthrax is not clear.

C. perfringens β- and ε-toxins. Infection with type B and C *C. perfringens* causes severe enteritis, diarrhea, and dysentery in lambs, calves, piglets, and foals; the most important of these are lamb dysentery (caused by type B strains), struck (type C strains), and hemorrhagic enterotoxemia (type C strains). Type B strains produce α-, β-, and ε-toxins, and type C strains produce α- and β-toxins, but the β-toxin is thought to be the most significant in the production of hemorrhagic enteritis and ulceration of the intestinal mucosa seen in lamb dysentery and hemorrhagic enterotoxemia (7). β-Toxin from a type B strain isolated from necrotic enteritis in humans is a single polypeptide chain of molecular weight 30,000; it is heat liable and trypsin sensitive (48), but its biochemical activity has not been characterized.

Pulpy kidney is an acute toxemia of ruminants that is caused by proliferation of type D *C. perfringens* in the intestines and liberation of ε-toxin. The clinical signs of enterotoxemia may not be seen, because there is a sudden onset of illness and death, but they include neurological signs, convulsions, and diarrhea. Large numbers of sheep in a normal flock may have ε-antitoxin in their sera, so that clearly the organism is widespread and sheep come into frequent contact with the toxin. ε-Toxin is lethal, necrotizing, and activated by trypsin, 100 ng of activated toxin being the minimum lethal dose for mice (20). When large concentrations of toxin are present in the intestine for long periods it is absorbed and the sheep dies with a marked hyperglycemia and glycosuria (10). A key feature of the disease is the presence of conditions that allow proliferation of type D strains of *C. perfringens* in the gut with elaboration of large amounts of ε-toxin. This appears to be related to changes in the diet and overeating of lush pasture. The disease can be controlled by vaccination with toxoid containing ε-antigen, and losses of up to 30% in unvaccinated lambs can be considerably reduced. In the light of new knowledge of bacterial toxins, *C. perfringens* ε-toxin merits further examination.

Toxins causing turbinate atrophy in pigs. Atrophic rhinitis is an important disease of pigs and is characterized by rhinitis, atrophy or hypoplasia of the nasal turbinate bones, snout deformation, and poor growth rates. Recent investigations have shown that the progressive changes in the snout and turbinate bones can be reproduced by using toxigenic strains of type D and A *P. multocida* and that a novel protein toxin is the major virulence factor (44). *B. bronchiseptica* also causes turbinate atrophy in pigs, but its effect is less severe, and in uncomplicated infections the atrophy is not progressive. *B. bronchiseptica* is an important animal pathogen, which also causes kennel cough in dogs. In pigs, in addition to causing moderately severe turbinate atrophy, *B. bronchiseptica* damages the nasal epithelium and enhances colonization by toxigenic *P. multocida*, which can lead to the progressive form of atrophic rhinitis.

Crude toxin, prepared by sonication of phase I strains of *B. bronchiseptica*, is lethal for mice and pigs, causes a dermonecrotic lesion in skin tests, and is cytotoxic for monolayers of embryo bovine lung fibroblast (EBL) cells

(44). Toxin from porcine isolates was more toxic for mice than that from phase I isolates from other species (15). The toxin may well be responsible for turbinate atrophy in pigs, because a phase I strain of *B. bronchiseptica* that produced hemolysin, hemagglutinin, adenylate cyclase, and cytotoxin colonized the nasal cavities of gnotobiotic piglets as efficiently as did a naturally occurring variant strain that produced the first three factors but not the EBL cytotoxin; however, only the cytotoxic strain caused turbinate atrophy in gnotobiotic pigs (T. Magyar, personal communication). A calmodulin-sensitive adenylate cyclase has been associated with the virulence of *B. pertussis* in mice, but the above results indicate that in pigs, production of cytotoxin rather than adenylate cyclase is associated with turbinate atrophy. The dermonecrotic toxin of *B. bronchiseptica* has been reported to have a molecular weight of 190,000, with subunits of molecular weight 118,000 and 75,000 (29), and an LT has been reported to have a molecular weight of 102,000 with subunits of molecular weight 30,000 and 20,000 (18). However, the relationships of these toxins to each other and to that causing turbinate atrophy in pigs have not been determined.

The toxin of *P. multocida* is lethal, causes a skin lesion in guinea pigs, is cytotoxic for EBL cells, and produces turbinate atrophy and snout deformation after injection in pigs (44). It is produced by type D and A isolates, it can be detected inside bacterial cells during the logarithmic phase of growth, and it is released into the medium toward the end of growth (46). The toxin is a polypeptide with a molecular weight of 150,000 to 155,000 which appears to be released in the active form. Storage in the absence of enzyme inhibitors results in the appearance of subunits of molecular weight 65,000 to 70,000 and accompanying loss of toxicity (13). Experimental infection or parenteral injection of the toxin into pigs causes turbinate atrophy consistently and, less frequently, shortening of the snout. The mode of action of the toxin on these cartilaginous and osseous tissue is not known, but other osseous tissues, e.g., long bones and costochondral junctions, do not appear to be significantly affected by the toxin (47). The cytotoxic effect of the toxin is most pronounced on EBL cells, although other cells are affected at lower titers (46). The toxin causes EBL cells in culture to change shape and become rounded, although this is not associated with obvious morphological changes as seen by electron microscopy; assays of nucleic acid synthesis and adenylate cyclase activity in EBL cells treated with toxin showed no significant changes, but protein synthesis measured by incorporation of [^{3}H]leucine was reduced by 50% (N. Chanter, personal communication). Whether this toxin conforms to the A-B structure and what its target receptors and activity are remain to be determined. The toxin gene has recently been cloned in *E. coli* for the first time, which should assist further characterization (A. J. Lax, personal communication). Protection studies have indicated that hyperimmune sera raised against purified toxoid will protect pigs against the turbinate atrophy produced by toxigenic *P. multocida* in gnotobiotic pigs (Chanter, personal communication).

Although there are similarities between *P. multocida* and *B. bronchiseptica* toxins (e.g., they cause turbinate atrophy in pigs and are cytotoxic for EBL cells), there are important differences. In pigs, the turbinate atrophy caused by *B. bronchiseptica* is reversible in uncomplicated infections, whereas the atrophy caused by *P. multocida* infection is irreversible and progressive. Furthermore, the effects on EBL cells can be differentiated morphologically, and cross-neutralization of the cytotoxic effects with hyperimmune sera does not occur. Thus, the two toxins appear to be distinct.

CURRENT AND FUTURE PERSPECTIVES

It is clear that bacterial toxicology has advanced a long way since the pioneer demonstrations 100 years ago that toxins were essential virulence determinants of some bacterial infections. As a result of these studies, a great

deal of knowledge has accumulated about the structure and mode of action of toxins that kill laboratory animals or affect cells in vitro; a general toxin model has been proposed against which both uncharacterized and new toxins can be compared; and fundamental new information has been obtained from studies of the effect of toxins on cell membrane structure and function, regulation of cell metabolism by cAMP, and protein synthesis. In some diseases, e.g., clostridial diseases of sheep, diarrhea caused by enterotoxigenic *E. coli*, and atrophic rhinitis of pigs, there is good evidence as a result of experimental infections in the target species that toxins are major virulence determinants; these can be termed bacterial virulence toxins, to differentiate them from bacterial toxins whose role in virulence has not been established. Clearly this approach is more difficult for human pathogens, and laboratory animal models, cell culture, or cell-free systems must frequently be used to elucidate mechanisms of pathogenicity. The need to relate such in vitro observations to the clinical signs seen in the target species is crucial to ascertain their significance, and the ability of toxoid preparations to protect against the clinical signs of disease provides additional support in this area.

The advent of new technology for gene cloning and monoclonal antibody production provides powerful new tools for the study of bacterial toxins and for the production of new and improved biological products for disease control. Clearly control of a toxigenic bacterial infection can occur at various stages; control mechanisms include (i) prevention of bacterial multiplication, (ii) neutralization of the toxin produced before it can bind to the receptor, and (iii) reversing of the enzymatic change on the target molecule in the cell. Most toxoid vaccines are relatively crude and involve antigens that use mechanisms (i) and (ii). However, a number of factors will determine whether new products derived by molecular biology and using mechanisms (ii) and (iii) will be attractive in the control of animal disease. These factors include efficacy and cost of the current crude product, the degree of reaction induced, the question of whether control of the toxic effects is more important or desirable than the control of infection which may be achieved by the more crude toxoid, and, finally, the market for such products, given the current methods of animal production.

There are obvious advantages associated with genetically engineered products. The prospect of linking together a number of toxin genes from clostridia for production in a single expression vector rather than having to culture seven or eight different strains of clostridia to produce a multivalent vaccine is very attractive. The possibility of linking molecules to the B subunit of a bacterial toxin to target them specifically at a cell receptor or cell type is also attractive and could have a variety of uses, e.g., to manipulate the immune system by eliminating or enhancing subsets of immune cells. In addition, a number of bacterial infections are still important in veterinary medicine, e.g., mastitis, salmonellosis, swine dysentery caused by *Treponema hyodysenteriae*, and pneumonia caused by *Haemophilus pleuropneumoniae*, in which the possible role of toxins as determinants of virulence is unclear. These merit further study in light of the new knowledge and new technology that are now available.

LITERATURE CITED

1. Arbuthnott, J. P. 1982. Bacterial cytolysins (membrane damaging toxins), p. 107–129. *In* P. Cohen and S. van Heyningen (ed.), *Molecular Action of Toxins and Viruses*. Elsevier Biomedical Press, Amsterdam.
2. Baluyut, C. S., R. R. Simonson, W. J. Bemrick, and S. K. Maheswaran. 1981. Interaction of *Pasteurella haemolytica* with bovine neutrophils: identification and partial characterization of a cytotoxin. *Am. J. Vet. Res.* 42:1920–1926.
3. Benson, M. L., R. G. Thomson, and V. E. O. Valli. 1978. The bovine alveolar macrophage. II. In vitro studies with *Pasteurella haemolytica. Can J. Comp. Med.* 42:368–369.
4. Berggren, K. A., C. S. Baluyut, R. R. Simonson, W. J. Bemrick, and S. K. Maheswaran. 1981. Cytotoxic effects of *Pasteurella haemolytica* on bovine neutrophils. *Am. J. Vet. Res.* 42:1383–1388.
5. Bernheimer, A. W. 1970. Cytolytic toxins of bacteria, p. 183–212. *In* S. J. Ajl, S. Kadis, and T. C. Montie (ed.), *Microbial Toxins: a Comprehensive Treatise*, vol. I. Academic Press, Inc., New York.
6. Bizzini, B. 1979. Tetanus toxin. *Microbiol. Rev.* 43:224–240.
7. Blood, D. C., O. M. Radostits, and J. A. Henderson. 1983. *Veterinary Medicine*, 6th ed., p. 550–556. Bailliere Tindall, London.
8. Boivin, A., and L. Mesrobeanu. 1935. Recherches sur les antigenes somatiques et sur les endotoxines des bacteries. I. Consideration generales, et exposé des techniques utilisés. *Rev. Immunol.* 1:553–569.
9. Bradley, S. G. 1979. Cellular and molecular mechanisms of action of bacterial endotoxins. *Annu. Rev. Microbiol.* 33:67–94.
10. Bullen, J. J. 1970. Role of toxins in host-parasite relationships, p. 233–276. *In* S. J. Ajl, S. Kadis, and T. C. Montie (ed.), *Microbial Toxins: a Comprehensive Treatise*, vol. I. Academic Press, Inc., New York.
11. Cantey, R. J. 1985. Shiga toxin—an expanding role in the pathogenesis of infectious diseases. *J. Infect. Dis.* 151:766–771.
12. Chanter, N., G. A. Hall, A. P. Bland, A. J. Hayle, and K. R. Parsons. 1986. Dysentery in calves caused by an atypical strain of *Escherichia coli* (S102-9). *Vet. Microbiol.* 12:241–253.
13. Chanter, N., J. M. Rutter, and A. Mackenzie. 1986. Partial purification of an osteolytic toxin from *Pasteurella multocida. J. Gen. Microbiol.* 132:1089–1097.
14. Cho, H. J., J. G. Bohac, W. D. G. Yates, and H. B. Ohmann. 1984. Anticytotoxin activity of bovine sera and body fluids against *Pasteurella haemolytica* A1 cytotoxin. *Can. J. Comp. Med.* 48:151–155.
15. Collings, L. A., and J. M. Rutter. 1985. The virulence of *Bordetella bronchiseptica* in the porcine respiratory tract. *J. Med. Microbiol.* 19:247–258.
16. Donowitz, M., T. G. Kreusch, and H. J. Binder. 1975. Effect of shigella enterotoxin on electrolyte transport in rabbit ileum. *Gastroenterology* 69:1230–1237.
17. Eidels, L., R. L. Proia, and D. A. Hart. 1983. Membrane receptors for bacterial toxins. *Microbiol. Rev.* 47:596–620.
18. Endoh, M., M. Amitani, and Y. Nakase. 1986. Purification and characterisation of heat-labile toxin from *Bordetella bronchiseptica. Microbiol. Immunol.* 30:659–673.
19. Gentry, M. J., A. W. Confer, and R. J. Panciera. 1985. Serum neutralisation of cytotoxin from *Pasteurella haemolytica* serotype 1 and resistance to experimental bovine pneumonic pasteurellosis. *Vet. Immunol. Immunopathol.* 9:239–250.
20. Gill, D. M. 1982. Bacterial toxins: a table of lethal amounts. *Microbiol. Rev.* 46:86–94.
21. Gill, D. M., J. D. Clements, D. C. Robertson,

and R. A. Finkelstein. 1981. Subunit structure and arrangement in *Escherichia coli* heat-labile enterotoxin. *Infect. Immun.* 33:677–682.

22. Gladstone, G. P., and J. G. Glencross. 1960. Growth and toxin production of staphylococci in cellophane sacs in vivo. *Br. J. Exp. Pathol.* 41:313–333.

23. Green, B. A., R. J. Neil, W. T. Ruyechan, and R. K. Holmes. 1983. Evidence that a new enterotoxin of *Escherichia coli* which activates adenylate cyclase in eucaryotic target cells is not plasmid mediated. *Infect. Immun.* 41:383–390.

24. Hase, S., and E. T. Rietschel. 1976. Isolation and analysis of the lipid A backbone: lipid A structure of lipopolysaccharides from various bacterial groups. *Eur. J. Biochem.* 63:101–107.

25. Himmel, M. E., M. D. Yates, L. H. Lauerman, and P. G. Squire. 1982. Purification and partial characterization of a macrophage cytotoxin from *Pasteurella haemolytica*. *Am. J. Vet. Res.* 43:764–767.

26. Holmes, R. K., E. M. Twiddy, and C. L. Pickett. 1986. Purification and characterization of type II heat-labile enterotoxin of *Escherichia coli*. *Infect. Immun.* 53:464–473.

27. Kaehler, K. L., R. J. F. Markham, C. C. Muscoplat, and D. W. Johnson. 1980. Evidence of cytocidal effects of *Pasteurella haemolytica* on bovine peripheral blood mononuclear leukocytes. *Am. J. Vet. Res.* 41:1690–1693.

28. Klipstein, F. A., R. F. Engert, and R. A. Houghton. 1984. Properties of cross-linked toxoid vaccines made with hyperantigenic forms of synthetic *Escherichia coli* heat-stable toxin. *Infect. Immun.* 44:268–273.

29. Kume, K., T. Nakai, Y. Samejima, and C. Sugimoto. 1986. Properties of dermonecrotic toxin prepared from swine extracts of *Bordetella bronchiseptica*. *Infect. Immun.* 52:370–377.

30. Leppla, S. H. 1982. Anthrax toxin oedema factor: a bacterial adenylate cyclase that increases cAMP concentrations in eukaryotic cells. *Proc. Natl. Acad. Sci. USA* 79:3162–3166.

31. Lincoln, R. E., and D. C. Fish. 1970. Anthrax toxin, p. 361–414. *In* T. C. Montie, S. Kadis, and S. J. Ajl (ed.), *Microbial Toxins: a Comprehensive Treatise,* vol. III. Academic Press, Inc., New York.

32. Macfarlane, M. G., and B. C. J. G. Knight. 1941. The biochemistry of bacterial toxins. 1. The lecithinase activity of *Cl. welchii* toxins. *Biochem. J.* 35:884–902.

33. Markham, R. J. F., and B. N. Wilkie. 1980. Interaction between *Pasteurella haemolytica* and bovine alveolar macrophages: cytotoxic effect on macrophages and impaired phagocytosis. *Am. J. Vet. Res.* 41:18–22.

34. Masure, H. R., R. L. Shattuck, and D. R. Storm. 1987. Mechanisms of bacterial pathogenicity that involve production of calmodulin-sensitive adenylate cyclases. *Microbiol. Rev.* 51:60–65.

35. Middlebrook, J. L., and R. B. Dorland. 1984. Bacterial toxins: cellular mechanisms of action. *Microbiol. Rev.* 48:199–221.

36. Mollby, R. 1978. Bacterial phospholipases, p. 367–424. *In* J. Jeljaszewicz and T. Wadstrom (ed.), *Bacterial Toxins and Cell Membranes*. Academic Press, Inc., New York.

37. Morrison, D. C. 1983. Bacterial endotoxins and pathogenesis. *Rev. Infect. Dis.* 5:S733–S747.

38. Oakley, C. L., and G. H. Warrack. 1959. The soluble antigens of *Clostridium oedematiens* type D *(Cl. haemolyticum)*. *J. Pathol. Bacteriol.* 78:543–551.

39. Onon, E. O. 1979. Purification and partial characterization of the exotoxin of *Corynebacterium ovis*. *Biochem. J.* 177:181–186.

40. Petric, M., M. A. Karmali, S. Richardson, and R. Cheung. 1987. Purification and biological properties of *Escherichia coli* verocytotoxin. *FEMS Microbiol. Lett.* 41:63–68.

41. Pfeiffer, R. 1892. Untersuchungen uber das Cholera gift. *Z. Hyg. Infektionskr.* 11:393–412.

42. Rogers, D. E., and R. Tompsett. 1952. The survival of staphylocci within human leucocytes. *J. Exp. Med.* 95:209–230.

43. Rogolsky, M. 1979. Non-enteric toxins of *Staphylococcus aureus*. *Microbiol. Rev.* 43:320–360.

44. Rutter, J. M. 1985. Atrophic rhinitis in swine. *Adv. Vet. Sci. Comp. Med.* 29:239–279.

45. Rutter, J. M., and J. G. Collee. 1969. Studies on the soluble antigens of *Clostridium oedematiens (Cl. novyi)*. *J. Med. Microbiol.* 2:395–417.

46. Rutter, J. M., and P. D. Luther. 1984. Cell culture assay for toxigenic *Pasteurella multocida* from atrophic rhinitis of pigs. *Vet. Rec.* 144:393–396.

47. Rutter, J. M., and A. Mackenzie. 1984. Pathogenesis of atrophic rhinitis in pigs: a new perspective. *Vet. Rec.* 144:89–90.

48. Sakurai, J., and C. L. Duncan. 1978. Some properties of beta-toxin produced by *Clostridium perfringens* type C. *Infect. Immun.* 21:678–680.

49. Shewen, P. E., and B. N. Wilkie. 1983. *Pasteurella haemolytica* cytotoxin: production by recognized serotypes and neutralization by type-specific rabbit antisera. *Am. J. Vet. Res.* 44:715–719.

50. Smith, H. W., P. Green, and Z. Parsell. 1983. Vero cell toxins in *Escherichia coli* and related bacteria: transfer by phage and conjugation and toxic action in laboratory animals, chickens and pigs. *J. Gen. Microbiol.* 129:3121–3137.

51. Smith, H. W., and C. L. Gyles. 1970. The relationship between two apparently different enterotoxins produced by enteropathogenic strains of *Escherichia coli* of porcine origin. *J. Med. Microbiol.* 3:387–401.

52. Smyth, C. J., and J. L. Duncan. 1978. Thiol-activated (oxygen-labile) cytolysins, p. 130–183. *In* J.

Jeljaszewicz and T. Wadstrom (ed.), *Bacterial Toxins and Cell Membranes.* Academic Press, Inc. (London), Ltd., London.

53. **Strockbine, N. A., L. R. M. Marques, J. W. Newland, H. W. Smith, R. K. Holmes, and A. D. O'Brien.** 1986. Two toxin-converting phages from *Escherichia coli* O157:H7 strain 933 encode antigenically distinct toxins with similar biologic activities. *Infect. Immun.* 53:135–140.

54. **Sugiyama, H.** 1980. *Clostridium botulinum* neurotoxin. *Microbiol. Rev.* 44:419–448.

55. **Tamura, M., K. Nogimori, S. Murai, M. Yajima, K. Ito, T. Katada, M. Ui, and S. Ishii.** 1982. Subunit structure of islet-activating protein of pertussis toxin in conformity with the A-B model. *Biochemistry* 21:5516–5522.

56. **Thelestam, M., and R. Mollby.** 1975. Determination of toxin-induced leakage of different size nucleotides through the plasma membrane of human diploid fibroblasts. *Infect. Immun.* 11:640–648.

57. **Thomas, L. H., E. J. Stott, C. J. Howard, and R. N. Gourlay.** 1986. The development of a multivalent vaccine against calf respiratory disease, p. 691–696. *In* P. J. Hartigan and M. L. Monaghan (ed.), *Proceedings of the 14th World Congress on Diseases of Cattle,* vol. 1. University College, Dublin.

58. **van Heyningen, W. E.** 1955. The role of toxins in pathology, p. 17–39. *In* J. W. Howie and A. J. O'Hea (ed.), *Mechanisms of Microbial Pathogenicity.* Cambridge University Press, Cambridge.

59. **Vawter, L. R., and E. Records.** 1926. Recent studies on icterochaemoglobinuria of cattle. *J. Am. Vet. Med. Assoc.* 68:494–512.

60. **Wannamaker, L. W.** 1983. Streptococcal toxins. *Rev. Infect. Dis.* 5:S723–S732.

61. **Westphal, O., J. Gmeiner, O. Luderitz, A. Tanaka, and E. Eichenberger.** 1969. Chemistry and biology of the lipid A component A of enterobacterial lipopolysaccharides. *Colloq. Int. Cent. Natl. Rech. Sci.* 174:69–78.

62. **Westphal, O., and O. Luderitz.** 1954. Chemische Erforschung von Lipopolysaccharide gram negativer Bakterien. *Angew. Chem. Int. Ed. Engl.* 66:404–417.

63. **Westphal, O., O. Luderitz, and F. Bister.** 1952. Uber der Extraction von Bakterien mit Phenol Wasser. *Z. Naturforsch.* 76:148–155.

64. **Wilkinson, P. C.** 1975. Inhibition of leukocyte locomotion and chemotaxis by lipid-specific bacterial toxins. *Nature* (London) 255:485–487.

65. **Woodin, A. M.** 1972. Leucocodin, p. 281–299. *In* J. O. Cohen (ed.), *The Staphylococci.* John Wiley & Sons, Inc., New York.

66. **Woodin, A. M.** 1972. Adenylate cyclase and the function of cyclic adenosine 3′:5′-monophosphate in the leucocidin treated leucocyte. *Biochim. Biophys. Acta* 286:406–413.

67. **Woods, D. E., and B. H. Iglewski.** 1983. Toxins of *Pseudomonas aeruginosa:* new perspectives. *Rev. Infect. Dis.* 5:S715–S722.

Chapter 14

Cytocidal Toxins of Gram-Negative Rods

PATRICIA E. SHEWEN

Department of Veterinary Microbiology and Immunology
University of Guelph
Guelph, Ontario, Canada N1G 2W1

INTRODUCTION

Toxin production is a well-recognized virulence attribute of pathogenic bacteria. For many organisms, particulary those infecting mucosal surfaces, a combination of the factors which permit colonization with the ability to release cytotoxin is the key to disease production, and the study of these virulence mechanisms has been very active in recent years. Activity has been particularly vigorous with regard to cytocidal toxins produced by certain gram-negative rods. The following is a brief review of recent information regarding the Shiga toxin of *Shigella dysenteriae* and the related verotoxins (VT) of *Escherichia coli,* the dermonecrotic toxins of *Pasteurella multocida* and *Bordetella bronchiseptica,* the cytocidal toxins of the pneumonic pathogens *Haemophilus pleuropneumoniae* and *Pasteurella haemolytica,* and the alpha-hemolysin of *E. coli.*

SHIGA TOXIN

The production by *S. dysenteriae* type 1 of a potent exotoxin with neurotoxic effects was first described by Conradi in 1903 (17). Early studies reported that neurotoxicity, recognized as limb paralysis, was a typical finding in le-thal intoxications of animals given filtered extracts of *S. dysenteriae* parenterally. Later it was shown that several primate cell lines of epithelial origin, including HeLa cells, were killed by a toxin that could be neutralized with antiserum raised to crude neurotoxin (91). Subsequently the enterotoxic effects of this exotoxin were demonstrated by using rabbit ileal loops, and its potential relevance to human enteric disease was recognized (36). More recently, evaluations of purified Shiga toxin have shown that the neurotoxic, cytotoxic, and enterotoxic properties are due to one toxin (20).

The structure and mechanism of action of Shiga toxin have been well characterized. The toxin is heat labile (80°C for 30 min), has a molecular weight of ca. 64,000, and consists of two kinds of noncovalently bound polypeptide chains (65). Its toxic action involves binding of the B chains, which are present in five to seven copies per molecule (molecular weight ca. 6,500), to cell surface receptors identified as an N-linked glycoprotein on HeLa cells (37) and a glycolipid on rabbit intestinal microvillous membrane (24). This permits entry of the active A chain (molecular weight ca. 32,000), which on proteolysis and reduction gives rise to an enzymatically active A_1 fragment that inhibits protein synthesis by inactivating 60S ribosomal subunits (73). Entry of

Shiga toxin into cells appears to require Ca^{2+} flux through naturally occurring calcium channels (79). In vitro, high concentrations of toxin strongly reduce protein synthesis within 30 min, but lower concentrations require longer times, and overnight incubation is usual before cytocidal effects are observed (21).

The actual role of Shiga toxin in the pathogenesis of shigellosis has remained undefined. Animals that die after receiving injection of Shiga toxin have tissue lesions compatible with ischemic injury, and it has been postulated that in vivo the toxin exerts its effect primarily on endothelial cells of small vessels (20). After injection of Shiga toxin, the intestinal mucosa often contains hemorrhages which are not found after treatment with cholera toxin or E. coli heat-labile enterotoxin. Also, hemorrhages into the spinal cord as a result of a toxic effect on endothelial cells could account for observed neurotoxic effects.

The production of Shiga toxin in several Shigella strains has been reported; however, only invasive strains (those that are able to enter and multiply in the epithelial cells of the colonic mucosa) are pathogenic (25). Noninvasive strains fail to colonize the host and are therefore unable to exert their pathogenic effect. Shigella species also differ in the ability to produce Shiga toxin. S. dysenteriae type 1 is more frequently associated with severe disease and dysenteric symptoms than with other forms of shigellosis. Recent in vitro studies have shown that strains of S. dysenteriae type 1 produce highly active toxin that is neuralized by antiserum to purified Shiga toxin, while non-type 1 S. dysenteriae and other Shigella species are 1,000-fold less toxic and produce nonneutralizable toxin instead of or as well as Shiga toxin (2). A role for this as yet uncharacterized nonneutralizable toxin in traveler's diarrhea has been proposed (71).

VEROTOXIGENIC ESCHERICHIA COLI

Cytotoxins similar to Shiga toxin have been detected in various enteropathogenic E. coli, in Vibrio cholerae and Vibrio parahaemolyticus, in Salmonella typhimurium, and in E. coli isolates associated with hemolytic uremic syndrome: the enterohemorrhagic E. coli. Konowalchuk et al. (39) first described E. coli strains that produced a cytotoxin active on Vero cells (an African green monkey kidney cell line). This heat-labile VT, or Shiga-like toxin, was found to be distinct from the recognized heat-labile and heat-stable cytotonic enterotoxins of E. coli, but was neutralized by antibodies raised against purified Shiga toxin from S. dysenteriae type 1 (64). The toxin has biological activities (cytotoxic, neurotoxic, and enterotoxic) and an A-B subunit structure similar to those of Shiga toxin with one A fragment of molecular weight ca. 31,500 and probably four B subunits, each of molecular weight 4,000 to 15,000 (63). It is bacteriophage encoded and is found in culture supernatants as well as bacterial lysates and sonic extracts (64, 88). Verotoxigenic E. coli strains have been implicated as a cause of diarrhea, hemorrhagic colitis, and hemolytic uremic syndrome in humans; diarrhea in calves; and diarrhea and edema disease in pigs (51). Food-borne infection in humans has been documented, and zoonotic transfer is a possibility. Recently, E. coli O157:H7, a common vertotoxigenic strain isolated in humans, was identified in bovine feces (8).

At least two different antigenic forms of VT are now recognized, and the one neutralized by antibody to Shiga toxin is designated VT_1 or SLT_1 (35). VT_2 is genetically related but antigenically distinct, and although the two toxins may be present in the same bacterial cell, they are encoded by two different toxin-converting phages (90).

As mentioned above, E. coli strains isolated during edema disease of weaned pigs have been shown to produce a heat-labile VT (19, 89). Edema disease is a generalized disease of the vasculature and affects small arteries and arterioles; cardinal signs are neurologic: ataxia, convulsions, and paralysis, which may lead to death, and edema of the subcutis, forehead, and eyelids (80). The disease can be reproduced experimentally by intravenous inoculation of sterile bacterial lysates which contain the toxic factor edema disease principle (EDP) (16). EDP has been shown to be the verotoxic factor, and the verotoxic effect can be neutralized by anti-EDP serum but not by anti-VT (VT$_1$) or anti-heat-labile toxin serum (19). EDP is partially neutralized by antiserum prepared against VT$_2$, and likewise VT$_2$ is partially neutralized by anti-EDP serum. Therefore, EDP may represent an additional antigenic type (VTE), which cross-reacts with VT$_2$ (V. P. J. Gannon and C. L. Gyles, submitted for publication).

The natural occurrence of VT-neutralizing antibodies in infected humans and of anti-EDP serum in infected swine has led to suggestions that the measurement of antibody may be useful diagnostically and that vaccination may be effective in prophylaxis. These possibilities must await clarification of the antigenic variability of VTs and the potential for cross-reactivity and cross-neutralization.

DERMONECROTIC TOXINS OF *P. MULTOCIDA* AND *B. BRONCHISEPTICA*

Atrophic rhinitis of pigs is a multifactorial disease in which infection, environment, management, and genotype all contribute to the prevalence and severity in individual herds. It is now recognized that severe disease, characterized by epistaxis, marked turbinate atrophy, nasal distortion, and reduced growth rates, results often from combined infection of the nasal turbinates with *B. bronchiseptica* and toxigenic strains of *P. multocida* type D (66). Infection with *B. bronchiseptica* alone or in combination with nontoxigenic *P. multocida* produces only mild to moderate lesions and nonprogressive turbinate hypoplasia followed by turbinate regeneration (78).

The pathogenicity of *P. multocida* in atrophic rhinitis is correlated with the production of a heat-labile exotoxin, dermonecrotic toxin (DNT), which is dermonecrotic in guinea pigs, lethal for mice, and cytotoxic for Vero cells (18). Vero cell toxicity is distinct from the cytotoxic effect of *E. coli* and requires 48

h of incubation before it is observed (68). The *P. multocida* toxin enhances osteoclastic resorption and impairs osteoblastic synthesis of the turbinate osseous core (67). Irreversible changes are produced within a few days, the epithelium and submucosa undergo secondary atrophy, and turbinates may disappear almost completely within 10 to 14 days.

The toxin is produced in the late-logarithmic and stationary growth phases of the bacterium and is found both in culture supernatants and as cell-associated toxin released from bacterial sonic extracts (76). Nakai et al. (61) purified DNT from *P. multocida* by using a combination of serial anion exchange and gel chromatography, as well as polyacrylamide gel electrophoresis. The molecular weight of the toxin was ca. 160,000, and it was heat labile and sensitive to trypsin, Formalin, and glutaraldehyde treatment. Further studies showed that it was composed of three polypeptide chains linked by disulfide bridges and noncovalent bonds (41). Its mechanism of action is unknown; however, intranasal or parenteral administration of crude exotoxin to gnotobiotic piglets results in clinical atrophic rhinitis (77).

P. multocida type D is primarily implicated in atrophic rhinitis. Toxigenic *P. multocida* type A has also been isolated infrequently from swine (67), and toxigenic *P. multocida* types D and A have occasionally been recovered from calves, cats, dogs, rabbits, and turkeys (62). The role of these isolates in disease is undetermined, although transmission by species other than pigs should be considered in control of atrophic rhinitis. DNT production is not considered of importance in swine pneumonia, in which most isolates are nontoxigenic *P. multocida* type A (67), and *P. multocida* type D is found only rarely (70). Furthermore, DNT apparently has no in vivo effect on swine alveolar macrophages, the primary defense mechanism of the lungs (69).

Although transient atrophic rhinitis has been produced in pigs infected with only *B. bronchiseptica*, this bacterium is thought to act principally by assisting colonization of the nasal mucosa by toxigenic *P. multocida* and enhancing the toxigenic effects (66, 78). It has been shown that B. bronchiseptica caused marked loss of cilia accompanied by degeneration and desquamation of nasal epithelial cells after intranasal inoculation in specific-pathogen-free neonatal pigs, whereas P. multocida induced no such effect (57), and it is reasonable to conclude that B. bronchiseptica-mediated mucosal damage may predispose pigs to P. multocida infection.

Organisms belonging to the genus Bordetella include B. bronchiseptica, which can infect humans, dogs, swine, and other animals, and the human pathogens Bordetella parapertussis and Bordetella pertussis, the causative agent of whooping cough. All have been shown to produce a heat-labile DNT which is similar in activity, as well as antigenically similar, among Bordetella species, but is antigenically distinct from the DNT of P. multocida (22, 60). Using methods similar to those used for purification of P. multocida DNT, Kume et al. (42) have purified DNT from B. bronchiseptica. It has a molecular weight of ca. 190,000 ± 5,000 and can be dissociated into two polypeptide chains of molecular weight ca. 75,000 ± 4,000 and 118,000 ± 5,000. Although the mechanism of action of DNT is also unknown, its production by B. bronchiseptica strains can be directly correlated with the induction of nasal and lung lesions in neonatal pigs (75).

Pertussis toxin, a major virulence factor of B. pertussis that induces increased cellular GMP, is not produced by either B. parapertussis or B. bronchiseptica, although some strains of these two bacteria have been shown by DNA and RNA hybridization studies to possess but not express the gene coding for pertussis toxin (46).

Commercial vaccines are available and in use for prevention of atrophic rhinitis. The use of Bordetella bacterins reduces the incidence of but does not completely control disease. P. multocida bacterins by themselves provide incomplete or poor protection. Newer combination products incorporating formalinized B. bronchiseptica and P. multocida and enriched with P. multocida DNT show promise. Theoretically an immune response to the Bordetella bacterin

would prevent colonization and mucosal destruction by this organism and thereby inhibit P. multocida colonization; anti-DNT antibody would neutralize the effect of any toxin that was produced.

P. HAEMOLYTICA LEUKOTOXIN

P. haemolytica is a commensal of the nasopharynges of ruminants and an important cause of fibrinous pneumonia in cattle, particularly feedlot cattle, and sheep. In 1978 Benson et al. (5) described cytotoxic changes in bovine alveolar macrophages incubated in vivo for 30 to 45 min with P. haemolytica. The effect was similar for four serotypes of P. haemolytica, serotypes 1, 2, 7, and 12, but was not seen with P. multocida (two strains), Serratia marcescens, Listeria monocytogenes, or Staphylococcus aureus. The toxic factor was present in bacterium-free culture filtrates and was heat labile after treatment at 60°C for 30 min. It has subsequently been shown that sublethal concentrations of crude toxin induce impaired phagocytosis (50), reduce chemotaxin production in pulmonary macrophages (49), and inhibit the luminol-dependent chemiluminescent response of bovine neutrophils (13).

The cytotoxic effect is specific for ruminant leukocytes (34, 82), including alveolar macrophages, cultured blood monocytes, lymphocytes, and neutrophils; hence the more current reference to this factor as a leukotoxin. The specificity for ruminant cells is relevant because P. haemolytica is an important pathogen of ruminants, but reports of infection in other species are rare. The toxin is a true extracellular product of metabolically active bacteria, since it is produced in vitro during the logarithmic growth phase and is not found in bacterial lysates or sonic extracts (85). The presence of iron on a suitable carrier molecule such as transferrin encourages optimal toxigenesis (28). All serotypes of P. haemolytica are toxigenic (14, 83), although not all are pathogenic. Toxin production is not affected by repeated (128 serial) passage of the organism (25).

The gene coding for leukotoxin production has been cloned (44) and shown to be chromosomally located (14, 44). It bears close sequence homology with the alpha-hemolysin of *E. coli* (44a), the implications of which are discussed in more detail below.

Although leukotoxic culture supernatant is readily obtained from logarithmic-phase cultures of *P. haemolytica* in serum-containing medium, attempts to purify the leukotoxin have mostly been unsuccessful. Partial characterization has demonstrated that it is a protein (30), but attempts to purify it have resulted in loss of activity (1, 30), perhaps owing to removal of stabilizing or carrier serum proteins (28; P. E. Shewen and B. N. Wilkie, unpublished observations). Molecular weight estimates have varied from 50,000 to 300,000 depending upon the purification methods used. Using a series of chromatographic techniques, Mosier et al. (55) found a 160-kilodalton (kDa) cytotoxic protein which could be broken down into 66-, 57-, and 23-kDa fragments. This agreed with the earlier work of Himmel et al. (30), who found a toxic 150-kDa protein that was resolved into 50- and 20-kDa fragments. Recent sequence analysis of the leukotoxin gene isolated from recombinant clones suggests that it codes for two molecules: a larger, approximately 100-kDa, protein which is antigenic and may act as the binding molecule and a smaller, 20-kDa, nonantigenic protein which may be the actual cytotoxic moiety or contribute to cytotoxicity of the larger molecule (44, 44a). It has been speculated that the 50-kDa fragments obtained from native toxin (30, 55) may represent fragments of the 100-kDa cloned product, that the native 23- and 20-kDa fragments correspond to the cloned 20-kDa protein, and that higher-molecular-mass estimates of 150, 160, or 300 kDa for the toxin represent binding to serum proteins such as albumin and/or aggregation of toxin molecules.

In cattle the leukotoxin may contribute to the pathogenesis of pneumonia by impairing phagocytic lung defenses and the subsequent immune response and by inducing inflammation and fibrosis as a consequence of leukocyte lysis. Slocombe et al. (86) demonstrated that calves depleted of neutrophils by prior administration of hydroxyurea were resistant to intratracheal challenge with live *P. haemolytica* A1, while normal calves developed severe exudative and necrotizing bronchopneumonia. These observations are consistent with the hypothesis that leukotoxin-induced lysis of neutrophils and macrophages results in the release of intracellular enzymes which are responsible for the acute lesions of fibrinous pneumonia.

The *P. haemolytica* leukotoxin is immunogenic, and toxin-neutralizing antibodies have been found in adult bovine serum samples (1, 15, 84) and serum samples from immunized rabbits (44, 83) and calves (P. E. Shewen and B. N. Wilkie, submitted for publication). In retrospective studies the capacity of bovine sera to neutralize leukotoxin has been correlated with resistance to fibrinous pneumonia in feedlot cattle (15, 84). However, it would seem that the protective immune response to *P. haemolytica* is complex and involves stimulation of antibodies to bacterial surface antigens which may act to inhibit colonization of the respiratory epithelium or to overcome the antiphagocytic effects of bacterial capsule, as well as the development of antitoxic activity. The importance of colonization factors is emphasized by the fact that although all serotypes produce leukotoxin, type 1 is almost exclusively associated with bovine pneumonia. Vaccination with formalinized bacterins, available for over 60 years, fails to stimulate antitoxic immunity (27; Shewen and Wilkie, submitted) and is ineffective in disease prevention (4, 53). Experimental exposure of calves to live *P. haemolytica* induces both toxin-neutralizing activity and antibodies to surface antigens and is protective against experimental challenge (27, 97). Recently introduced live vaccines have the potential to protect against pneumonic pasteurellosis; however, the limited number of field trials conducted have not demonstrated a beneficial effect (72). This may reflect the inappropriate handling and storage of the live product or be due to the frequent practice of incorporating antibiotics in cattle feed or water. In experimental trials, vaccination of calves with leu-kotoxic culture supernatant was shown to induce both serospecific agglutinating activity and toxin-neutralizing antibodies, and both were found necessary for protection (Shewen and Wilkie, submitted). Production of a commercial vaccine incorporating bacterium-free culture supernatant is imminent; its usefulness in the field remains to be assessed.

H. PLEUROPNEUMONIAE LEUKOTOXIC HEMOLYSIN

Haemophilus (Actinobacillus) pleuropneumoniae is the major cause of pleuropneumonia, an economically important disease of pigs worldwide (81). The rapid clinical course of acute pleuropneumonia and the fibrin exudation and hemorrhagic lesions observed suggest that a potent toxin or toxins may be produced early in the infection. Endobronchial administration to pigs of sonicated nonviable H. pleuropneumoniae organisms or sterile logarithmic-phase culture supernatant results in lesions grossly and histologically similar to those produced in the natural disease (S. Rosendal, W. R. Mitchell, M. Weber, M. R. Wilson, and M. R. Zaman, Abstr. Proc. 5th Int. Pig Vet. Soc. Congr. 1980, p. 221).

Live H. pleuropneumoniae type 1 has been shown to be toxic for porcine alveolar macrophages and blood monocytes, causing cell death after 1 h of incubation at 37°C (3). The cytotoxic effect was not exerted by heat-killed bacteria but was present in a heat-stable form in cell-free culture supernatant from the late-logarithmic growth phase (3, 69). In addition, H. pleuropneumoniae strains, on primary isolation, characteristically exhibit hemolytic activity on blood agar medium, and Nakai et al. (58) have demonstrated release of hemolysin into the culture supernatant during logarithmic growth (1 to 5 h) of shaking cultures and the late stationary phase (5 days) of static cultures. Hemolytic activity was shown to be trypsin resistant and heat stable (121°C for 2 h), but although not clearly stated, it appears that the

5-day culture material was used to assess stability. Furthermore, these workers have shown that intratracheal inoculation of heat-stable hemolytic culture supernatant from 5-day static cultures induces severe hemorrhagic lesions in piglets (59), and that such preparations have in vitro antiphagocytic and cytocidal effects on pulmonary macrophages obtained from pigs (43). They propose that production of hemolysin by H. pleuropneumoniae in the lungs of infected pigs and subsequent macrophage lysis may account for the pneumonic lesions.

Other workers (52) have demonstrated the production of an unstable, heat-labile hemolysin which is sensitive to degradation by pronase, trypsin, and chymotrypsin during logarithmic growth (7 h) of H. pleuropneumoniae in the presence of RNA. Heat-labile, trypsin-sensitive hemolysin was also found by Maudsley and Kadis (54) during the early- to mid-logarithmic growth phase of H. pleuropneumoniae in chemically defined medium. Recently Rosendal et al. demonstrated the presence of hemolysin and cytotoxicity for porcine and bovine neutrophils in logarithmic-phase culture supernatant from several strains of H. pleuropneumoniae (S. Rosendal, J. Devenish, J. I. MacInnes, J. H. Lumsden, S. Watson, and H. Xun, submitted for publication). Both activities were sensitive to heat, trypsin, oxygen, and cholesterol. All strains of H. pleuropneumoniae with hemolytic activity were also cytotoxic; however, some cytotoxic strains were not hemolytic.

Apparently, live H. pleuropneumoniae may release into the culture medium material which is hemolytic and leukotoxic and may therefore be important in the pathogenesis of pleuropneumonia. Whether heat-stable hemolysin, heat-labile hemolysin, and leukotoxic activities reside in the same toxin remains to be determined. These may represent different characteristics of the same substance produced or assayed under differing conditions, varying activities of a single toxin undergoing enzymatic digestion or stabilization, or the effects of two or more distinct bacterial products. Nevertheless, it has been shown that macrophage-monocyte cytotoxicity (3) and heat-labile leukotoxin-hemolysin activity (Rosendal et al., submitted) can be neutralized by sera from convalescent swine and that parenteral injection of the corresponding culture supernatant stimulates the production of antibodies which neutralize heat-stable hemolysin (43) or heat-labile neutrophil cytotoxic and hemolytic activities (Rosendal et al., submitted). Furthermore, it was shown that formalinized bacterins, which are recognized to be inefficient in disease prevention, induced little neutralizing activity in either of the experiments referred to above. Therefore, the potential to produce effective vaccines by using toxin-containing culture supernatant warrants further investigation.

THE ALPHA-HEMOLYSIN OF E. COLI

In 1976 Jorgensen et al. (33) described the alpha-hemolysin of *E. coli* as a filterable, heat-labile (56°C for 30 min) macromolecule, produced by several strains of *E. coli* during logarithmic-phase growth in media containing blood, serum, or meat extract. Investigations by several groups have demonstrated that hemolysin production correlates with virulence in human extraintestinal infections (31, 93). In animals hemolysin production is a frequent characteristic of *E. coli* strains that cause diarrhea, but no clear correlation with virulence has been established (9). In addition to lysis of erythrocytes, partially purified alpha-hemolysin has been shown to exert heat-labile cytocidal effects on human leukocytes (10) and, at sublethal doses, to impair the ability of these cells to undergo phagocytosis and chemotaxis (11). Recent work has demonstrated induction of histamine release from rat mast cells and leukotriene and enzyme release from neutrophils (38), as well as impairment of membrane receptor function (95). Thus, hemolysin production by virulent *E. coli* cells may amplify inflammatory reactions and compromise leukocyte-mediated defense mechanisms.

The hemolysins commonly found among animal isolates of *E. coli* are encoded on transferable plasmids, which confer virulence when transferred to avirulent strains of *E. coli* (89). However, the hemolysin genes of human *E. coli* isolates reside on the bacterial chromosome (32). The chromosomal and plasmid hemolysin genes have been shown to have regions of sequence homology, suggesting a common origin (56). However, there is little similarity in noncoding flanking sequences, and three distinct classes of promoter regions have been recognized (29). Differences in promoters result in different levels of hemolysin expression, which in turn may affect the level of hemolysin-associated virulence in vivo (94). Recombinant DNA technology has permitted analysis and understanding of the location and functions of the cistrons coding for alpha-hemolysin production and secretion. The synthesis and secretion of hemolysin from *E. coli* require the four genes *hlyC*, *hlyA*, *hlyB*, and *hlyD*, which are clustered in that order on the bacterial plasmid or chromosome (6, 96). *hlyA* is the structural gene for hemolysin and codes for a 110-kDa protein that is transported across the double membrane of *E. coli* when *hlyB* and *hlyD* are provided (47, 92). *hlyD* is transcribed separately from *hlyC*-*hlyA*-*hlyB*, and its absence results in production of hemolysin that is trapped in the periplasmic space. The *hlyC* gene is highly conserved and codes for a 19-kDa protein required to render *hlyA* hemolytically active, although the mechanism of activation is as yet unknown (48, 92). *hlyA* lacks a typical leader sequence for transport and is transported across both the cytoplasmic and outer membranes of *E. coli* without processing (23). It is now known that export does not involve use of a conventional N-terminal signal sequence, as is the case for transport of enterotoxins, nor does it proceed by way of cell lysis, as is the case for colicin E release. Thus, the extracellular release of alpha-hemolysin represents genuine secretion, a phenomenon once considered to be impossible for gram-negative bacteria.

Recent evidence suggests that the hemolysin damages cell membranes by partial insertion of monomeric molecules into the target cell lipid bilayer and formation of discrete, hydrophilic transmembrane pores which permit rapid efflux of cellular K^+ and influx of Ca^{2+}, spherocyte formation, and subsequent lysis (7). A single hit of alpha-hemolysin is sufficient to cause cell death. By using mutagenesis it has been shown that one hydrophobic domain in *hlyA* is essential for hemolytic activity (45). These observations are consistent with the molecular structure and mode of action proposed from sequence analysis of cloned DNA (95), wherein the hydrophilic N-terminal domain was envisioned as initiating binding to the membrane by electrostatic interaction, the adjacent region took on a globular structure, and a mid-hydrophobic region was inserted into the membrane, leaving an acidic hydrophilic half of the polypeptide extending out on the external side of the target cell, where it might interact with divalent cations such as Ca^{2+}.

Structural predictions for the hemolysin molecule further indicate that it contains a basic, hydrophilic N-terminal domain and a large acidic hydrophilic C-terminal region (23, 95). Thus, the molecule would tend to aggregate in solution or readily bind to other bacterial or medium components in culture supernatant. This may account for difficulties encountered in attempts to purify native hemolysin and further help explain the apparent discrepancies in molecular mass estimates which have varied from 50 to 580 kDa (9). It may also explain the presence of carbohydrate in hemolysin prepared in certain media (12).

Recombinant DNA technology may also have resolved a long-standing controversy in studies of *E. coli* hemolysin. Mutagenesis has shown that removal of the last 37 amino acids from the C-terminal end of HlyA leads to a truncated hemolysin that retains hemolytic activity but remains cell associated (45). Much earlier it was recognized that *E. coli* produced at least two hemolysins: the alpha hemolysin that was heat labile and extracellular and a cell-associated beta-hemolysin (87). Both produced beta-hemolysis (clear zone of lysis) on blood agar. It now appears possible that beta-hemolysin

represents an incomplete form of alpha-hemolysin, produced without the C-terminal amino acids needed for excretion or, alternately, produced by *E. coli* lacking the *hlyB* and *hlyD* genes needed for transport. The two hemolysins do not cross-neutralize; however, this was explained some time ago by Rennie and Arbuthnott (74), who suggested that the structural conformation of beta-hemolysin changed when it was released into fluid medium as alpha-hemolysin. Others (9) have described a heat-stable hemolysin found particularly in culture supernatant from late-logarithmic- or stationary-phase cultures. This has a high molecular weight and associated carbohydrate and may be the result of lytic release of membrane-bound hemolysin or, alternatively, stabilization of heat-labile hemolysin (usually most apparent earlier in the growth curve) by association with solubilized bacterial carbohydrate.

Thus, molecular cloning of the alpha-hemolysins of *E. coli* has permitted rapid advances in the study of hemolysin production, excretion, function, and relation to virulence and may also have resolved several longstanding controversial questions about the relationships between various *E. coli* hemolysins. These investigations may also provide clues about the same mechanisms with regard to cytolytic exotoxins produced by other gram-negative bacteria.

RELATIONSHIP OF THE *E. COLI* ALPHA-HEMOLYSIN TO CYTOLYTIC TOXINS OF OTHER GRAM-NEGATIVE BACTERIA

Very recently, Koronakis et al. (40) reported clear but incomplete homology between the cloned *E. coli* alpha-hemolysin determinants and DNA extracted from hemolytic isolates of *Proteus mirabilis, Proteus vulgaris,* and *Morganella* (formerly *Proteus*) *morganii.* The *E. coli hlyD* secretion gene hybridized only with DNA from *Proteus vulgaris* and *M. morganella,* which produced cell-free hemolysins, but not with DNA from *Proteus mirabilis,* which has only

cell-associated activity. The four *hly* genes of
E. coli had a G+C content of 39%, rather than
the expected 50% of the *E. coli* genome (23,
29), leading Koronakis et al. to suggest that
the *E. coli* genes originated in *Proteus* species.

Also very recently, my colleagues have
discovered extensive homology between recombinant genes coding for the *P. haemolytica* A1
leukotoxin and the *hlyC* and *hlyA* genes of *E.
coli* (44a). They observed close correspondence
between *hlyC* and the *P. haemolytica* gene coding for a nonantigenic 20-kDa protein and
named this protein LktC. LktA, a 101.9-kDa
protein coded for by *P. haemolytica*, was dis-
continuously homologous with HlyA, but had
a remarkably similar hydropathy profile and
contained a series of tandemly repeated sequences, believed to be important in alpha-
hemolysin in interaction with the target cell
membrane and/or calcium (95). The observed
lack of homology in other regions may reflect
differing target cell specificities of the two cytotoxins.

The cloned leukotoxin genes *lktC* and *lktA*
code for production of active leukotoxin (44),
which is confined to the cytoplasm of *E. coli*
K-12 strains, and analysis of DNA adjacent to
lktA has failed to reveal sequences analogous to
hlyB and *hlyD* that are needed for secretion of
alpha-hemolysin. The remainder of the *P. haemolytica* genome is now being screened to determine whether these genes are present at a
remote site. Like the alpha-hemolysin, *P. haemolytica* leukotoxin is a genuine exotoxin, suggesting that secretion sequences would be expected. To date no relationship has been
established between the *P. haemolytica* leukotoxin and the as yet uncharacterized hemolysin
of *P. haemolytica*. Attempts to induce hemolysis by using native or cloned leukotoxin have
so far been unsuccessful (82; unpublished observations). Hemolysis that is confined to the
area immediately below colonies grown on sheep
blood agar is characteristic of *P. haemolytica*. In
view of the observed relationships between the
hemolytic and leukotoxic activities of *E. coli*
and *H. pleuropneumoniae,* it may be supposed
that one toxin mediates these functions in *P.*

haemolytica as well. Perhaps the hemolytic characteristic is a function of cell-bound leukotoxin.

The G+C content of *P. haemolytica* is 39
to 45%, and that of the leukotoxin gene is 42%,
making it tempting to speculate, as Koronakis
et al. (40) did, that the hemolysin gene of *E.
coli* was donated from *P. haemolytica* as a transmissible plasmid to *E. coli* animal strains and
was subsequently incorporated into the chromosomal DNA of human *E. coli* isolates.
Whether this is so or whether *E. coli, P. haemolytica,* and *Proteus* spp. all acquired their toxin
genes from a common donor is perhaps less important than recognition that the toxigenic
phenotype appears to have been conserved among
these gram-negative organisms.

In this context it may be worthwhile to
note that all three cytolytic toxins described in
this paper, *P. haemolytica* leukotoxin, *H. pleuropneumoniae* cytotoxin, and *E. coli* alpha-hemolysin, produce a heat-labile cytolysin during
the logarithmic growth phase, particularly in
serum-enriched media (33, 58, 85), all release
a heat-stable cytolysin during the stationary
growth phase (9, 33, 58, 85), and all have hemolytic and leukotoxic activities that may be
related to virulence. It is conceivable that the
rapid advances now being made with recombinant DNA technology will resolve several of
the unanswered questions about these toxins,
their relationship to each other, and their importance in virulence mechanisms.

LITERATURE CITED

1. **Baluyut, C. S., R. R. Simonson, W. J. Bemrick,
   and S. K. Maheswaran.** 1981. Interaction of *Pasteurella haemolytica* with bovine neutrophils: identification and partial characterization of a cytotoxin.
   Am. J. Vet. Res. 42:1920–1926.
2. **Bartlett, A. V., D. Prado, T. G. Clecry, and L.
   K. Pickering.** 1986. Production of Shiga toxin and
   other cytotoxins by serogroups of *Shigella. J. Infect.
   Dis.* 6:996–1002.
3. **Bendixen, P. H., P. E. Shewen, S. Rosendal,
   and B. N. Wilkie.** 1981. Toxicity of *Haemophilus
   pleuropneumoniae* for porcine lung macrophages, peripheral blood monocytes, and testicular cells. *Infect.
   Immun.* 33:673–676.

4. Bennett, B. W. 1982. Efficacy of pasteurella bacterins for yearling feedlot cattle. *Bovine Pract.* 3:26–30.

5. Benson, M. L., R. G. Thomson, and V. E. O. Valli. 1978. The bovine alveolar macrophage. II. In vitro studies with *Pasteurella haemolytica. Can. J. Comp. Med.* 42:368–369.

6. Berger, H., J. Hacker, A. Juarez, C. Hughes, and W. Goebel. 1982. Cloning of the chromosomal determinants encoding hemolysin production and mannose-resistant hemagglutination in *Escherichia coli. J. Bacteriol.* 163:88 93.

7. Bhakdi, S., N. Mackman, J.-M. Nicaud, and I. B. Holland. 1986. *Escherichia coli* hemolysin may damage target cell membranes by generating transmembrane pores. *Infect. Immun.* 52:63–69.

8. Borczyk, A. A., M. A. Karmali, H. Lior, and L. M. Duncan. 1987. Bovine reservoir for verotoxin-producing *Escherichai coli* O157:H7. *Lancet* i:98.

9. Cavalieri, S. J., G. A. Bohach, and I. S. Snyder. 1984. *Escherichia coli* alpha-hemolysin: characteristics and probable role in pathogenicity. *Microbiol. Rev.* 48:326–343.

10. Cavalieri, S. J., and I. S. Snyder. 1982. Effect of *Escherichia coli* alpha-hemolysin on human peripheral leukocyte viability in vitro. *Infect. Immun.* 36:455–461.

11. Cavalieri, S. J., and I. S. Snyder. 1982. Effect of *Escherichia coli* alpha-hemolysin on human peripheral leukocyte function in vitro. *Infect. Immun.* 37:966–974.

12. Cavalieri, S. J., and I. S. Snyder. 1982. Cytotoxic activity of partially purified *Escherichia coli* alpha hemolysin. *J. Med. Microbiol.* 15:11–21.

13. Chang, Y.-F., H. W. Renshaw, and J. L. Augustine. 1985. Bovine pneumonic pasteurellosis: chemiluminescent response of bovine peripheral blood leukocytes to living and killed *Pasteurella haemolytica, Pasteurella multocida* and *Escherichia coli. Am. J. Vet. Res.* 46:2266–2271.

14. Chang, Y.-F., H. Renshaw, and R. Young. 1987. Pneumonic pasteurellosis. Examination of typable and untypable *Pasteurella haemolytica* strains for leukotoxin production, plasmid content, and anti-microbial susceptibility. *Am. J. Vet. Res.* 48:378–384.

15. Cho, H. J., J. G. Bohac, W. D. G. Yates, and H. Bielefeldt Ohman. 1984. Anticytotoxin activity of bovine sera and body fluids against *Pasteurella haemolytica* A1 cytotoxin. *Can. J. Comp. Med.* 48:151–155.

16. Clugston, R. E., and N. O. Nielsen. 1974. Experimental edema disease of swine (*E. coli* enterotoxemia). 1. Detection and preparation of an active principle. *Can. J. Comp. Med.* 38:22–28.

17. Conradi, H. 1903. Ueber losliche durch aseptische Autolyse erhaltene Giftstoffe von Ruhr- und Typhusbazillen. *Dtsch. Med. Wochenschr.* 29:26–28.

18. DeJong, M. F., H. L. Oei, and G. J. Tetenburg. 1980. AR-pathogenicity-tests for *Pasteurella multocida* isolates, p. 211. *In Proceedings of the International Pig Veterinary Society.* International Pig Veterinary Society, Copenhagen.

19. Dobescu, L. 1983. New biological effect of edema disease principle (*Escherichia coli*-neurotoxin) and its use as an in vitro assay for this toxin. *Am. J. Vet. Res.* 44:31–34.

20. Eiklid, K., and S. Olsnes. 1983. Animal toxicity of *Shigella dysenteriae* cytotoxin: evidence that the neurotoxic, enterotoxic and cytotoxic activities are due to one toxin. *J. Immunol.* 130:380–384.

21. Eiklid, K., and S. Olsnes. 1983. Entry of *Shigella dysenteriae* toxin into HeLa cells. *Infect. Immun.* 42:771–777.

22. Evans, D. G., and H. B. Maitland. 1939. The toxin of *Br. bronchiseptica* and the relationship of the organism to *H. pertussis. J. Pathol. Bacteriol.* 48:67–78.

23. Felmlee, T., S. Pellett, and R. A. Welch. 1985. *Escherichia coli* hemolysin is released extracellularly without cleavage of a signal peptide. *J. Bacteriol.* 163:88–93.

24. Fuchs, G., M. Mobassaleh, A. Donohue-Rolfe, R. K. Montgomery, R. J. Grand, and G. T. Keusch. 1986. Pathogenesis of *Shigella* diarrhea: rabbit intestinal cell microvillus membrane-binding site for *Shigella* toxin. *Infect. Immun.* 53:372–377.

25. Gemski, P., A. Takeuchi, O. Washington, and S. B. Formal. 1972. Shigellosis due to *Shigella dysenteriae* 1: relative importance of mucosal invasion versus toxin production in pathogenesis. *J. Infect. Dis.* 126:523–530.

26. Gentry, M. J., A. W. Confer, and P. C. Craven. 1987. Effect of repeated in vitro transfer of *Pasteurella haemolytica* A1 on encapsulation, leukotoxin production and virulence. *J. Clin. Microbiol.* 25:142–145.

27. Gentry, M. J., A. W. Confer, and R. J. Panciera. 1985. Serum neutralization of cytotoxin from *Pasteurella haemolytica* serotype 1 and resistance to experimental bovine pneumonic pasteurellosis. *Vet. Immunol. Immunopathol.* 9:239–250.

28. Gentry, M. J., A. W. Confer, E. D. Weinberg, and J. T. Homer. 1986. Cytotoxin (leukotoxin) production by *Pasteurella haemolytica:* requirement for an iron-containing compound. *Am. J. Vet. Res.* 47:1919–1923.

29. Hess, J., W. Wels, M. Vogel, and W. Goebel. 1986. Nucleotide sequence of a plasmid-encoded hemolysin determinant and its comparison with a corresponding chromosomal hemolysin sequence. *FEMS Microbiol. Lett.* 34:1–11.

30. Himmel, M. E., M. D. Yates, L. H. Lauerman, and P. G. Squire. 1982. Purification and partial characterization of a macrophage cytotoxin from *Pas-*

teurella haemolytica. Am. J. Vet. Res. 43:764–767.

31. **Hughes, C., J. Hacker, A. Roberts, and W. Goebel.** 1983. Hemolysin production as a virulence marker in symptomatic and asymptomatic urinary tract infections caused by *Escherichia coli. Infect. Immun.* 39:546–551.

32. **Hull, S. I., R. A. Hull, B. H. Minshew, and S. Falkow.** 1982. Genetics of hemolysin of *Escherichia coli. J. Bacteriol.* 151:1006–1012.

33. **Jorgensen, S. E., E. C. Short, H. J. Hurtz, H. K. Mussen, and G. K. Wu.** 1976. Studies on the origin of the alpha-haemolysin produced by *Escherichia coli. J. Med. Microbiol.* 9:173–189.

34. **Kaehler, K. L., R. J. F. Markham, C. C. Muscoplat, and D. W. Johnson.** 1980. Evidence of species specificity in the cytocidal effects of *Pasteurella haemolytica. Infect. Immun.* 30:615–616.

35. **Karmali, M. A., M. Petrie, S. Louie, and R. Cheung.** 1986. Antigenic heterogeneity of *Escherichia coli* verotoxins. *Lancet* i:164–165.

36. **Keusch, G. T., G. F. Grady, A. Takeuchi, and H. Sprinz.** 1972. The pathogenesis of shigella diarrhea. I. Enterotoxin-induced acute enteritis in the rabbit ileum. *J. Infect. Dis.* 126:92–95.

37. **Keusch, G. T., M. Jacewicz, and A. Donohue-Rolfe.** 1986. Pathogenesis of shigella diarrhea: evidence of an N-linked glycoprotein shigella toxin receptor and receptor modulation by β-galactosidase. *J. Infect. Dis.* 153:238–248.

38. **Konig, B., W. Konig, J. Scheffer, J. Hacker, and W. Goebel.** 1986. Role of *Escherichia coli* alpha-hemolysin and bacterial adherence in infection: requirement for the release of inflammatory mediators from granulocytes and mast cells. *Infect. Immun.* 54:886–892.

39. **Konowalchuk, J., J. I. Speirs, and S. Stavric.** 1977. Vero response to a cytotoxin of *Escherichia coli. Infect. Immun.* 18:775–779.

40. **Koronakis, V., M. Cross, B. Senior, E. Koronakis, and C. Hughes.** 1987. The secreted hemolysins of *Proteus mirabilis, Proteus vulgaris,* and *Morganella morganii* are genetically related to each other and to the alpha-hemolysin of *Escherichia coli. J. Bacteriol.* 169:1509–1515.

41. **Kume, K., and T. Nakai.** 1985. Dissociation of *Pasteurella multocida* dermonecrotic toxin into three polypeptide fragments. *Jpn. J. Vet. Sci.* 47:829–833.

42. **Kume, K., T. Nakai, Y. Samejima, and C. Sugimoto.** 1986. Properties of dermonecrotic toxin prepared from sonic extracts of *Bordetella bronchiseptica. Infect. Immun.* 52:370–377.

43. **Kume, K., T. Nakai, and A. Sawata.** 1986. Interaction between heat-stable hemolytic substance from *Haemophilus pleuropneumoniae* and porcine pulmonary macrophages in vitro. *Infect. Immun.* 51:563–570.

44. **Lo, R. Y. C., P. E. Shewen, C. A. Strathdee,**

and **C. N. Greer.** 1985. Cloning and expression of the leukotoxin genes of *Pasteurella haemolytica* A1 in *Escherichia coli* K-12. *Infect. Immun.* 50:667–671.

44a. **Lo, R. Y. C., C. A. Strathdee, and P. E. Shewen.** 1987. Nucleotide sequence of the leukotoxin genes of *Pasteurella haemolytica* A1. *Infect. Immun.* 55:1987–1996.

45. **Ludwig, A., M. Vogel, and W. Goebel.** 1987. Mutations affecting activity and transport of haemolysin in *Escherichia coli. Mol. Gen. Genet.* 206:238–245.

46. **Machitto, K. S., S. G. Smith, C. Locht, and J. M. Keith.** 1987. Nucleotide sequence homology to pertussis toxin gene in *Bordetella bronchiseptica* and *Bordetella parapertussis. Infect. Immun.* 55:497–501.

47. **Mackman, N., and I. B. Holland.** 1984. Functional characterization of a cloned haemolysin determinant from *Escherichia coli* of human origin, encoding information for the secretion of a 107 kD polypeptide. *Mol. Gen. Genet.* 196:129–134.

48. **Mackman, N., J. M. Nicaud, L. Gray, and I. B. Holland.** 1985. Genetical and functional organization of the *Escherichia coli* haemolysin determinant 2001. *Mol. Gen. Genet.* 201:282–288.

49. **Markham, R. J. F., M. L. R. Ramnaraine, and C. C. Muscoplat.** 1982. Cytotoxic effect of *Pasteurella haemolytica* on bovine polymorphnuclear leukocytes and impaired production of chemotactic factors by *Pasteurella haemolytica*-infected alveolar macrophages. *Am. J. Vet. Res.* 43:285–288.

50. **Markham, R. J. F., and B. N. Wilkie.** 1980. Interaction between *Pasteurella haemolytica* and bovine alveolar macrophages. Cytotoxic effect on macrophages and impaired phagocytosis. *Am. J. Vet. Res.* 41:18–22.

51. **Marques, L. R. M., M. A. Moore, J. G. Wells, I. K. Wachsmith, and A. D. O'Brien.** 1986. Production of Shiga-like toxin by *Escherichia coli. J. Infect. Dis.* 154:338–341.

52. **Martin, P. G., P. Lachance, and D. F. Niven.** 1985. Production of RNA-dependent haemolysin by *Haemophilus pleuropneumoniae. Can. J. Microbiol.* 31:456–462.

53. **Martin, S. W., A. H. Meek, D. G. Davis, J. A. Johnson, and R. A. Curtis.** 1981. Factors associated with morbidity and mortality in feedlot calves: the Bruce County beef project, year two. *Can. J. Comp. Med.* 45:103–112.

54. **Maudsley, J. R., and S. Kadis.** 1986. Growth and haemolysin production by *Haemophilus pleuropneumoniae* cultivated in a chemically defined medium. *Can. J. Microbiol.* 32:801–805.

55. **Mosier, D. A., B. A. Lessley, A. W. Confer, S. M. Antone, and M. J. Gentry.** 1986. Chromatographic separation and characterization of *Pasteurella haemolytica* cytotoxin. *Am. J. Vet. Res.* 47:2233–2241.

56. **Muller, D., C. Hughes, and W. Goebel.** 1983.

Relationship between plasmid and chromosomal hemolysin determinants of *Escherichia coli*. *J. Bacteriol.* 153:846–851.

57. Nakai, T., K. Kume, H. Yoshikawa, T. Oyamada, and T. Yoshikawa. 1986. Changes in the nasal mucosa of specific-pathogen-free neonatal pigs infected with *Pasteurella multocida* or *Bordetella bronchiseptica*. *Jpn. J. Vet. Sci.* 48:693–701.

58. Nakai, T., A. Sawata, and K. Kume. 1983. Characterization of hemolysin produced by *Haemophilus pleuropneumoniae*. *Am. J. Vet. Res.* 44:344–347.

59. Nakai, T., A. Sawata, and K. Kume. 1984. Pathogenicity of *Haemophilus pleuropneumoniae* for laboratory animals and possible role for its hemolysin for production of pleuropneumoniae. *Jpn. J. Vet. Res.* 46:851–858.

60. Nakai, T., A. Sawata, M. Tsuji, and K. Kume. 1984. Characterization of dermonecrotic toxin produced by serotype D strains of *Pasteurella multocida*. *Am. J. Vet. Res.* 45:2410–2413.

61. Nakai, T., A. Sawata, M. Tsuji, Y. Samejima, and K. Kume. 1984. Purification of dermonecrotic toxin from a sonic extract of *Pasteurella multocida* SP-72 serotype D. *Infect. Immun.* 46:429–434.

62. Nielsen, J. P., M. Bisgaard, and K. B. Pedersen. 1986. Production of toxin in strains previously classified as *Pasteurella multocida*. *Acta Pathol. Microbiol. Immunol. Scand. Sect. B* 94:203–204.

63. O'Brien, A. D., and G. D. LaVeck. 1983. Purification and characterization of *Shigella dysenteriae* 1-like toxin produced by *Escherichia coli*. *Infect. Immun.* 40:675–683.

64. O'Brien, A. D., G. D. LaVeck, M. R. Thompson, and S. B. Formal. 1982. Production of *Shigella dysenteriae* type 1 like cytotoxin by *Escherichia coli*. *J. Infect. Dis.* 146:763–769.

65. Olsnes, S., R. Reisbig, and K. Eiklid. 1981. Subunit structure of *Shigella* cytotoxin. *J. Biol. Chem.* 256:8732–8738.

66. Pedersen, K. B., and K. Barford. 1981. The aetological significance of *Bordetella bronchiseptica* and *Pasteurella multocida* in atrophic rhinitis in swine. *Nord. Veterinaermed.* 33:513–522.

67. Pedersen, K. B., and F. Elling. 1984. The pathogenesis of atrophic rhinitis in pigs induced by toxigenic *Pasteurella multocida*. *J. Comp. Pathol.* 94:203–214.

68. Pennings, A. M. M. A., and P. K. Storm. 1984. A test in Vero cell monolayers for toxin production by strains of *Pasteurella multocida* isolated from pigs suspected of having atrophic rhinitis. *Vet. Microbiol.* 9:503–508.

69. Pijoan, C. 1986. Effect of *Pasteurella multocida* and *Haemophilus pleuropneumoniae* toxins on swine alveolar macrophages. *Vet. Immunol. Immunopathol.* 13:141–149.

70. Pijoan, C., R. B. Morrison, and H. D. Hilley.

1983. Serotyping of *Pasteurella multocida* isolated from swine lungs collected at slaughter. *J. Clin. Microbiol.* 17:1074–1076.

71. Prado, D., T. C. Cleary, L. K. Pickering, C. D. Ericsson, A. V. Bartlett, H. L. DuPont, and P. C. Johnson. 1986. The relation between production of cytotoxin and clinical features of shigellosis. *J. Infect. Dis.* 154:149–155.

72. Purdy, C. W., C. W. Livingston, G. H. Frank, J. M. Cummins, N. A. Cole, and R. W. Loan. 1986. A live *Pasteurella haemolytica* vaccine efficacy trial. *J. Am. Vet. Med. Assoc.* 188:589–591.

73. Reisbig, R., S. Olnes, and K. Eiklid. 1981. The cytotoxic activity of *Shigella* toxin. Evidence for catalytic inactivation of the 60S ribosomal subunit. *J. Biol. Chem.* 256:8739–8744.

74. Rennie, R. P., and J. P. Arbuthnott. 1974. Partial characterization of *Escherichia coli* haemolysin. *J. Med. Microbiol.* 7:179–188.

75. Roop, R. M., H. P. Veit, R. J. Sinsky, S. P. Viet, E. L. Hewlett, and E. T. Kornegay. 1987. Virulence factors of *Bordetella bronchiseptica* associated with the production of infectious atrophic rhinitis and pneumonia in experimentally infected neonatal swine. *Infect. Immun.* 55:217–222.

76. Rutter, J. M., and P. D. Luther. 1984. Cell culture assay for toxigenic *Pasteurella multocida* from atrophic rhinitis of pigs. *Vet. Rec.* 114:393–396.

77. Rutter, J. M., and A. MacKenzie. 1984. Pathogenesis of atrophic rhinitis in pigs. A new perspective. *Vet. Rec.* 114:87–90.

78. Rutter, J. M., and X. Rojas. 1982. Atrophic rhinitis in gnotobiotic piglets: differences in the pathogenicity of *Pasteurella multocida* in combined infections with *Bordetella bronchiseptica*. *Vet. Rec.* 110:531–535.

79. Sandvig, K., and E. Brown. 1987. Ionic requirements for entry of Shiga toxin from *Shigella dysenteriae* 1 into cells. *Infect. Immun.* 55:298–303.

80. Schimmelpfenning, H. 1970. Untersuchungen zur Aetiologie der Oedemkrankheit des Schweines. *Fortschr. Veterinaermed.* 13:1–80.

81. Sebunya, T. N. K., and J. R. Saunders. 1983. *Haemophilus pleuropneumoniae* infection in swine: a review. *J. Am. Vet. Med. Assoc.* 182:1331–1337.

82. Shewen, P. E., and B. N. Wilkie. 1982. Cytotoxin of *Pasteurella haemolytica* acting on bovine leukocytes. *Infect. Immun.* 35:91–94.

83. Shewen, P. E., and B. N. Wilkie. 1983. *Pasteurella haemolytica* cytotoxin: production by recognized serotypes and neutralization by type-specific rabbit antisera. *Am. J. Vet. Res.* 44:715–719.

84. Shewen, P. E., and B. N. Wilkie. 1983. *Pasteurella haemolytica* cytotoxin neutralizing activity in sera from Ontario beef cattle. *Can. J. Comp. Med.* 47:497–498.

85. Shewen, P. E., and B. N. Wilkie. 1985. Evi-

dence for *Pasteurella haemolytica* cytotoxin as a product of actively growing bacteria. *Am. J. Vet. Res.* 46:1212–1214.

86. Slocombe, R. F., J. Malark, R. Ingersoll, F. J. Derksen, and N. E. Robinson. 1985. Importance of neutrophils in the pathogenesis of acute pneumonic pasteurellosis in calves. *Am. J. Vet. Res.* 46:2253–2258.

87. Smith, H. W. 1963. The hemolysins of *Escherichia coli. J. Pathol. Bacteriol.* 85:197–211.

88. Smith, H. W., P. Green, and Z. Parsell. 1983. Vero cell toxins in *Escherichia coli* and related bacteria: transfer by phage and conjugation and toxic action in laboratory animals, chickens and pigs. *J. Gen. Microbiol.* 129:3121–3137.

89. Smith, H. W., and S. Halls. 1967. The transmissible nature of the genetic factor in *Escherichia coli* that controls haemolysin production. *J. Gen. Microbiol.* 47:153–161.

90. Strockbine, N. A., L. R. M. Marques, J. W. Newland, H. W. Smith, R. K. Holmes, and A. D. O'Brien. 1986. Two toxin-converting phages from *Escherichia coli* O157:H7 strain 933 encode antigenically distinct toxins with similar biologic activities. *Infect. Immun.* 53.135–140.

91. Vicari, G., A. L. Olitzki, and Z. Olitzki. 1960. The action of the thermolabile toxin of *Shigella dysenteriae* on cells cultivated in vivo. *Br. J. Exp. Pathol.* 41:179–189.

92. Wagner, W., M. Vogel, and W. Goebel. 1983. Transport of hemolysin across the outer membrane of *Escherichia coli* requires two functions. *J. Bacteriol.* 154:200–210.

93. Welch, R. A., A. P. Dellinger, B. Minshew, and S. Falkow. 1981. Hemolysin contributes to virulence of extra intestinal *E. coli* infections. *Nature* (London) 294:665–667.

94. Welch, R. A., and S. Falkow. 1984. Characterization of *Escherichia coli* hemolysins conferring quantitative differences in virulence. *Infect. Immun.* 43:156–160.

95. Welch, R. A., T. Felmlee, S. Pellett, and D. E. Chenoweth. 1986. The *Escherichia coli* haemolysin: its gene organization and interaction with neutrophil receptors, p. 431–438. *In* D. L. Lark, S. Normark, B. E. Uhlin, and H. Wolf-Watz (ed.), *Protein-Carbohydrate Interactions in Biological Systems.* Academic Press, Inc. (London), Ltd., London.

96. Welch, R. A., R. Hull, and S. Falkow. 1983. Molecular cloning and physical characterization of a chromosomal hemolysin from *Escherichia coli. Infect. Immun.* 42:178–186.

97. Yates, W. D. G., P. H. G. Stockdale, L. A. Babiuk, and R. J. Smith. 1983. Prevention of experimental bovine pneumonic pasteurellosis with an extract of *Pasteurella haemolytica. Can. J. Comp. Med.* 47:250–256.

Chapter 15

Pathogenesis and Enterotoxins of Diarrheagenic *Escherichia coli*

DONALD C. ROBERTSON

Department of Microbiology
University of Kansas
Lawrence, Kansas 66045

INTRODUCTION

The role(s) of enterotoxins in pathogenesis of diarrheal diseases varies widely, and it is often difficult to establish their relative importance as virulence factors unless the toxin is the primary cause of disease. For example, all symptoms of clinical cholera can be induced by administration of the purified enterotoxin under appropriate conditions (12, 43). Also, the role of enterotoxins as virulence factors depends largely on whether diarrheal disease results from intoxication or infection. Bacteria such as *Staphylococcus aureus* (15, 49), *Bacillus cereus* (175), and *Clostridium perfringens* (114) produce potent toxins in a variety of foods which, upon ingestion, cause nausea, emesis, abdominal pain, and diarrhea. In contrast, the enteric bacilli usually cause disease in humans and animals after being ingested and then colonizing either the large or small intestine, subsequently producing enterotoxins which influence either absorption or secretion in the intestines.

The bacterial enterotoxins listed below can be conveniently grouped into two major types based on biological activity against cell cultures (9, 90). Cytotonic enterotoxins include *Vibrio cholerae* cholera toxin (CT), enterotoxi-genic *Escherichia coli* (ETEC) heat-labile toxin (LT) and heat-stable toxins (ST_a and ST_b), and toxins from NAG vibrios, *Salmonella* spp., *Aeromonas hydrophila*, *Campylobacter jejuni*, *Clostridium difficile* (toxin A), and *Staphylococcus aureus*. Cytotoxic enterotoxins include *Shigella dysenteriae* type 1 toxin (Shiga toxin), ETEC Shiga-like toxin (Vero toxin), and toxins from NAG vibrios, *Salmonella* spp. (possibly), *A. hydrophila*, *Campylobacter jejuni*, *C. difficile* (toxin B), *C. perfringens*, *C. perfringens* type E (iota toxin), and *B. cereus*. The prototype of cytotonic enterotoxins, which do not damage cell membranes and effect some type of physiological response, is cholera toxin produced by *V. cholerae* (43, 46, 100, 120). Cytotonic enterotoxins can increase intracellular levels of cyclic nucleotides in cell cultures and intestinal epithelial cells or induce other metabolic changes with no cellular damage. In contrast, cytotoxic enterotoxins (e.g., *C. perfringens* enterotoxin and Shiga toxin) cause cell death by damage to membranes or inhibition of protein synthesis, which induces a marked inflammatory response (19, 114, 127).

Several of the bacterial species listed above produce both cytotoxic and cytotonic enterotoxins, which complicates interpretation of the role of each enterotoxin in the disease process. For example, *A. hydrophila* (23, 26) produces a cytotoxic activity, a cytotonic activity similar to CT, and a hemolysin. The precise role of each virulence factor is still in question. Other examples of bacterial pathogens which produce both cytotonic and cytotoxic enterotoxins include NAG vibrios (146), *Campylobacter jejuni* (87), *Salmonella typhimurium* (134), and *C. difficile* (24). It may not be appropriate to include the staphylococcal enterotoxins with other cytotonic enterotoxins, since these toxins do not appear to be active against cell cultures (21). Recent evidence suggests that staphylococcal enterotoxin B stimulates the release of histamine from mast cells (Chapter 17 of this volume).

STRUCTURE-FUNCTION RELATIONSHIPS OF BACTERIAL ENTEROTOXINS

Bacterial enterotoxins are characterized by three major kinds of subunit structures (Table 1). Staphylococcal enterotoxins (15, 49) and *C. perfringens* enterotoxin (114) consist of a single polypeptide chain. The biological activity of *C. perfringens* ι-toxin (159) and *B. cereus* enterotoxin (175) results from the interaction of two or more proteins which differ with respect to molecular weight, isoelectric point, and immunological properties. The ι-toxin has been implicated in cases of fetal calf, lamb, and guinea pig enterotoxemias (17, 111). Other examples of binary toxins include the Panton-Valentine leukocidin produced by *Staphylococcus aureus* (124, 181), the C_2 enterotoxin of *C. botulinum* (129–131, 150), and anthrax toxin (103).

A significant number of bacterial enterotoxins consist of an A-B subunit structure (43, 46, 100, 120, 169, 182). The B components of bacterial toxins consist of one to five subunits and bind the toxins to specific receptors on cell surfaces (182). The receptor for CT and *E. coli* LT is G_{M1} ganglioside (121, 140); however, *E. coli* LT also binds to a galactoprotein (66, 81). In contrast to CT and *E. coli* LT, Shiga toxin appears to bind to a disaccharide (Galα1–4Galβ) on cell surfaces (108). The A,

TABLE 1
Structure-function relationships of bacterial enterotoxins

Enterotoxin	Subunit structure	Mol wt	Mode of action	Receptor
CT	A5B	82,000 (A = 28,500, B = 11,500)	ADP ribosylation of $G_{S\alpha}$	G_{M1} ganglioside
E. coli LT	A5B	Same as CT	Same as CT	G_{M1} ganglioside and galactoproteins
Shiga toxin	A5B	70,000 (A = 32,000, B = 7,700)	Inhibition of EF-1[a] function	Galα1–4Galβ (galabiose)
Shiga-like toxin	A5B	Same as Shiga toxin	Probably like Shiga toxin	Unknown
C. perfringens (type E), ι-toxin	Binary	ι_a = 48,000, ι_b = 71,000	Unknown	Unknown
B. cereus enterotoxin	Binary	575 = 43,000, 577 = 39,500, 580 = 38,000	Unknown	Unknown
C. perfringens enterotoxin	Single chain	35,000	Disrupts membranes	Unknown
Staphylococcus aureus enterotoxin (A, B, C_1, C_2, D, E)	Single chain	27,400–34,000	Unknown	Unknown

[a]EF-1, Elongation factor 1.

or active, subunit exhibits enzymatic activity, usually NAD-glycohydrolase and ADP-ribosyltransferase activities (120, 121). The A subunit is internalized by eucaryotic cells and mediates an ADP ribosylation reaction with different essential amino acid residues of target proteins as substrates (177). The net result is inhibition of a key enzymatic activity, for example, elongation factor 2 by diphtheria toxin, which inhibits protein synthesis (133). CT ADP ribosylates a guanine nucleotide-binding protein (G_s) associated with the catalytic subunit of adenylate cyclase (22, 88, 182). Inactivation of GTPase activity associated with the G_s protein inhibits the normal turn-off control and maintains the enzyme in an activated state. Pertussis toxin ADP ribosylates a different G protein (G_i) associated with regulation of adenylate cyclase (88, 89, 182). Many hormone receptors act through specific guanine nucleotide proteins which couple receptors and an enzyme system in the plasma membrane (33). Cytotoxic enterotoxins such as Shiga toxin cause cell death and inhibit protein synthesis by blocking the function of elongation factor 1 (19, 126, 127). Obrig et al. (127) found that Shiga toxin does not affect elongation factor 2-dependent reactions, analogous to diphtheria toxin, but acts by direct inhibition of elongation factor 1-dependent binding of aminoacyl-tRNA binding to ribosomes. The exact role of Shiga toxin in the pathogenesis of mild diarrhea associated with shigellosis remains open to speculation, but may be related to decreased absorption after the death of intestinal epithelial cells (125).

PATHOGENESIS OF DIARRHEAGENIC E. COLI

History of Colibacillosis

The ability of E. coli to cause diarrheal disease in humans and animals was recognized in the latter part of the 19th century. The major cause of infant mortality was "summer diarrhea" due to Bacterium coli, a normal inhabitant of the small bowel of humans and animals (2).

A group of veterinarians working on diarrheal disease in calves reported in 1925 that Bacterium coli appeared to be responsible for watery diarrhea (156). There was some suggestion that adsorption of toxin(s) produced by the bacteria was responsible for the pathophysiology of the disease.

The etiologic relationship between E. coli and diarrheal disease in piglets, calves, and lambs was firmly established in the late 1960s. A role for an enterotoxin in pathogenesis of piglet diarrhea was suggested by several investigators (73, 95, 153, 170). Both whole-cell lysates and culture supernatants of porcine ETEC strains caused fluid accumulation in ligated porcine intestinal loops (73). At least two enterotoxic activities were shown to be associated with diarrhea in piglets (151). Also, the genes which coded for the enterotoxins were detected on transmissible plasmids (154). The differential heat stability of the two enterotoxic activites forms the basis for the nomenclature used today (71). The LT produced by ETEC is inactivated by being heated at 70°C for 30 min and is similar to CT produced by V. cholerae with respect to amino acid composition, subunit structure, receptor binding, and immunological properties (43, 46, 100, 120, 140). The ST, which is stable to heating, has been found to exist as two major types (20, 128), one which activates particulate intestinal guanylate cyclase (ST_a or STI) (42, 67, 69) and a second with an unknown mechanism of action (ST_b or STII) (179).

Pathogenesis of EPEC

Strains of E. coli associated with diarrheal disease exhibit at least four pathogenic mechanisms based on virulence properties: association with intestinal mucosa, production of clinical symptoms, etiology, and distinct O:H serotypes (104, 115, 143, 144). Despite differences in pathogenic mechanisms, E. coli strains associated with diarrheal disease in humans and animals exhibit several common properties: (i) the genes for virulence factors are often located on transmissible plasmids; (ii) specific receptors in the intestine bind each group of *E. coli* and determine host specificities; (iii) multiple cytotoxic and cytotonic enterotoxins may be produced; and (iv) each pathogenic group is characterized by distinctive O:H serotypes. Several serotypes of enteropathogenic *E. coli* (EPEC) were first recognized as the etiologic agent of infantile diarrhea in the 1940s. Serotyping is useful for identification and characterization of the *E. coli* strains associated with diarrhea (104, 144). Classical EPEC strains cause diarrheal disease by a mechanism not involving synthesis of LT or ST or *Shigella*-like invasiveness (104, 143). Several recent observations have significantly expanded our understanding of the pathogenesis and virulence factors of EPEC: (i) distinctive histopathological lesions were observed in human intestines not associated with ETEC strains (104); (ii) the strains can be divided into two groups on the basis of adherence to HEp-2 cells (31); (iii) adherence to HEp-2 cells is coded by a 60-megadalton (MDa) plasmid (11); and (iv) some EPEC strains elaborate moderate amounts of a cytotoxin similar to Shiga toxin produced by *S. dysenteriae* type 1 (113, 126). The EPEC adherence factor plasmid encodes a 94-kDa outer membrane protein; however, its role in pathogenesis remains to be defined (106).

Pathogenesis of ETEC

The pathogenesis of ETEC is mediated by at least two kinds of virulence factors (140, 143): fimbriae which bind to intestinal receptors and determine species specificity, and at least two kinds of cytotonic enterotoxins, LT and ST. Genes for fimbriae, referred to as adhesins, and enterotoxins are often present on transmissible plasmids. At least four distinct antigenic fimbrial adhesins have been identified on ETEC strains isolated from animals (K88, K99, 987P, and F41) and three different colonization factors have been found to be associated with human ETEC strains (CFA/I, CFA/II, and E8775) (39, 41, 117, 173). The CFA/II colonization

factor has been shown to be composed of three distinct antigenic proteins, CS1, CS2, and CS3 (107). The hydrophobic properties of surface fimbriae probably supply the driving force necessary to overcome the negative charge on bacterial and intestinal cell surfaces before adherence and subsequent colonization (157). As noted above, a good correlation exists between serotype and major pathogenic groups of *E. coli* associated with diarrheal disease. For example, even though over 10,000 O:K:H serotypes are possible, approximately 12 serotypes are responsible for ETEC disease in piglets, and 8 serotypes have been found associated with ETEC disease in calves (132). Distinctive patterns of enterotoxin loss have been correlated with serotype, which is probably explained by plasmid incompatibilities (41). The role of adherence in pathogenesis of ETEC is the subject of several recent reviews (38, 50, 51, 116; Chapter 2 of this volume).

Pathogenesis of EIEC

The pathogenesis of enteroinvasive *E. coli* (EIEC) is remarkably similar to that of *Shigella* spp., since both exhibit the capacity to specifically bind, invade, and survive within epithelial cells (104, 125, 126). A marked inflammatory response is typically observed as a result of epithelial cell death and influx of polymorphonuclear leukocytes. Although shigellosis is an acute infectious enteritis affecting only humans, EIEC are of considerable importance in both human and veterinary medicine. EIEC strains produce multiple cytotoxins referred to as Shiga-like toxins or Vero toxins, which are immunologically related, but not identical, to Shiga toxin (96, 126, 147). Shiga-like cytotoxins have been implicated in human diseases such as hemorrhagic colitis or hemolytic uremic syndrome, and in edema disease in swine (126; Chapter 14 of this volume). Invasiveness of both EIEC and *Shigella* spp. is due to the presence of a 140-MDa plasmid which codes for several outer membrane proteins (Chapter 4 of this volume). Recent developments in studies on Shiga toxin and Shiga-like toxins have been recently reviewed (126).

Pathogenesis of EHEC

An outbreak of hemorrhagic colitis caused by enterohemorrhagic *E. coli* O157:H77 (EHEC) was first noted in 1982 (137). The outbreak was unusual because the serotype had not been recognized as being associated with human diarrheal disease and the clinical presentation was characterized by bloody but copious diarrhea, which distinguished the clinical picture from bacillary dysentery due to *Shigella* spp. or EIEC. Strains isolated from patients with hemorrhagic colitis or hemolytic uremic syndrome elaborate high levels of a cytotoxin similar to Shiga toxin produced by *S. dysenteriae* type 1 (113). The Shiga-like toxin produced in high levels has also been referred to as Vero toxin I (96) and may be identical to Shiga toxin (126). Some strains also produce a second potent cytotoxin, referred to as Shiga-like toxin II or Vero toxin II, that is not neutralized by antibody to Shiga toxin (126). More important, similar strains have been implicated in edema disease of swine and may produce related cytotoxins (chapter 14 of this volume). Immunologic diversity among the immunodominant B subunit of cytotonic and cytotoxic enterotoxins with an A-B subunit structure appears to be common to the cholera-coli family of enterotoxins.

E. COLI LT

Purification, Characterization, and Chemical Properties

Even though CT and *E. coli* LT are similar with respect to chemical properties, subunit structure, and mechanisms of action, purification of LT was more difficult than that of CT because the LT protein is not exported and accumulates in the periplasmic space (76, 77). Also, significant amounts of LT remain associated with the outer membrane after disruption of bacteria (140). Several purification schemes for *E. coli* LT have been described (29, 30, 78, 98, 140); however, most involve at least one hydrophobic interaction chromatography step which resolves LT from lipopoly-saccharides and other outer membrane components.

Numerous factors influence the synthesis and release of LT by ETEC (58, 97). The amino acids methionine and lysine stimulate LT synthesis, whereas branched-chain amino acids inhibit LT synthesis. In contrast to effects on ST synthesis (6, 7), glucose is required for synthesis of maximal levels of LT. The toxin is not exported below pH 7.3 and cannot be detected in culture supernatants when bacteria are grown below 26°C. Protease inhibitors block release of LT if added before the pH of culture supernatants is adjusted (97). Divalent cations are not required and do not inhibit LT synthesis, which is unique compared with synthesis of Shiga-like toxins by EIEC (126).

The molecular weight of *E. coli* LT determined by gel electrophoresis and sedimentation equilibrium ranged from 73,000 to 93,000 (29, 30, 78, 98). Recent studies on the nucleotide sequence of the LT-A and LT-B genes showed that the A subunit of holotoxin produced by human ETEC strains consists of 240 amino acids and the B subunit contains 103 amino acids (183–185). Thus, the molecular weight of the holotoxin, based on the nucleotide sequence, is 87,866.

CT and *E. coli* LT both consist of a single A subunit and five identical B subunits (57) and exhibit NAD-glycohydrolase and ADP-ribosyltransferase activities that are stimulated by dithiothreitol (121). In contrast to that of CT, ADP-ribosyltransferase activity of *E. coli* LT was increased by over 200% by use of trypsin. When recombinant plasmids encoding *E. coli* LT were expressed in a *V. cholerae* host, the toxin was secreted into culture supernatants but remained unnicked (74). These results showed that protease cleavage is not required for export of the toxin and that the A subunit of LT is not susceptible to the protease produced by *V. cholerae*. Both CT and *E. coli* LT bind to G_{M1} ganglioside on cell surfaces (120, 121, 140); however, LT also binds to a glycoprotein associated with human and rabbit intestinal epithelial cells (66, 82).

Immunological Relationships between *E. coli* LTs and CT

Strains of ETEC isolated from piglets and humans exhibit species-specific binding owing to the presence of antigenically distinct fimbrial adhesins (114, 115). In addition to fimbrial adhesins, LTs produced by ETEC are antigenically diverse. The LTs produced by human and porcine isolates that share antigenic cross-reactivity with CT are referred to as type I LTs (LT-I), whereas a second antigenic type, originally isolated from a water buffalo, is not neutralized by anti-CT, does not bind to G_{M1} ganglioside, and has been designated type II LT (LT-II) (79, 80). The type I LTs produced by porcine and human strains are designated LTp and LTh, respectively (84, 167). When the two kinds of *E. coli* type I LTs are compared with each other and with CT, several important points can be noted: (i) the homology between the two kinds of LTs ranges from 93 to 96% for the A and B subunits (183), respectively; (ii) LTh is more closely related to CT than is LTp (83, 183); and (iii) only four amino acid substitutions determine the immunological diversity of the immunodominant B subunits (45).

Studies with Polyclonal Antisera

The immunological cross-reactivity between *E. coli* LTs and CT has been described by several investigators (27, 28, 59, 72, 83–85, 112, 155, 176). Studies with polyclonal antisera raised in rabbits and goats have revealed the following: (i) each enterotoxin contains unique and shared antigenic determinants, and the unique antigenic determinants are usually immunodominant (59, 140); (ii) sensitive solid-phase radioimmunoassays showed that the unique and shared determinants are localized in distinct antigenic domains, since heterologous subunits do not compete with radiolabeled subunits in tubes coated with antibodies raised against the radiolabeled homologous subunit (59, 140); (iii) rabbits immunized with CT were not protected when challenged with ETEC (16); and (iv) neutralization of homologous antigens is always greater than neu-

TABLE 2

Neutralization of pH extracts from strains of ETEC by anti-386C₂ LT

Strain	Origin	Toxin	Antitoxin units[a,b]
286C₂	Human	LT	9,720 ± 279
334	Human	LT-STₐ	267 ± 66
408-3	Human	LT-STₐ	665 ± 190
H-10407	Human	LT-STₐ	746 ± 77
263	Porcine	LT	334 ± 3
1288	Porcine	LT-STₐ	206 ± 34
1291	Porcine	LT-STₐ	280 ± 44
1362	Porcine	LT-STₐ	174 ± 28

[a] Presented as the mean ± standard error of quadruplicate experiments.

[b] The neutralizing titer of antisera was determined by twofold serial dilutions and is expressed as the reciprocal of the highest dilution which caused less than a 50% rounding response. The neutralization coefficient was determined for the same dilution of antiserum by comparing the reduction in toxin-induced steroidogenesis with that of controls lacking antisera. The neutralization coefficient (NC) was calculated as follows: NC = [1 − nanomoles of steroid (experimental)]/nanomoles of steroid (control). An NC of zero indicates no neutralization, while an NC of unity indicates complete neutralization of toxin activity. Antitoxin units were calculated by multiplication of the NC with the neutralization titer.

tralization of heterologous antigens by polyclonal antisera (Table 2). When antisera raised against strain 286C2 LT were used in neutralization experiments, neutralization activity was highest against homologous 286C2 LT, intermediate with LTh's produced by two human strains (408-3 and H-10407), and low against four LTp's and one LTh produced by an ETEC strain (strain 334) isolated in Calcutta, India. These data point to potential problems in developing a vaccine against *E. coli* diarrhea and cholera (105). Protective epitopes must be identified and the appropriate carrier must be developed to produce protective antitoxic immunity.

Antigenic analysis by Ouchterlony-type immunodiffusion assays with polyclonal antisera (83, 84, 167, 176) showed that (i) each enterotoxin has at least one unique antigenic determinant; (ii) at least one antigenic determinant is common to all three kinds of enterotoxins; (iii) LTh and CT share one antigenic determinant not present on LTp; (iv) LTh and LTp possess at least one antigenic determinant

TABLE 3
Amino acid composition of human and porcine LT-B subunits

Amino acid	Amt[a] in LTh-B from:			Amt[a] in LTp-B from:		
	286C$_2$	K108C$_3$	LTh[b]	263	8203	LTp[c]
Asp	10	10	10	10	10	10
Thr	11	11	11	12	11 (−1)	12
Ser	10 (+1)	10 (+1)	9	9 (+1)	9 (+1)	8
Pro	2 (−1)	3	3	2 (−1)	3	3
Gly	4 (+1)	4 (+1)	3	4 (+1)	4 (+1)	3
Ala	6	6	6	5	5	5
Çys	2	2	2	2	2	2
Val	4	4	4	4	4	4
Met	4	4	4	4	3 (−1)	4
Ile	11 (−1)	11 (−1)	12	11 (−1)	10 (−2)	12
Leu	5	5	5	5	5	5
Tyr	4	4	4	4	4	4
Phe	2	2	2	2	2	2
His	1	1	1	1	1	1
Lys	9	9	9	10	9 (−1)	10
Arg	3 (−1)	4	4	4	4	4
Try	1	1	1	1	1	1
Total	102	104	103	103	99	103

[a]Expressed as residues of each amino acid per mole of B subunit.
[b]Reference 185.
[c]Reference 183.

not present on CT; and (v) no shared determinant unique to CT and LTp has been detected, which may be due to the lower nucleotide sequence homology compared with that of the other pairs of enterotoxins (184).

The homogeneity of the B subunits of LTp and LTh is shown by the data in Table 3. The subunits of each holotoxin were separated by acid urea gel filtration (44) and subjected to amino acid analysis. Two human strains (286C2 and K108C3) were compared with two porcine strains (263 and 8203). Consistent differences were found for some amino acids (serine, glycine, and isoleucine), possibly as a result of problems with calibration standards; however, the data with different standards were consistently within the accuracy of the amino acid analyzer (±3 to 5%). We have no explanation about why the number of amino acids was low in the B subunit of strain 8203. The data show that differences are minor and that the nucleotide sequence of B subunits must be deter-

mined to identify LT variants. The amino acid sequences deduced from the subunit B genes of LTh, LTp, and CT are shown in Fig. 1. The LTs differ by only four amino acids at positions 4, 13, 46, and 102.

To determine the neutralization capacity of heterologous LTs by antisera raised against porcine and human LTs, the antigenic equivalent of 10 doses of LT which induced 50% rounding of Y-1 adrenal cells and twofold serial dilutions of antisera were incubated for 2 h at 37°C. Aliquots of reaction mixtures were transferred to 24-well clusters containing Y-1 adrenal cells to measure residual enterotoxin activity. The data in Table 4 are in good agreement with the results of others (45); that is, anti-LTp sera exhibits a low neutralization activity against CT, and the amount of neutralization activity exhibited by anti-CT sera against E. coli LTs and CT is higher, but depends on the animal species and immunization conditions. The neutralization assays described in Table 4 were done at high concentrations of antigens and antisera to maximize the contribution of unique and shared antigenic determinants, and to provide a sharp titration endpoint. At the low concentrations present in solid-phase radioimmunoassays, there was minimal competition by heterologous LTs when radiolabeled LTs or CT was used (unpublished observations).

Studies with Monoclonal Antibodies

In an attempt to characterize the major and minor cross-reacting epitopes of E. coli LTs and CT, several investigators have raised monoclonal antibodies to each enterotoxin (LTp, LTh, and CT). Early studies focused on the cross-reactivity between LTh and CT, since CT was used as the immunogen (45, 79, 109). A panel of anti-CT monoclonal antibodies was classified into seven different groups based on their binding to homologous and heterologous enterotoxins or their subunits in solid-phase radioimmunoassays. All monoclonal antibodies against CT-B had high neutralizing titers; however, there was no direct correlation be-

```
CT    Thr         Asn           Asp       Ala                         His   Leu
H-LT  Ala Pro Gln Ser Ile 5 Thr Glu Leu Cys Ser10 Glu Tyr His Asn Thr15 Gln Ile Tyr Thr Ile20
P-LT          Thr                                   Arg
```

```
CT          Asn        Phe                    Leu                  Ala
H-LT  Asn Asp Lys Ile Leu25 Ser Tyr Thr Glu Ser30 Met Ala Gly Lys Arg35 Glu Met Val Ile Ile40
P-LT
```

```
CT                Asn
H-LT  Thr Phe Lys Ser Gly45 Ala Thr Phe Gln Val50 Glu Val Pro Gly Ser55 Gln His Ile Asp Ser60
P-LT              Glu
```

```
CT                            Asn              Ala                    Ala
H-LT  Gln Lys Lys Ala Ile65 Glu Arg Met Lys Asp70 Thr Leu Arg Ile Thr75 Tyr Leu Thr Glu Thr80
P-LT
```

```
CT    Val Glu                          His Ala
H-LT  Lys Ile Asp Lys Leu85 Cys Val Trp Asn Asn90 Lys Thr Pro Asn Ser95 Ile Ala Ala Ile Ser100
P-LT
```

```
CT          Ala
H-LT  Met Glu Asn103
P-LT        Lys
```

FIGURE 1. Amino acid sequences of B subunits of human *E. coli* LT (H-LT), porcine *E. coli* LT (P-LT), and CT. Sequences are adapted from references 45 and 183–185.

tween the ability of monoclonal antibodies to neutralize CT and to cross-react with LTh and LTp. Lindholm et al. (109) observed that about two-thirds of a panel of anti-CT-B antibodies did not react with *E. coli* LT. About one-half of the remaining 30% of cross-reacting anti-CT-B monoclonal antibodies reacted equally well with LT, and the remaining half reacted poorly with the heterologous toxin. These data were interpreted to show the presence of at least one identical and one nonidentical cross-reactive

determinant in addition to specific anti-CT-B determinants. Monoclonal anti-CT-B antibodies which reacted equally well with CT and *E. coli* LT were strongly neutralizing.

Similar results have been observed with LTh and LTp as immunogens (13, 14, 45, 161; M. D. Wuenscher and D. C. Robertson, unpublished observations). Neutralizing and nonneutralizing antibodies that recognize the unique cross-reacting epitopes of LTh have been isolated. Some monoclonal antibodies were against

TABLE 4
Neutralization of homologous and heterologous *E. coli* LTs

Enterotoxin	Antiserum dilution[a]				
	Anti-CT	Anti-286C$_2$	Anti-K108C$_3$	Anti-263	Anti-8203
CT	1:10	1:5	1:5	1:2.5	1:2.5
286C$_2$ LT[b]	1:10	1:40	1:40	1:40	1:20
K108C$_3$ LT[b]	1:10	1:40	1:40	1:40	1:20
263 LT[c]	1:5	1:20	1:10	1:80	1:40
8203 LT[c]	1:5	1:20	1:20	1:40	1:40

[a]Dilution of antisera with a percent rounding of less than 50.
[b]LTh antigen.
[c]LTp antigen.

conformational epitopes, yet at least one bound to the monomeric form of LT-B as determined by Western blot (immunoblot) analyses (13, 14). Cross-neutralization of LTh, LTp, and CT by monoclonal anti-LTh and anti-CT antibodies showed that the epitopes involved in neutralization of LTh and LTp are not shared by CT (161). Most of the neutralizing antibodies against LTh reacted with determinants common to LTh and LTp.

We raised a panel of monoclonal antibodies against both types of *E. coli* LTs and identified antibodies reacting with unique and shared LT epitopes (Table 5). No hybridoma clones producing anti-LT-A were detected when holotoxins were used as immunogens, which supports other observations that the A subunit is

a weak immunogen (59, 140). Twenty-five monoclonal antibodies have been characterized on the basis of their reactivity with each subunit and cross-linked forms of the holotoxins. All 25 monoclonal antibodies reacted with the B subunit; however, only about half exhibited neutralizing activity. The unique epitopes of LTh appear to be immunodominant compared with cross-reacting epitopes, whereas the cross-reacting epitopes of LTp-B and LTh-B appear to be immunodominant. The panel of monoclonal antibodies did not react with LT-B monomers, but did react with dimers, trimers, tetramers, and the pentameric form of LT-B. These data suggest that the monoclonal antibodies reacting with the LT-B subunit are against conformational epitopes and not against

TABLE 5
Properties of monoclonal antibodies to LTh and LTp

Monoclonal antibody	Immunogen	Isotype[a]	Neutralization	ELISA[b] reaction		
				LTh	LTp	CT
9.7B5	LTh	IgG3	+	+	−	−
9.4D2	LTh	IgG3	−	+	−	−
9.4B7	LTh	IgG1	−	+	−	−
6.4B3	LTh	IgG1	+	+	−	−
3.1F4[c]	LTh	IgG1	ND[d]	+	−	−
4.3F8	LTh	IgG1	+	+	−	−
6.2B7	LTh	IgG1	−	+	−	−
6.7E9	LTh	IgM	+	+	−	−
6.9F6	LTh	IgG1	+	+	+	−
6.2G7	LTh	IgM	+	+	+	−
9.1E6	LTh	IgG3	+	+	+	−
6.7D2	LTh	IgM	−	+	−	+
4.1E2	LTh	IgM	−	+	−	+
7.6G5	LTh	IgM	−	+	−	+
9.4G9	LTh	IgM	−	+	−	+
9.5E6	LTh	IgM	+	+	−	+
9.4C2	LTh	IgG2a	−	+	+	+
6.4E5	LTh	IgG1	−	+	+	+
6.6F10	LTh	IgM	−	+	+	+
10.3F6	LTp	IgG1	−	−	+	−
10.5E5	LTp	IgM	±	+	+	−
10.5F11	LTp	IgM	±	+	+	−
10.5D8	LTp	IgM	−	+	+	−
10.6G8	LTp	IgG1	−	+	+	−
10.1B10	LTp	IgG2a	−	+	+	−

[a] IgG, Immunoglobulin G; IgM, immunoglobulin M.
[b] ELISA, Enzyme-linked immunosorbent assay.
[c] Monoclonal antibody 3.1F4 did not bind biotinylated LT.
[d] ND, Not done.

linear epitopes; thus, it is impossible to isolate peptide fragments and identify more precise amino acid sequences which constitute each epitope.

E. COLI ST

Background

As noted previously, several years before being implicated in human disease, ETEC were recognized as an etiologic agent of diarrheal disease in neonatal animals (139, 140). Clinical strains of ETEC which produce only ST have been shown to cause disease in neonatal animals (70, 95, 151) and human infants (55) and to cause traveler's diarrhea in adults (60, 119, 149). Smith and Halls (153) observed that heating bacterium-free culture filtrates for 30 min at 100°C did not decrease their enterotoxin activity. Two different enterotoxin activities, one heat labile and one heat stable, were detected in ligated piglet intestinal loops by Smith and Gyles (151). The biological activity of E. coli ST in suckling mice (48) and in ligated intestinal loops of rabbits (40, 118, 152), piglets (72, 118, 152), dogs (123), and calves (122, 152) has been assayed. Enzyme-linked immunosorbent assays have been developed (93, 110, 141, 160, 174) which make it unnecessary to use cumbersome bioassays. The suckling-mouse assay can be used to study structure-function relationships, and immunological assays can be used for detection and quantitation.

It is now well established that two kinds of STs are produced by porcine ETEC strains (20, 102, 128, 135): (i) a methanol-soluble molecule with biological activity in suckling mice, rats, rabbits, and piglets, referred to as ST_a or STI, and (ii) a methanol-insoluble molecule with biological activity in piglets, referred to as ST_b or STII. The biological activity of ST_a is mediated by stimulation of particulate intestinal guanylate cyclase (42, 67, 69, 136). The mechanism of action and molecular properties of ST_b are unknown; however, ST_b does not elevate intracellular cyclic nucleotide levels

(R. N. Greenberg, D. J. Kennedy, A. H. Stephenson, A. J. Lonigro, F. Murad, and R. L. Guerrant, *Clin. Res.* **30**:367A, 1982; L. A. Dreyfus, L. Jaso-Friedmann, and D. C. Robertson, unpublished observations) and appears to stimulate a nonchloride anion secretion by intestinal cells (180). Initially it appeared that ST_b was active only in ligated porcine intestinal loops; however, recent evidence demonstrates that in contrast to ST_a, ST_b is sensitive to proteases (S. Whipp, personal communication). Protease inhibitors must be added to detect biological activity in other animal species such as the rat.

The ST_as produced by human and animal strains of ETEC are remarkably homogeneous, yet two types, referred to as STh and STp, have been described (5, 162). The nomenclature is somewhat confusing, because STp is produced by both human and animal ETEC strains, whereas STh is produced only by human strains. In addition to *E. coli,* NAG vibrios (10, 163), *Yersinia entercolitica* (164, 165), *Klebsiella pneumoniae* (92), *Citrobacter freundii* (68), and *Enterobacter aerogenes* (91) produce ST_as.

Purification and Structure

Several purification schemes have been described which yield *E. coli* ST_a in high yield and homogenous form (5, 8, 35, 101, 142, 145, 158). Most of the purification schemes involve an initial step based on hydrophobic interactions such as XAD-2 or octyl-Sepharose and a combination of gel filtration, ion-exchange chromatography, and reverse-phase high-performance liquid chromatography.

The amino acid sequences shown in Fig. 2 illustrate the unique chemical properties of ST_as. The enterotoxins range in size from 17 to 30 amino acid residues, and most contain 10 or 11 of the amino acids commonly found in proteins. The form of ST_a noted as STp contains 18 amino acids, while STh contains 19 amino acids. All ST_as contain three disulfide bonds within the characteristic sequence of 13 amino acids, which is the smallest form of the toxin which exhibits biological activity. The

E. coli ST$_p$ H$_2$N-ASN-THR-PHE-TYR-CYS-CYS-GLU-LEU-CYS-CYS-ASN-PRO-ALA-CYS-ALA-GLY-CYS-TYR-COOH^a

E. coli ST$_h$ H$_2$N-ASN-SER-SER-ASN- - - - - - - - - - - - - -THR-GLY-CYS-TYR-COOH^b

E. coli 213 ST$_a$ H$_2$N-ASN-THR-SER- - - - - - - - - - - - - - - -SER-GLY-CYS-TYR-COOH^c

V. Cholerae non-01 ST   H$_2$N-ILE-ASP- - - -ILE- - - - - - -PHE- - -LEU-ASN-COOH^d

Y. enterocolitica STs   ⌐ CYS-CYS-ASP-VAL-CYS-CYS-ASN-PRO-ALA-CYS-ALA-GLY-CYS-COOH
                          ∟ ASP-TRY-ASP-SER-SER-VAL-GLU-NH$_2$^{e}
                                     ↑   ↑   ↑   ↑

FIGURE 2. Amino acid sequences of STs, with suckling mouse activity. References: a (162), b (5), c (35), d (10, 163), e (164, 165). The arrows in the bottom line depict the multiple forms isolated from culture supernatants.

arrangement of the disulfide linkages has recently been determined (54, 148). Conservative amino acid substitutions are possible within the sequence of 13 amino acids; for example, Dreyfus et al. (35) isolated a form of STp produced by a human ETEC strain in which the phenylalanine and alanine residues at positions 3 and 15 were replaced by serine. Replacement of the glutamic acid-leucine sequence in *E. coli* ST$_a$ by aspartic acid and valine in *Y. enterocolitica* ST reduces the biological activity in suckling mice 25-fold (165). Five ST$_a$s ranging from 16 to 20 amino acids have been purified from culture supernatants of *Y. enterocolitica* (165). Most STs specifically stimulate guanylate cyclase associated with intestinal cells, except for *Y. enterocolitica* ST, which also activates the particulate enzyme in cultured cells (86).

Binding Properties of *E. coli* ST$_a$

Specific binding of ^{125}I-labeled ST$_a$ has been observed with rat and porcine intestinal epithelial cells and intestinal brush border membranes (BBM) from each species (47, 56). The binding was found to be saturable, time and temperature dependent, and mediated by a single class of receptors. Intestinal cells contain about 50,000 ST$_a$ receptors per cell, which appears to be a glycoprotein (47). Binding of ST$_a$ to its receptor is stimulated by monovalent cations such as Na$^+$ and divalent cations such as Mg^{2+} to a lesser extent. Dissociation of ^{125}I-labeled ST$_a$ from its receptor ranges from 20

to 50% depending on several factors (e.g., composition of the reaction medium, age of the ^{125}I-labeled ST$_a$, whether ^{125}I-labeled ST$_a$ is purified by high-performance liquid chromatography, age of the animal, etc.). Despite the observation that the effects of ST$_a$ are reversible in perfusion experiments (55), it is not clear whether ST$_a$ receptors must remain occupied after binding to maintain the activated form of guanylate cyclase, or whether the effects of ST$_a$ are completely reversible at the molecular level. It must be determined whether guanylate cyclase returns to basal levels of activity after ST$_a$ is chemically removed from its receptor. The significance of the dissociation of ^{125}I-labeled ST$_a$ from BBM depends on whether the 50 ± 10% which dissociates is more or less important than the 40 to 60% which remains bound. It cannot be ignored that a significant amount of ST$_a$ remains associated with its receptor and can be used to radiolabel the receptor during polyacrylamide gel electrophoresis and gel filtration chromatography. The association of ST$_a$ with its receptor is not a typical reversible binding system as is observed with several polypeptide hormones (53).

Piglets develop resistance to some strains of ETEC (class 2), but remain susceptible to others referred to as class 1 strains (80). To determine whether age susceptibility is due to differences in intestinal receptors for fimbrial adhesins or enterotoxin receptors, porcine intestinal epithelial cells and BBM were incubated with ST$_a$s produced by both classes of

ETEC strains (35; L. Jaso-Friedmann, A. Dreyfus, S. C. Whipp, and D. C. Robertson, manuscript in preparation). There were no differences in the stimulation of guanylate cyclase associated with porcine BBM of 7-day-old or 7-week-old piglets (Fig. 3). Also, there were no differences in levels of intracellular cyclic GMP in epithelial cells treated with ST_a. Thus, differences in fimbrial adhesin receptors and other environmental factors appear to determine age susceptibility, not sensitivity to ST_as.

Mechanism of Action of *E. coli* ST_a

In contrast to *E. coli* LT and CT, which mediate intestinal secretion by activation of adenylate cyclase, *E. coli* ST_a specifically stimulates the particulate form of intestinal guanylate cyclase (42, 69). Guanylate cyclase is present in soluble and particulate fractions of most tissues, and the chemical properties of the two forms of the enzyme are different (52). The unique tissue specificity exhibited by *E. coli* ST_a is explained by the observation that the ST_a re-

ceptor is not associated with other tissues (37). Only intestinal membranes exhibited specific binding of ^{125}I-labeled ST_a and increased guanylate cyclase activity after treatment with the toxin. Binding to a specific receptor by ST_a must occur before activation of guanylate cyclase, but few additional details are available on the mechanism of action. The toxin may act by two possible mechanisms (Fig. 4): (i) generation of a transmembrane signal observed in other stimulus-response systems mediated by hormones, or (ii) direct interaction in which the ST_a receptor and guanylate cyclase exist as a single transmembrane protein or separate proteins coupled by a regulatory protein (33). De Jonge (32) has referred to these mechanisms as the cascade and direct coupling models, respectively.

The transmembrane signal or cascade model initially appeared attractive as a mechanism of action, since inhibitors of prostaglandin biosynthesis and calmodulin-mediated reactions blocked fluid secretion induced in suckling mice by submaximal doses of ST_a, but had no effect

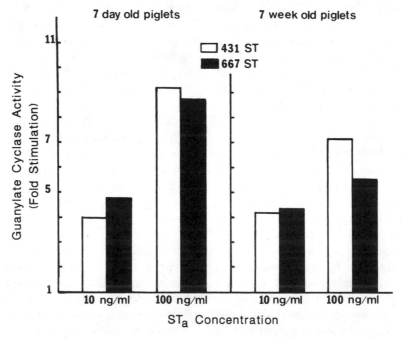

FIGURE 3. Stimulation of particulate porcine intestinal guanylate cyclase by *E. coli* ST_as. BBM were incubated in the reaction mixture described by Dreyfus et al. (36).

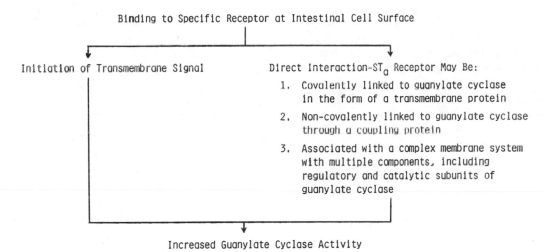

Binding to Specific Receptor at Intestinal Cell Surface

Initiation of Transmembrane Signal

Direct Interaction-ST_a Receptor May Be:

1. Covalently linked to guanylate cyclase in the form of a transmembrane protein
2. Non-covalently linked to guanylate cyclase through a coupling protein
3. Associated with a complex membrane system with multiple components, including regulatory and catalytic subunits of guanylate cyclase

Increased Guanylate Cyclase Activity

FIGURE 4. Proposed mechanism(s) of action of *E. coli* ST_a.

when animals were challenged with maximal doses of enterotoxin (1, 63–65, 94, 171). Indomethacin decreased the secretory affect of ST_a when administered to suckling mice (64), but had no effect in porcine jejunal segments (3). Chlorpromazine also decreased the secretory response of suckling mice to low doses of ST_a (138); however, the inhibition was later shown to be nonspecific (168). Quinacrine, a specific inhibitor of phospholipase A_2, decreased rat intestinal guanylate cyclase activity and ST_a-induced chloride secretion in suckling mice (63, 171). Also, inhibitors of calcium transport and calmodulin-mediated reactions (nifedipine, diltiazem, cromolyn sodium, lanthanum, and lodoxamide tromethamine) decreased the ST_a-mediated fluid response in suckling mice (171) and the release of histamine by rat basophilic leukemia cells (172). The α-adrenergic agonists clonadine, L-phenylephrine, and morphine reduced the secretory response induced by ST_a in perfused porcine jejunal segments and stimulated absorption in the normal porcine jejunum (4). Berberine also reduced the secretory response of porcine jejunal segments to ST_a and enhanced water and electrolyte absorption in control segments (186). Thus, a model was proposed that ST_a activated phospholipase A_2 with the subsequent release of arachidonic acid and synthesis of prostaglandins (62).

To test some of the pharmacological observations noted above, isolated rat intestinal cells and rat BBM were used to study activation of intestinal guanylate cyclase to avoid the complex cause-and-effect relationships observed with whole animals (36). Experiments with isolated rat intestinal cells supported previous data obtained with suckling mice; that is, quinacrine, a specific inhibitor of phospholipase A_2, and the cyclooxygenase inhibitor 5,8,11,14-eicosatetraynoic acid inhibited ST_a-induced formation of intracellular cyclic GMP. Several contradictory observations indicated that the effects were not specific for ST_a: (i) the rate of release of [^{3}H]arachidonic acid by prelabeled cells incubated with ST_a was identical to that of cells in reaction mixtures which did not contain ST_a; (ii) there were no major differences in the distribution of radioactivity in major classes of lipids extracted from intestinal epithelial cells incubated with ST_a compared with controls (no ST_a); and (iii) levels of prostaglandins E_2, $F_{2\alpha}$, and TXB_2 did not increase in supernatants of cells or BBM treated with ST_a.

Purified BBM were incubated with various pharmacological agents which inhibit prostaglandin biosynthesis. Without exception, bromophenacyl bromide, indomethacin, and 5,8,11,14-eicosatetraynoic acid inhibited both activation of guanylate cyclase by ST_a and basal levels of the enzyme assayed in the presence of either Mg^{2+} or Mn^{2+}. Since calcium has been proposed as a second messenger in stimulus-response coupling (25, 34), several pharmacological agents which inhibit calcium- or calmodulin-mediated reactions were incubated with BBM and other components of the guanylate cyclase reaction mixture. As observed with the anti-inflammatory agents, inhibitors of calcium–calmodulin-mediated reactions (trifluoperazine and chlorpromazine) and calcium channel blockers (verapamil and nifedipine) inhibited both basal and ST_a-stimulated guanylate cyclase activity associated with BBM.

Free radicals activate soluble guanylate cyclase, and the activity of both soluble and particulate guanylate cyclase depends on vicinal thiol groups at the active site (18). Enzymatic activity may also be regulated by the oxidation state of the enzyme; thus, the role of molecular oxygen in the ST_a-induced activation of guanylate cyclase was examined. When argon was substituted for air, the guanylate cyclase activity associated with BBM and induced by ST_a was identical to that in the air atmosphere. Other potential stimulus-secretion response mechanisms have also been eliminated from consideration as a mechanism of action of ST_a, e.g., (i) methylation and demethylation of membrane phospholipids, (ii) phosphorylation coupled with dephosphorylation, and (iii) activation of phospholipase C measured by the turnover of phosphatidylinositol.

Several lines of evidence suggest that a thiol-disulfide exchange reaction may be the first in a series of reactions leading to activation of particulate guanylate cyclase: (i) reduction of the disulfide bonds of ST_a destroys all biological activity (8, 35, 158); (ii) thiols and disulfides reduce the secretory response of ST_a in suckling mice (61); (iii) thiol-reactive compounds [cysteine, N-ethylmaleimide, and 5,5'dithio-bis(2-nitrobenzoic acid)] inhibit the binding of ST_a to BBM (36); and (iv) ST_a receptor bound to ST_a affinity columns is eluted only with 4 M urea containing 50 mM dithiothreitol (L. Jaso-Friedmann and D. C. Robertson, unpublished observations).

Properties of Detergent-Solubilized ST_a Receptor

The ST_a receptor and guanylate cyclase might exist as a single transmembrane protein or as separate proteins in a complex containing regulatory proteins analogous to the adenylate cyclase system. To distinguish between the two mechanisms, both activities were extracted from brush border membranes by using several detergents (37; Jaso-Friedmann et al., in preparation). The zwitterionic detergent 3-[(3-cholamidopropyl)dimethylammonio]-1-propane sulfonate (CHAPS) solubilized about 50% of the ST_a receptor and guanylate cyclase activities without nonspecific activation of guanylate cyclase. CHAPS detergent exhibits the high critical micelle concentration and low aggregation number typical of bile salt detergents without having the denaturing effects of ionic detergents (75). The complex formed between ^{125}I-labeled ST_a and its receptor did not dissociate when treated at room temperature with high salt concentrations, chaotropic agents, or detergents. Boiling in the presence of 1% sodium dodecyl sulfate or incubation with sodium dodecyl sulfate–50 mM dithiothreitol resolved ^{125}I-labeled ST_a from its receptor (37). The ^{125}I-labeled ST_a-receptor complex migrated during sodium dodecyl sulfate-polyacrylamide gel electrophoresis with a mobility corresponding to about 100,000 Da.

Detergent extracts of rat BBM have been fractionated on the basis of size, guanylate cyclase activity, ion-exchange chromatography, and ST_a-affinity columns in an attempt to resolve the two activities (L. Jaso-Friedmann, M. Chakrabarti, and D. C. Robertson, manuscript in preparation). Fractionation of detergent extracts of BBM on 5 to 20% sucrose density gradients (Fig. 5) and gel filtration on Superose 12 columns (FPLC; Pharmacia, Inc.) did not separate ST_a receptor and guanylate cyclase activities. Results presented in Fig. 5 show that the ST_a receptor and guanylate cyclase comigrated at a rate corresponding to a molecular weight of 135,000. Similar results were obtained by using a mono-Q anion-exchange col-

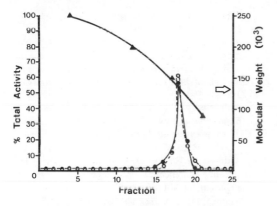

FIGURE 5. Sucrose density gradient fractionation of the CHAPS-soluble fraction of rat BBM. For details on the preparation of detergent extract, see reference 37. Samples (0.3 ml) of detergent extract were applied to 11.2-ml sucrose gradients (5 to 20%) containing 10 mM HEPES (*N*-2-hydroxyethylpiperazine-*N'*-2-ethanesulfonic acid; pH 7.4) and 2.5 mM CHAPS. Marker proteins (▲) were catalase (250 kDa), β-amylase (200 kDa), alcohol dehydrogenase (150 kDa), and bovine serum albumin (67 kDa). Fractions were collected and assayed for A_{280}, ST_a receptor activity, and guanylate cyclase activity. Symbols: ○, ST_a receptor activity; ●, guanylate cyclase activity.

TABLE 6
Affinity chromatography of ST_a receptor

Elution conditions	ST_a receptor activity eluted (%)
Run buffer[a]	7–20[b]
Run buffer–50 mM DTT[c]	<1.0
Run buffer–4 M urea	<1.0
Run buffer–4 M urea–50 mM DTT ...	22.7
Run buffer–3 M MgCl₂	<1.0
0.05 M sodium acetate (pH 4.5)–1 M NaCl–5 mM CHAPS	<1.0
0.05 M Na₂CO₃ (pH 11.0)–0.5 M NaCl–50 mM DTT–5 mM CHAPS	<1.0

[a]Run buffer is composed of 10 mM Tris hydrochloride, 150 mM NaCl, 2.5 mM CHAPS, and 25% propylene glycol.
[b]Range of ST_a receptor activity which did not bind to the column during five runs.
[c]DTT, Dithiothreitol.

umn, concanavalin A-Sepharose, and GTP-affinity columns. Results with GTP-affinity columns were complicated by the low recoveries of guanylate cyclase activity. Guanylate cyclase is a labile enzyme associated either with BBM or with detergent extracts. Activity is completely lost by incubation at room temperature for 10 min. Several storage conditions were tested and did not improve stability properties at 4°C (e.g., GTP, protease inhibitors, divalent cations, reducing agents, and EDTA). Stability was improved by addition of 20% glycerol or propylene glycol.

The ST_a receptor is present in low numbers on surfaces of intestinal cells (about 50,000 ST_a receptors per cell), and a specific affinity column would facilitate purification. Affinity columns of ST_a covalently linked to Affi-Gel 15 (Bio-Rad Laboratories, Richmond, Calif.) were used to purify and characterize the ST_a receptor (Jaso-Friedmann and Robertson, unpublished observations). In a typical experiment, 80 to 95% of the ST_a receptor activity bound to the affinity column and was not eluted by conditions used to isolate hormone receptors (Table 6). The ST_a receptor could be recovered in about 20% yield by elution with 4 M urea containing 50 mM dithiothreitol. Fractions containing receptor activity were dialyzed overnight against run buffer to remove urea and were concentrated 10-fold for assay. The specificity of the ST_a column was shown by reducing toxin bound to the gel with dithiothreitol followed by reaction with iodoacetic acid. Less than 1% of the receptor activity was retained by the carboxymethyl-ST_a-affinity column. In contrast to ST_a receptor activity, guanylate cyclase activity was not retained by the ST_a-affinity column. Thus, the bulk of the evidence favors a single transmembrane protein containing ST_a receptor and guanylate cyclase activity, yet data from the ST_a-affinity column and other sources (99, 178) suggest that the two activities are associated with distinct membrane proteins.

More work is necessary to understand the interactions of the ST_a receptor and guanylate cyclase and to establish the mechanism of action of *E. coli* ST_a. It is likely that each membrane component will have to be purified and reconstituted in liposomes to study the reaction mechanism as it occurs in the membrane. The ST_a receptor may exist in two forms, one covalently linked to guanylate cyclase and a second in which the enzyme is not covalently associated with guanylate cyclase, as found with the atrial natriuretic factor receptor purified from bovine adrenal cortex (166). Alternatively, the ST_a receptor and guanylate cyclase proteins may form a stable complex in membranes owing to hydrophobic interactions that are not disrupted by detergents which maintain the biological activity of each component. The solubilized form of guanylate cyclase is not stimulated by ST_a; thus, a critical component may have been left behind in the membranes or inactivated when the ST_a receptor and guanylate cyclase were solubilized from BBM. The next few years will probably bring exciting developments in studies on the mechanism of stimulation of guanylate cyclase by ST_a, much like the adenylate cyclase system in the late 1970s.

ACKNOWLEDGMENTS.   This research was supported by Public Health Service grant AI-12357 under the U.S.-Japan Cooperative Medical Science Program administered by the National Institute of Allergy and Infectious Diseases.

I thank Sharon Mason for secretarial assistance and for typing the manuscript.

LITERATURE CITED

1. Abbey, D. M., and F. C. Knoop. 1979. Effect of chlorpromazine on the secretory activity of *Escherichia coli* heat-stable enterotoxin. *Infect. Immun.* 26:1000–1003.

2. Adam, A. 1923. Uber die Biologie der Dyspepsie coli und ihre Bezhiehung zur Pathogenese der Dyspepsie und Intoxikation. *J. Kinderheilk.* (Berlin) 3. F. LI:295–314.

3. Ahrens, F. A., and B. Zhu. 1982. Effects of indomethacin, acetazolamide, ethacrynate sodium, and atropine on intestinal secretion mediated by *Escherichia coli* heat-stable enterotoxin in pig jejunum. *Can. J. Physiol. Pharmacol.* 60:1281–1286.

4. Ahrens, F. A., and B. L. Zhu. 1982. Effects of epinephrine, clonidine, L-phenylephrine, and morphine on intestinal secretion mediated by *Escherichia coli* heat-stable enterotoxin in pig jejunum. *Can. J. Physiol. Pharmacol.* 60:1680–1685.

5. Aimoto, S., T. Takao, Y. Shimonishi, S. Hara, T. Takeda, Y. Takeda, and T. Miwatani. 1982. Amino acid sequence of heat-stable enterotoxin pro-

duced by human enterotoxigenic *Escherichia coli. Eur. J. Biochem.* 129:257–263.

6. Alderete, J. F., and D. C. Robertson. 1977. Nutrition and enterotoxin synthesis by enterotoxigenic strains of *Escherichia coli:* defined medium for production of heat-stable enterotoxin. *Infect. Immun.* 15:781–788.

7. Alderete, J. F., and D. C. Robertson. 1977. Repression of heat-stable enterotoxin and synthesis in enterotoxigenic *Escherichia coli. Infect. Immun.* 17:629–633.

8. Alderete, J. F., and D. C. Robertson. 1978. Purification and chemical characterization of the heat-stable enterotoxin produced by porcine strains of enterotoxigenic *Escherichia coli. Infect. Immun.* 19:1021–1030.

9. Alouf, J. E. 1982. Bacterial toxins: an outlook. *Toxicon* 20:211–216.

10. Arita, M., T. Takeda, T. Honda, and T. Miwatani. 1986. Purification and characterization of *Vibrio cholerae* non-O1 heat-stable enterotoxin. *Infect. Immun.* 52:45–49.

11. Baldini, M. M., J. B. Kaper, M. M. Levine, D. C. A. Candy, and H. W. Moon. 1983. Plasmid-mediated adhesin in enteropathogenic *Escherichia coli. J. Pediatr. Gastroenterol. Nutr.* 2:534–538.

12. Banwell, J. G. 1973. Effect of bacterial enterotoxins on the gastrointestinal tract. *Gastroenterology* 64:467–497.

13. Belisle, B. W., E. M. Twiddy, and R. K. Holmes. 1984. Monoclonal antibodies with an expanded repertoire of specificities and potent neutralizing activity for *Escherichia coli* heat-labile enterotoxin. *Infect. Immun.* 46:759–764.

14. Belisle, B. W., E. M. Twiddy, and R. K. Holmes. 1984. Characterization of monoclonal antibodies to heat-labile enterotoxin encoded by a plasmid from a clinical isolate of *Escherichia coli. Infect. Immun.* 43:1027–1032.

15. Bergdoll, M. 1983. Enterotoxins, p. 559–598. *In* C. Easman and C. Adlam (ed.), *Staphylococci and Staphylococcal Infections,* vol. II. Academic Press, Inc., New York.

16. Boseman-Finkelstein, M., and R. A. Finkelstein. 1982. Protection in rabbits induced by the Texas star-SR attenuated A^-B^+ mutant candidate live oral cholera vaccine. *Infect. Immun.* 36:221–226.

17. Bosworth, T. J. 1943. On a new type of toxin produced by *Clostridium welchii. J. Comp. Pathol.* 53:245–255.

18. Brandwein, H. J., J. A. Lewicki, and F. Murad. 1981. Reversible inactivation of guanylate cyclase by mixed disulfide formation. *J. Biol. Chem.* 256:2958–2962.

19. Brown, J. E., T. G. Obrig, M. A. Ussery, and T. P. Moran. 1986. Shiga toxin from *Shigella dysenteriae* 1 inhibits protein synthesis in reticulocyte

lysates by inactivation of aminoacyl-tRNA binding. *Microb. Pathogenesis* 1:325–334.

20. **Burgess, M. N., R. J. Bywater, C. M. Cowley, N. A. Mullan, and P. M. Newsome.** 1978. Biological evaluation of a methanol-soluble, heat-stable *Escherichia coli* enterotoxin in infant mice, pigs, rabbits, and calves. *Infect. Immun.* 21:526–531.

21. **Buxser, S., and P. F. Bonventre.** 1981. Staphylococcal enterotoxins fail to disrupt membrane integrity or synthetic functions of Henle 407 intestinal cells. *Infect. Immun.* 31:929–934.

22. **Cassel, D., and T. Pfeuffer.** 1978. Mechanism of cholera toxin action: covalent modification of the guanyl nucleotide-binding protein of the adenylate cyclase system. *Proc. Natl. Acad. Sci. USA* 75:2669–2673.

23. **Chakaborty, T., M. A. Montenegro, S. C. Sanyal, R. Helmuth, E. Bulling, and K. N. Timmis.** 1984. Cloning of enterotoxin gene from *Aeromonas hydrophila* provides conclusive evidence of production of a cytotonic enterotoxin. *Infect. Immun.* 46:435–441.

24. **Chang, T.-W., J. G. Bartlett, and N. M. Sullivan, and T. D. Wilkins.** 1986. *Clostridium difficile* toxin, p. 571–580. *In* F. Dorner and J. Drews (ed.), *International Encyclopedia of Pharmacology and Therapeutics*, sect. 119. *Pharmacology of Bacterial Toxins*. Pergamon Press, Inc., Elmsford, N.Y.

25. **Cheung, W. Y.** 1982. Calmodulin: an overview. *Fed. Proc.* 41:2253–2257.

26. **Chopra, A. K., C. W. Houston, C. T. Genaux, J. D. Dixon, and A. Kurosky.** 1986. Evidence for production of an enterotoxin and cholera toxin cross-reactive factor by *Aeromonas hydrophila*. *J. Clin. Microbiol.* 24:661–664.

27. **Clements, J. D., and R. A. Finkelstein.** 1978. Immunological cross-reactivity between a heat-labile enterotoxin(s) of *Escherichia coli* and subunits of *Vibrio cholerae* enterotoxin. *Infect. Immun.* 21:1036–1039.

28. **Clements, J. D., and R. A. Finkelstein.** 1978. Demonstration of shared and unique immunological determinants in enterotoxins from *Vibrio cholerae* and *Escherichia coli* cultures. *Infect. Immun.* 22:709–713.

29. **Clements, J. D., and R. A. Finkelstein.** 1979. Isolation and characterization of homogeneous heat-labile enterotoxins with high specific activity from *Escherichia coli* cultures. *Infect. Immun.* 24:760–769.

30. **Clements, J. D., R. J. Yancey, and R. A. Finkelstein.** 1980. Properties of homogeneous heat-labile enterotoxin from *Escherichia coli*. *Infect. Immun.* 23:91–97.

31. **Cravioto, A., S. M. Scotland, and B. Rowe.** 1982. Hemagglutination activity and colonization factor antigens I and II in enterotoxigenic and non-enterotoxigenic strains of *Escherichia coli* isolated from humans. *Infect. Immun.* 36:189–197.

32. **de Jonge, H. R.** 1984. The mechanism of action of *Escherichia coli* heat-stable toxin. *Biochem. Soc. Trans.* 12:180–184.

33. **Dohlman, H. G., M. C. Caron, and R. J. Lefkowitz.** 1987. A family of receptors coupled to guanine nucleotide regulatory proteins. *Biochemistry* 26:2657–2664.

34. **Donowitz, M., and J. L. Madara.** 1982. Effect of extracellular calcium depletion on epithelial structure and function in rabbit ileum: a model for selective crypt or villus epithelial cell damage and suggestion of secretion by villus epithelial cells. *Gastroenterology* 83:1231–1243.

35. **Dreyfus, L. A., J. C. Frantz, and D. C. Robertson.** 1983. Chemical properties of heat-stable enterotoxins produced by enterotoxigenic *Escherichia coli* of different host origins. *Infect. Immun.* 42:539–548.

36. **Dreyfus, L. A., L. Jaso-Friedmann, and D. C. Robertson.** 1984. Characterization of the mechanism of action of *Escherichia coli* heat-stable enterotoxin. *Infect. Immun.* 44:493–501.

37. **Dreyfus, L. A., and D. C. Robertson.** 1984. Solubilization and partial characterization of the intestinal receptor for *Escherichia coli* heat-stable enterotoxin. *Infect. Immun.* 46:537–543.

38. **Duguid, J. P., and D. C. Old.** 1980. Adhesive properties of enterobacteriaceae, p. 185–218. *In* E. Beachey (ed.), *Bacterial Adherence, Receptors and Recognition*, series B, vol. 6. Chapman & Hall, Ltd., London.

39. **Evans, D. G., and D. J. Evans, Jr.** 1978. New surface-associated heat-labile colonization factor antigen (CFA/II) produced by enterotoxigenic *Escherichia coli* of serogroups O6 and O8. *Infect. Immun.* 21:638–648.

40. **Evans, D. G., D. J. Evans, Jr., and N. F. Pierce.** 1973. Differences in the response of rabbit small intestine to heat-labile and heat-stable enterotoxins of *Escherichia coli*. *Infect. Immun.* 7:873–880.

41. **Evans, D. J., D. G. Evans, H. L. DuPont, F. Ørskov, and I. Ørskov.** 1977. Patterns of loss of enterotoxigenicity by *Escherichia coli* isolated from adults with diarrhea: suggestive evidence for an interrelationship with serotype. *Infect. Immun.* 17:105–111.

42. **Field, M., L. H. Graf, Jr., W. J. Laird, and P. L. Smith.** 1978. Heat-stable enterotoxin of *Escherichia coli*: in vitro effects on guanylate cyclase activity, cyclic GMP concentration, and ion transport in small intestine. *Proc. Natl. Acad. Sci. USA* 75:2800–2804.

43. **Finkelstein, R. A.** 1973. Cholera. *Crit. Rev. Microbiol.* 2:553–623.

44. **Finkelstein, R. A., M. Boseman, S. H. Neoh, M. LaRue, and R. Delaney.** 1974. Dissociation

and recombination of the subunits of cholera entero-toxin (choleragen). *J. Immunol.* 113:145–150.

45. Finkelstein, R. A., M. F. Burks, A. Zupan, W. S. Dallas, C. O. Jacob, and D. S. Ludwig. 1987. Epitopes of the cholera family of enterotoxins. *Rev. Infect.Dis.* 9:544–561.

46. Finkelstein, R. A., and F. Dorner. 1985. Cholera enterotoxin (choleragen). *Pharmacol. Ther.* 27:34–47.

47. Frantz, J. C., L. Jaso-Friedmann, and D. C. Robertson. 1984. Binding of *Escherichia coli* heat-stable enterotoxin to rat intestinal cells and brush border membranes. *Infect. Immun.* 43:622–630.

48. Frantz, J. C., and D. C. Robertson. 1981. Immunological properties of *Escherichia coli* heat-stable enterotoxins: development of a radioimmunoassay specific for heat-stable enterotoxins with suckling mouse activity. *Infect. Immun.* 33:193–198.

49. Freer, J. A., and J. P. Arbuthnott. 1983. Toxins of *Staphylococcus aureus*. *Pharmacol. Ther.* 19:55–106.

50. Freter, R. 1978. Association of enterotoxigenic bacteria with the mucosa of the small intestine: mechanisms and pathogenic implications, p. 155–170. *In* O. Ouchterlony and J. Holmgren (ed.), *Cholera and Related Diarrheas*. S. Karger, Basel.

51. Gaastra, W., and F. de Graaf. 1982. Host-specific fimbrial adhesins of noninvasive enterotoxigenic *Escherichia coli* strains. *Microbiol. Rev.* 46:129–161.

52. Garbers, D. L., and E. W. Radany. 1981. Characteristics of the soluble and particulate forms of guanylate cyclase. *Adv. Cyclic Nucleotide Res.* 14:241–254.

53. Gardner, J. D. 1979. Receptors for gastrointestinal hormones. *Gastroenterology* 76:202–214.

54. Gariepy, J., A. Lane, F. Frayman, D. Wilbur, W. Robien, G. K. Schoolnik, and O. Jardetsky. 1986. Structure of the toxic domain of the *Escherichia coli* heat-stable enterotoxin ST I. *Biochemistry* 25:7854–7866.

55. Giannella, R. A. 1981. Pathogenesis of acute bacterial diarrheal disorders. *Annu. Rev. Med.* 32:341–357.

56. Giannella, R. A., M. Luttrell, and M. Thompson. 1983. Binding of *Escherichia coli* heat-stable enterotoxin to receptors on rat intestinal cells. *Am. J. Physiol.* 254:G492–G498.

57. Gill, D. M., J. D. Clements, D. C. Robertson, and R. A. Finkelstein. 1981. Subunit number and arrangement in the heat-labile enterotoxin of *Escherichia coli*. *Infect. Immun.* 33:677–682.

58. Gilligan, P. H., and D. C. Robertson. 1979. Nutritional requirements for synthesis of heat-labile enterotoxin by enterotoxigenic strains of *Escherichia coli*. *Infect. Immun.* 23:99–107.

59. Gilligan, P. H., J. C. Brown, and D. C. Robertson. 1983. Immunological relationships between cholera toxin and *Escherichia coli* heat-labile enterotoxin. *Infect. Immun.* 42:683–691.

60. Gorbach, S. L., B. H. Kean, D. G. Evans, D. J. Evans, Jr., and D. Bessudo. 1975. Travelers' diarrhea and toxigenic *Escherichia coli*. *N. Engl. J. Med.* 292:933–936.

61. Greenberg, R. N., J. A. Dunn, and R. L. Guerrant. 1983. Reduction of the secretory response to *Escherichia coli* heat-stable enterotoxin by thiol and disulfide compounds. *Infect. Immun.* 41:174–180.

62. Greenberg, R. N., and R. L. Guerrant. 1981. *E. coli* heat-stable enterotoxin. *Pharmacol. Ther.* 13:507–531.

63. Greenberg, R. N., R. L. Guerrant, B. Chang, D. C. Robertson, and F. Murad. 1982. Inhibition of *Escherichia coli* heat-stable enterotoxin effects on intestinal guanylate cyclase and fluid secretion by quinacrine. *Biochem. Pharmacol.* 31:2005–2009.

64. Greenberg, R. N., F. Murad, B. Chang, D. C. Robertson, and R. L. Guerrant. 1980. Inhibition of *Escherichia coli* heat-stable enterotoxin by indomethacin and chlorpromazine. *Infect. Immun.* 29:908–913.

65. Greenberg, R. N., F. Murad, and R. L. Guerrant. 1982. Lanthanum chloride inhibition of the secretory response to *Escherichia coli* heat-stable enterotoxin. *Infect. Immun.* 35:483–488.

66. Griffiths, S. L., R. A. Finkelstein, and D. R. Critchley. 1986. Characterization of the receptor for cholera toxin and *Escherichia coli* heat-labile toxin in rabbit intestinal brush borders. *Biochem J.* 238:313–322.

67. Guandalini, S., M. C. Rao, P. L. Smith, and M. Field. 1982. cGMP modulation of ileal ion transport: *in vitro* effects of *Escherichia coli* heat-stable enterotoxin. *Am. J. Physiol.* 243:G36–G41.

68. Guarino, A., G. Capano, B. Malamisura, M. Alessio, S. Guandalini, and A. Rubino. 1987. Production of *Escherichia coli* ST_a-like heat-stable enterotoxin by *Citrobacter freundii* isolated from humans. *J. Clin. Microbiol.* 25:110–114.

69. Guerrant, R. L., J. M. Hughes, B. Chang, D. C. Robertson, and F. Murad. 1980. Activation of intestinal guanylate cyclase by heat-stable enterotoxin of *Escherichia coli*: studies of tissue specificity, potential receptor and intermediates. *J. Infect. Dis.* 142:220–228.

70. Guth, B. E. C., E. M. Twiddy, L. R. Trabulsi, and R. K. Holmes. 1986. Variation in chemical properties and antigenic determinants among type II heat-labile enterotoxins of *Escherichia coli*. *Infect. Immun.* 54:529–536.

71. Gyles, C. L. 1971. Heat-labile and heat-stable forms of the enterotoxin from *E. coli* strains enteropathogenic for pigs. *Ann. N.Y. Acad. Sci.* 176:314–316.

72. Gyles, C. L. 1974. Relationships among heat-labile enterotoxins of *Escherichia coli* and *Vibrio cholerae*. *J. Infect. Dis.* 129:277–283.

73. Gyles, C. L., and D. A. Barnum. 1967. *Esche-richia coli* in ligated segments of pig intestine. *J. Pathol. Bacteriol.* 94:189–194.

74. Hirst, T. R., J. Sanchez, J. B. Kaper, S. J. S. Hardy, and J. Holmgren. 1984. Mechanism of toxin secretion by *Vibrio cholerae* investigated in strains harboring plasmids that encode heat-labile enterotoxins of *Escherichia coli. Proc. Natl. Acad. Sci. USA* 81:7752–7756.

75. Hjelmeland, L. M. 1980. A nondenaturing zwitterionic detergent for membrane biochemistry: design and synthesis. *Proc. Natl. Acad. Sci. USA* 77: 6368–6370.

76. Hofstra, H., and B. Witholt. 1984. Kinetics of synthesis, processing, and membrane transport of heat-labile enterotoxin, a periplasmic protein in *Escherichia coli. J. Biol. Chem.* 259:15182–15187.

77. Hofstra, H., and B. Witholt. 1985. Heat-labile enterotoxin in *Escherichia coli:* kinetics of association of subunits into periplasmic holotoxin. *J. Biol. Chem.* 260:16037–16044.

78. Holmes, R., M. G. Bramucci, and E. M. Twiddy. 1979. Genetic and biochemical studies of heat-labile enterotoxin of *Escherichia coli,* p. 187–201. *In Proceedings of the 15th Joint Conference, U.S.–Japan Cooperative Medical Science Program.* Publication no. 80-2003. National Institutes of Health, Bethesda, Md.

79. Holmes, R. K., and E. M. Twiddy. 1983. Characterization of monoclonal antibodies that react with unique and cross-reacting determinants of cholera enterotoxin and its subunits. *Infect. Immun.* 42:914–923.

80. Holmes, R. K., E. M. Twiddy, and C. L. Pickett. 1986. Purification and characterization of type II heat-labile enterotoxin of *Escherichia coli. Infect. Immun.* 53:464–473.

81. Holmgren, J., P. Fredman, M. Lindblad, A.-M. Svennerholm, and L. Svennerholm. 1982. Rabbit intestinal glycoprotein receptor for *Escherichia coli* heat-labile enterotoxin lacking affinity for cholera toxin. *Infect. Immun.* 38:424–433.

82. Holmgren, J., and A.-M. Svennerholm. 1979. Immunological cross-reactivity between *Escherichia coli* heat-labile enterotoxin and cholera toxin A and B subunits. *Curr. Microbiol.* 2:55–58.

83. Honda, T., Y. Takeda, and T. Miwatani. 1981. Isolation of special antibodies which react only with homologous enterotoxins from *Vibrio cholerae* and enterotoxigenic *Escherichia coli. Infect. Immun.* 34:333–336.

84. Honda, T., T. Tsuji, Y. Takeda, and T. Miwatani. 1981. Immunological nonidentity of heat-labile enterotoxins from human and porcine enterotoxigenic *Escherichia coli. Infect. Immun.* 34:337–340.

85. Hsia, J. A., J. Moss, E. L. Hewlett, and M. Vaughn. 1984. ADP-ribosylation of adenylate cy-clase by pertussis toxin: effects on inhibitory agonist binding. *J. Biol. Chem.* 259:1086–1090.

86. Inoue, T., T. Kobayashi, Y. Fujisawa, Y. Kawamoto, and A. Miyama. 1984. Effect of heat-stable enterotoxins of *Escherichia coli* and *Yersinia enterocolitica* on cyclic guanosine 3',5'-monophosphate levels of cultured cells. *FEMS Microbiol. Lett.* 22:219–221.

87. Johnson, W. M., and C. Lior. 1986. Cytotoxic and cytotonic factors produced by *Campylobacter jejuni, Campylobacter coli,* and *Campylobacter laridis. J. Clin. Microbiol.* 24:275–261.

88. Katada, T., G. M. Bokoch, J. K. Northup, M. Ui, and A. G. Gilman. 1984. The inhibitory guanine nucleotide-binding regulatory component of adenylate cyclase: properties and function of the purified protein. *J. Biol. Chem.* 259:3568–3577.

89. Katada, T., and M. Ui. 1982. Direct modification of the membrane adenylate cyclase system by islet-activating protein due to ADP-ribosylation of a membrane protein. *Proc. Natl. Acad. Sci. USA* 79:3129–3133.

90. Keusch, G. T., and S. T. Donta. 1975. Classification of enterotoxins on the basis of activity in cell culture. *J. Infect. Dis.* 131:58–63.

91. Klipstein, F. A., and R. F. Engert. 1976. Partial purification of *Enterobacter aerogenes* heat-stable enterotoxin. *Infect. Immun.* 13:1307–1314.

92. Klipstein, F. A., R. F. Engert, and R. A. Houghten. 1983. Immunological properties of purified *Klebsiella pneumoniae* heat-stable enterotoxin. *Infect. Immun.* 42:838–841.

93. Klipstein, F. A., R. F. Engert, R. A. Houghten, and B. Rowe. 1984. Enzyme-linked immunosorbent assay for *Escherichia coli* heat-stable enterotoxin. *J. Clin. Microbiol.* 19:798–803.

94. Knoop, F. C., and D. M. Abbey. 1981. Effect of chemical and pharmacological agents on the secretory activity induced by *Escherichia coli* heat-stable enterotoxin. *Can. J. Microbiol.* 27:754–758.

95. Kohler, E. M. 1968. Enterotoxic activity of filtrates of *Escherichia coli* in young pigs. *Am. J. Vet. Res.* 29:2263–2274.

96. Konowalchuk, J., N. Dickie, S. Stavric, and J. I. Speirs. 1978. Comparative studies of five heat-labile toxic products of *Escherichia coli. Infect. Immun.* 22:644–648.

97. Kunkel, S. L., and D. C. Robertson. 1979. Factors affecting release of heat-labile enterotoxin by enterotoxigenic *Escherichia coli. Infect. Immun.* 23:652–659.

98. Kunkel, S. L., and D. C. Robertson. 1979. Purification and chemical characterization of the heat-labile enterotoxin produced by enterotoxigenic *Escherichia coli. Infect. Immun.* 25:586–596.

99. Kuno, T., Y. Kamisaki, S. A. Waldman, J. Gariepy, G. Schoolnik, and F. Murad. 1986.

Characterization of the receptor for heat-stable enterotoxin from *Escherichia coli* in rat intestine. *J. Biol. Chem.* 261:1470–1476.

100. Lai, C. Y. 1980. The chemistry and biology of cholera toxin. *Crit. Rev. Biochem.* 9:171–206.

101. Lallier, R., F. Bernard, M. Gendreau, C. Lazure, N. G. Seidah, M. Chretien, and S. A. St.Pierre. 1982. Isolation and purification of *Escherichia coli* heat-stable enterotoxin of porcine origin. *Anal. Biochem.* 127:267–275.

102. Lee, C. H., S. L. Moseley, H. W. Moon, S. C. Whipp, C. L. Gyles, and M. So. 1983. Characterization of the gene encoding heat-stable toxin II and preliminary molecular epidemiological studies of enterotoxigenic *Escherichia coli* heat-stable toxin II. *Infect. Immun.* 42:264–268.

103. Leppla, S. H. 1982. Anthrax toxin edema factor: a bacterial adenylate cyclase that increases cyclic AMP concentrations in eukaryotic cells. *Proc. Natl. Acad. Sci. USA* 79:3162–3166.

104. Levine, M. M. 1987. *Escherichia coli* that cause diarrhea: enterotoxigenic, enteropathogenic, enteroinvasive, enterohemorrhagic, and enteroadherent. *J. Infect. Dis.* 155:377–389.

105. Levine, M. M., J. B. Kaper, R. E. Black, and M. L. Clements. 1983. New knowledge on pathogenesis of bacterial enteric infections as applied to vaccine development. *Microbiol. Rev.* 47:510–550.

106. Levine, M. M., J. P. Nataro, H. Karch, M. M. Baldini, J. B. Kaper, R. E. Black, M. L. Clements, and A. D. O'Brien. 1985. The diarrheal response of humans to some classic serotypes of enteropathogenic *Escherichia coli* is dependent on a plasmid encoding an enteroadhesiveness factor. *J. Infect. Dis.* 152:550–559.

107. Levine, M. M., P. Ristaino, G. Marley, C. Smyth, S. Knutton, E. Boedeker, R. Black, C. Young, M. L. Clements, C. Cheney, and R. Patnaik. 1984. Coli surface antigens 1 and 3 of colonization factor antigen II-positive enterotoxigenic *Escherichia coli*: morphology, purification, and immune responses in humans. *Infect. Immun.* 44:409–420.

108. Lindberg, A. A., J. E. Brown, N. Stromberg, M. Westling-Ryd, J. E. Schultz, and K.-A. Karlsson. 1987. Identification of the carbohydrate receptor for Shiga toxin produced by *Shigella dysenteriae* type I. *J. Biol. Chem.* 262:1779–1785.

109. Lindholm, L., J. Holmgren, M. Wikstrom, U. Karlsson, K. Andersson, and N. Lycke. 1983. Monoclonal antibodies to cholera toxin with special reference to cross reactions with *Escherichia coli* heat-labile enterotoxin. *Infect. Immun.* 40:570–576.

110. Lockwood, D. E., and D. C. Robertson. 1984. Development of a competitive enzyme-linked immunosorbent assay (ELISA) for *Escherichia coli* heat-stable enterotoxin (ST$_a$). *J. Immunol. Methods* 75:295–307.

111. Madden, D. L., R. E. Horton, and N. B. McCullough. 1970. Spontaneous infection in germ-free guinea pigs due to *Clostridium perfringens*. *Lab. Anim. Care* 20:454–455.

112. Marchlewicz, B. A., and R. A. Finkelstein. 1983. Immunologic differences among the cholera/coli family of enterotoxins. *Diagn. Microbiol. Infect. Dis.* 1:129–138.

113. Marques, L. R. M., M. A. Moore, J. G. Wells, I. K. Wachmuth, and A. D. O'Brien. 1986. Production of Shiga-like toxin by *Escherichia coli*. *J. Infect. Dis.* 154:338–341.

114. McDonel, J. L. 1980. *Clostridium perfringens* toxins (type A, B, C, D, E). *Pharmacol. Ther.* 10:617–656.

115. Merson, M. H., F. Ørskov, I. Ørskov, R. B. Sack, I. Hug, and F. T. Koster. 1979. Relationship between enterotoxin production and serotypes in enterotoxigenic *Escherichia coli*. *Infect. Immun.* 23:325–329.

116. Moon, H. W. 1978. Mechanisms in pathogenesis of diarrhea—review. *J. Am. Vet. Med. Assoc.* 172:443–448.

117. Moon, H. W., E. M. Kohler, R. A. Schneider, and S. C. Whipp. 1980. Prevalence of pilus antigens, enterotoxin types, and enteropathogenicity among K88-negative enterotoxigenic *Escherichia coli* from neonatal pigs. *Infect. Immun.* 27:222–230.

118. Moon, H. W., and S. C. Whipp. 1971. Systems for testing the enteropathogenicity of *Escherichia coli*. *Ann. N.Y. Acad. Sci.* 176:197–211.

119. Morris, G. K., M. H. Merson, D. A. Sack, J. G. Wells, W. T. Martin, W. E. DeWitt, J. C. Feeley, R. B. Sack, and D. M. Bessudo. 1976. Laboratory investigation of diarrhea in travelers to Mexico: evaluation of methods for detecting enterotoxigenic *Escherichia coli*. *J. Clin. Microbiol.* 3:486–495.

120. Moss, J., and M. Vaughn. 1979. Activation of adenylate cyclase by choleragen. *Annu. Rev. Biochem.* 48:581–600.

121. Moss, J. M., J. C. Osborne, P. H. Fishman, S. Nakaya, and D. C. Robertson. 1981. *Escherichia coli* heat-labile enterotoxin: ganglioside specificity and ADP-ribosyltransferase activity. *J. Biol. Chem.* 256:12861–12865.

122. Meyers, L. L., F. S. Newman, G. R. Warren, J. E. Catlin, and C. L. Anderson. 1975. Calf ligated intestinal segment test to detect enterotoxigenic *E. coli*. *Infect. Immun.* 11:588–591.

123. Nalin, D. R., A. K. Bhattacharjee, and S. H. Richardson. 1974. Cholera-like toxin effect of culture filtrates of *Escherichia coli*. *J. Infect Dis.* 130:595–601.

124. Noda, M., I. Kato, F. Matsuda, and T. Mirayama. 1981. Mode of action of staphylococcal leukocidin: relationship between binding of ^{125}I-la-

beled S and F components of leukocidin to rabbit polymorphonuclear leukocytes and leukocidin activity. *Infect. Immun.* 34:362–367.

125. O'Brien, A. D., M. K. Gentry, M. R. Thompson, B. P. Doctor, P. Gemski, and S. B. Formal. 1979. Shigellosis and *Escherichia coli* diarrhea: relative importance of invasive and toxigenic mechanisms. *Am. J. Clin. Nutr.* 32:229–233.

126. O'Brien, A. D., and R. K. Holmes. 1987. Shiga and shiga-like toxins. *Microbiol. Rev.* 51:206–220.

127. Obrig, T. G., T. P. Moran, and J. E. Brown. 1987. The mode of action of Shiga toxin on peptide elongation of eukaryotic protein synthesis. *Biochem. J.* 244:287–294.

128. Olsson, E., and O. Soderlind. 1980. Comparison of different assays for definition of heat-stable enterotoxigenicity of *Escherichia coli* porcine strains. *J. Clin. Microbiol.* 11:6–15.

129. Ohashi, Y., and S. Narumiya. 1987. ADP-ribosylation of a M_r 21,000 membrane protein by type D botulinum toxin. *J. Biol. Chem.* 262:1430–1433.

130. Ohishi, I., and M. Miyake. 1985. Binding of the two components of C_2 toxin to epithelial cells and brush borders of mouse intestine. *Infect. Immun.* 48:769–775.

131. Ohishi, I., and S. Tsuyama. 1986. ADP-ribosylation of nonmuscle actin with component I of C_2 toxin. *Biochem. Biophys. Res. Commun.* 138:802–806.

132. Ørskov, F., and I. Ørskov. 1979. Special *Escherichia coli* serotypes from enteropathies in domestic animals and man. *Adv. Vet. Med.* 29:7–14.

133. Pappenheimer, A. M., Jr. 1977. Diphtheria toxin. *Annu. Rev. Biochem.* 46:69–95.

134. Peterson, J. W. 1986. *Salmonella* toxins, p. 227–234. *In* F. Dorner and J. Drews (ed.), *International Encyclopedia of Pharmacology and Therapeutics*, section 119. *Pharmacology of Bacterial Toxins.* Pergamon Press, Inc., Elmsford, N.Y.

135. Picken, R. N., A. J. Mazaitus, W. K. Maas, M. Rey, and H. Heyneker. 1983. Nucleotide sequence of the gene for heat-stable enterotoxin II of *Escherichia coli. Infect. Immun.* 42:269–275.

136. Rao, M. C., S. Guandalini, P. L. Smith, and M. Field. 1980. Mode of action of heat-stable *Escherichia coli* enterotoxin: tissue and subcellular specificities and role of cyclic GMP. *Biochim. Biophys. Acta* 632:35–46.

137. Riley, L. W., R. S. Remis, S. D. Helgerson, H. B. McGee, J. G. Wells, B. R. Davis, R. J. Herbert, E. S. Olcott, L. M. Johnson, N. T. Hargrett, P. A. Balke, and M. L. Cohen. 1982. Hemorrhagic colitis associated with a rare *Escherichia coli* serotype. *N. Engl. J. Med.* 308:681–685.

138. Robbins-Browne, R. M., and M. M. Levine. 1981. Effect of chlorpromazine on intestinal secretion mediated by *Escherichia coli* heat-stable enterotoxin and 8-Br-cyclic GMP in infant mice. *Gastroenterology* 80:321–326.

139. Robertson, D. C. 1978. Chemistry and biology of the heat-stable *Escherichia coli* enterotoxin, p. 115–126. *In* O. Ouchterlony and J. Holmgren (ed.), *Cholera and Related Diarrheas.* S. Karger, Basel.

140. Robertson, D. C., J. L. McDonel, and F. Dorner. 1985. *E. coli* heat-labile enterotoxin. *Pharmacol. Ther.* 28:303–339.

141. Ronnberg, B., J. Carlsson, and T. Wadstrom. 1984. Development of an enzyme linked immunosorbent assay for detection of *Escherichia coli* heat-stable enterotoxin. *FEMS Microbiol. Lett.* 23:275–279.

142. Ronnberg, B., T. Wadstrom, and H. Jornvall. 1983. Structure of heat-stable enterotoxin produced by a human strain of *Escherichia coli*: differences from the toxin of another human strain suggest the presence of compensated amino acid exchanges. *FEBS Lett.* 155:183–185.

143. Sack, R. B. 1975. Human diarrheal disease caused by enterotoxigenic *Escherichia coli. Annu. Rev. Microbiol.* 29:333–353.

144. Sack, R. B. 1980. Enterotoxigenic *Escherichia coli*. Identification and characterization. *J. Infect. Dis.* 142:279–286.

145. Saeed, A. M. K., N. Sriranganathan, W. Cosand, and D. Burger. 1983. Purification and characterization of heat-stable enterotoxin from bovine enterotoxigenic *Escherichia coli. Infect. Immun.* 40:701–707.

146. Sanyal, S. C. 1983. NAG vibrio toxin. *Pharmacol. Ther.* 20:183–202.

147. Scotland, S. M., N. P. Day, and B. Rowe. 1980. Production of a cytotoxin affecting Vero cells by strains of *Escherichia coli* belonging to traditional enteropathogenic serogroups. *FEMS Microbiol. Lett.* 7:15–17.

148. Shimonishi, Y., Y. Hidaka, M. Koizumi, M. Hane, S. Aimoto, T. Takeda, T. Miwatani, and Y. Takeda. 1987. Mode of disulfide bond formation of a heat-stable enterotoxin (ST_h) produced by a human strain of enterotoxigenic *Escherichia coli. FEBS Lett.* 215:165–170.

149. Shore, E. G., A. G. Dean, K. J. Holik, and B. R. Davis. 1974. Enterotoxin-producing *Escherichia coli* and diarrheal disease in adult travelers: a prospective study. *J. Infect. Dis.* 129:577–582.

150. Simpson, L. L. 1984. Molecular basis for the pharmacological actions of *Clostridium botulinum* type C_2 toxin. *J. Pharmacol. Exp. Ther.* 230:665–669.

151. Smith, H. W., and C. L. Gyles. 1970. The relationship between two apparently different enterotoxins produced by enteropathogenic strains of *Escherichia coli. J. Med. Microbiol.* 3:387–401.

152. Smith, H. W., and S. Halls. 1967. Observations by the ligated intestinal segment and oral inoculation methods on *Escherichia coli* infections in pigs, calves, lambs and rabbits. *J. Pathol. Bacteriol.* 93:499–529.

153. Smith, H. W., and S. Halls. 1967. Studies on *Escherichia coli* enterotoxin. *J. Pathol. Bateriol.* 93:531–543.

154. Smith, H. W., and S. Halls. 1968. The transmissible nature of the genetic factor in *Escherichia coli* that controls enterotoxin production. *J. Gen. Microbiol.* 52:319–334.

155. Smith, N. M., and R. B. Sack. 1973. Immunologic cross-reactions of enterotoxins from *Escherichia coli* and *Vibrio cholerae*. *J. Infect. Dis.* 127:164–170.

156. Smith, T., and M. L. Orcutt. 1925. The bacteriology of the intestinal tract of young calves with special reference to the early diarrhea ("scours"). *J. Exp. Med.* 41:89–106.

157. Smyth, C. J., P. Johnsson, E. Olsson, O. Soderlind, J. Rosengren, S. Hjerten, and T. Wadstrom. 1978. Differences in hydrophobic surface characteristics of porcine enteropathogenic *Escherichia coli* with or without K-88 antigen as revealed by hydrophobic interaction chromatography. *Infect. Immun.* 22:462–472.

158. Staples, S. J., S. E. Asher, and R. A. Giannella. 1980. Purification and characterization of heat-stable enterotoxin produced by a strain of *Escherichia coli* pathogenic for man. *J. Biol. Chem.* 255:4716–4721.

159. Stiles, B. G., and T. D. Wilkins. 1986. Purification and characterization of *Clostridium perfringens* iota toxin: dependence on two nonlinked proteins for biological activity. *Infect. Immun.* 54:683–688.

160. Svennerholm, A.-M., and M. Lindblad. 1985. G_{m1} ELISA method for demonstration of *Escherichia coli* heat-stable enterotoxin. *FEMS Microbiol. Lett.* 30:1–6.

161. Svennerholm, A.-M., M. Wikstrom, M. Lindblad, and J. Holmgren. 1986. Monoclonal antibodies to *Escherichia coli* heat-labile enterotoxins. Neutralizing activity and differentiation of human and porcine LTs and cholera toxin. *Med. Biol.* 64:23–30.

162. Takao, T., T. Hitouji, S. Aimoto, Y. Shimonishi, S. Hara, T. Takeda, Y. Takeda, and T. Miwatani. 1983. Amino acid sequence of a heat-stable enterotoxin isolated from enterotoxigenic *Escherichia coli* strain 18D. *FEBS Lett.* 152:1–5.

163. Takao, T., Y. Shimonishi, M. Kobayashi, O. Nishimura, M. Arita, T. Takeda, T. Honda, and T. Miwatani. 1985. Amino acid sequence of heat-stable enterotoxin produced by *Vibrio cholerae* non-O1. *FEBS Lett.* 193:250–254.

164. Takao, T., N. Tominaga, Y. Shimonishi, S. Hara, T. Inoue, and A. Miyama. 1984. Primary structure of heat-stable enterotoxin produced by *Yersinia enterocolitica*. *Biochem. Biophys. Res. Commun.* 125:845–851.

165. Takao, T., N. Tominaga, S. Yosimura, Y. Shimonishi, S. Hara, T. Inoue, and A. Miyama. 1985. Isolation, primary structure and synthesis of heat-stable enterotoxin produced by *Yersinia enterocolitica*. *Eur. J. Biochem.* 152:199–206.

166. Takayanagi, R., R. M. Snajdar, T. Imada, M. Tamura, K. N. Pandey, K. S. Misono, and T. Inagami. 1987. Purification and characterization of two types of atrial natriuretic factor receptors from bovine adrenal cortex: guanylate cyclase-linked and cyclase-free receptors. *Biochem. Biophys. Res. Comun.* 144:244–250.

167. Takeda, T., T. Honda, H. Sima, T. Tsuji, and T. Miwatani. 1983. Analysis of antigenic determinants in cholera enterotoxin and heat-labile enterotoxins from human and porcine enterotoxigenic *Escherichia coli*. *Infect. Immun.* 41:50–53.

168. Takeda, T., T. Honda, Y. Takeda, and T. Miwatani. 1981. Failure of chlorpromazine to inhibit fluid accumulation caused by *Escherichia coli* heat-stable enterotoxin in suckling mice. *Infect. Immun.* 32:480–483.

169. Tamura, M., K. Nogimori, S. Murai, M. Yajima, K. Ito, K. Katada, M. Ui, and S. Ishii. 1982. Subunit structure of islet-activating protein, pertussis toxin, in conformity with the A-B model. *Biochemistry* 21:5516–5522.

170. Taylor, I., and K. A. Bettelheim. 1966. The action of chloroform-killed enteropathogenic *Escherichia coli* on ligated rabbit-gut segments. *J. Gen. Microbiol.* 42:309–313.

171. Thomas, D. D., and F. C. Knoop. 1982. The effect of calcium and prostaglandin inhibitors on the intestinal fluid response to heat-stable enterotoxin of *Escherichia coli*. *J. Infect. Dis.* 145:141–147.

172. Thomas, D. D., and F. C. Knoop. 1983. Effect of heat-stable enterotoxin of *Escherichia coli* on cultured mammalian cells. *J. Infect. Dis.* 147:450–459.

173. Thomas, L. V., A. Cravioto, S. M. Scotland, and B. Rowe. 1982. New fimbrial type (E8775) that may represent a colonization factor in enterotoxigenic *Escherichia coli* in humans. *Infect. Immun.* 35:1119–1124.

174. Thompson, M., H. J. Brandwein, M. LaBine-Racke, and R. A. Giannella. 1984. Simple and reliable enzyme-linked immunosorbent assay with monoclonal antibodies for detection of *Escherichia coli* heat-stable enterotoxins. *J. Clin. Microbiol.* 20:59–64.

175. Thompson, N. E., M. Ketterhagen, M. Bergdoll, and E. J. Schantz. 1984. Isolation and some properties of an enterotoxin produced by *Bacillus cereus*. *Infect. Immun.* 43:887–894.

176. Tsuji, T., S. Taga, T. Honda, Y. Takeda, and T. Miwatani. 1982. Molecular heterogeneity of heat-labile enterotoxins from human and porcine enterotoxigenic *Escherichia coli*. *Infect. Immun.* 38:444–448.

177. Ueda, K., and O. Hayaishi. 1985. ADP-ribosylation. *Annu. Rev. Biochem.* 54:73–100.

178. Waldman, S. A., T. Kuno, Y. Kamisaki, L. Y. Chang, J. Gariepy, and P. O'Hanley. 1986. Intestinal receptor for heat-stable enterotoxin of *Escherichia coli* is tightly coupled to a novel form of particulate guanylate cyclase. *Infect. Immun.* 51:320–326.

179. Weikel, C. S., H. N. Nellans, and R. L. Guerrant. 1986. *In vivo* and *in vitro* effects of a novel enterotoxin, ST$_b$, produced by *Escherichia coli*. *J. Infect. Dis.* 153:893–901.

180. Whipp, S. C., H. W. Moon, and R. A. Argenzio. 1981. Comparison of enterotoxigenic activities of heat-stable enterotoxins from class I and class II *Escherichia coli* of swine origin. *Infect. Immun.* 31:245–251.

181. Woodin, A., and A. A. Wieneke. 1966. The interaction of leucocidin with the cell membrane of the polymorphonuclear leukocyte. *Biochem. J.* 99:479–492.

182. Wreggett, K. A. 1986. Bacterial toxins and the role of ADP-ribosylation. *J. Recept. Res.* 6:95–126.

183. Yamamoto, T., T. Tamura, and T. Yokota. 1984. Primary structure of heat-labile enterotoxin produced by *Escherichia coli* pathogenic for humans. *J. Biol. Chem.* 259:5037–5044.

184. Yamamoto, T., T.-A. Tamura, M. Ryoji, A. Kaji, T. Yokota, and T. Takano. 1982. Sequence analysis of the heat-labile enterotoxin subunit B gene originating in human enterotoxigenic *Escherichia coli*. *J. Bacteriol.* 152:506–509.

185. Yamamoto, T., and T. Yokota. 1983. Sequence of heat-labile enterotoxin of *Escherichia coli* pathogenic for humans. *J. Bacteriol.* 155:728–733.

186. Zhu, B., and F. A. Ahrens. 1982. Effect of berberine on intestinal secretion mediated by *Escherichia coli* heat-stable enterotoxin in jejunum of pigs. *Am. J. Vet. Res.* 43:1594–1598.

Chapter 16

Toxins as Virulence Factors of Gram-Positive Pathogenic Bacteria of Veterinary Importance

JOHN H. FREER

Department of Microbiology
University of Glasgow
Glasgow G11 6NU
Scotland

INTRODUCTION

The first attempts to demonstrate extracellular diffusible toxins (sepsins) in sterile culture broths were made by Klebbs in 1872, who proposed that chemical substances released by bacteria, sepsins, were responsible for the lesions caused by staphylococci. This was soon followed by suggestions by Koch and by Loeffler in 1884 that cholera and diphtheria were consequences of extracellular toxins produced by bacteria. Indeed, Loeffler showed that in experimental animals infected with the diphtheria bacillus, the lesions in the major organs were bacterium free and suggested that a diffusible poison was the likely explanation for the observed tissue damage. In the following year, Roux and Yersin isolated a crude protein fraction from old culture filtrates that was lethal for guinea pigs at low doses and, in what proved to be a remarkably accurate guess, suggested that this substance, which they referred to as a toxin, was a kind of enzyme (see reference 100 for a fuller account). This was the beginning of the era of bacterial toxinology, which has expanded to the present multidisciplinary subject in the intervening century.

Because of the diversity in structure, mode of action, specificity, and immunogenicity and the wide variation in the degree of detailed knowledge of different bacterial toxins, a precise definition is not possible, and we must fall back on the working definition suggested by Bernheimer in 1976 (12): "a collection of bacterial products whose principal common feature is their capacity to produce injury or kill when administered in relatively small quantities in living entities."

Bacterial toxins fall naturally into two broad classes: the so-called endotoxins of the gram-negative species, which consist of lipopolysaccharide cell envelope components, and the second group, consisting predominantly of protein and peptide toxins. The endotoxins are similar in terms of structure and mode of action in vivo; this has been the subject of much attention and is not considered further here. For a recent comprehensive review, see reference 64.

In the second group about 220 bacterial toxins have been described in the scientific literature up to 1986; they are extremely diverse in structure and mode of toxicity (J. E. Alouf, *in* M. Veron and L. le Minor, ed., *Traite de*

Bactériologie Médicale, in press). More than 100 were first described between 1979 and 1985, illustrating the pace of the subject under review. About 100 of the total number of toxins described are produced by species of gram-positive bacteria, many of which are important pathogens in animals other than humans. These toxins are the subject of this chapter. Except for the classical monotoxic diseases, such as botulism, tetanus, and staphylococcal food poisoning, evidence for an essential role for toxins in the pathogenesis of infection is often lacking or at best tenuous, since the etiology is usually complex and in most cases the pathogenetic process is multifactorial, often involving pathogens which produce more than one toxin or even involving more than one infecting species.

In this review I consider the important gram-positive genera in turn, describe the toxins produced by species pathogenic for animals, and discuss available data pertaining to their role in pathogenesis. Because of limitations on space, many aspects which warrant fuller discussion have been covered only superficially, but I have attempted to cite recent reviews in which more detailed consideration is given.

GENUS *BACILLUS*

Toxigenic species in the genus *Bacillus* include *Bacillus anthracis, Bacillus cereus, Bacillus subtilis, Bacillus thuringiensis, Bacillus alvei,* and *Bacillus laterosporus.*

B. anthracis

B. anthracis produces a single, multicomponent, lethal toxin and is responsible for anthrax, the once common and rapidly fatal disease of domestic livestock. The toxin is of major importance in this highly invasive disease, but pathogenesis is multifactorial, with the capsule playing a major role in virulence. Toxin is synthesized only in strains possessing a large plasmid (pX01) of 170 kilobase pairs, which can be eliminated by passage at $42.5°C$. Whether the plasmid contains both structural and regulatory genes for toxin production is not absolutely clear (71). However, the loss of plasmid together with toxigenicity after passage at the elevated temperature and the regaining of toxigenesis in cured strains coincident with transfer of the large plasmid from toxigenic strains established an absolute relationship between the two properties and provided a rational explanation for the creation of live attenuated vaccine strains (Pasteur strains) by growth at elevated temperatures as originally described by Pasteur (see reference 71).

Recently it has been established that the DNA coding region for capsule production, the other major virulence determinant in this bacterium, is located on a second, smaller plasmid (pX02) of 90 kilobase pairs (43).

The toxin consists of three clearly separable components, namely edema factor (factor I; EF), protective antigen (factor II; PA), and lethal factor (factor III; LF), which can be recovered separately from the culture medium by salting out and hydroxyapatite chromatography. EF is a nontoxic protein of M_r 89,000, which has potent intracellular calmodulin-dependent adenylate cyclase activity (58) but requires the presence of PA (a protein of M_r 85,000) for induction of elevated cyclic AMP levels in a variety of cell lines (e.g., CHO cells). Also, injection of PA along with EF is necessary for induction of edema in guinea pigs and rabbits. LF is a protein of M_r 83,000, which also requires coinjection of PA for lethal activity in experimental animals. Although LF is not generally cytotoxic in vitro, when injected with PA in the rat it rapidly causes pulmonary edema, and death can follow within 40 min. Following the suggestion of Molnar and Altenbern (73) that PA binds to tissue receptors and facilitates the activity of EF and LF, it now seems likely that anthrax toxin represents a novel type of complex toxin with structural characteristics similar to those of the so-called A-B toxins (e.g., diphtheria toxin, tetanus toxin, cholera toxin, etc.), which consist of an active (A) subunit (often catalytic) and a binding (B) subunit(s), which facilitates binding and entry

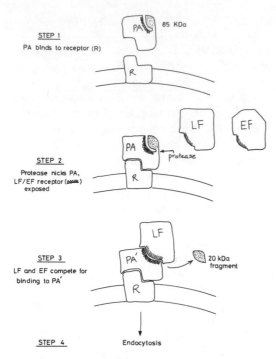

STEP 1
PA binds to receptor (R)

STEP 2
Protease nicks PA,
LF/EF receptor (⌇⌇⌇)
exposed

STEP 3
LF and EF compete for
binding to PA'

STEP 4
Endocytosis

FIGURE 1. Postulated roles of factor I (EF), factor II (PA), and factor III (LF) in the interaction of anthrax toxin with target cells. PA binds to its cell surface receptor (step 1) and is nicked by a cell surface protease (step 2). This results in the release of a 20-kilodalton fragment from PA, exposing a high-affinity receptor on PA' for either LF or EF (step 3). After competitive binding of either LF or EF to the binary complex on the membrane, the ternary toxic complex is internalized by endocytosis. Adapted from references 39 and 95 and S. H. Leppla, A. M. Friedlander, and E. M. Cora, personal communication.

of the A subunit to its intracellular target. Generally the A subunit is nontoxic alone and requires the B subunit for toxic activity in intact cells or experimental animals. It seems that in anthrax toxin, PA is functionally equivalent to the B, or binding, subunit of the A-B toxins, facilitating the binding and activation of either of two different A-type subunits, one being EF and the other being LF (Fig. 1). Inherent in this postulate is the possibility that EF and LF may compete for PA in terms of binding, the outcome of which would modulate their biological activities. This hypothesis

is in keeping with the experimental observations that (i) factor II is indeed a protective antigen and presumably elicits antibodies which block its own binding to receptors on target cells and/or block the binding of EF or LF or both to PA and that (ii) addition of LF to a mixture of EF and PA reduces the ratio of edema to lethality (for full discussion, see reference 95).

The kinetics of binary complex and ternary complex formation are not known and probably differ for different target cell receptors. Binding of the PA-EF complex to its receptor somehow facilitates the exposure of all or part of the EF on the intracellular surface of the cell in such a manner that it can be activated by intracellular calmodulin and calcium ions and thus catalyze the conversion of ATP to cyclic AMP. One of the consequences of such elevated levels of intracellular cyclic AMP, a powerful secretagogue, is edema, which manifests itself as a raised blister surrounding the necrotic black center of the lesion in the cutaneous form of the disease; hence the name malignant pustule.

The precise relationships and relative contributions of the various combinations of these three factors to virulence in the natural infection have yet to be defined, but there is no doubt that they are major virulence determinants, since mutants lacking these factors are avirulent (Pasteur strains). Recently, Leppla et al. (59) reported the cloning of PA from BamHI digests of plasmid pXO1 into Escherichia coli. Restriction analysis showed that the gene for PA was located on a 6-kilobase-pair fragment and was expressed in E. coli at a level about 10^3-fold less than in B. anthracis. However, extracts of E. coli harboring the recombinant plasmid contained a protein which cross-reacted immunologically with PA and, when combined with purified EF, induced elongation of CHO cells, indicating the presence of biologically active PA. In a second cloning experiment, immunological screening resulted in the isolation of two LF-positive clones and several that produced small amounts of EF. Cloning of these toxin genes will allow (i) further development of live vaccine strains with, for example, toxins inactivated by site-directed mutagenesis and (ii) elucidation of the mechanisms of control and expression of the toxin genes and the relative contribution of their products in the pathogenesis of anthrax.

Although the mode of action of LF is not understood, Freidlander (39) recently reported experiments on the mode of entry of the toxin into cells. In that study, LF-PA cytotoxicity for mouse peritoneal exudate macrophages was totally abrogated by amines or monensin, both of which dissipate proton gradients and result in elevated pH values in intracellular vesicles. Such results indicate that the lethal toxin is internalized via passage through an acidic endocytotic vesicle before exerting its toxic effects. This mechanism of entry via receptor-mediated endocytosis and entry into the cytoplasm from internal cell compartments is similar to the mechanisms which are thought to operate for several other bacterial toxins which exert their effects on intracellular targets (e.g., diphtheria toxin, Shiga toxin, *Clostridium difficile* toxin B, and *Pseudomonas* exotoxin A) (88).

B. cereus

B. cereus has been associated with a wide range of human lesions and diseases including abscesses, bacteremia and septicemia, cellulitis, ear and eye infections, endocarditis, gastroenteritis, meningitis, kidney and urinary tract infections, osteomyelitis, puerperal sepsis, pulmonary infections, and wound infections (for a review, see reference 99). It is also well recognized as a cause of bovine mastitis and has been identified as the causative agent in bovine abortion and caprine mastitis (53). It has been identified as a causative agent in food poisoning episodes in humans (see below) and has also been strongly implicated in similar episodes in dogs fed canned dog food which, upon bacteriological examination, was shown to be heavily contaminated with *B. cereus* and probably contained preformed toxin (D. Taylor, personal

communication). Wet sugar beet pulp fed to cattle and pigs and later shown to be heavily contaminated with *B. cereus* resulted in intoxication, presumably caused by preformed toxins, and was also associated with cases of abortion (Taylor, personal communication).

There are seven different toxins or toxic factors of *B. cereus* reported in the literature, five of which are clearly distinct toxins and two of which are possibly related to each other and in turn to the lethal toxin (Table 1).

Lethal Toxin

Partially purified lethal toxin (mouse lethal factor I) increases vascular permeability in rabbit or guinea pig skin when injected intradermally and causes fluid accumulation in ligated rabbit ileal loops. Necrosis also occurs at both sites as a result of large enough doses. Present evidence suggests that the lethal toxin is a protein of M_r ca. 50,000 which exists as two charge isomers of pI 5.1 and 5.6. Lethality for mice is thought to arise by direct cardiotoxic effects.

Emetic Toxin

Emetic toxin is a low-molecular-weight ($M_r < 10,000$) heat stable (survives autoclaving) toxin commonly associated with cooked-rice dishes contaminated with *B. cereus*. Some evidence suggests that it may be sporulation associated, occurring almost exclusively in serotype 1 strains, which have a highly heat-resistant spore. It induces emesis in monkeys and humans. Its significance in vomiting episodes in cats and dogs after consumption of food contaminated by *B. cereus* is not known.

Cereolysin

Cereolysin (mouse lethal factor II, hemolysin I) is one of a well-characterized group of SH-activated toxins (hemolysins), typified by streptolysin O (SLO) (see below), that share many properties and yet are produced by a relatively diverse group of bacteria (Table 2). The

TABLE 1
Toxins of bacilli[a]

Strain	Toxin
B. alvei	Alveolysin
B. anthracis	Anthrax toxin (EF, PA, LF)
B. cereus	Cereolysin O; hemolysin II, lethal toxin, emetic toxin, diarrheagenic toxin
B. laterosporus	Laterosporolysin
B. pumilu	Cytotoxin
B. sphaericus	Larvicidal toxin
B. subtilis	Surfactin
B. thuringiensis	
subsp. kurstaki and berliner	Crystal protoxin and active δ-endotoxin (larval), thuringiolysin, α-toxin
subsp. israelensis	Crystal protoxin and insecticidal toxin, cytolytic toxin
subsp. tenebrionis	Crystal protoxin and insecticidal toxin

[a]Abstracted from references 65 and 99 and from Alouf (in press).

common properties include lethality (cardiotoxicity) for animals; cytolysis of eucaryotic cells; necessity for prior reduction for biological activity; inactivation by oxygen or SH-group reagents; antigenic relatedness and stimulation of cross-reacting precipitating and neutralizing antibodies; inactivation by cholesterol and related 3-β-hydroxy sterols; and possible damage of cell membranes by interaction with sterols. All these toxins consist of single polypeptide

TABLE 2
SH-activated toxins of bacteria[a]

Strain	Toxin
Streptococcus types A, C, G	SLO[b]
S. pneumoniae	Pneumolysin[b]
B. cereus	Cereolysin[b]
B. thuringiensis	Thuringiolysin[b]
B. alvei	Alveolysin[b]
B. laterosporus	Laterosporolysin
C. bifermentans	Bifermentolysin
C. botulinum	Botulinolysin
C. histolyticum	Histolyticolysin
C. novyi type A	Edematolysin O
C. perfringens	Perfringolysin O[b]
C. septicum	Septicolysin
C. tetani	Tetanolysin[b]
C. chauvoei	Chauveolysin
L. monocytogenes	Listeriolysin[b]
K. pneumoniae	Hemolysin (?)

[a]Abstracted from reference 92 and from Alouf (in press).
[b]Purified to apparent homogeneity.

chains in the range 48 to 68 kilodaltons (the reduced form of cereolysin has M_r 55,000 and consists of 518 amino acid residues), with pIs ranging from 4.9 to 7.8 (cereolysin pI, 6.6), reflecting considerable differences in amino acid composition (for a review, see reference 92). Work with both erythrocytes and artificial membranes in the form of liposomes showed that lysis is accompanied by the formation of ring- and arc-shaped structures both on the membranes and released into the supernatants, which measure 35 to 38 nm in diameter. This feature is common to all SH-activated toxins examined so far, even those from the large sea anemone Metridium senile (14). (For a fuller discussion on the mechanism of membrane damage of this group of toxins, see the discussion of Streptococcus SLO below.)

There is no doubt that cereolysin is responsible for part of the lethal and cardiotoxic activity present in B. cereus culture supernatant that can be demonstrated in experimental animals. However, its contribution to the establishment of lesions in the cases of bovine mastitis attributable to this species is not clear (49). The ability of some SH-activated toxins (SLO, alveolysin, and perfringolysin) to induce leukotriene generation in human polymorphs, and thereby induce the inflammatory response (23), and to circulate as immune complexes (SLO), activating complement formation of C5b-9 assemblies on autologous cells (17), may be very relevant in this context if such properties are shared by all members of this class of toxins.

Hemolysin II

A second heat-stable hemolysin, distinct from hemolysin I (which is now known to be identical with cereolysin, being heat labile with no activity remaining after 2 min at 60°C), was described in some detail by Coolbaugh and Williams (28) following the earlier report by Fossum (34). Both were distinct from the phospholipases produced by this species. Hemolysin II has M_r 29,000 to 31,000 and shows the Arrhenius effect when heated (increasing inactivation up to 60°C and then decreasing inactivation between 70 and 100°C). It is not cholesterol sensitive and is acidic, with a pI of 5.3 (56). More recently, Chakraborty et al. (26) and Gilmore (41) cloned a hemolysin (cereolysin II or cereolysin AB) which consisted of two proteins of molecular mass 32.3 kilodaltons (component A) and 36.7 kilodaltons (component B). Component B was thought to be responsible for binding component A to membrane receptors, thus eliciting hemolysis. Exactly how this hemolysin relates to hemolysin II is not clear, although the relationship may resemble that found in *Staphylococcus aureus* gamma toxin, for which a two-component toxin was originally reported, although more recently it has been shown that there is one hemolysin which is potentiated by a second component, with very low hemolytic activity (see below for *S. aureus* γ-toxin and CAMP factor of *Streptococcus agalactiae*).

B. cereus also produces three phopholipases C which differ in substrate specificity, the best characterized, a zinc metalloenzyme, hydrolyzing a variety of glycerophosphatides. The other two are of very narrow substrate specificity, one being restricted to sphingomyelin and the other to phosphatidylinositol. However, although these enzymes may well be classed as aggressins, there is no convincing case for them to be regarded as toxins.

Apart from reports of possible toxemia and abortion mentioned above (53, 99) and well-documented cases of mastitis in cattle, there is a dearth of reports on natural *B. cereus* infections in animals other than humans. A notable exception is that of septicemia and death in a tiger, with this bacterial species being isolated in pure culture from blood and viscera post mortem (21).

B. thuringiensis

It is only by the presence of the parasporal crystal protein that *B. thuringiensis* can be differentiated from *B. cereus*. By all other criteria the two species are extremely closely related, if not identical. Indeed, *B. thuringiensis* produces a (mouse) lethal toxin, the so-called α-exotoxin, apparently identical to lethal toxin I of *B. cereus*. It also produces two hemolysins, one of which is SH activated (thuringiolysin) and belongs to the group typified by SLO. The other is thought to be equivalent to hemolysin II of *B. cereus*. The β-exotoxin is a nucleotide excreted into the medium during exponential growth but not produced by all strains (for a review, see reference 65).

The toxin of most interest, the δ-endotoxin, is that derived from the parasporal crystal protein after partial hydrolysis by enzymes in the insect gut. This is a lethal enterotoxin for larvae of members of the orders Lepidoptera and Diptera, which stop feeding and moving a few minutes after crystals are consumed. The histopathological changes in the midgut epithelium include swelling, with consequent shortening and vacuolation of microvilli, which eventually disappear in the swollen cells as they become progressively vacuolated. The endoplasmic reticulum and mitochondria eventually disintegrate, and the loss of vital function in the gut results in fluid imbalance and death. Toxins from different bacterial strains show different potencies against the same insect type, and larval species differ in susceptibility to δ-endotoxins from different bacterial serovars (66).

The crystal protein gene is usually carried on a large plasmid, but can occur as a second copy on the chromosome in a few strains and only on the chromosome in *B. entomocidus* and

B. dendrolimus strains. The gene has been cloned and sequenced by several groups. Lereclus et al. (60), in a structural analysis of crystal genes from several strains, showed that the crystal gene of strain *Berliner* was flanked by inverted repeats and suggested that this transposonlike structure might explain the ubiquity of the crystal gene in the different serotypes of *B. thuringiensis*.

The use of crystal suspensions or mixtures of viable spores and crystals as commercial biological control agents against insects is not seen as constituting any threat to animal or public health by licensing authorities, even though *B. thuringiensis* is capable of producing the α-exotoxin under appropriate conditions. Lack of toxicity per os leaves only the development of wound infection or septicemia as a possible consequential risk, and since neither *B. thuringiensis* nor *B. cereus* is significantly invasive (cf. *B. anthracis*), this risk is theoretically very low. Indeed, after extensive safety testing, both organisms have been declared noninfective in vertebrates by any route (see discussion in reference 99).

GENUS *CLOSTRIDIUM*

Species of the genus *Clostridium* constitute many of the most important animal pathogens and account for a wide range of animal diseases. Important pathogenic species include *Clostridium perfringens* types A, B, C, D, and E, *Clostridium botulinum*, *Clostridium tetani*, *Clostridium chauvoei*, *Clostridium difficile*, *Clostridium septicum*, *Clostridium novyi*, *Clostridium haemolyticum*, *Clostridium histolyticum*, *Clostridium sordellii*, and several other less-common pathogenic species such as *Clostridium spiroforme* and *Clostridium colinum*. The potential of each species to produce the various toxins is summarized in Table 3. Space does not allow consideration of each species in terms of the range of toxins produced. However, the main toxins of the genus are reviewed under *C. perfringens*, *C. botulinum*, *C. tetani*, and *C. difficile*.

C. perfringens

C. perfringens types A to E produce 13 different toxins (Table 3) and are responsible for or implicated in a wide variety of diseases in animals (Table 4).

C. perfringens α-Toxin

C. perfringens α-toxin was the first toxin recognized as an enzyme (phosphatidylcholine cholinephosphohydrolase; EC 3.1.4.3) (69). It is a zinc metalloenzyme, a phospholipase C stimulated by calcium ions that hydrolyzes sphingomyelin, phosphatidylcholine, phosphatidylethanolamine, phosphatidylserine, and the lyso derivatives of phosphatidylcholine and phosphatidylethanolamine, releasing water-soluble phosphorylamines and leaving the insoluble diacylglyceride in the membrane. Consequently the enzyme hydrolyzes most of the lipid species found in eucaryotic cell membranes and is lethal, necrotizing, hemolytic, and cytolytic. It is a protein of M_r 43,000 (404 amino acid residues) and pI 5.6 (Alouf, in press).

The hemolytic activity of α-toxin can be demonstrated easily against a variety of erythrocyte types (e.g., bovine or mouse erythrocytes) in vitro and is characterized by the hot-cold effect. This is a property shared with the sphingomyelinase of *S. aureus* (β-toxin) and is manifested by a large increase (several orders of magnitude) in the hemolytic zone (blood agar plates) or hemolytic titer (erythrocyte suspensions) when the temperature of the incubation mixture of toxin and eythrocytes is lowered below 10°C after an initial period of incubation at 37°C. This enhanced release of hemoglobin occurs as a result of temperature-induced destabilization of the membrane, already damaged by hydrolysis of substantial amounts of choline-containing phospholipids which are located exclusively in the outer leaflet of the membrane lipid bilayer. The lowering of temperature is one of several physical and chemical stresses causing lysis via disruption of the stabilizing interactions between cations and membrane lipids (93). Addition of zinc ions protects erythrocytes against the lytic activity of

TABLE 3
Toxins of clostridia[a]

Strain	Toxins
C. botulinum	Neurotoxins A, B, C1, D, E, F, C2 toxin (C2I and C2II), botulinolysin
C. difficile	Toxin A, toxin B
C. perfringens	β-Toxin, δ-toxin, ε-toxin, θ-toxin (perfringolysin), ι-toxin components A and B, enterotoxin
C. sordellii	Lethal toxin, hemorrhagic toxin
C. tetani	Tetanus neurotoxin (tetanospasmin), tetanolysin
C. septicum	α-Toxin, related to that of C. histolyticum and C. chauvoei, septicolysin
C. chauvoei	α-Toxin, SH-activated δ-toxin, chauveolysin
C. novyi	α-Toxin (edema inducing toxin); SH-activated δ-toxin (edematolysin), ε-toxin

[a]Abstracted from references 91 and 95 and from Alouf (in press).

α-toxin as well as numerous other cytolytic toxins (9).

Not surprisingly, α-toxin also damages membranes and alters behavior in a variety of cell types, including fibroblasts, muscle cells, and platelets. An early effect after application of α-toxin to rat mesentery was the occurrence of thrombi in small vessels, and this was thought to be a prelude to necrosis and possibly induction of toxemia in later stages of gas gangrene (for a review, see reference 67).

Apart from its almost certain involvement, along with other toxins and *Clostridium* species, in the disease syndrome of gas gangrene, the α-toxin is thought to be centrally involved in chicken necrotic enteritis caused by *C. perfringens* type A; enterotoxemias also occur in lambs, with accompanying symptoms of massive intravascular hemolysis and capillary wall destruction, a possible consequence of α-toxin activity. Ulcerative enteritis in quail and possibly in chickens as a result of type C strains, as well as enteritis in piglets, shares symptoms of villus tip necrosis and is thought to result in part at least from the activity of α-toxin (D. J. Taylor and A. E. Estrada, personal communication). However, the relative contribution of α-toxin and other potent toxins secreted by the clostridia during such diseases has yet to be defined.

TABLE 4
Some animal diseases caused by clostridia[a]

Strain	Disease
C. perfringens	
Type A	Enterotoxemia in cattle, sheep, and horses
Type B	Lamb dysentery (α, β, ε-toxins)
Type C	Struck (sheep) (α and β-toxins)
Type D	Enterotoxemia (sheep) (α and ε-toxins)
Type E	Associated with sheep and cattle diseases. Pathogenicity? (α and ι-toxins)
C. novyi	
Type A	Big head in rams (α, γ, and ε-toxins)
Type B	Black disease (sheep) (α, β, ζ, and η-toxins)
Type D	Redwater disease (bacilliary hemoglobinuria) in cattle (β, η, and θ-toxins)
C. septicum	Braxy (sheep) (α-toxin)
C. chauvoei	Blackquarter (sheep, cattle) (α-toxin)
C. colinum	Ulcerative enteritis (birds)
C. spiroforme	Enterotoxemia (rabbits)
C. sordellii	Enteritis and enterotoxemia (sheep and cattle) (lethal toxin and hemorrhagic toxin)

[a]Abstracted from references 80, 91, and 95.

C. perfringens β-Toxin

C. perfringens β-toxin is plasmid encoded and is found only in type B and C strains, which are important agents of enterotoxemias (lamb dysentery for type B strains and struck for type C strains) and necrotic enteritis in domestic animals. The toxin is partially characterized and is a single-chain protein of M_r 28,000 and pI 5.5; the minimal lethal dose for mice is ca. 4 μg, and the toxin is paralytic when injected intravenously. It is sensitive to trypsin, and the native toxin is dermonecrotizing in guinea pig skin and causes a pronounced hemorrhagic effect with severe necrosis of the villi and mucosa but no accumulation of fluid in ligated intestinal loops. The toxin had no effect on a range of cell lines except CHO cells, which were killed by 0.1 μg of toxin per ml, without any evidence of cytolysis (52).

The interpretation of previous work on β-toxin (and many of the other clostridial toxins) is problematical, owing to lack of stringency in defining purity. A comprehensive review has been written by McDonel (67). The trypsin sensitivity of the β-toxin is an important factor in destruction of the toxin in vivo and is likely to be highly relevant in cases of necrotic enteritis caused by type C strains in neonatal pigs and in pigs fed on soya-based protein supplements which contain natural anti-trypsin factors.

C. perfringens δ-Toxin

C. perfringens δ-toxin is produced by some strains of types B and C in exponential growth phase. It is a single-chain basic protein (pI, 9.1) of M_r 42,000, comprises 391 amino acid residues, and is lethal and hemolytic for erythrocytes of even-toed ungulates (4). It is selectively cytotoxic for a subpopulation of rabbit leukocytes and platelets from humans, horses, rabbits, and guinea pigs. The hemolytic activity is inhibited by GM2 ganglioside, which suggests that it is part of the receptor structure, although this has not yet been identified (25).

The role of δ-toxin in disease is poorly understood. Certainly, type C strains produce δ- and θ-toxins as well as β-toxin, and δ-toxin causes an acute fluid accumulation in guinea pig ileal loops. Although β-toxin is thought to be of paramount importance in necrotic enteritis, evidence for involvement of δ-toxin is still lacking.

C. perfringens ε-Toxin

C. perfringens ε-toxin is produced as an inative protoxin of 311 amino acid residues, M_r 35,600, and pI ca. 8.0 by type B and D strains and is activated by tryptic cleavage of the highly basic N-terminal peptide of 14 residues to yield a potent, lethal, and necrotizing toxin with pI ca. 5.5. It is responsible for a rapidly fatal enterotoxemia (pulpy kidney disease, overeating disease) of sheep and other herbivores suddenly supplied with a diet which apparently results in passage of undigested food into the intestine along with C. perfringens spores, which then germinate and grow, synthesizing protoxin. This is activated by intestinal proteases, thus generating active toxin. This enters the bloodstream and results in swollen hyperemic kidneys, lung edema, and pericardial fluid accumulation followed by death. The toxin also appears to cause brain intoxication by binding to the vascular endothelium (for a review, see ref. 67).

C. perfringens ι-Toxin

C. perfringens ι-toxin is restricted to type E strains, and early reports of its being a protoxin which needs activation by cleavage in a manner similar to ε-toxin have not been confirmed. Indeed, Stiles and Wilkins (96) and Simpson et al. (90) provide evidence that it is a two-component toxin, consisting of quite separate and nonrelated proteins (ι_a and ι_b) which act synergistically to yield active toxin that is lethal and dermonecrotizing. Their molecular weights are 47,500 to 48,000 and 67,000 to 71,500, respectively, and their pI values are 5.2 and 4.2, respectively. The ι_a component possesses ADP ribosylating activity against polyarginine, but the physiological acceptor has not yet been identified.

The toxin has been implicated in fatal enterotoxemias in calves, lambs and guinea pigs. It is interesting that *C. spiroforme* also produces an ι-like toxin, which can be neutralized by type E ι-toxin antiserum and is implicated as a causative agent of fatal enterotoxemia in ranched rabbits (46, 80).

C. perfringens θ-Toxin

C. perfringens θ-toxin (perfringolysin) belongs to the group of SH-activated toxins typified by SLO and is produced by all types of *C. perfringens* (see above for cereolysin of *B. cereus* and below for *Streptococcus* SLO). It is hemolytic, lethal, and necrotizing, has M_r 60,000, and contains 465 amino acid residues. The pI is about 6.9. Besides its effects on erythrocytes, it has a wide spectrum of activity against other cell types. Its primary membrane receptor appears to be cholesterol and other β-hydroxy sterols, and it produces clearly defined membrane lesions in a wide variety of cell types, as do the other members of this group of toxins when present in high enough concentration. However, it is still not clear whether the lesions bordered by the ring- and arc-shaped structures (as for SLO) seen in erythrocyte membranes treated with this class of toxins are the only type of lesion or indeed the most significant. Inoue et al. (51) claimed that θ-toxin requires only two or three hits to effect lysis, and Mitsui et al. (72) raised the estimate to seven. This is an order of magnitude below the estimated number of toxin monomers (70 to 80) present in the ring structures observed by electron microscopy on SLO-treated membranes (18). However, for SLO, calculations by Alouf and Raynaud (5) indicated that the minimum number of toxin molecules required for erythrocyte lysis was 114.

A precise role for θ-toxin in disease is not evident at present, but it seems inescapable to conclude that such a potent toxin with wide-ranging activities against mammalian cells, if produced in significant quantities in vivo, must play an important accessory role in the pathogenesis of clostridial infections (see below for SLO).

Enterotoxin

Enterotoxin is produced by type A, C, and D strains and is responsible for the diarrheagenic response. It is membrane damaging, cytoxic, and lethal and is produced in the gut in association with sporulation stages II and III. It is a precursor of spore coat protein and is produced in vast excess of requirements for sporulation in enterotoxigenic strains which are thought to be deregulated in production of this component. The toxin consists of a single peptide of 309 amino acid residues with M_r 34,262 and pI 4.3 (42). The brush border of the intestinal epithelial cells is the target for the toxin, and in rats a membrane protein receptor of 50,000 daltons is involved. After nicking and interaction with target cells, the toxin induces changes in permeability of the epithelial cells, in which the net uptake of sodium, chloride, and water is reversed, amino acid transport is inhibited, and the uptake of glucose is much reduced. The result is diarrhea (42) (see Chapter 15 of this volume).

In addition to the above toxins, *C. perfringens* produces a range of hydrolytic enzymes which are, in general, poorly defined in terms of toxicity. These include κ-toxin (collagenase), λ-toxin (protease), μ-toxin (hyaluronidase), and ν-toxin (DNase). These may more correctly be regarded as aggressins rather than toxins. It is well recognized that much of the previous work reporting toxicity or lethality in such enzymes may be accounted for by minor contamination with more potent and classical toxins of this species. Unless rigorous criteria for defining purity and freedom from other detectable toxins are applied, reports of toxicity in preparations of undefined purity must be regarded with suspicion.

C. botulinum

C. botulinum produces seven serologically related neurotoxins, A1, B, C1, D, E, F, and G. These are among the most potent toxins

known. Types C1 and D are coded for by lysogenic bacteriophages.

C. botulinum Type A to G Toxins

Toxins of types A, B, and D occur in
spoiled food as very high-molecular-weight
complexes (e.g., 900,000 for type A) which
have both toxic and hemagglutinating activity.
However, all these related neurotoxin types
consist of a common toxin component of approximately the same size. The reported molecular weights for the different serotypes are
as follows: type A, 145,000 (1,302 amino acid
residues); type B, 155,000 (1,322 residues);
type C1, 141,000; type D, 170,000; type E,
147,000 (1,317 residues); and type F, 155,000.

In addition to the neurotoxin component,
type C strains produce a second toxin, C2 toxin,
of M_r 141,000, which consists of two components, C2I and C2II, with molecular weight
51,000 and 90,000, respectively. The toxin has
mouse lethal and guinea pig erythemal and
hemagglutinating activity (78) and is a two-
component (A-B) toxin. The binding component (C2II) requires activation by nicking before it binds to the target cell receptor, and it
facilitates the binding and access of the A component (C2I) to its substrate, where it effects
the enzymatic transfer of an ADP-ribose moiety
to actin (77).

The botulinum neurotoxins are synthesized as single-chain inactive protoxins which
are cleaved during activation by clostridial proteases (except type E strains, which lack appropriate protease activity) to yield a heavy (M_r
ca. 100,000) and a light (M_r ca. 50,000) chain
linked by a disulfide bridge. The heavy chain
is thought to be a binding component and
competes with native toxin for binding, whereas
the light chain is thought to be equivalent in
function to the A component of the A-B toxins
exemplified by diphtheria toxin and cholera
toxin (for reviews, see reference 86 and Alouf
et al., in press). The catalytic activity of the
light chain (A component) and its substrate have
not yet been defined, although ADP-ribosylat-
ing activity in type C1 neurotoxin has recently

been reported (76). The toxin acts presynaptically at the neuromuscular junctions affecting
motor and parasympathetic nerves and results
in flaccid paralysis (cf. tetanus toxin). Although the molecular detail of its mode of action is not known, its site of action is presynaptic, and the action results in the inhibition
of calcium-dependent exocytosis of presynaptic
vesicles containing the neurotransmitter acetylcholine (86).

The disease in animals is often of spectacular proportions. Examples of mass deaths of
farmed trout as a result of ingestion of water
containing toxin derived from fish food carrying type E spores, which have germinated in
bottom sludge, have been described. Also, large-
scale deaths of farmed mink after ingestion of
food (low-grade animal offal, etc.) containing
type C toxin have occurred. Widespread outbreaks of type C botulism have also occurred
in wild duck populations after ingestion of fly
larvae containing toxin derived from rotting
carcasses. Similar spread of disease can occur
among cattle after ingestion of feed contaminated from carcasses of animals killed by type
D botulism. Broiler chickens may also be affected by type C botulism after ingestion of
spores in feed, etc.; the spores are thought to
germinate in the gut and release toxin which
may accumulate to critical levels in the gut as
a result of constant coprophagy. Such cases are
discussed in the excellent review by Sakaguchi
(86).

Cases of botulism in herbivores are thought
to occur via ingestion of preformed toxin in
contaminated pastures, particularly after alkaline fermentation of rotting vegetable matter.
Also, recent cases in herbivores have been reported after they had been fed with big-bale
silage, possibly contaminated with rotting carcasses of small rodents. The potency of this toxin
is illustrated in a recent report of a fatal case
of botulism in a dog that had swum in a lake
where an outbreak of the disease had occurred
in water fowl. Type C1 toxin was detected in
a serum sample taken from the dog after death
(102).

Botulinolysin

Botulinolysin, an SH-activated toxin belonging to the group described above for cereolysin and below for SLO, is also produced by *C. botulinum*, with properties similar to toxins in that group. Its role in disease, like that of C2 toxin, is not known.

C. tetani

C. tetani produces a single immunological species of neurotoxin of M_r 150,700, the genes of which have been cloned and sequenced (32). The peptide, of 1,315 amino acid residues, is often nicked by bacterial proteases when purified. Thiol reduction gives a light chain (M_r 52,288) and a heavy chain (M_r 98,300). The characteristics of in vitro binding and transmembrane channel-forming activity of the heavy chain are reviewed by Habermann and Dreyer (45). The disease is characterized by spastic paralysis due to blockade of inhibitory neurotransmitter (γ-aminobutyric acid and glycine) release at inhibitory neurons in the central nervous system, although the toxin can effect blockade at neuromuscular junctions also (local tetanus). It passes, by retrograde axonal transport of toxin-containing vesicles, along the motor nerve fibers from the neuromuscular junctions near the site of infection to the central nervous system, where it acts presynaptically, causing tetanic spasms. The disease in animals is characterized by spastic paralysis, and horses are highly sensitive to the neurotoxin, whereas it is rarely found in dogs or pigs and even more rarely in cats. Birds are also relatively resistant. Occurrence of the disease is associated mainly with contamination of castration wounds in cattle and lambs, umbilical infections in lambs, and vaginal infections in sheep. In contrast to the clear role of the neurotoxin in disease, that of the SH-activated toxin tetanolysin (compare cereolysin and SLO) produced by this species is not known, although like all toxins in this group, it is membrane damaging, cardiotoxic, and lethal in experimental animals.

C. difficile

C. difficile produces two toxins: toxin A, which is enterotoxic and lethal, causes fluid accumulation in ligated rabbit intestinal loops, and induces hemorrhagic diarrhea, and toxin B, which is lethal and highly cytotoxic for cultured mammalian cells but has no effect in ligated loops. The molecular weight of toxin A is 440,000, and subunits of 230,000, 41,000, and 16,000 have been reported. Toxin B has M_r 500,000 with subunits of 50,000 (Alouf, in press).

Although the biochemical basis for the activities of these toxins is not known, toxin B appears to act intracellularly and induces its uptake via receptor-mediated endocytosis through acidic vesicles (33). Toxin A has been found in dog, cat, and calf feces, and the organism has been strongly implicated in a natural disease (Taylor, personal communication) in hares and ulcerative colitis, which may have been induced by antibiotic therapy, in pigs (22).

C. sordellii

C. sordellii produces a lethal toxin of M_r 250,000 and pI 4.5, containing 2,179 amino acid residues, which cross-reacts immunologically with the cytotoxin (toxin B) of *C. difficile*. This species also produces a poorly characterized hemorrhagic toxin, which is associated with sporulation, is dermonecrotizing in guinea pig skin, and has caused acute hemorrhagic necrosis in the loop test. This species is the etiological agent of enteritis and enterotoxemia in sheep and cattle (81).

C. chauvoei

Although a number of toxins of *C. chauvoei* have been reported, they are as yet poorly characterized. However, they are likely to play significant roles in myelonecrotic diseases caused by this important pathogen, e.g., blackquarter in cattle and sheep. The α-toxin is thought to be the major toxin. It is lethal, necrotizing, and hemolytic and is reported to be similar to that of *C. septicum*. Early reports give a molecular weight of 27,000 (see reference 91).

Other Toxigenic Clostridia

Other toxigenic clostridia include the following. *C. septicum* causes braxy in sheep; this is an acute, fatal disease involving hemorrhagic inflammatory lesions in the abomasum and is preventable by vaccination with *C. septicum* toxoids. *C. novyi* produces a range of toxins and aggressins (enzymes) which include the lethal and necrotizing α-toxin produced by type A and B strains and the SH-activated δ-toxin produced by type A strains. The α-toxin, thought to be the most significant in pathogenesis, with lethal and edema-inducing activity resulting from endothelial damage (91), is bacteriophage encoded. Type B strains are responsible for black disease in sheep; this is an infectious necrotic hepatitis associated with fluke infestation; liver damage by the parasite is a prerequisite for germination of latent spores in areas of necrotic liver tissue, and vegetative growth results in the synthesis and release of lethal α-toxin. Type D strains cause a somewhat similar disease in cattle (redwater disease, bacilliary hemoglobinuria), which is characterized by jaundice, subcutaneous hemorrhage, and edema at various sites in the thorax, as well as an intense hemorrhagic enteritis and lymphadenitis. The liver appears to be particularly affected, with large anemic infarcts due to blockage of branches of the portal vein. Only the β-toxin (phospholipase C) is produced in culture in these strains.

GENUS *CORYNEBACTERIUM*

Five *Corynebacterium* species are recognized as potential animal pathogens: *Corynebacterium pseudotuberculosis* ("*Corynebacterium ovis*") *Corynebacterium ulcerans, Corynebacterium renale, Corynebacterium equi,* and *Corynebacterium pyogenes.* Two of these are now classified elsewhere; *C. equi* is now renamed *Rhodococcus equi,* and *C. pyogenes* is now renamed *Actinomyces pyogenes.*

C. pseudotuberculosis produces an exotoxin which has phospholipase D activity, with substrate specificity for sphingomyelin and M_r

14,500. It is lethal, dermonecrotizing, and weakly hemolytic. By virtue of its phospholipase D activity, it inhibits hemolysis caused by sphingomyelinase C (β-toxin) of *S. aureus* (61). Toxigenic strains can be detected by inhibition of hemolytic activity of β-toxigenic staphylococci after being cross-streaked on sheep blood agar plates. There is strong evidence that the *C. pseudotuberculosis* toxin plays a major role in caseous lymphadenitis (cheesey gland), an economically important disease in sheep and goats. The toxin is thought to cause its effect through endothelial damage in vivo, and considerable protection can be afforded by vaccination of animals with toxoid vaccine (24).

Selected strains have been reported to produce diphtheria toxin (104), a property also reported for *C. ulcerans,* which also produces the lethal, dermonecrotizing toxin with phospholipase D activity (10).

A. pyogenes

A. pyogenes produces an exotoxin which is cytolytic and lethal but poorly characterized. The toxin is thought to be produced in abscesses, although it probably plays no major role in abscess formation per se. It is probably absorbed from there to cause generalized symptoms in cattle, sheep, and pigs. It may also be involved in abortions in pigs, since the toxin can be found in the placenta after abortion associated with infection by this species (Taylor, personal communication).

C. renale

C. renale is an agent of cystitis and pyelitis in cattle and produces a protein factor (renalin) which potentiates hemolytic activity due to sphingomyelinase C (β-toxin) of *S. aureus.* This factor and the CAMP factor of *S. agalactiae,* although not toxins sensu stricto, are both thought to potentiate β-toxin by binding to ceramide, a product of hydrolysis of sphingomyelin (13). Whether renalin has a role in the generation of disease by this species is not known.

R. equi

R. equi is recognized primarily as the agent of lung abscesses in foals. Although it is nonhemolytic and no toxins have been detected in pathogenic isolates, these isolates do produce phospholipase and cholesterol oxidase, both of which may act as aggressins (48). Cholesterol oxidase has demonstrated potentiating activity against the phospholipases of S. aureus, Listeria monocytogenes, and C. pseudotuberculosis (61). Whether such agents can potentiate endogenous phospholipases is not clear.

GENUS LISTERIA

The genus Listeria contains two toxigenic species, L. monocytogenes and Listeria ivanovi. Each produces two hemolytic toxins with closely similar activities and properties. α-Listeriolysin belongs to the SH-activated group typified by streptolysin O. It is lethal, cytolytic, and of M_r 60,000. The second lysin is unrelated to the SH-activated toxin but is hemolytic and may vary in molecular detail from species to species (26). These species are implicated in meningeal septicemia and encephalitis in sheep, abscesses of the central nervous system in cattle and sheep, and instances of infectious abortion. Listeria species are the suspected causative agents, but the role of toxins in the diseases caused by these species awaits further clarification; however, it has recently been shown that the hemolysin is essential for virulence in the mouse (40).

GENUS STAPHYLOCOCCUS

Three species are important in the pathogenesis of animal diseases, the coagulase-positive S. aureus and the coagulase-negative Staphylococcus intermedius and Staphylococcus hyicus. Like the clostridia and streptococci, the staphylococci in general produce a considerable array of toxins and aggressins, and apart from several notable exceptions (e.g., enterotoxemias, toxic shock syndrome, and scalded-skin syndrome), the pathogenesis of infection is al-

most certainly multifactorial, so that the precise contribution of individual toxins is not known. Diseases of importance in animals include bovine mastitis, although this can also occur in sheep, goats, pigs, and rabbits (the incidence in dogs, cats, and horses is low), exudative epidermitis in pigs, pyoderma in dogs, tick pyemia in lambs, staphylococcosis in poultry, and endometritis in various species (6).

α-Toxin

α-Toxin is a single-chain protein of M_r 33,000 and pI 8.5 and consists of 293 residues; the gene coding for the toxin has been cloned and sequenced, and the peptide as synthesized intracellularly contains an additional 26-residue signal peptide (reviewed in reference 36). The toxin is mitogenic, lethal, dermonecrotizing, and cytolytic and probably plays a major role in staphylococcal disease by acting with other virulence factors (e.g., coagulase, leukocidin, and other cytolysins and hydrolytic enzymes) to cause local necrosis, promoting the spread of the infection. It has also been demonstrated that subtoxic levels of α-toxin inhibit host defense cells in vitro (85) and are neurotoxic in vivo, directly affecting brain bioelectric activity as well as interacting with proteolipid protein in myelin (47).

The membrane-damaging activity of α-toxin has been examined in considerable detail (35), and it is now established that in black lipid membranes, the toxin forms gated ion-selective channels that display voltage-dependent closure in the presence of divalent cations such as Ca^{2+} (70). Such channels, consisting of hexameric rings of toxin complexes, evident in both natural and artificial membranes (37), have since been isolated from detergent micelles and erythrocyte membranes and have an effective pore size of about 3 nm (16). The cytolytic activity of the toxin almost certainly results from its ability to form such transmembrane channels in eucaryotic cells, damaging the membrane selectivity. In erythrocytes, high doses elicit lysis via a colloid-osmotic mechanism (36). The paralytic activity of α-toxin on smooth muscle that was noted by Lominski et al. (62) is thought to result from a direct spasmogenic effect of the toxin (for a discussion, see reference 101).

S. aureus plays a major role in herbivore mastitis and is particularly relevant to infections in dairy cows, since it results in considerable economic losses. The disease is usually chronic, but occasionally a fatal gangrenous disease may develop, particularly in sheep. Both forms have been studied in the rabbit, in which they occur naturally. In an extensive study of the role of toxins in the disease and the protective effects of immunization with toxoids, Adlam et al. (1) demonstrated that prior immunization with α-toxoid reduces the gangrenous form of the disease to the more confined and milder form, indicating that the α-toxin is essential for the development of spreading gangrenous lesions.

β-Toxin

β-Toxin is, like the α-toxin of *C. perfringens,* a magnesium-requiring phospholipase C, but with a substrate range restricted to sphingomyelin and lysophosphatidylcholine (sphingomyelin cholinephosphohydrolase; EC 3.1.4.12). It is produced with high frequency in animal isolates but less so in human isolates and is a single-chain protein of M_r 30,000 and pI ca. 9.5 and consists of 256 residues. It is hemolytic, and the sensitivity of erythrocytes correlates with their sphingomyelin content; sheep, goat, and bovine cells are highly susceptible. Hemolysis displays the hot-cold effect like that induced by *C. perfringens* α-toxin (see above). The purified toxin lyses guinea pig macrophages and human platelets, inhibits chemotaxis of human monocytes, and causes marked necrosis in lactating mammary tissue (101). Its role in pathogenesis is not clear, although it may be important in staphylococcal mastitis.

Coleman et al. (27) reported the cloning and mapping of the β-toxin gene. The toxin is encoded in a 1,250-base-pair sequence. These authors showed that the acquisition or loss of

β-toxin production depends upon a lysogenic converting phage which inactivates toxin production by insertion at a locus in the coding region for the structural gene. A similar insertional inactivation occurs with lipase in this species. More recent data from Coleman's group (D. Coleman, *J. Gen. Microbiol.,* in press) shows that most bovine isolates which are deficient in β-toxin production harbor lysogenic phages located in or very close to the β-toxin structural gene in the chromosome. Mitomycin C induction often results in reversion of the strain to β-toxin production, and all of the serotype F converting phages also convert positively for staphylokinase production. The structural determinant for staphylokinase (*sak*) is adjacent to the phage attachment site in several cases examined. Such studies illustrate the importance of phage conversion in the expression of virulence determinants in this species, which include (in addition to β-toxin) lipase, staphylokinase, and enterotoxin A, the last two products being coded for on the phage genome (see below).

γ-Toxin

γ-Toxin is commonly produced in vivo and in vitro in coagulase-positive human strains and is thought to be involved in bone disease. Its distribution in animal isolates is poorly documented, probably because its hemolytic activity is inactivated by sulfonated polymers such as agar. It is reported to be a two-component toxin, γ1 (consisting of a protein of M_r 29,000 and pI 9.8) and γ2 (consisting of a protein of M_r 26,000 and pI 9.9) (97). However, more recent data (I. McNiven and T. H. Birkbeck, personal communication) agree with previous observations that it is a single-component lysin, with component 2 (γ2; M_r 33,400) having hemolytic activity which is most active against rabbit erythrocytes, the hemolytic titer being unaffected by the presence of component 1 (γ1; M_r 35,000). However, when component 2 was tested against human or sheep erythrocytes, hemolytic activity was potentiated but not totally dependent on the presence of component

1. The relationship between the two components of γ-toxin may be similar to that noted between renalin or CAMP factor and staphylococcal β-toxin (see above).

γ-Toxin is mitogenic and cytolytic for a range of cell types including rabbit peritoneal granulocytes, in which it induces a similar pattern of release of hydrolytic lysosomal enzymes to that induced by the α-toxin. It is lethal for guinea pigs, with consequent massive intravascular hemolysis and hemorrhaging of the kidneys and serosal surface of the intestine. Lethality for rabbits and mice has also been reported (36). Its significance in animal disease is not known, although it is produced by the majority of strains of S. aureus isolated from cases of tick pyemia (T. H. Birkbeck, personal communication).

δ-Toxin

δ-Toxin is a small, amphiphilic peptide of M_r 2,977 and pI ca. 5.0, which is produced by almost all coagulase-positive as well as a high proportion of coagulase-negative isolates. It consists of 26 amino acid residues, the sequence of which is known and differs slightly in human or bovine strains and canine isolates. A similar peptide (antigonococcal substance) is produced by S. haemolyticus (19). In aqueous solution the toxin occurs as a mixture of aggregates of relatively high molecular weight.

The toxin is characterized by its low lytic potency and wide spectrum of activity. A wide variety of cell types are susceptible, and in relatively high concentrations the toxin is thought to bring about membrane disruption by a detergentlike insertion into the hydrophobic interior of the target membrane, leading to altered permeability and eventual lysis by membrane solubilization (35, 38). The possibility that the toxin initially forms transmembrane channels is suggested by its tertiary structure, which consists of a laterally amphipathic rod with a rigid α-helical domain between residues 2 and 20 (A. Pastore, M. J. Tappin, R. S. Norton, J. H. Freer, and I. D. Campbell, *Biochemistry,* in press) when solubilized in methanol. A similar rigid α-helical rod structure from residues 5 to 23, with pronounced lateral amphipathicity, has also been demonstrated in the molecular form bound to lipid micelles (57).

The toxin also activates endogenous phospholipases A2 in several cell lines and is thought to bring about lysis by generation of lysolipids in situ (31). It is reported as lethal at high doses (10 to 100 mg) for small experimental animals, although this could be accounted for by low levels of contamination with, for example, the more potent α-toxin. It is erythrogenic but not necrotizing in rabbit skin and causes increased vascular permeability detectable by the blueing test. Stimulation of fluid accumulation in loops of guinea pig ileum has been reported, but this is thought to result from direct stimulation of ion pumps rather than by a cyclic AMP effect (36).

The role of the toxin in staphylococcal disease is not defined, although its lytic activity is so effectively inactivated by interaction with phospholipids in normal serum (serum lipoproteins, etc.) that a central role in systemic disease is not likely. It potentiates the lytic activity of the α- and β-toxins and may act as a virulence factor in localized lesions by virtue of its membrane-damaging properties, although direct proof is lacking.

Leucocidin

Leucocidin is a two-component mitogenic toxin, consisting of the so-called F (fast) and S (slow) proteins, which together were reported as having leukotoxic activity for a relatively narrow range of cell types including polymorphonuclear leucocytes, macrophages, and mast cells of both humans and rabbits (105). More recently it was reinvestigated by Noda et al. (75), who reported that F consists of a peptide of 275 residues with M_r 32,000 and pI 9.08 and S has 269 residues with M_r 31,000 and pI 9.39. The leucocidin is thought to bring about membrane damage by binding of S to a GM1-containing receptor on the leukocyte membrane. This is accompanied by increased activity of methyltransferase and synthesis of phosphatidylcholine, which is thought to act as the receptor for F. The binding of F is accompanied by activation of endogenous phospholipase A2, resulting in generation of lysophospholipid and free fatty acid, the initiation of the arachidonic acid cascade, and cytolysis.

Leucocidin is not a lethal toxin, although there is no doubt that it is produced in vivo in natural infections. Recently, potent necrotizing activity in rabbit skin and lactating mammary tissue has been demonstrated. Paradoxically, immunization with leucocidin gives no protection against experimental mastitis in rabbits, despite high levels of circulating antibody (2). Although a role in disease by virtue of its cytotoxic effects is likely, direct proof is still lacking.

Enterotoxins

S. auereus produces seven low-molecular-weight proteins which have common modes of action and yet can be differentiated immunologically. They are classified as enterotoxins A, B, C_1, C_2, C_3, D, and E with M_r 27,500 (240 residues), 28,494 (243 residues), 27,500 (239 residues), 26,900 (236 residues), 27,111 (236 residues), 27,197 (236 residues), and 26,900 (259 residues), respectively. The coding regions for enterotoxins A, B, and C_1 have been cloned and sequenced; enterotoxin A can be encoded by either phage or chromosomal determinants, whereas enterotoxin B genes are carried on a transposon (11, 15). Also, enterotoxins A, B, and C_1 are mitogenic (36).

The toxins are solely responsible for the rapid emetic and diarrheal response characteristic of the staphylococcal enterotoxemia which follows ingestion of preformed toxin. The toxins are apparently less potent in animals than humans; animals tested experimentally include monkeys (the animals of choice in experimentation), pigs, cats, dogs, rabbits, chinchillas, rats, and mice. Although the rodents lack a vomiting mechanism, they do respond to the toxin. Unlike enterotoxins of other species, those of staphylococci also induce vomiting and diarrhea when administered intravenously. Evidence from studies with rhesus monkeys suggests that the site of emetic action is the abdominal viscera and that the vomiting center in the central nervous system is stimulated via the vagus nerve. The diarrheal response probably arises from both inhibition of fluid absorption in the colon and increased transmucosal fluid flux. In addition, enterotoxins at relatively high doses (150 μg) induce gastroenteritis in monkeys, with damage evident at the villus tips and degenerative changes evident in the epithelial cells of the jejunum (for a review, see reference 11). It seems likely that enterotoxigenic *S. aureus* can induce enteric disease in a wide range of animal species. Enterotoxins have been detected in cheeses contaminated by animal strains, and, indeed, animals strains can induce food poisoning in humans. Anecdotal evidence exists for cases of enterotoxemia of staphylococcal etiology in dogs fed dried milk powder containing enterotoxins (Taylor, personal communication).

Pyrogenic Exotoxins A and B

Pyrogenic exotoxins A and B are proteins of M_r 12,000 and 18,000, respectively, which induce interleukin-1 production, resulting in fever. The role of these toxins in animal disease is undefined, but the toxin formerly referred to as pyrogenic exotoxin C and now known as toxic shock syndrome toxin 1 (TSST 1) (see below) has been shown to potentiate the effects of lipopolysaccharide endotoxins up to 50,000-fold (89) in vivo (in the rabbit model).

Epidermolytic Toxins

Epidermolytic toxins (exfoliatin A and B) are single-chain proteins of M_r 27,000 (242 residues) and 27,492 (243 residues), respectively, with pI 7.0 and 6.9, respectively. The toxins have common properties but differ serologically. The coding region for epidermolytic toxin B is carried on a plasmid. Strains producing epidermolytic toxin A or epidermolytic toxins A and B usually belong to phage group II (7). The consequences of infection with toxigenic strains is the scalded-skin syndrome, typified by separation of the cells in the stratum granulosum and the formation of an intraepidermal cleft. When this occurs over extensive areas of skin, the skin becomes loose if gently stroked (positive Nikolsky sign) and may slough off over large areas if disturbed, leaving a glistening, raw area with the appearance of a scald. Animal species sensitive to the effects of these toxins include mice, monkeys, and hamsters. The symptoms can be reproduced most conveniently by subcutaneous injection of pure toxin in infant or adult nude mice. The toxin may be implicated in canine pyoderma and in greasy-pig disease (exudative epidermitis, caused by the coagulase-negative species *S. hyicus* subsp. *hyicus*) in young piglets (6).

TSST 1

TSST1 is a single-chain mitogenic protein of M_r 22,049 (194 residues). The coding region has been cloned and sequenced (20). Originally described as enterotoxin F and pyrogenic exotoxin C, this toxin causes a syndrome in humans which begins with headache, fever, myalgia, vomiting, and watery diarrhea and progresses rapidly to a systemic illness involving symptoms of clinical shock. Bacteremia is characteristically absent, and the condition has been frequently associated with the use by women of tampons in which conditions are favorable for multiplication of toxigenic *S. aureus*. Recently Arbuthnott et al. (8) have developed a rabbit uterine model with which they are attempting to assess the role of TSST 1 and endotoxins in this interesting syndrome.

Clearly, the only equivalent situation in animals may include the use of intravaginal sponges as hormonal implants in sheep and goats to synchronize estrous cycle. Although such implants are not in widespread use, the occurrence of TSST 1-producing strains in goats and cattle (see below) serves as a notice for increasing vigilance for toxic shock-type symptoms in these situations.

Morgan et al. (74) recently reported an outbreak of dermatitis in a herd of goats from which a TSST 1- (and enterotoxin C)-producing strain of *S. aureus* was isolated from the skin lesions of several of the affected animals. The skin lesions were reported as being similar in appearance to those seen in scalded-skin syndrome in humans, although no epidermolytic toxins were detectable in cultures. TSST 1- (and enterotoxin C)-producing bovine strains of *S. aureus* (lysed by phage 78) have also been isolated from cases of severe bovine mastitis (54), but the role of this toxin in the disease, which appears to be multifactorial, is not clear.

GENUS *STREPTOCOCCUS*

The genus *Streptococcus* contains a number of pyogenic hemolytic species of importance in animal disease. These include *S. agalactiae* (group B), a major cause of bovine mastitis; *Streptococcus equi* (group C), the agent of strangles in horses, which involves acute pharyngitis and septicemia, resulting in swollen lymph nodes with abscess formation and hence obstruction of the windpipe and death by asphyxia; and *Streptococcus dysgalactiae* (group C), an agent of bovine mastitis.

Related group C organisms (previously known as *Streptococcus equisimilis, Streptococcus pseudogalactiae,* and *Streptococcus zooepidemicus*) are associated with septicemia in cattle, rabbits, and pigs; they have been isolated from wound infections in horses and are associated with avian disease. In addition, they are perhaps best recognized for their involvement in acute mastitis in cows and polyarthritis (joint-ill) in lambs. They are now grouped in a single unnamed taxon (83).

Other, as yet unnamed, groups of pyogenic strains are classified under group G (isolated from skin lesions and inflammatory exudates in dogs and cats and associated with puppy fading), group E (associated with lymphadenitis in pigs), or groups P, V, and U (causative organisms similar to those in group E; organisms of groups E, P, V, and U are collectively termed *Streptococcus porcinus*), groups L and M (associated with skin lesions and exudates and with urogenital infections in dogs), and group P (associated with pharyngeal abscesses in pigs).

Streptococcus uberis is a heterogeneous group of organisms associated with bovine mastitis, and *Streptococcus bovis* and *Enterococcus durans* ("*Streptococcus durans*") (group D enterococci) have been associated with cases of enteritis. *Streptococcus iniae* is not assigned to any of the Lancefield groups. It appears to be nonpathogenic for mice, guinea pigs, and rabbits, but was isolated from subcutaneous abscesses in freshwater dolphins in the Amazon (83).

The pyogenic streptococci generally show zones of beta-hemolysis on blood agar, and the group D species are characterized by alpha-hemolytic activity.

The two major cytolytic toxins, SLS and SLO, are likely candidates for the hemolytic activity, although *S. agalactiae* and other group B strains are characterized by their ability to produce CAMP factor, which, although nonhemolytic itself, potentiates the lytic activity of staphylococcal β-toxin (sphingomyelinase C) against bovine or sheep erythrocytes. In addition to its production by group B strains, CAMP factor is produced by some strains belonging to groups C, F, G, P, and V.

Streptococcus Toxins

SLO

SLO is one of a relatively large group of lethal, cytolytic (hemolytic) toxins with mitogenic activity that are produced by *Bacillus, Clostridium, Streptococcus,* and *Listeria* species. These SH-activated toxins are remarkably similar in properties (92) and induce cross-reacting, precipitating, and neutralizing antibodies, yet appear to lack appreciable sequence homology in their DNA coding regions (55). It is likely that their modes of membrane damage are identical or at least closely similar and depend on the presence of cholesterol or similar β-hydroxysterols in the membrane. These toxins have been authoritatively reviewed by Smyth and Duncan (92).

SLO is produced by most group A strains, as well as by many strains belonging to groups C and G. It is lethal and a potent cardiotoxin, but its biological activity is reversibly sensitive to oxidation (hence the former name for this type of toxin: oxygen-labile hemolysin) and to the presence of small amounts of cholesterol. As mentioned above for cereolysin, membrane lesions induced by these toxins are associated with the appearance of arc and ring structures 35 to 38 nm in diameter, which were originally thought to represent complexes of lysin and sterol. Earlier suggestions for the mechanism of lysis induced by SLO and related toxins included transmembrane holes surrounded by the postulated sterol-toxin complexes in the form of rings or arcs (29); sequestration of sterol by the toxin, leading to sterol-enriched areas (rings and arcs); and sterol-depleted areas of membrane. Resulting destabilization of the bilayer in these areas was thought to lead to lysis, although no evidence to support the suggestions was available at the time (30). However, ring- and arc-shaped structures occur in purified tetanolysin (84), perfringolysin (93), and probably other SH-activated toxins in the absence of sterols if the protein concentration is high enough and almost certainly represent toxin polymers. Polymerization appears to be facilitated at the membrane surface by sterols. Rings and arcs recovered from membranes after treatment with SLO do not contain sterols, and recently convincing evidence has been presented by Bhakdi et al. that the rings and arcs are in fact toxin polymer lining transmembrane lesions induced by the action of active toxin on susceptible cells and sterol-containing liposomes (18). For a fuller discussion, see reference 35.

There is no doubt that SLO is produced in vivo in some streptococcal infections, and it is likely that it rapidly combines with antibody as it is formed, establishing an equilibrium of constant formation and slow dissociation of antigen-antibody complexes. This may establish a slow-release reservoir of active SLO during chronic infections, with progressive accumulation to toxic levels in susceptible tissues such as the heart (3). The role of SLO in animal disease is uncertain, although because of its high cardiotoxicity in experimental animals it is likely to be an important virulence factor once the infection is established. There is little doubt that like *S. aureus* and *C. perfringens*, *S. pyogenes* has a large repertoire of virulence factors available, including toxins, enzymes, and aggressins.

SLS

SLS is a lethal, highly potent cytolysin that is responsible for the familiar zones of beta-hemolysis produced by almost all members of groups A, C, and G and by some strains belonging to groups E, H, and L. Members of groups B and D do not produce SLS.

This toxic peptide is produced in association with a carrier molecule and is active only in the carrier-bound state. A variety of different carriers can induce its release from streptococci, and some of those of possible significance in vivo include serum albumin, α-lipoprotein, and RNA. It is cytolytic for a wide range of cell types in vitro, including leukocytes and erythrocytes from a wide range of species, platelets, tumor cells, heart cells of rabbits and rats, renal cells, and a variety of established cell lines (for a review, see reference 3). SLS (M_r 1,800; pI 9.2) has recently been isolated for the first time free of carrier (63). This small cytolytic peptide resembles staphylococcal δ-toxin in its sensitivity to inhibition by serum and phospholipids. However, its labile nature and its extraordinary potency (about 10^5 times that of δ-toxin) contrast strongly with those of δ-toxin. It is likely that the streptococcal leukotoxicity, in which mammalian leucocytes are killed after ingestion of streptococci, is a consequence of release of SLS (14). However, the role of this toxin in animal disease is still not understood. Indeed, because the toxin is nonimmunogenic, it is still not known whether it is produced in vivo. This fact, together with the ability of the toxin to transfer from one carrier to another, may enable it to circulate freely and cause its deleterious effects at sites distant from its release in localized lesions.

Erythrogenic Toxins

Erythrogenic toxins (pyrogenic exotoxins) are synthesized by group A streptococci and exist as three distinct serological forms (A, B, and C). They are single-chain proteins with M_r 25,805, 17,500, and 13,200, respectively. Toxigenic strains carry lysogenic phages associated with toxin production, and phage conversion has been demonstrated by numerous workers (3). The toxins (responsible for scarlet fever in humans) have a wide range of biological effects, demonstrable in experimental animals (mostly rabbits). These include pyrogenicity, enhancement of lethal endotoxic shock, depression of the reticuloendothelial system and antibody production, mitogenicity, and induction of skin reactions. These properties closely resemble many of those of the staphylococcal enterotoxins, and recently, Hynes et al. (50) have shown antigenic cross-reactivity between streptococcal erythrogenic toxin A and staphylococcal enterotoxins B and C_1, indicating that a common ancestral gene may be involved.

Although they are clearly responsible for disease in humans, the role, if any, of these toxins in streptococcal disease in animals is not known.

CONCLUSION

The brief survey of toxins produced by bacteria involved in animal disease illustrates clearly our state of ignorance about the role of such agents in many important diseases. Fortunately, a knowledge of the precise role of toxins in diseases is not a condition of their use as protective antigens in vaccines, nor is it usually necessary to purify and characterize them before such use. Sometimes, empirical vaccines consisting of mixtures of relatively crude culture fractions (made into toxoid) are extremely effective protective agents (e.g., multivalent clostridial vaccines) against a variety of organisms and diseases. However, in other instances, little protection is afforded by vaccination by using this approach, or indeed by vaccination with relatively well-characterized toxoid vaccines (e.g., staphylococcal mastitis vaccine). In such instances it is more essential to dissect the process of pathogenesis and attempt to evaluate the individual contribution of each virulence factor in the overall process. In these instances, well-characterized toxins are prerequisites, not only for assessment of immune status and evaluation of the protective efficacy of single-component vaccines, but also as an aid to the use of gene manipulation to construct strains which are defective in production of individual virulence components. The relative virulence of such engineered strains can then be assessed, and this may provide an indication of importance of each component in the pathogenetic process.

ACKNOWLEDGMENTS.   I am grateful to David Coleman, Harry Birkbeck, and Joseph Alouf for making available information prior to publication, to David Taylor and Harry Birkbeck for their comments on the manuscript, and to my wife, Jo, for help with editing the manuscript.

LITERATURE CITED

1. Adlam, C., P. D. Ward, A. C. McCartney, J. P. Arbuthnott, and C. M. Thorley. 1977. Effect of immunization with highly purified alpha- and beta-toxins on staphylococcal mastitis in rabbits. *Infect. Immun.* 17:250–256.

2. Adlam, C., P. D. Ward, and W. H. Turner. 1980. Effect of immunisation with highly purified Panton-Valentine leucocidin and delta toxin on staphylococcal mastitis in rabbits. *J. Comp. Pathol.* 90:265–274.

3. Alouf, J. E. 1986. Streptococcal toxins (streptolysin O, streptolysin S and erythrogenic toxin), p. 635–691. *In* F. Dorner and J. Drews (ed.), *Pharmacology of Bacterial Toxins.* Pergamon Press, London.

4. Alouf, J. E., and C. Jolivet-Reynaud. 1981. Purification and characterization of *Clostridium perfringens* delta toxin. *Infect. Immun.* 31:535–546.

5. Alouf, J. E., and M. Raynaud. 1968. Action de la streptolisine O sur les membranes cellulaires. I. Fixation sur la membrane erythrocytaire. *Ann. Inst. Pasteur* (Paris) 114:812–827.

6. Anderson, J. C. 1983. Veterinary aspects of staph-

ylococci, p. 193–225. *In* C. S. F. Easmon and C. Adlam (ed.), *Staphylococci and Staphylococcal Infections,* vol. 1. Academic Press, Inc. (London), Ltd., London.

7. Arbuthnott, J. P. 1983. Epidermolytic toxins, p. 599–615. *In* C. S. F. Easmon and C. Adlam (ed.), *Staphylococci and Staphylococcal Infections,* vol. 1. Academic Press, Inc. (London), Ltd., London.

8. Arbuthnott, J. P., J. C. S. de Azavedo, T. J. Foster, and A. M. Drumm. 1986. Models for the study of staphylococcal toxic shock syndrome toxin 1, p. 141–144. *In* P. Falmange, J. E. Alouf, F. J. Fehrenbach, J. Jeljaszewicz, and M. Thelestam (ed.), *Bacterial Protein Toxins.* Gustav Fischer Verlag, Stuttgart, Federal Republic of Germany.

9. Avigad, L., and A. W. Bernheimer. 1976. Inhibition by zinc of hemolysis induced by bacterial and other cytolytic agents. *Infect. Immun.* 13:1378–1381.

10. Barkesdale, L., R. Linder, I. T. Sulea, and M. Pollice. 1981. Phopholipase D activity of *Corynebacteruim pseudotuberculosis (Corynebacterium ovis)* and *Corynebacterium ulcerans,* a distinctive marker within the genus *Corynebacterium. J. Clin. Microbiol.* 13:335–343.

11. Bergdol, M. S. 1983.Enterotoxins, p. 559–598. *In* C. S. F. Easmon and C. Adlam (ed.), *Staphylococci and Staphylococcal Infections,* vol. 2. Academic Press, Inc. (London), Ltd., London.

12. Bernheimer, A. W. 1976. Introduction, p. ix. *In* A. W. Bernheimer (ed.), *Mechanisms in Bacterial Toxinology.* John Wiley & Sons, Inc., New York.

13. Bernheimer, A. W., and L. Avigad. 1982. Mechanism of hemolysis by renalin, a CAMP-like protein from *Corynebacterium renale. Infect. Immun.* 36:1253–1256.

14. Bernheimer, A. W., and B. Rudy. 1986. Interactions between membranes and cytolytic peptides. *Biochim. Biophys. Acta* 864:123–141.

15. Betley, M. J., V. L. Miller, and J. J. Mekalanos. 1986. Genetics of bacterial enterotoxins. *Annu. Rev. Microbiol.* 40:577–605.

16. Bhakdi, S., and J. Tranum-Jensen. 1983. Membrane damage by channel-forming proteins. Trans. Biochem. Sci. 1983(April):134–136.

17. Bhakdi, S., and J. Tranum-Jensen. 1985. Complement activation attack on autologous cell membranes induced by streptolysin O. *Infect. Immun.* 48:713–719.

18. Bhakdi, S., J. Tranum-Jensen, and A. Sziegoleit. 1985. Mechanism of membrane damage by streptolysin O. *Infect. Immun.* 47:62–70.

19. Birkbeck, T. H., R. J. Basaillon, and R. Beaudet. 1986. *Staphylococcus haemolyticus* anti-gonococcal substance: a third type of staphylococcal delta haemolysin, p. 51–52. *In* P. Falmange, J. E. Alouf, F. J. Fehrenbach, J. Jeljaszewicz, and M. Thelestam

(ed.), *Bacterial Protein Toxins*. Gustav Fischer Verlag, Stuttgart, Federal Rebpulic of Germany.

20. Blomster-Hautamaa, D. A., B. N. Kreiswirth, J. S. Kornblum, R. P. Novick, and P. M. Schleivert. 1986. The nucleotide and partial amino acid sequence of toxic shock syndrome toxin 1. *J. Biol. Chem.* 261:15783–15786.

21. Bonventre, P. F., and C. E. Johnson. 1970. *Bacillus cereus* toxin, p. 415–435. *In* T. C. Montie, S. Kadis, and S. J. Ajl (ed.), *Microbial Toxins,* vol. 3. Academic Press, Inc., New York.

22. Boriello, S. P., and R. J. Carman. 1985. Clostridial diseases of the gastrointestinal tract in animals, p. 196–221. *In* S. P. Boriello (ed.), *Clostridia and Gastrointestinal Diseases.* CRC Press, Inc., Boca Raton, Fla.

23. Bremm, K. D., W. Konig, P. Pfeiffer, I. Rauschen, K. Theobald, M. Thelestam, and J. E. Alouf. 1985. Effect of thiol-activated toxins (streptolysin O, alveolysin, and theta toxin) on the generation of leukotrienes and leukotriene-inducing and -metabolizing enzymes from human polymorphonuclear granulocytes. *Infect. Immun.* 50:844–851.

24. Brown, C. C., H. J. Olander, E. L. Biberstein, and S. M. Morse. 1986. Use of a toxoid vaccine to protect goats against intradermal challenge exposure to *Corynebacterium pseudotuberculosis. Am. J. Vet. Res.* 47:1116–1119.

25. Cavaillon, J.-M., C. Jolivet-Reynaud, C. Fitting, B. David, and J. E. Alouf. 1986. Ganglioside identification on human monocyte membrane with *Clostridium perfringens* delta-toxin. *J. Leukocyte Biol.* 40:65–72.

26. Chakraborty, T., M. Gilmore, J. Hacker, B. Huhle, S. Katharion, S. Knapp, J. Kreft, B. Muller, M. Leimeister, J. Parrisius, W. Wagner, and W. Goebel. 1986. Genetic approaches to study haemolytic toxins in bacteria, p. 241–252. *In* P. Falmange, J. E. Alouf, F. J. Fehrenbach, J. Jeljaszewicz, and M. Thelestam (ed.), *Bacterial Protein Toxins.* Gustav Fischer Verlag, Stuttgart, Federal Republic of Germany.

27. Coleman, D. C., J. P. Arbuthnott, H. M. Pomeroy, and T. H. Birkbeck. 1986. Cloning and expression in *Escherichia coli* and *Staphylococcus aureus* of the beta lysin determinant from *Staphylococcus aureus*: evidence that bacteriophage conversion of beta lysin activity is caused by insertional inactivation of the beta lysin determinant. *Microb. Pathogenesis* 1:549–564.

28. Coolbaugh, J. C., and R. P. Williams. 1978. Production and characterisation of two haemolysins of *Bacillus cereus. Can. J. Microbiol.* 24:1289–1295.

29. Dourmashkin, R. R., and W. F. Rosse. 1966. Morphology changes in the membranes of red blood cells undergoing hemolysis. *Am. J. Med.* 41:699–710.

30. Duncan, J. L., and R. Schlegel. 1975. Effect of streptolysin O on erythrocyte membranes, liposomes and lipid dispersions. A protein cholesterol interaction. *J. Cell Biol.* 67:160–173.

31. Durkin, J. P., and W. T. Shier. 1981. Staphylococcal delta toxin stimulates endogenous phospholipase A_2 activity and prostaglandin synthesis in fibroblasts. *Biochim. Biophys. Acta* 663:467–479.

32. Fairweather, N. F., and V. A. Lyness. 1986. The complete nucleotide sequence of tetanus toxin. *Nucleic Acids Res.* 14:7809–7812.

33. Florin, I., and M. Thelestam. 1986. Lysosomal involvement in cellular internalisation of *Clostridium difficile* toxin B, p. 229–230. *In* P. Falmange, J. E. Alouf, F. J. Fehrenbach, J. Jeljaszewicz, and M. Thelestam (ed.), *Bacterial Protein Toxins.* Gustav Fischer Verlag, Stuttgart, Federal Republic of Germany.

34. Fossum, K. 1963. Separation of haemolysin and egg yolk turbidity factor in cell-free extracts of *Bacillus cereus. Acta Pathol. Microbiol. Scand.* 59:400–406.

35. Freer, J. H. 1986. Membrane damage caused by bacterial toxins, p. 189–211. *In* J. B. Harris (ed.), *Natural Toxins, Animal, Plant and Microbial.* Oxford University Press, Oxford.

36. Freer, J. H., and J. P. Arbuthnott. 1986. Toxins of *Staphylococcus aureus*, p. 581–633. *In* F. Dorner and J. Drews (ed.). *Pharmacology of Bacterial Toxins.* Pergamon Press, Oxford.

37. Freer, J. H., J. P. Arbuthnott, and A. W. Bernheimer. 1968. Interaction of staphylococcal α-toxin with artificial and natural membranes. *J. Bacteriol.* 95:1153–1168.

38. Freer, J. H., T. H. Birkbeck, and M. Bhakoo. 1984. Interaction of staphylococcal delta-lysin with phospholipid monolayers and bilayers—a short review, p. 181–190. *In* J. E. Alouf, F. J. Fehrenbach, J. H. Freer, and J. Jeljaszewicz (ed.), *Bacterial Protein Toxins.* Academic Press, Inc. (London), Ltd., London.

39. Freidlander, A. M. 1986. Macrophages are sensitive to anthrax lethal toxin through an acid-dependent process. *J. Biol. Chem.* 261:7123–7126.

40. Gaillard, J.-L., P. Berche, and P. Sansonetti. 1986. Transposon mutagenesis as a tool to study the role of hemolysin in the virulence of *Listeria monocytogenes. Infect. Immun.* 52:50–55.

41. Gilmore, M. S. 1985. Molecular cloning of genes encoding Gram–positive virulence factors. *Curr. Top. Microbiol. Immunol.* 118:219–234.

42. Granum, E. 1986. Structure and mechanism of action of the enterotoxin from *Clostridium perfringens,* p. 327–334. *In* P. Falmange, J. E. Alouf, F. J. Fehrenbach, J. Jeljaszewicz, and M. Thelestam (ed.), *Bacterial Protein Toxins.* Gustav Fischer Verlag, Stuttgart, Federal Republic of Germany.

43. Green, B. D., L. Battisti, T. M. Koehler, and C. B. Thorne. 1985. Demonstration of a capsule plasmid in *Bacillus anthracis*. *Infect. Immun.* 49:291–297.

44. Habeeb, A. F. S. A. 1975. Studies on ε-protoxin of *Clostridium perfringens* type D: physicochemical and chemical properties of ε-protoxin. *Biochim. Biophys. Acta* 412:62–69.

45. Habermann, E., and F. Dreyer. 1986. Clostridial neurotoxins: handling and action at the cellular level. *Curr. Top. Microbiol. Immunol.* 29:94–179.

46. Harris, I. E., and B. H. Portas. 1985. Enterotoxaemia in rabbits caused by *Clostridium spiroforme*. *Aust. Vet. J.* 62:342–343.

47. Harshman, S., and N. Sugg. 1986. Studies on the staphylococcal alpha-toxin receptor on myelin and RB-RBC, p. 213–219. *In* P. Falmange, J. E. Alouf, F. J. Fehrenbach, J. Jeljaszewicz, and M. Thelestam (ed.), *Bacterial Protein Toxins,* Gustav Fischer Verlag, Stuttgart, Federal Republic of Germany.

48. Hillage, C. J. 1986. Review of *Corynebacterium (Rhodococcus) equi* lung abscesses in foals: pathogenesis, diagnosis and treatment. *Vet. Rec.* 119:261–264.

49. Horvath, G., E. Toth-Marton, J. M. Meszaros, and L. Quarini. 1986. Experimental *Bacillus cereus* mastitis in cows. *Acta Vet. Hung.* 34:29–35.

50. Hynes, W. L., C. R. Weeks, J. J. Iandolo, and J. J. Ferretti. 1987. Immunologic cross-reactivity of type A streptococcal exotoxin (erythrogenic toxin) and staphylococcal enterotoxins B and C_1. *Infect. Immun.* 55:837–838.

51. Inoue, K., Y. Akiyama, T. Kinshita, Y. Higashi, and T. Amano. 1976. Evidence for a one-hit theory in the immune bactericidal reaction and demonstration of a multi-hit response for hemolysis by streptolysin O and *Clostridium perfringens* theta toxin. *Infect. Immun.* 13:337–344.

52. Jolivet-Reynaud, C., M. R. Popoff, M.-A. Vinit, P. Ravisse, H. Moreau, and J. E. Alouf. 1986. Enteropathogenicity of *Clostridium perfringens* beta toxin and other clostridial toxins, p. 145–151. *In* P. Falmange, J. E. Alouf, F. J. Fehrenbach, J. Jeljaszewicz, and M. Thelestam (ed.), *Bacterial Protein Toxins*. Gustav Fischer Verlag, Stuttgart, Federal Republic of Germany.

53. Jones, T. O., and P. C. B. Turnbull. 1981. Bovine mastitis caused by *Bacillus cereus*. *Vet. Rec.* 108:272–274.

54. Jones, T. O., and A. A. Wienecke. 1986. Staphylococcal toxic shock syndrome. *Vet. Rec.* 119:435–436.

55. Kehoe, M., and K. N. Timmis. 1984. Cloning and expression in *Escherichia coli* of streptolysin O determinant from *Streptococcus pyogenes*: characterization of the cloned streptolysin O determinant and demonstration of the absence of substantial homology with determinants of other thiol-activated toxins. *Infect. Immun.* 43:804–810.

56. Kramer, J. M. 1984. *Bacillus cereus* exotoxins: production, isolation, detection and properties. p. 385–386. *In* J. E. Alouf, F. J. Fehrebach, J. H. Freer, and J. Jeljaszewicz (ed.), *Bacterial Protein Toxins*. Academic Press, Inc. (London), Ltd., London.

57. Lee, K. H., J. E. Fitton, and K. Wuthrich. 1987. Nuclear magnetic resonance investigation of the conformation of δ-haemolysin bound to dodecylphosphocholine micelles. *Biochim. Biophys. Acta* 911:144–153.

58. Leppla, S. H. 1982. Anthrax toxin edema factor: a bacterial adenylate cyclase that increases cyclic AMP concentrations in eukaryotic cells. *Proc. Natl. Acad. Sci. USA* 79:3162–3166.

59. Leppla, S. H., D. L. Robertson, S. L. Welkos, L. A. Smith, and M. H. Vodkin. 1986. Cloning and analysis of genes for anthrax toxin components, p. 275–278. *In* P. Falmange, J. E. Alouf, F. J. Fehrenbach, J. Jeljaszewicz, and M. Thelestam (ed.), *Bacterial Protein Toxins*. Gustav Fischer Verlag, Stuttgart, Federal Republic of Germany.

60. Lereclus, D., A. Klier, J. Ribier, G. Menon, M.-M. Lecadet, C. Bourgouin, and G. Rapoport. 1986. Structural organisation of the crystal toxin genes from different serotypes. p. 285–288. *In* P. Falmange, J. E. Alouf, F. J. Fehrenbach, J. Jeljaszewicz, and M. Thelestam (ed.), *Bacterial Protein Toxins*. Gustav Fischer Verlag, Stuttgart, Federal Republic of Germany.

61. Linder, R. 1984. Alteration of mammalian membranes by the cooperative and antagonistic actions of bacterial proteins. *Biochim. Biophys. Acta* 779:423–435.

62. Lominski, I., J. P. Arbuthnott, A. C. Scott, and H. M. McCallum. 1962. Effect of staphylococcal alpha toxin on striated muscle in mice. *Lancet* ii:590.

63. Loridan, C., and J. E. Alouf. 1986. Purification of RNA-core induced streptolysin S and isolation and haemolytic characteristics of the carrier-free toxin. *J. Gen. Microbiol.* 132:307–315.

64. Luderitz, O., and C. Galanos. 1986. Endotoxins of Gram-negative bacteria, p. 307–321. *In* F. Dorner and J. Drews (ed.), *Pharamacology of Bacterial Toxins*. Pergamon Press, Oxford.

65. Luthy, P., and H. R. Ebersold. 1986. The entomocidal toxins of *Bacillus thuringiensis*. p. 449–475. *In* F. Dorner and J. Drews (ed.), *Pharmacology of Bacterial Toxins*. Pergamon Press, Oxford.

66. Luthy, P., F. Jaquet, C. Hofmann, M. Huber-Lukac, and M. G. Wolfsberger. 1986. Pathogenic actions of *Bacillus thuringiensis* toxin, p. 161–166. *In* P. Falmange, J. E. Alouf, F. J. Fehrenbach, J. Jeljaszewicz, and M. Thelestam (ed.), *Bacterial Protein Toxins*. Gustav Fischer Verlag, Stutt-

gart, Federal Republic of Germany.

67. **McDonel, J. L.** 1986. Toxins of Clostridium perfringens types A, B, C, D, and E, p. 477–517. *In* F. Dorner and J. Drews (ed.), *Pharmacology of Bacterial Toxins*. Pergamon Press, Oxford.

68. **McDonel, J. L., F. Dorner, and J. Drews.** 1986. The role of toxins in bacterial pathogenesis, p. 1–4. *In* F. Dorner and J. Drews (ed.), *Pharmacology of Bacterial Toxins*. Pergamon Press, Oxford.

69. **McFarlane, M. G., and B. C. J. G. Knight.** 1941. The biochemistry of bacterial toxins I. The lecithinase activity of *Cl. welchii* toxins. *Biochem. J.* 35:884–902.

70. **Menestrina, G.** 1986. Ionic channels formed by *Staphylococcus aureus* alpha toxin: voltage dependent inhibition by di- and trivalent cations. *J. Membr. Biol.* 90:177–190.

71. **Mikesell, P., B. E. Ivins, J. D. Ristroph, and T. M. Dreier.** 1983. Evidence for plasmid-mediated toxin production in *Bacillus anthracis*. *Infect. Immun.* 39:371–376.

72. **Mitsui, K., T. Kekiya, Y. Nozawa, and J. Hase.** 1979. Alteration of human erythrocyte plasma membranes by perfringolysin O as revealed by freeze fracture electron microscopy. Studies on *Cl. perfringens* exotoxins V. *Biochim. Biophys. Acta* 554:68–75.

73. **Molnar, D. M., and R. A. Altenbern.** 1963. Alterations in the biological activity and protective antigen of *Bacillus anthracis* toxin. *Proc. Soc. Exp. Biol. Med.* 114:294–297.

74. **Morgan, K. L., E. Gruffydd-Jones, A. A. Wienecke, J. de Azavedo, P. J. Carroll, and L. P. Stevenson.** 1986. Staphylococcal toxic shock syndrome. *Vet. Rec.* 119:559.

75. **Noda, M., T. Hirayama, I. Kato, and F. Matsuda.** 1980. Crystallisation and properties of staphylococcal leucocidin. *Jpn. J. Bacteriol.* 35:137–144.

76. **Ohashi, Y., T. Kamiya, and M. Fijiwara.** 1987. ADP-ribosylation by type C1 botulinum neurotoxins: stimulation by guanine nucleotides and inhibition by guanidino containing compounds. *Biochem. Biophys. Res. Commun.* 142:1032–1038.

77. **Ohishi, I.** 1987. Activation of botulinum C_2 toxin by trypsin. *Infect. Immun.* 55:1461–1465.

78. **Ohishi, I., M. Iwasaki, and G. Sakaguchi.** 1980. Vascular permeability activity of botulinum C2 toxin elicited by cooperation of two dissimilar protein components. *Infect. Immun.* 31:890–895.

79. **Ohsaka, A., M. Tsuchiya, C. Oshio, M. Miyaira, K. Suzuki, and Y. Yamakawa.** 1978. Aggregation of platelets in the mesenteric microcirculation of the rat induced by α-toxin (phospholipase C) of *Clostridium perfringens*. *Toxicon* 16:333–341.

80. **Peeters, J. E., R. Geeroms, R. J. Carman, and T. D. Wilkins.** 1986. Significance of *Clostridium spiroforme* in the enteritis complex of commercial rabbits. *Vet. Microbiol.* 12:25–31.

81. **Popoff, M. R.** 1987. Purification and characterization of *Clostridium sordellii* lethal toxin and cross-reactivity with *Clostridium difficile* cytotoxin. *Infect. Immun.* 55:35–43.

82. **Raynaud, M., and J. E. Alouf.** 1970. Intracellular versus extracellular toxins, p. 67–112. *In* S. J. Ajl, S. Kadis, and T. C. Montie (ed.), *Microbial Toxins*, vol. I. Academic Press, Inc., New York.

83. **Rotta, J.** 1986. Pyogenic hemolytic streptococci, p. 1047–1054. *In* P. H. A. Sneath, N. S. Mair, M. E. Sharpe, and J. G. Holt (ed.), *Bergey's Manual of Systematic Bacteriology*, vol. 2. The Williams & Wilkins Co., Baltimore.

84. **Rottem, S., R. M. Cole, W. H. Habig, M. F. Barile, and M. C. Hardigree.** 1982. Structural characteristics of tetanolysin and its binding to lipid vesicles. *J. Bacteriol.* 152:888–892.

85. **Russell, R. J., P. C. Wilkinson, R. J. McInroy, S. McKay, A. C. McCartney, and J. P. Arbuthnott.** 1976. Effect of staphylococcal products on locomotion and chemotaxis of human blood neutrophils and monocytes. *J. Med. Microbiol.* 8:433–449.

86. **Sakaguchi, G.** 1986. Clostridium botulinum toxins, p. 519–548. *In* F. Dorner and J. Drews (ed.), *Pharmacology of Bacterial Toxins*. Pergamon Press, Oxford.

87. **Sakurai, J., and M. Nagahama.** 1985. Tryptophan content of *Clostridium perfringens* epsilon toxin. *Infect. Immun.* 47:260–263.

88. **Sandvig, K., and S. Olsnes.** 1986. Mechanisms of intoxication by protein toxins, p. 175–188. *In* J. B. Harris (ed.), *Natural Toxins, Animal, Plant and Microbial*. Oxford University Press, Oxford.

89. **Schlievert, P. M.** 1982. Enhancement of host susceptibility to lethal endotoxin shock by staphylococcal pyrogenic exotoxin type C. *Infect. Immun.* 36:123–128.

90. **Simpson, L. L., B. G. Stiles, H. H. Zepeda, and T. D. Wilkins.** 1987. Molecular basis for the pathological action of *Clostridium perfringens* iota toxin. *Infect. Immun.* 55:118–122.

91. **Smith, L. D. S., and B. L. Williams.** 1984. *The Pathogenic Anaerobic Bacteria*, 3rd ed., p. 70. Charles C Thomas, Publisher, Springfield, Ill.

92. **Smyth, C. J., and J. L. Duncan.** 1978. Thiol-activated (oxygen-labile) cytolysins, p. 129–183. *In* J. Jeljaszewicz and T. Wadstrom (ed.), *Bacterial Toxins and Cell Membranes*. Academic Press, Inc. (London), Ltd., London.

93. **Smyth, C. J., J. H. Freer, and J. P. Arbuthnott.** 1975. Interaction of *Clostridium perfringens* theta haemolysin, a contaminant of commercial phospholipase C, with erythrocyte ghost membranes and lipid dispersions. *Biochim. Biophys. Acta* 382:479–493.

94. **Smyth, C. J., R. Mollby, and T. Wadstrom.** 1975. Phenomenon of hot-cold hemolysis: chelator-induced lysis of sphingomyelinase-treated erythro-

cytes. *Infect. Immun.* 12:1104–1111.

95. **Stephen, J.** 1986. Anthrax toxin, p. 281–295. *In* F. Dorner and J. Drews (ed.), *Pharmacology of Bacterial Toxins.* Pergamon Press, Oxford.

96. **Stiles, B. G., and T. D. Wilkins.** 1986. Purification and characterization of *Clostridium perfringens* iota toxin: dependence on two non-linked proteins for biological activity. *Infect. Immun.* 54:683–688.

97. **Taylor, A. G., and A. W. Bernheimer.** 1974. Further characteristics of staphylococcal gamma hemolysin. *Infect. Immun.* 10:54–59.

98. **Thorne, G. M., and S. L. Gorbach.** 1986. General characteristics: nomenclature of microbial toxins, p. 5–14. *In* F. Dorner and J. Drews (ed.), *Pharmacology of Bacterial Toxins.* Pergamon Press, Oxford.

99. **Turnbull, P. C. B.** 1986. *Bacillus cereus* toxins, p. 397–448. *In* F. Dorner and J. Drews (ed.), *Pharmacology of Bacterial Toxins.* Pergamon Press, Oxford.

100. **van Heyningen, W. E.** 1970. General characteristics, p. 1–26. *In* S. J. Ajl, S. Kadis, and T. C. Montie (ed.), *Microbial Toxins,* vol. I. Academic Press, Inc., New York.

101. **Wadstrom, T.** 1983. Biological effects of cell damaging toxins, p. 671–704. *In* C. S. F. Easmon and C. Adlam (ed.), *Staphylococci and Staphylococcal Infections,* vol. 1. Academic Press, Inc. (London), Ltd., London.

102. **Wallace, V., and D. M. McDowell.** 1986. Botulism in a dog—first confirmed case in New Zealand. *N.Z. Vet. J.* 34:149–150.

103. **Ward, P. D., C. Adlam, and W. Turner.** 1981. A comparison of the intradermal effects of some hemolytic and leukocidic toxins from *Staphylococcus aureus,* p. 281–285. *In* J. Jeljaszewicz (ed.), *Staphylococci and Staphylococcal Infections. Zentralblatt fuer Bakteriologie* Suppl. 10. Gustav Fischer Verlag, New York.

104. **Wong, T. P., and N. Groman.** 1984. Production of diphtheria toxin by selected strains of *Corynebacterium ulcerans* and *Corynebacterium pseudotuberculosis. Infect. Immun.* 43:1114–1116.

105. **Woodin, A. M.** 1972. Staphylococcal leucocidin, p. 281–299. *In* J. O. Cohen (ed.), *The Staphylococci.* John Wiley & Sons, Inc., New York.

Chapter 17

New Pathophysiological Aspects in the Action of Staphylococcal Enterotoxin B in the Monkey

PETER H. SCHEUBER,[1] JOCHEN R. GOLECKI,[2] CLAUDIO DENZLINGER,[3] DIETMAR WILKER,[4] BARBARA SAILER-KRAMER,[1] DIETRICH KEPPLER,[3] AND DIETRICH K. HAMMER[1]

Max-Planck-Institut für Immunbiologie,[1] Institut Biologie II, Mikrobiologie,[2] and Biochemisches Institut,[3] Universität Freiburg, D-7800 Freiburg, and Chirurgische Klinik Innenstadt der Universität München, D-8000 München,[4] Federal Republic of Germany

INTRODUCTION

Staphylococcal enterotoxin (SE) is the causative agent of a prevalent type of food-borne debilitating enteric intoxication in humans. The most common clinical manifestations after peroral challenge to human volunteers and other primates are emesis and diarrhea (2), whereas nonprimate laboratory animals show little if any response. So far, sequential morphologic (10) and ultrastructural (12) alterations associated with the peroral administration of SE have been described, suggesting that the site of emetic action lies within the gastrointestinal tract (5) and that the toxin-induced vomiting response via stimulation of local neural receptors in the gastrointestinal tract follows vagal and sympathetic afferents (18).

Although considerable effort has been expended on attempts to define the pathophysiology of enterotoxemia, the target cells and their mediators involved in the intestinal site of SE type B (SEB) action still remain obscure. In this report a new in vivo model is described for studies of SEB function by an immediate-type hypersensitivity reaction in the skin of monkeys (15). A series of experiments provides evidence that SEB administered intradermally causes skin reactions by degranulation of mast cells (15). Finally, both pharmacological studies and the strongly enhanced generation of cysteinyl leukotrienes upon SEB challenge indicate that these mediators play an important role in the pathophysiology of the toxin-induced actions in vivo.

IN VIVO MODEL

SEB Challenge of Monkeys

In basic experiments, cynomolgus monkeys (*Macaca fascicularis*) used for skin tests or gastric intubation were anesthetized and maintained unconscious for 15 min. Enteric intoxication was induced by administration of 5 µg of SEB per kg in 5 ml of phosphate-buffered saline by gastric tube, and the clinical response was monitored for 24 h.

Prior to any form of intradermal challenge, unsensitized monkeys received 2 ml of 1% Evans blue intravenously. Immediately after this, duplicate samples of various concentrations of SEB (0.1 to 10 μg) and phosphate-buffered saline as control were injected intradermally into the anterior aspect of the thorax and abdomen of each monkey. The size of any blueing reaction evoking a threshold of 5 mm in diameter was noted 15 min after injection.

Carboxymethylation of SEB

The chemical modification of histidine residues in highly purified SEB (6) with bromoacetic acid has been used to study the influence of bromoacetic acid on the biological activity of the toxin. After carboxymethylation of the six histidine residues present in our SEB (cSEB) preparation, 4.96 residues were derivatized to 3-monocarboxymethyl histidine and 1.05 residues were modified to 1,3-carboxymethyl histidine (15). This chemical modification of SEB caused a conversion from alkaline components to more acidic species and an increase in microheterogeneity (15). A comparison of the emetic efficiency of SEB and cSEB showed that the emetic 100% effective dose of SEB upon challenge by gastric intubation was even less than 5 μg/kg (Table 1). cSEB, however, consistently failed to evoke emetic responses even when five times the effective dose of SEB was used (Table 1).

Immediate-Type Skin Reactions Elicited by SEB

In an attempt to define the mechanisms involved in the toxin action, the capability of SEB to induce an immediate-type hypersensi-tivity reaction in the skin of unsensitized monkeys when challenged intradermally was used as a model system (Table 2). It was apparent that SEB and cSEB were almost equally effective in provoking immediate-type reactions in skin sites of monkeys presensitized with rat anti-SEB immunoglobulin E (IgE). Of particular importance, however, was the finding that even 10^{-9} M SEB was highly efficient in promoting immediate-type hypersensitivity reactions in the skin of unsensitized monkeys, whereas cSEB consistently failed to do so (Table 2). To determine whether cSEB, which is incapable of evoking immediate-type hypersensitivity reactions in unsensitized skin sites, shares with SEB the ability to interact with functional domains of a putative receptor on the target cell, inhibition experiments were performed. From the data in Table 2 it can be inferred that immediate-type skin reactions following challenge with 5 μg of SEB were completely antagonized by cSEB, when used at fivefold molar excess.

To establish whether SEB behaves as a nonimmunological stimulus such as basic polypeptides (16), bypassing the regular two-stage mast cell IgE antibody-antigen interaction by acting directly on a putative receptor, we took advantage of the observation that mast cells initially exposed to a mast cell-degranulating agent become unresponsive to a subsequent exposure to a second challenging agent. From the results in Table 2 it is apparent that the immediate-type reaction in unsensitized monkeys was completely abolished by pretreatment of skin sites with the histamine liberator 48/80 24 h before SEB challenge. In this context, it was ascertained that vascular reactivity was not significantly reduced by comparing the hista-

TABLE 1

Effect of carboxymethylation on the emetic response to SEB in the monkey

No. of histidine residues modified	Method of modification	SEB dose (μg/kg)	Emetic response
0	None	5	6/6[a]
6	Carboxymethylation[b]	5	0/3
6	Carboxymethylation[b]	25	0/3

[a]Number vomiting/number challenged.
[b]Carboxymethylation with bromoacetic acid.

TABLE 2
Effect of cSEB and compound 48/80 on SEB-provoked immediate-type skin reactions in monkeys[a]

Skin sites sensitized with IgE antibody to:	Pretreatment	Challenge	Skin reaction[b] (mm diameter ± SE)
SEB	None	SEB	25.0 ± 1.0
SEB	None	cSEB	20.0 ± 1.0
None	None	SEB	18.0 ± 1.0
None	None	cSEB	<1.0
None	None	cSEB + SEB (5:1)[c]	<1.0
None	48/80[d]	SEB	<1.0

[a] Sensitized sites were prepared by intradermal injection of rat anti-SEB IgE, and after 72 h monkeys were challenged with SEB (5 µg).
[b] Means ± standard error of the mean of four separate experiments.
[c] cSEB and SEB were injected simultaneously at a molar ratio of 5:1 into unsensitized skin sites.
[d] Compound 48/80 (25 µg) was injected into unsensitized skin sites; sites were challenged with SEB after 24 h.

mine-induced response at a pretreated site with that at a control site. This argues against the possibility that a histamine liberator-induced inhibition of vascular response contributes to the demonstrated abrogation of the immediate-type skin reaction following exposure to SEB.

The data reviewed here favor the hypothesis that mast cells are triggered by SEB only when the active peptide carries a positive charge. Chemical modification of SEB by carboxymethylation, causing a loss in toxicity, completely abrogated skin-sensitizing activity and protected against the emetic response without changing the immunological specificity of the molecule. Most important, however, is the fact that cSEB competitively antagonizes the action of native SEB on binding sites of target cells but is incapable of promoting activation signals by itself.

Ultrastructural Changes in Skin Reactions after SEB Challenge

That SEB acts by affecting mast cells is reflected in the ultrastructural morphology at sites of skin reactions. The cytoplasm of mast cells in control biopsies is packed with typical electron-dense granules of uniform size but variable shape (Fig. 1A). Mast cell granules from SEB-challenged skin sites, however, show alterations including limited fusion of adjacent granules and some loss of dense contents (Fig.

1B). Many of these cells have prominent mitochondria and ribosomes and many vesicles, indicating active synthesis. These observations suggest that SEB-induced triggering of mast cells is accompanied by synthetic and metabolic activity. Mast cells of skin sites challenged with cSEB, however, had no distinctly different morphology from those of control skin sites (Fig. 1C).

Massive extrusion of granules from cells, as occurs in anaphylactic degranulation of mast cells, was rarely observed.

Effect of Anti-Id on SEB-Induced Skin Reactions

It must be shown whether SEB exerts its effect on mast cells by binding to specific cell surface receptors or whether some less-specific type of ligand-cell membrane interaction is involved. It has been demonstrated previously that hormone or neurotransmitter receptors share with antibodies a number of conceptual analogies which may be reflected in structural similarities (17). Studies of antibodies raised against the binding sites of these hormone-specific antibodies have confirmed the conservation of structures, since anti-idiotypic antibodies (anti-Id) directed against the active site of the ligand-specific antibody were able to interact with hormone receptors. Such an approach might be successfully applied with SEB, a more complex

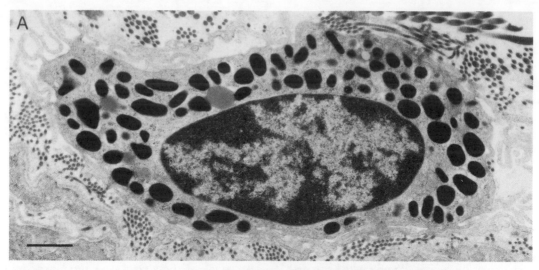

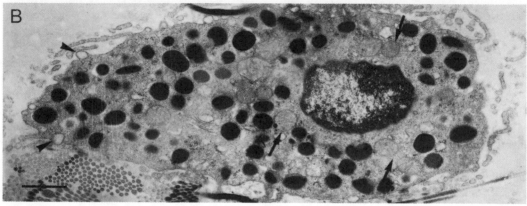

FIGURE 1. (A) Electron micrograph of a dermal mast cell from a control skin site of an unsensitized monkey injected with phosphate-buffered saline 15 min prior to sample fixation. (B) Mast cell from the skin site challenged with SEB. Note the occasional granule fusion, numerous mitochondria in the cytoplasma (arrows), and vesicles (arrowhead) partially associated with the granules. (C) Mast cell from the skin site challenged with cSEB does not appear to be distinctly different from that of control sites. Bars in all panels represent 1 μm.

ligand than hormones, to identify whether ligand-specific receptors actually exist on the target cell membrane (Fig. 2). Anti-Id against monoclonal anti-SEB antibodies (anti-SEB) were raised in BALB/c mice and purified by idiotype (anti-SEB) affinity chromatography (1). Anti-Id did not contain any contamination with anti-SEB or anti-IgG antibodies. To show that purified anti-Id was indeed directed against the idiotype of monoclonal anti-SEB, the inhibition of ^{125}I-labeled anti-SEB binding to solid-phase SEB in microtiter plates was used. Even

2 nM anti-Id was able to effect 50% inhibition of anti-SEB binding, whereas preimmune BALB/c IgG consistently lacked any capacity to compete for binding (Fig. 3A).

A competitive inhibition analysis in which increasing concentrations of SEB were used to impede the binding of ^{125}I-labeled anti-SEB to anti-Id showed that inhibition of the interaction of these two species by 10 μM SEB approached 80%, whereas SEA and SEC$_1$ lacked any inhibitory capacity (Fig. 3B). This indicated that the purification of anti-Id results in

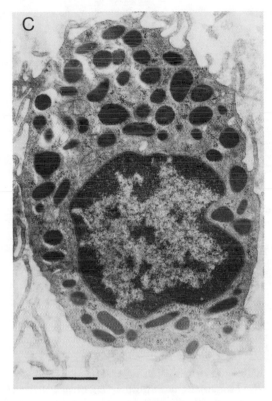

FIGURE 1. *Continued.*

a high degree of binding-site selectivity (1).

To determine whether anti-Id were able to recognize SEB-specific receptors on the target cell membrane, we examined the influence of anti-Id in an inhibition analysis in which increasing concentrations of purified anti-Id (10^{-6} to 10^{-11} M) were used to compete with the action of SEB at different doses (0.02 to 2 µg) on the target cell. For this purpose, anti-Id were added to SEB and the mixture (0.1 ml) was tested for its ability to elicit immediate-type reactions in unsensitized skin sites. Anti-Id at 1 to 100 nM impedes the immediate-type skin reaction in a concentration-dependent manner following challenge with SEB (1) (Fig. 4). No such inhibition was found when preimmune IgG was used, suggesting that it was indeed the anti-Id against anti-SEB competing with the ligand for binding to the target cell membrane.

Analogously, anti-Id administered intra-dermally 48 h before challenge with SEB also antagonized the immediate-type skin reaction (data not shown), indicating that the anti-Id-mediated prolonged blocking effect reflects a rather considerable affinity of these antibodies for the target cell receptor. The evidence presented indicates that anti-Id to monoclonal anti-SEB display the characteristics of a potent SEB antagonist without triggering biologic function themselves. Thus, anti-Id may potentially be of therapeutic value in SEB-induced intestinal disorders.

Effect of Drugs on SEB-Induced Actions

The ability of SEB to elicit, besides enteric intoxication, immediate-type hypersensitivity reactions in the skin of unsensitized monkeys was more closely examined in an attempt to define the type of mediators involved by using selective antagonists and by measuring the endogenous generation of mediators in vivo.

For potential inhibition of immediate-type skin reactions and intestinal disorders following challenge with SEB, pharmacologic agents such as diphenhydramine, an H1 receptor antagonist of histamine, and cimetidine, an H2 receptor antihistamine, were injected at 1 mg/kg intravenously 1 h before intradermal injection and 15 min before and 1, 2 and 3 h after intragastric intubation with SEB. Methysergide, a serotonin antagonist, was administered by gastric tube at 30 µg/kg 15 min before exposure with SEB. Additionally, the following calcium channel blockers were delivered by gastric tube 15 min before SEB challenge, at the dosages indicated: diltiazem, 0.3 mg/kg, and nifedipine, 0.07 mg/kg.

Diphenhydramine caused a substantial inhibition of the immediate-type skin reaction in unsensitized monkeys, but failed to have any influence on the emetic response following challenge with SEB by gastric tube (Table 3). Pretreatment with cimetidine, a selective blocker of the H2 receptor, however, totally abrogated the immediate-type skin response and completely and consistently prevented emesis and

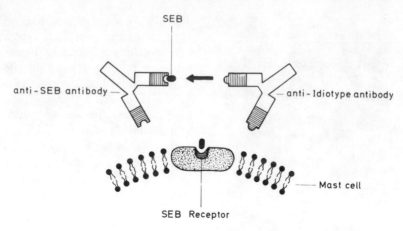

FIGURE 2. Interacting components of an Id–anti-Id network involving SEB, SEB receptor, and anti-SEB as well as anti-Id. Antibodies specific for SEB display binding sites which are similar to those found on the SEB receptor. Anti-Id recognize determinants on anti-SEB and the receptor which are complementary to the SEB combining site.

diarrhea. Methysergide at 30 μg/kg, which gives optimal therapeutic levels in human plasma (11), did not have any inhibitory effect when administered 15 min prior to SEB challenge by gastric tube. Most interestingly, the immediate-type skin reaction, as well as the emetic response, following exposure to SEB was totally abrogated by the calcium channel blockers diltiazem and nifedipine.

On the basis of these studies, the use of pharmacologic agents provided a more complete assessment of the skin reactivity upon challenge with SEB in unsensitized monkeys.

The apparent inhibitory effect of calcium channel blockers on both skin reaction and emetic response suggests that a predominant step in the sequence of biochemical events following SEB challenge is the role of calcium as

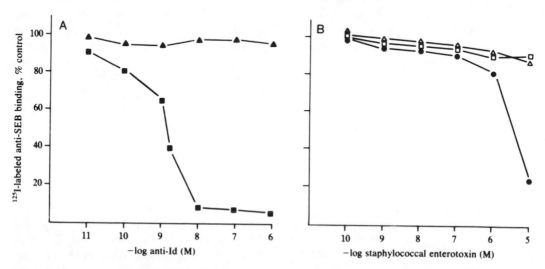

FIGURE 3. Assessment of anti-Id binding activity. (A) Effect of anti-Id (■) or preimmune IgG (▲) on binding of ^{125}I-labeled anti-SEB to the solid-phase SEB. (B) Influence of SEB (●), SEA (□), or SEC$_1$ (△) on the binding of ^{125}I-labeled anti-SEB to solid-phase anti-Id.

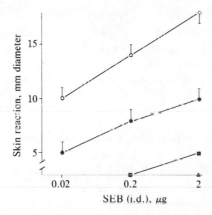

FIGURE 4. Effect of anti-Id on immediate-type hypersensitivity reaction in the skin of unsensitized monkeys upon SEB challenge. Anti-Id at 1 nM (●), 10 nM (■), or 100 nM (▲) or preimmune IgG (○) was mixed with various concentrations of SEB in a total volume of 0.1 ml, and the incubation mixture was injected intradermally. Each point is the mean and standard deviation of quadruplicate determinations.

a second messenger mediating the action of the toxin. Furthermore, treatment of monkeys with H2 but not with H1 antihistamines notably inhibited immediate-type skin reactions; it also completely protected against the emetic response following SEB challenge. Although SEB-induced skin response is consistent with mast cell triggering, there is no definite proof so far that histamine is the principal mediator of these reactions. Rather, the lack of ability of H2 receptor antagonists alone to inhibit the skin response to histamine or passive cutaneous anaphylaxis reactions to antigen in monkeys (9) argues against the predominance of histamine as mediator of these reactions.

Another group of mediators released by mast cells are the products of the 5-lipoxygenase pathway, which include the cysteinyl leukotrienes (LTs) LTC_4, LTD_4, and LTE_4, the major elements of slow-reacting substance of anaphylaxis (13). LTs constitute a newly recognized family of metabolites of arachidonic acid with very potent functions in inflammation and immediate-type hypersensitivity reactions (13) and provoke many of the pathophysiologic sequelae of endotoxic shock (8). Further studies were therefore designed to obtain information about the potential role of LTs in immediate-type hypersensitivity reactions in the skin and enteric intoxication in unsensitized monkeys upon SEB challenge.

The mediator function of cysteinyl LTs in SEB-induced disorders was investigated by using inhibitors of prostanoid synthesis and LT action and by measuring LT generation in vivo. To examine potential inhibition of skin reactions and emetic responses, the following pharmacologic agents were administered 30 min before SEB challenge: indomethacin (3 mg/kg intravenously), aspirin (4 mg/kg intravenously), both inhibitors of prostanoid formation (19), and LY171883 (0.1 to 1 mg/kg by

TABLE 3

Effects of pharmacologically active agents on skin reactions and emetic response in unsensitized monkeys upon SEB challenge[a]

Drug treatment	No. of animals	Skin reaction[b] (mm diameter ± SE)	Emetic response[c]
None	10	18.0 ± 1.0	10/10
Diphenhydramine	6	6.0 ± 1.0	6/6
Cimetidine	6	<1.0	0/6
Methysergide	4	18.0 ± 1.0	4/4
Diltiazem	6	<1.0	0/6
Nifedipine	4	<1.0	0/4

[a]Monkeys were injected intravenously with Evans blue and subsequently challenged with 5 μg of SEB intradermally. Intestinal intoxication was induced by 5 μg of SEB per kg, administered by gastric tube. The animals were treated with the drugs and reactions were evaluated as described in the text.
[b]Means ± standard error of the mean of 4 to 10 separate experiments.
[c]Number of animals vomiting/number challenged.

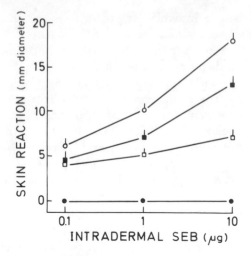

FIGURE 5. Effect of intradermal administration of LY171883 on immediate-type skin reactions in unsensitized monkeys after intradermal SEB challenge. Untreated monkeys (○) or monkeys pretreated with the antagonist at 0.1 mg/kg (■), 0.3 mg/kg (□), or 1 mg/kg (●), injected with Evans blue 15 min later, and subsequently challenged with SEB intradermally in a dose range of 0.1 to 10 μg. The means and the standard errors of the mean for six separate experiments are presented.

gastric tube), a potent and selective LTD_4/LTE_4 receptor antagonist (7).

Pretreatment with LY171883 at 1 mg/kg completely and consistently abrogated immediate-type skin reactions and protected against emesis and diarrhea in a concentration-dependent manner (Fig. 5 and Table 4). Intragastric intubation of LY171883 at 0.3 mg/kg, how-

ever, impeded skin reactions and the vomiting response only by 50% (Fig. 5). In contrast, the cyclooxygenase inhibitors indomethacin and aspirin did not have any effect on skin reactions and emetic responses when compared with controls (Table 4).

Generation of Cysteinyl LTs upon SEB Challenge

Cysteinyl LT levels in blood plasma, bile, and urine of anesthetized monkeys were measured as described in detail previously (3). One week before bile sampling for analysis, a subcutaneously looped biliary bypass was implanted. By choledochotomy a catheter was inserted into the bile duct and oriented toward the liver. A subcutaneous loop was then created, and the catheter was inserted into the same choledochotomy site and advanced toward the duodenum. The gall bladder was removed (3). The subcutaneous loop allowed access to bile without surgical trauma, preventing interference by LTs produced by tissue injury (4).

On the day of experiment, monkeys received SEB (10 to 30 μg/kg) under anesthesia. Blood was withdrawn from a venous catheter or by puncture of the femoral artery. Bile was collected by tapping the subcutaneous part of the biliary bypass, and urine was collected from a catheter introduced into the urinary bladder. Endogenous cysteinyl LTs were measured by the sequential use of high-performance liquid

TABLE 4

Effects on the LTD_4-LTE_4 receptor antagonist LY171883 and cyclooxygenase inhibitors on skin reactions and emetic response upon challenge with SEB[a]

Drug treatment	Dose (mg/kg)	No. of animals	Skin reaction[b] (mm diameter ± SE)	Emetic response[c]
None		10	18.0 ± 1.0	10/10
LY171883	1.0	6	<1.0	0/6
LY171883	0.3	6	7.0 ± 1.0	3/6
Aspirin	4.0	4	18.0 ± 1.0	4/4
Indomethacin	3.0	4	18.0 ± 1.0	4/4

[a]Monkeys were pretreated with the agents, or with buffer as control, intragastrically, and then challenged with SEB. Reactions were evaluated as described in the text.
[b]Means ± standard error of the mean of 4 to 10 separate experiments.
[c]Enteric intoxication was inducted by 5 μg of SEB per kg, administered by gastric tube. Data represent number of animals with vomiting and diarrhea/number challenged.

chromatography and radioimmunoassay.

Generation of cysteinyl LTs in blood plasma upon SEB challenge could not be demonstrated; i.e., LTC_4, LTD_4, and LTE_4 were all below 15 pmol/liter of blood plasma. LTE_4 was the major biliary cysteinyl LT after intragastric intubation of SEB (Fig. 6). Its concentration averaged 1 nmol/liter before administration of the toxin and rose in a biphasic course to 10 nmol/liter after SEB challenge. The second increase in biliary LTE_4 concentration correlates with the time course of emetic response, occurring about 4 h after intragastric SEB administration in unanesthetized monkeys. In addition to LTE_4, LTD_4 was found in concentrations of up to 6 nmol/liter at 2 to 4 h after the 30-μg/kg SEB dose, whereas in control bile the LTD_4 level was below 0.2 nmol/liter (14).

Urinary concentrations of LTC_4, LTD_4, LTE_4, and N-acetyl-LTE_4 were all below 50 pmol/liter before as well as after SEB admin-

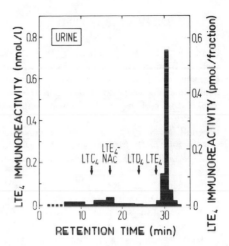

FIGURE 7. LTE_4 immunoreactivity in monkey urine collected 90 to 180 min after intragastric administration of SEB (10 μg/kg). Separation by high-pressure liquid chromatography and subsequent determination of LTE_4 immunoreactivity demonstrate a cysteinyl LT metabolite less polar than LTE_4. Arrows indicate retention times of internally added [3H]-labeled standards. LTE_4NAc, N-Acetyl-LTE_4.

istration. However, a single immunoreactive metabolite was observed following intragastric SEB challenge (Fig. 7). This metabolite was less polar than LTE_4, resisted chemical N-acetylation, and coeluted with a radioactive cysteinyl LT derivative observed after intraduodenal [3H]LTC_4 (3). The data presented demonstrate abolition of SEB actions by a selective LTD_4-LTE_4 receptor antagonist and a remarkable increase of cysteinyl LTs in bile and urine following SEB challenge, indicating that these mediators play a significant role in the pathophysiology of SEB-induced reactions in vivo. This is the first evidence for a convincing correlation between the in vivo inhibition of LT action and amelioration of the symptoms.

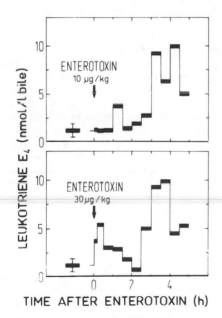

FIGURE 6. LTE_4 concentrations in bile of monkeys before (mean and standard error of the mean for four animals) and after intragastric intubation of SEB (10 or 30 μg/kg). LTE_4 concentrations in bile fractions were determined by sequential use of high-performance liquid chromatography and radioimmunoassay as described in the text.

ACKNOWLEDGMENTS. This work was supported by grants from the Fraunhofer-Gesellschaft, Munich, Federal Republic of Germany, and the Deutsche Forschungsgemeinschaft Bonn, through SFB 154, Freiburg, Federal Republic of Germany.

LITERATURE CITED

1. Bamberger, U., P. H. Scheuber, B. Sailer-Kramer, K. Bartsch, A. Hartmann, G. Beck, and D. K. Hammer. 1986. Anti-idiotypic antibodies that inhibit immediate-type skin reactions in unsensitized monkeys on challenge with staphylococcal enterotoxin. *Proc. Natl. Acad. Sci. USA* **83**:7054–7058.

2. Bergdoll, M. S. 1979. Staphylococcal intoxications, p. 443–494. *In* H. Riemann and F. L. Bryan (ed.), *Staphylococcal Intoxication.* Academic Press, Inc., New York.

3. Denzlinger, C., A. Guhlmann, P. H. Scheuber, D. Wilker, D. K. Hammer, and D. Keppler. 1986. Metabolism and analysis of cysteinyl leukotrienes in the monkey. *J. Biol. Chem.* **261**:15601–15606.

4. Denzlinger, C., S. Rapp, W. Hagmann, and D. Keppler. 1985. Leukotrienes as mediators in tissue trauma. *Science* **230**:330–332.

5. Elwell, M. R., C. T. Liu, R. O. Spertzel, and W. R. Beisel. 1975. Mechanisms of oral staphylococcal enterotoxin B-induced emesis in the monkey. *Proc. Soc. Exp. Biol. Med.* **148**:424–427.

6. Ende, I., G. Terplan, B. Kickhöfen, and D. K. Hammer. 1983. Chromatofocusing: a new method for purification of staphylococcal enterotoxin B and C_1. *Appl. Environ. Microbiol.* **46**:1323–1330.

7. Fleisch, J. H., L. E. Rinkema, K. D. Haisch, D. Swanson-Bean, T. Goodson, P. P. K. Ho, and W. S. Marshall. 1985. LY171883 1-[2-hydroxy-3-propyl-4-[4-(1H-tetrazol-5-yl)butoxy]phenyl]ethanone, an orally active leukotriene D_4 antagonist. *J. Pharmacol. Exp. Ther.* **233**:148–157.

8. Hagmann, W., C. Denzlinger, and D. Keppler. 1984. Role of peptide leukotrienes and their hepatobiliary elimination in endotoxin action. *Circ. Shock* **14**:223–235.

9. Hutchcroft, B. J., E. G. Moore, and R. P. Orange. 1979. The effects of H_1 and H_2 receptor antagonism on the response of monkey skin to intradermal histamine, reverse-type anaphylaxis, and passive cutaneous anaphylaxis. *J. Allergy Clin. Immunol.* **63**:376–382.

10. Kent, T. H. 1966. Staphylococcal enterotoxin gastroenteritis in rhesus monkeys. *Am. J. Pathol.* **48**:387–398.

11. Meier, J., and E. Schreier. 1976. Human plasma levels of some antimigraine drugs. *Headache* **16**:96–104.

12. Merrill, T. G., and H. Sprinz. 1968. The effect of staphylococcal enterotoxin on the fine structure of the monkey jejunum. *Lab. Invest.* **18**:114–123.

13. Samuelsson, B. 1983. Leukotrienes: mediators of immediate hypersensitivity reactions and inflammation. *Science* **220**:568–575.

14. Scheuber, P. H., C. Denzlinger, D. Wilker, G. Beck, D. Keppler, and D. K. Hammer. 1987. Staphylococcal enterotoxin B as a nonimmunological mast cell stimulus in primates: the role of endogenous cysteinyl leukotrienes. *Int. Arch. Allergy Appl. Immunol.* **82**:289–291.

15. Scheuber, P. H., J. R. Golecki, B. Kickhöfen, D. Scheel, G. Beck, and D. K. Hammer. 1985. Skin reactivity of unsensitized monkeys upon challenge with staphylococcal enterotoxin B: a new approach for investigating the site of toxin action. *Infect. Immun.* **50**:869–876.

16. Stanworth, D. R. 1984. The role of non-antigen receptors in mast cell signalling processes. *Mol. Immunol.* **21**:1183–1190.

17. Strosberg, A. D., P.-O. Courand, and A. B. Schreiber. 1981. Immunological studies of hormone receptors: a two-way approach. *Immunol. Today* **2**:75–79.

18. Sugiyama, H., and T. Hayama. 1965. Abdominal viscera as site of emetic action for staphylococcal enterotoxin in the monkey. *J. Infect. Dis.* **115**:330–336.

19. Vane, J. R. 1971. Inhibition of prostaglandin synthesis as a mechanism of action for aspirin-like drugs. *Nature (London) New Biol.* **231**:232–235.

Section V: Strategies to Overcome Bacterial Virulence Mechanisms

Chapter 18

Strategies to Overcome Bacterial Virulence Mechanisms: an Overview

LYNETTE B. CORBEIL

Department of Pathology
University of California, San Diego, Medical Center
San Diego, California 92103

INTRODUCTION

Strategies to overcome bacterial virulence mechanisms include many different approaches, several of which have been discussed in earlier chapters of this volume. Because of the breadth of the topic, only strategies involving host defense mechanisms are addressed here, although chemotherapeutic measures could be considered under this heading if time and space allowed. Even with this limitation, the subject is broad indeed. Many examples of each strategy could be given. However, to give an overview of the topic, I will discuss various approaches to overcoming bacterial virulence mechanisms and dwell on only a few examples which may not be covered in other papers.

In a sense, our attempts to overcome bacterial virulence usually involve a study of the existing natural host defense mechanisms and the use or augmentation of those defenses to protect against bacterial disease. Such mechanisms can be categorized as nonimmune defenses (or natural immunity) and specific immune defenses. Both have been exploited for prophylaxis against disease.

NONSPECIFIC IMMUNITY

Nonimmune defenses include protective mechanisms which do not involve antigen-specific responses mediated by T or B lymphocytes. This could include everything from the protective barrier of the skin to the low pH of the stomach. In recent years, however, several strategies for manipulating nonspecific defenses have emerged which may lead to better protection against bacterial infection. It has long been known that the normal flora of the skin and mucous surfaces provides a microenvironment which may inhibit colonization by pathogens. Many studies show that isolates of the normal flora inhibit pathogens in vitro, but few have succeeded in causing these inhibitory flora to colonize people or animals to prevent disease. In human medicine, Sprunt et al. (40) were successful in producing nasopharyngeal colonization of 22 neonates in an intensive care unit with alpha-hemolytic streptococci from the normal flora of healthy infants. This colonization with normal flora inhibited colonization by potential pathogens (40). Similarly, colonization of the skin of infants with nonpathogenic staphylococci has been useful in controlling staphylococcal pyoderma in newborn children in nurseries (37). In veterinary medicine, colonization of the gut with normal flora has been reported to prevent colonization of poultry by pathogens (39, 43, 44) and to prevent neonatal diarrhea in pigs (12). This approach has also been used by Brooks and Barnum (6) to prevent mastitis in dairy cows by colonization of the udder with *Corynebacterium bovis*. The mechanism of protection against mastitis was thought to involve increasing the numbers of inflammatory cells in the udder, thus promoting phagocytosis and killing of bacterial pathogens before multiplication occurred. In our laboratory, Woodward et al. (47) were intrigued by this nonimmune, nonpharmacologic approach to control of mastitis. We decided that if it was possible to colonize the teat skin with isolates from the normal flora which inhibit the growth of mastitis pathogens, it may be possible to prevent mastitis without increasing inflammation, which is thought to decrease production (21). As a first step in the study, the ability of isolates of bacterial flora from normal teats to inhibit the growth of mastitis pathogens was determined (47). We found that some, but not all, *Bacillus, Corynebacterium, Staphylococcus,* and *Aerococcus* isolates inhibited gram-negative or gram-positive mastitis pathogens, or both, in vitro. Other bacterial normal flora isolates did not inhibit mastitis pathogens (Table 1). These results encouraged us to attempt to colonize teats with

inhibitor flora. Since most new cases of mastitis begin during the dry period or at parturition (27, 29, 31), it appeared that this would be the best time to colonize teats with bacterial inhibitors. We therefore attempted to colonize teats with normal flora isolates. First, we studied colonization by normal flora isolates which inhibited both gram-positive and gram-negative mastitis pathogens in vitro, but none persisted on the teats for more than an average of 10 days (Table 2). Because it is well known that it is difficult to manipulate a well-established normal flora (26) and because we found that staphylococci were the predominant organisms in teat flora (W. D. Woodward and L. B. Corbeil, unpublished data), we then compared colonization of neonatal calves with a *Staphylococcus hominis* 1 isolate which inhibited staphylococcal and streptococcal mastitis pathogens in vitro. Although neonatal calves remained colonized longer than dry cows in preliminary studies (Table 2), the mean colonization time of 15 days in dry cows was encouraging. Since many new infections occur during the dry period (27, 29), since our *S. hominis* 1 isolate inhibits gram-positive pathogens, and since staphylococci and *Streptococcus uberis* are found on the teat skin, colonization of the teat skin with this *S. hominis* 1 inhibitor isolate throughout the dry period may be protective. Although challenge studies have not yet been done, in the preliminary studies cited above *S. hominis* 1 of the inoculated biotype was often isolated from dry cow teats in pure culture. This provides some indication that in

TABLE 1
Normal bovine teat flora inhibitory for mastitis pathogens in vitro

Normal flora isolates[a]	No. tested	No. inhibitory for:	
		Gram-positive pathogens[b]	Gram-negative pathogens[c]
Corynebacterium	42	11	10
Bacillus spp.	21	11	8
Aerococcus spp.	2	2	2
Staphylococcus spp.	35	3	0

[a] *Acinetobacter* (36 isolates), *Micrococcus* (9 isolates), *Pseudomonas* (1 isolate), *Serratia* (1 isolate), *Streptobacillus* (1 isolate), *Streptococcus* (2 isolates), and *Streptomyces* (1 isolate) were tested also, but none were inhibitory.
[b] Gram-positive pathogens included *S. aureus* (two isolates), *S. epidermidis* (two isolates), and *Corynebacterium pyogenes* (one isolate).
[c] Gram-negative pathogens included *E. coli* (three isolates) and *Klebsiella* spp. (three isolates).

TABLE 2
Colonization of bovine teats with normal flora isolates which inhibit mastitis pathogens in vitro

Pathogen inhibitor	Animals[a]	No. treated	No. colonized	Mean duration of colonization (days)
Bacillus/Corynebacterium xerosis	Dry cows	3	3	5
Bacillus sp.	Dry cows	2	2	9.5
Aerococcus viridans	Dry cows	2	0	0
S. hominis 1	Dry cows	4	3	15
S. hominis 1	Neonatal calves	7	7	>36

[a]Dry cows, Colonization initiated at the beginning of the dry period. Neonatal calves, Colonization initiated in first 3 days of life.

vivo inhibition of other normal flora did occur. Since gram-positive organisms were the predominant normal teat flora in our studies, the deliberate use of S. hominis 1 inhibitor bacteria to colonize dry cow teats may be a useful adjunct to prevention of Staphylococcus and Streptococcus uberis mastitis.

Another approach to preventing colonization with pathogenic bacteria involves blocking receptor-ligand interactions at the epithelium. In both pigs and calves, enteric colibacillosis is mediated by several virulence factors (17). Attachment of Escherichia coli to the intestinal mucosa is critical to local multiplication, with resulting high population density of pathogens. Adherence to mucosal epithelium can be mediated by many specific adhesins, but in enteric disease caused by E. coli, pili are the key (17). The K88 pili in pigs have been studied most thoroughly, although other antigenic types including K99, 987P, and F41 are also found in porcine and bovine enterotoxigenic E. coli (ETEC). Colonization factors I and II (CFA/I and CFA/II) are the best-characterized of several pili of human ETEC (25). Similarly, pili are involved in the attachment of ovine and equine E. coli isolates associated with diarrhea. The K88 pili of porcine ETEC have been shown to attach to specific receptors of neonatal pig intestinal mucosa which are genetically controlled (17, 34). Piglets lacking the gene for the K88 receptor are resistant to disease due to K88 ETEC, whereas piglets with the gene are susceptible (34). Since the gene for the K88 receptor is dominant (34), it should be possible to select for homozygous recessive

animals as a strategy to overcome the adhesion virulence mechanism. This has become a little more complicated, since it is now clear that there are several different K88 variants, but because one of the pig phenotypes is resistant to all K88 variants (17), it should still be possible to select for resistance. However, screening for receptors in the small-intestinal brush border is cumbersome in that the piglets must be sacrificed or intestinal biopsies must be done to obtain brush border cells. This problem could be overcome by a method suggested by Atroshi et al. (3). They showed that fat globule membranes in sow milk or colostrum had K88 receptors derived from the apical epithelium of mammary secretory epithelium (4). These receptors were under the same genetic control as the intestinal epithelial cells (3); thus, milk fat globules could be used as a screening method to determine the phenotype of the sow to select for piglets without K88 receptors (3). A method for selecting resistant pigs is not the only application of this work, however. The above studies also present another means of interfering with receptor-ligand interaction to overcome the adhesin virulence mechanism. Since milk fat globules have receptors for K88 and K99 pili (32), the milk fat globules should interfere with the attachment of ETEC to the intestinal epithelium by competitive inhibition (3). This would be especially true in neonatal animals, since proteinase and lipase activities are very low in the upper gastrointestinal tract in neonatal piglets (3). Atroski et al. (4) have shown that fat globules from sow milk can be fractionated into several antiadhesive components. These include immunologically specific, high-molecular-weight immunoglobulin G (IgG) and IgA, the high-molecular-weight membrane fractions, and a low-molecular-weight (molecular weight 1,000) factor which bound K88 (4). They postulated that the low-molecular-weight inhibitor may be composed of released membrane surface determinants which may compete with brush border determinants. Thus, both fat globule membranes and released components may act as traps for K88-bearing ETEC, resulting in removal of the pathogens with the feces. Others have shown other food substances to be involved in adhesion inhibition. Recently Neeser et al. (30) demonstrated that some plant glycoproteins were potent inhibitors of adhesion mediated by type 1 pili of *E. coli*. In agreement with this, Freter (16) has suggested that many foodstuffs may act as competitive inhibitors for adherence by pathogens.

A third means of nonspecific defense against bacterial pathogens includes the whole area of stimulation of the cells of the immune system by various immunomodulators. Much has been done on the ability of such modulators as interferon, the interleukins, and bacterial products such as lipopolysaccharide (LPS) to stimulate immune cells in vitro. Less has been done showing protection against bacterial infection in vivo. Since this area is addressed in Chapter 20 of this volume, I will merely give a few examples here. Some of the early studies on the role of interferon in protection against bacterial infection showed that human leukocytic interferon reduced the number of *Salmonella* and *Shigella* organisms invading HEp-2 tissue culture cells (7). Later it was shown that human gamma interferon inhibited intracellular multiplication of *Legionella pneumophila* (5) or *Chlamydia psittaci* (33) in vitro. In vivo, protection of mice against *Listeria monocytogenes* infection has been accomplished with recombinant murine gamma interferon (23), demonstrating that interferon may be useful in protection of whole animals against some facultative intracellular bacterial infections.

SPECIFIC IMMUNITY

Since the days of Louis Pasteur, a commonly used strategy to overcome bacterial virulence has been via the specific immune response. His early contributions on immunization against pasteurellosis (fowl cholera) and anthrax laid the groundwork for modern immunoprophylaxis of bacterial infections. Both killed and attenuated live vaccines have been quite successful in preventing many bacterial infections, such as *Bordetella pertussis* infection in humans, vibriosis, anthrax, and brucellosis in cattle, and erysipelas in pigs, as well as leptospiral and clostridial infections in many domestic animal species, to mention only a few. However, whole-cell vaccines have not been ideal, because the required repeated high doses of killed vaccine often cause detrimental side effects, whereas attenuated live vaccines may revert to virulence or lose potency owing to bacterial death. Passive immunization, on the other hand, has been useful in the face of an outbreak or in cases of failure of passive transfer in neonates. Problems with passive immunization include the short duration of immunity and the problem of serum sickness which may result from systemic administration of whole serum. Thus, new strategies seemed to be required.

Two major approaches may be taken to develop new immunoprophylactic or immunotherapeutic measures. The first involves identification of an important virulence mechanism or combination of virulence mechanisms, followed by administration of the virulence factor(s) as a vaccine or use of antibodies against the factor(s) in passive-immunization regimens. The second approach involves demonstration of a protective immune response, followed by determination of the type of response which was crucial to protection (e.g., systemic or local antibody- or cell-mediated responses) and identification of the specificity of the protective response. Examples of these approaches are given below in the context of the several ways in which the identified immunogens and protective responses may be applied to prevention of bacterial disease.

Passive Immunity

Prophylaxis or immunotherapy by passive immunization has been useful in several special circumstances. The importance of colostrum in most domestic animals is well known, yet failure of passive transfer is a factor in many infectious diseases of neonates. Management procedures to minimize failure of passive transfer have helped considerably, but even in situations in which all precautions have been taken, up to 30% of calves are hypogammaglobulinemic (11). Such calves are very susceptible to enteric disease, pneumonia (11), and colisepticemia (45). It is known that in enteric colibacillosis, pili are involved in the pathogenesis and that antibody against the K99 pili of E. coli is protective (2). However, to protect the neonate, it is necessary to vaccinate the mother. In cases of failure of passive transfer, the neonate is still unprotected. Recently this problem has been addressed by oral treatment of calves with monoclonal antibodies to the K99 pili of E. coli. This was shown to prevent enteric colibacillosis (36), and the monoclonal antibody is now commercially available for use in the field. Hybridoma technology has been applied in other bacterial infections also. Monoclonal antibodies against type 1 fimbriae or the complementary D-mannose receptors have been shown to protect against E. coli-induced urinary tract infections in mice (1). A similar approach was taken in prevention of colisepticemia in calves. In this case, not one serotype but many can be etiologic agents. Thus identification of one immunogen for protection was difficult. A cross-reactive antibody was needed. Since antibodies to LPS core glycolipid protect against a variety of gram-negative infections in laboratory animals (48) and humans (49), this appeared to be a useful approach to control of colisepticemia in calves. Antiserum to a UDP-galactose-4-epimerase-deficient mutant of E. coli (strain J5) was produced in cattle and used to protect colostrum-deprived calves against an oral challenge with virulent E. coli JL9 originally obtained from a septicemic calf (45). In this study, we showed that such cross-reactive antibody delays the onset and decreases the magnitude of bacteremia (Table 3). The challenge dose in this study (10^{10} CFU) was probably higher than the dose received in nature, but the protection would still have to be maximized to be useful in the field. Since a mixture of specificities and immunoglobulin isotypes was given, it appeared that achieving a high titer of the most protective specificity and isotype may provide this maximal protection. Recently Teng et al. (42) demonstrated protection against lethal murine gram-negative bacteremia and dermal Shwartzman reactions with monoclonal IgM antibody against lipid A. Furthermore, Ziegler et al. (E. J. Ziegler, N. N. H. Teng, H. Douglas, A. Wunderlich, H. J. Berger, and S. D. Bolmer, Clin. Res. 35:619A, 1987) administered the same IgM monoclonal antibody (HA-1A) to neutropenic rabbits already infected by conjunctival inoculation of Pseudomonas aeruginosa. Treatment of rabbits with HA-1A prevented death in a situation similar to the bacteremia following mu-

TABLE 3

Antiserum to a UDP-galactose-4-epimerase-deficient mutant of E. coli (strain J5) for protection against colisepticemia in calves

Animal[a]	ELISA titer[b]			Mean hour of onset of bacteremia[c]	Mean hour of death[c]	Mean bacteremia level (CFU[d])
	IgG1	IgG2	IgM			
Control	<20	<10	<10	12	25	2.9×10^6
Treated	325	45	50	52	80	1.4×10^3

[a]Four colostrum-deprived calves per group were challenged orally with 10^{10} virulent E. coli JL9 5 h after being given 200 ml of saline (controls) or anti-J5 serum intravenously.
[b]Mean titers against heated J5 cells. ELISA, Enzyme-linked immunosorbent assay.
[c]Treated animals were significantly different from controls (P = 0.014).
[d]Mean CFU at peak of bacteremia.

cosal infection in immunocompromised neonatal calves. Thus monoclonal antibodies to LPS
core glycolipid (especially lipid A) hold great
promise in prevention and treatment of colisepticemia or endotoxemia. Others have shown
that passive (J. S. Cullor, B. W. Fenwick, M.
R. Williams, B. P. Smith, A. Kelly, K. Pel-
zer, and B. I. Osburn, *Conf. Res. Workers. Am.
Dis.* 1984, abstr. 48, p. 9) or active (14) immunization with *E. coli* J5 protects against *Salmonella* endotoxemia in calves and *Haemophilus*
pleuropneumonia in pigs. Thus, this approach
may have widespread application for use against
gram-negative infections of domestic animals
as well as humans.

Active Immunity

Active immunization has a long history.
Whole attenuated or killed bacteria have been
used successfully to prevent many bacterial infections or even to treat a few diseases such as
bovine venereal vibriosis (35). In cases in which
these straightforward approaches with whole-
cell vaccines have not been successful, many
strategies have been used to overcome the vaccine problems mentioned above.

Live Vaccines

To avoid reversion of attenuated live vaccines to virulence, genetically modified live
vaccines hold great promise. For example, non-
reverting aromatic-dependent *Salmonella* vaccines have been shown to protect calves against
challenge with *Salmonella typhimurium* or *Salmonella dublin* (38). Others have shown that
Salmonella dublin lacking an 80-kilobase plasmid is avirulent, whereas reintroduction of the
plasmid restores virulence for mice (8). The
plasmid-free derivative of *Salmonella dublin* (the
Lane strain) is an effective live oral vaccine in
mice (D. G. Guiney, J. Fierer, G. Chikami,
P. Beninger, E. J. Heffernan, and K. Tanabe,
UCLA Symp. Mol. Cell. Biol., in press). Such
avirulent *Salmonella* mutants (with the ability
to attach to and invade the gut epithelium) have
been further manipulated by recombinant DNA

technology to express genes for virulence antigens of other pathogens, resulting in bivalent
live vaccines (see Chapter 19 of this volume).
Formal et al. (15) used a similar approach for
protection against *Shigella flexneri*. They transferred both the *Shigella flexneri* plasmid which
confers the ability to invade and the chromosomal genes for the *Shigella flexneri* somatic antigen into *E. coli* K-12. This constructed oral
vaccine (which should have no potential to revert) protected monkeys against challenge with
virulent *Shigella flexneri* (15).

Subunit Vaccines

Aside from the above strategies to overcome problems with live attenuated vaccines,
there have been a series of strategies to avoid
problems with killed vaccines, whose high doses
and detrimental side effects have been major
obstacles. To overcome this, many investigators have resorted to subunit vaccines. Perhaps
the first subunit vaccine to be widely used was
tetanus toxoid. The success of this vaccine
encourages us to utilize new biotechnologic
methods to develop subunit vaccines for bacterial infections which are continuing problems. Recent examples of subunit vaccines include the capsular vaccines for *H. influenzae* type
b, *Neisseria meningitidis* groups A and C, and
Streptococcus pneumoniae. Furthermore, purified
pili of *E. coli* have been shown to protect against
enterotoxigenic colibacillosis in calves (2) and
pigs (28). Purified enterotoxins also protect
against enteric colibacillosis (24). Once such
subunit vaccines have been shown to protect,
it is then possible to characterize the subunit
structure and chemically synthesize the antigen. Using this rationale, Houghten et al. (20)
have developed a synthetic enterotoxin vaccine
that is effective against challenge with heterologous enterotoxigenic *E. coli*. When synthetic peptides are shown not only to protect shortly
after immunization, but also to provide good
anamnestic responses to bacterial challenge, this
should be a very economical approach. Use of
recombinants for purification of immunogens

is another approach for providing large amounts of antigen for vaccine production.

A variant of the subunit-vaccine strategy to avoid the whole-cell vaccine problems is the use of antibodies as immunogens. Over 10 years ago it was reported that immunity could be induced by immunization with anti-idiotypic antibodies (13). This has been applied to protection against several infectious agents, but only very recently have studies of anti-idiotypic immunogens been reported for bacterial infections. Stein and Söderström (41) produced monoclonal idiotypic and anti-idiotypic antibodies against an *E. coli* polysaccharide capsular antigen and against the anticapsular monoclonal antibody, respectively. Both antibodies were shown to prime weanling mice for protection against *E. coli* infection (41). This showed that monoclonal antibodies could not only passively protect the young but also contribute to long-term protection. It also demonstrated the effectiveness of anti-idiotypic immunogens in protection against bacterial infection. This may be especially useful for polysaccharide antigens, which are not always as immunogenic as proteins (especially in the young). A similar approach was taken by Kaufmann et al. (22) to protect against *L. monocytogenes* infection in mice, but since this is a facultative intracellular parasite, clonotypic antibodies were used rather than anti-idiotypic antibodies. Clonotypic antibodies have specificity for individual T-cell clones and thus can block or stimulate homologous T cells. Since cell-mediated immunity is crucial in protecting against listeriosis, the ability to stimulate a specific antilisterial T-cell response would be ideal. In the above study, antiserum against a T-cell clone specific for an epitope expressed by *L. monocytogenes* blocked antigen stimulation of the specific T-cell hybridoma but not concanavalin A stimulation. Mice immunized with this clonotypic antiserum were protected against challenge with homologous *L. monocytogenes* but not *L. monocytogenes* of a different serotype, suggesting that clonotypic antibodies may be useful in vaccination against facultative intracellular bacterial infections.

CHARACTERIZATION OF PROTECTIVE IMMUNE RESPONSE

The above examples were all based on the strategy of identification of a virulence factor (or factors) and development of a vaccine by using that virulence factor (with the partial exception of the clonotypic antibody study). The other major approach is to characterize the immune cell types, antibody isotypes, and specificity responsible for protection. Our work with *H. somnus* infections of cattle is an example of the latter approach. We first developed and characterized experimental infections of *H. somnus*-induced pneumonia (19) and abortion (46). In characterizing the immune responses of experimentally infected cattle, we found that IgG2 anti-*H. somnus* antibodies increased the most after infection and remained high the longest (46). Also, low IgG2 titers appeared to be somewhat correlated with susceptibility to abortion (46). We then attempted to confer passive protection with convalescent serum taken 6 weeks after induction of experimental pneumonia (18). Calves were inoculated by fiberoptic bronchoscopy with 10^7 CFU of *H. somnus* preincubated (for 5 min) in preimmune serum into one diaphragmatic lobe and with 10^7 CFU of *H. somnus* preincubated in convalescent-phase serum into the other lobe. At necropsy, 24 h later, viable bacterial counts were done on bronchoalveolar lavage fluid from each side. The volume of the pneumonic lung was determined in serial lung slices by computerized image analysis. There was a significant difference between the pneumonic lung volumes on the side with convalescent serum (0.9 cm^3) and that with preimmune serum (50.04 cm^3) at $P < 0.0005$ if lung volumes of each calf at each level of the lung were compared or at $P < 0.05$ if total volumes of pneumonic lung for each treatment were compared among all four calves. Viable *H. somnus* cell counts were also significantly different ($P < 0.05$) on the protected ($10^{7.1}$ CFU/ml of bronchoalveolar lavage fluid) and unprotected ($10^{4.1}$ CFU/ml) sides. Since this convalescent-phase serum was known to be protective, we then characterized its specificity

(18), as well as the specificity of convalescent-phase serum from animals in the experimental abortion study (9). Western blot (immunoblot) analysis showed that the sera obtained after abortion recognized 270,000-molecular-weight (270K), 76K, 60K, and 40K protein antigens most intensely, whereas serum from animals convalescent to pneumonia recognized 78K, 60K, 40K, and several low-molecular-weight protein antigens most intensely, although the 270K and 76K antigens could be detected at lower intensity. *H. somnus* LPS antigens were recognized also (18). Most of these antigens were present in outer membrane preparations, and the antibody reactivity to them could be absorbed out with whole live *H. somnus* organisms, demonstrating their surface location. Thus, one or a combination of these antigens may be candidates for a subunit vaccine, even though the role of the proteins as virulence factors is unknown and little is known of the role of *H. somnus* LPS, except that it does share the toxic properties of other LPSs (T. Inzana, personal communication).

In using the approach of characterizing a protective immune response to produce a vaccine, it is necessary to develop criteria for the choice of most likely candidate antigens. Our criteria included the following. (i) The antigen is recognized by a protective humoral or cellular immune response. (ii) The antigen is on the surface of the bacterium or is released from the bacterium (e.g., toxins, enzymes, etc.). (iii) The antigen does not undergo antigenic variation in vivo (as is the case with the superficial antigens of *Campylobacter fetus* [10]), because this would allow evasion of the protective response. (iv) The antigen is conserved among *H. somnus* isolates or at least among pathogenic *H. somnus* isolates. (v) The antigen is not widely distributed among other bacterial species, especially among normal flora isolates which may be beneficial to the host. (vi) The antigen is immunogenic for the host species which is to be protected.

On the basis of the above data and criteria, our approach is to purify and/or clone and express the genes for each *H. somnus* candidate antigen. Monospecific bovine polyclonal antisera are then prepared against each antigen and used to determine whether the antigen is shared by a wide variety of *H. somnus* isolates as well as whether it is shared by isolates of other bacteria. Monospecific sera for antigens which are secreted or located on the surface of *H. somnus,* do not undergo antigenic variation in vivo, are conserved among many *H. somnus* isolates, but are not widely cross-reactive with other bacteria will be used in passive protection experiments as described above. Thus, the knowledge that serum protects against *H. somnus* pneumonia, that the IgG2 antibody response is predominant, and that several surface antigens are recognized most intensely in Western blots has enabled us to progress toward development of subunits and recombinant vaccines for *H. somnus* infection in cattle.

ACKNOWLEDGMENTS. This work was supported in part by U.S. Department of Agriculture grants 83-CRSR-2-2282, 84-CRSR-2-2423, and 86-CRCR-1-2268.

LITERATURE CITED

1. **Abraham, S. N., J. P. Babu, C. S. Giampapa, D. L. Hasty, W. A. Simpson, and E. H. Beachey.** 1985. Protection against *Escherichia coli*-induced urinary tract infections with hybridoma antibodies directed against type 1 fimbriae or complementary D-mannose receptors. *Infect. Immun.* 48:625–628.

2. **Acres, S. D., R. E. Isaacson, L. A. Babiuk, and R. A. Kapitany.** 1979. Immunization of calves against enterotoxigenic colibacillosis by vaccinating dams with purified K99 antigen and whole cell bacteria. *Infect. Immun.* 25:121–126.

3. **Atroshi, F., T. Alavuhkola, R. Schildt, and M. Sandholm.** 1983. Fat globule membrane of sow milk as a target for adhesion of K88-positive *Escherichia coli. Comp. Immunol. Microbiol. Infect. Dis.* 6:235–245.

4. **Atroshi, F., R. Schildt, and M. Sandholm.** 1983. K88-mediated adhesion of *E. coli* inhibited by fractions in sow milk. *Zentralbl. Veterinaermed. Reihe B* 30:425–433.

5. **Bhardway, N., T. W. Nash, and M. A. Horwitz.** 1982. Interferon-γ-activated human monocytes inhibit the intracellular multiplication of *Legionella pneumophila. J. Immunol.* 137:2662–2669.

6. **Brooks, B. W., and D. A. Barnum.** 1984. The

susceptibility of bovine udder quarters colonized with *Corynebacterium bovis* to experimental infection with *Staphylococcus aureus* or *Streptococcus agalactiae*. *Can. J. Comp. Med.* 48:146–150.

7. Bukholm, G., and M. Degre. 1983. Effect of human leukocyte interferon on invasiveness of *Salmonella* species in HEp-2 cell cultures. *Infect. Immun.* 42:1198–1202.

8. Chikami, G. K., J. Fierer, and D. G. Guiney. 1985. Plasmid-mediated virulence in *Salmonella dublin* demonstrated by use of a Tn5-*oriT* construct. *Infect. Immun.* 50:420–424.

9. Corbeil, L. B., J. E. Arthur, P. R. Widders, J. W. Smith, and A. F. Barbet. 1987. Antigenic specificity of convalescent serum from cattle with *Haemophilus somnus* induced experimental abortion. *Infect. Immun.* 55:1381–1386.

10. Corbeil, L. B., G. C. D. Schurig, P. J. Bier, and A. J. Winter. 1975. Bovine veneral vibriosis: antigenic variation of the bacterium during infection. *Infect. Immun.* 11:240–244.

11. Corbeil, L. B., B. Watt, R. R. Corbeil, T. G. Betzer, R. K. Brownson, and J. L. Morrill. 1984. Immunoglobulin concentrations in serum and nasal secretions of calves at the onset of pneumonia. *Am. J. Vet. Res.* 45:773–778.

12. Davidson, J. N., and D. C. Hirsh. 1976. Bacterial competition as a means of preventing neonatal diarrhea in pigs. *Infect. Immun.* 13:1773–1774.

13. Eichmann, K., and K. Rajewsky. 1975. Induction of T and B cell immunity by anti-idiotypic antibody. *Eur. J. Immunol.* 5:661–666.

14. Fenwick, B. W., J. S. Cullor, B. I. Osburn, and H. J. Olander. 1986. Mechanisms involved in protection provided by immunization against core lipopolysaccharides of *Escherichia coli* J5 from lethal *Haemophilus pleuropneumoniae* infections in swine. *Infect. Immun.* 53:298–304.

15. Formal, S. B., T. L. Hale, C. Kapfer, J. P. Cogan, P. J. Snoy, R. Chung, M. E. Wingfield, B. L. Elisberg, and L. S. Baron. 1984. Oral vaccination of monkeys with an invasive *Escherichia coli* K-12 hybrid expressing *Shigella flexneri* 2a somatic antigen. *Infect. Immun.* 46:465–469.

16. Freter, R. 1980. Prospects for preventing the association of harmful bacteria with host mucosal surfaces, p. 441–458. *In* E. H. Beachey (ed.), *Bacterial Adherence. Receptors and Recognition,* series B, vol. 6. Chapman & Hall, Ltd., London.

17. Gaastra, W., and F. K. de Graaf. 1982. Host-specific fimbrial adhesins of noninvasive enterotoxigenic *Escherichia coli* strains. *Microbiol. Rev.* 46:129–161.

18. Gogolewski, R. P., S. A. Kania, T. J. Inzana, P. R. Widders, H. D. Liggitt, and L. B. Corbeil. 1987. Protective ability and specificity of convalescent serum from *Haemophilus somnus* pneumonia. *Infect. Immun.* 55:1403–1411.

19. Gogolewski, R. P., C. W. Leathers, H. D. Liggitt, and L. B. Corbeil. 1987. Experimental *Haemophilus somnus* pneumonia in calves and immunoperoxidase localization of bacteria. *Vet. Pathol.* 24:250–256.

20. Houghten, R. A., R. A. Lerner, S. R. Hoffman, P. A. Worrell, P. Wright, and F. A. Klipstein. 1985. Completely synthetic vaccine effective against heterologous enterotoxigenic *Escherichia coli*, p. 91–94. *In* R. A. Lerner, R. M. Charnock, and F. Brown (ed.), *Vaccines 85.* Cold Spring Harbor Laboratory, Cold Spring Harbor, N.Y.

21. Huston, G. E., and C. W. Heald. 1983. Effect of the intramammary device on milk infection status, yield and somatic cell count and on the morphological features of the lactiferous sinus of the bovine udder. *Am. J. Vet. Res.* 44:1856–1860.

22. Kaufmann, S. H. E., K. Eichmann, I. Muller, and L. J. Wragel. 1985. Vaccination against the intracellular bacterium *Listeria monocytogenes* with a clonotypic antiserum. *J. Immunol.* 134:4123–4127.

23. Kiderlen, A. F., S. H. E. Kaufmann, and M.-L. Lohmann-Matthes. 1984. Protection of mice against the intracellular bacterium *Listeria monocytogenes* by recombinant immune interferon. *Eur. J. Immunol.* 14:964–967.

24. Klipstein, F. A., R. F. Engert, and R. A. Houghten. 1983. Protection in rabbits immunized with a vaccine of *Escherichia coli* heat-stable toxin cross-linked to the heat-labile toxin B subunit. *Infect. Immun.* 40:888–893.

25. Knutton, S., D. R. Lloyd, and A. S. McNeish. 1987. Identification of a new fimbrial structure in enterotoxigenic *Escherichia coli* (ETEC) serotype O148:H28 which adheres to human intestinal mucosa: a potentially new human ETEC colonization factor. *Infect. Immun.* 55:86–92.

26. Mackowiak, P. A. 1982. Medical progress: the normal microbial flora. *N. Engl. J. Med.* 307:83–93.

27. McDonald, J. S. 1984. Streptococcal and staphylococcal mastitis. *Vet. Clin. North Am. Large Anim. Pract.* 6:269–285.

28. Morgan, R. L., R. E. Isaacson, H. W. Moon, C. C. Brinton, and C.-C. To. 1978. Immunization of suckling pigs against enterotoxigenic *Escherichia coli*-induced diarrheal disease by vaccinating dams with purified 987 or K99 pili: protection correlates with pilus homology of vaccine and challenge. *Infect. Immun.* 22:771–777.

29. Neave, F. K., F. H. Dodd, and E. Henriques. 1950. Udder infections in the 'dry period'. 1. *J. Dairy Res.* 17:37–49.

30. Neeser, J.-R., B. Koellreutter, and P. Wuersch. 1986. Oligomannoside-type glycopeptides inhibiting adhesion of *Escherichia coli* strains mediated by type 1 pili: preparation of potent inhibitors from plant gly-

coproteins. *Infect. Immun.* 52:428–436.

31. Oliver, S. P., and B. A. Mitchell. 1983. Susceptibility of bovine mammary gland to infections during the dry period. *J. Dairy Sci.* 66:1162–1166.

32. Reiter, B., and T. Brown. 1976. Inhibition of haemagglutination of red blood cells by K88 and K99 adhesion using milk fat and fat globule membrane. *Proc. Soc. Gen. Microbiol.* 3:109.

33. Rothermel, C. D., B. Y. Rubin, and H. W. Murray. 1983. γ-Interferon is the factor in lymphokine that activates human macrophages to inhibit intracellular *Chlamydia psittaci* replication. *J. Immunol.* 131:2542–2544.

34. Rutter, J. G., M. R. Burrows, R. Sellwood, and R. A. Giggons. 1975. A genetic basis for resistance to enteric disease caused by *Escherichia coli. Nature* (London) 257:135–136.

35. Schurig, G. G. D., C. E. Hall, L. B. Corbeil, J. R. Duncan, and A. J. Winter. 1975. Bovine venereal vibriosis: cure of genital infection in females by systemic immunization. *Infect. Immun.* 11:245–251.

36. Sherman, D. M., S. D. Acres, P. L. Sadowski, J. A. Springer, B. Bray, T. J. G. Raybould, and C. C. Muscoplat. 1983. Protection of calves against enteric colibacillosis by orally administered *Escherichia coli* K99-specific monoclonal antibody. *Infect. Immun.* 42:653–658.

37. Shinefield, H. R., J. C. Ribble, and M. Boris. 1971. Bacterial interference between strains of *Staphylococcus aureus* 1960–1970. *Am. J. Dis. Child.* 121:148–152.

38. Smith, B. P., M. Reina-Guerra, B. A. D. Stocker, S. K. Hoiseth, and E. Johnson. 1984. Aromatic dependent *Salmonella dublin* as a parenteral modified live vaccine for calves. *Am. J. Vet. Res.* 45:2231–2235.

39. Soerjadi, A. S., G. H. Snoeyenbos, and O. M. Weinack. 1982. Intestinal colonization and competitive exclusion of *Campylobacter fetus* subsp. *jejuni* in young chicks. *Avian Dis.* 26:520–524.

40. Sprunt, K., G. Leidy, and W. Redman. 1980. Abnormal colonization of neonates in an ICU: conversion to normal colonization by pharyngeal implantation of alpha hemolytic Streptococcus strain 215. *Pediatr. Res.* 14:308–313.

41. Stein, K. E., and T. Soderström. 1984. Neonatal administration of idiotype or antiidiotype primes for protection against *Escherichia coli* K13 infection in mice. *J. Exp. Med.* 160:1001–1011.

42. Teng, N. N. H., H. S. Kaplan, J. M. Herbert, C. Moore, H. Douglas, A. Wunderlich, and A. I. Braude. 1985. Protection against Gram negative bacteremia and endotoxemia with human monoclonal Ig M antibodies. *Proc. Natl. Acad. Sci. USA* 82:1790–1794.

43. Weinack, O. M., G. H. Snoeyenbos, E. P. Smyser, and A. S. Soerjadi. 1981. Competitive exclusion of intestinal colonization of *Escherichia coli* in chicks. *Avian Dis.* 25:696–705.

44. Weinack, O. M., G. H. Snoeyenbos, C. F. Smyser, and A. S. Soerjadi. 1982. Reciprocal competitive exclusion of *Salmonella* and *Escherichia coli* by native intestinal microflora of the chicken and turkey. *Avian Dis.* 26:585–595.

45. Wickstrom, M. L., C. C. Gay, J. L. Hodgson, P. R. Widders, D. Schaeffer, R. Lee, and L. B. Corbeil. 1987. Cross-reactive antibody in immunity to colisepticemia in calves. *Vet. Microbiol.* 13:259–271.

46. Widders, P. R., L. G. Paisley, R. P. Gogolewski, J. F. Evermann, J. W. Smith, and L. B. Corbeil. 1986. Experimental abortion and the systemic immune response in cattle to *Haemophilus somnus. Infect. Immun.* 54:555–560.

47. Woodward, W. D., T. E. Besser, A. C. S. Ward, and L. B. Corbeil. 1987. *In vitro* growth inhibition of mastitis pathogens by bovine teat skin normal flora. *Can. J. Vet. Res.* 51:27–31.

48. Ziegler, E. J. 1987. Passive immunization in gram-negative infections, p. 115–126. *In* J. Cash (ed.), *Progress in Transfusion Medicine,* vol. 2. Churchill Livingstone, Edinburgh.

49. Ziegler, E. J., J. A. McCutchan, J. Fierer, M. P. Glauser, J. C. Sadoff, H. Douglas, and A. I. Braude. 1982. Treatment of Gram negative bacteremia and shock with human antiserum to a mutant *Escherichia coli. N. Engl. J. Med.* 307:1225–1230.

Chapter 19

Avirulent Salmonellae Expressing Virulence Antigens from Other Pathogens for Use as Orally Administered Vaccines

Roy Curtiss III, Sandra M. Kelly, Paul A. Gulig,
Claudia R. Gentry-Weeks, and Jorge E. Galán

Department of Biology
Washington University
St. Louis, Missouri 63130

INTRODUCTION

With the advent of recombinant DNA techniques, scientists have increasingly used these techniques to study bacterial pathogens. A diversity of genetic, immunological, and biochemical approaches coupled with appropriate in vitro and in vivo assessments of virulence attributes have therefore been used to elucidate molecular mechanisms of bacterial pathogenicity.

Infectious disease is the product of a sequence of events. First, the microbial pathogen must make contact with a suitable portal of entry into the host. For example, this entry could be ingestion, inhalation, injection due to the bite of an insect vector, or wound infection. Second, most pathogens must locate and attach to a specific host receptor. Third, for pathogens that use surfaces as a portal of entry, the pathogen must either colonize the host surface or invade through the surface to multiply either intracellularly or extracellularly within the body. Fourth, the pathogen must then synthesize products (i.e., enzymes, toxins, acids, etc.) which act to overcome host defenses or cause damage to the host. The genetic control for this sequence of events has evolved for each pathogen-host combination and is undoubtedly very sophisticated. The expression of colonization and virulence attributes for some pathogens, at least, is temporally regulated in response to the environment, the host, or both. For example, some bacteria such as *Shigella* spp. do not express their colonization and virulence properties until they come in contact with their warm-blooded host (47). Thus, *Shigella* spp. do not synthesize the proteins needed for attachment to and invasion of cells at the ambient temperatures of contaminated water but only after ingestion by the human target (47). It appears also that many pathogens have multiple means to accomplish productive infection, which makes prevention of infection difficult. The basic information derived from studies of pathogenesis can be applied to the development of vaccines or therapeutic agents. Thus, if the mechanism by which a pathogen colonizes, invades, and overcomes the host can be defined in biochemical terms, it should be possible to develop a vaccine to prevent or a therapeutic agent to alleviate infection and disease.

IMMUNITY AND IMMUNIZATION

There are three branches of the immune system: the mucosal or secretory, humoral, and cellular branches.

A detailed study of mucosal immunity has only recently begun. Mucosal immunity is mediated primarily by secretory immunoglobulin A (IgA) present in secretions that bathe mucosal surfaces and produced by secretory glands in the body (10, 13, 48). Several mechanisms have been proposed by which secretory IgA exerts protective abilities: the blocking of attachment and colonization by pathogens on a mucosal surface (72), antibody-directed cell cytotoxicity (40), antitoxic activity (49), and neutralization of viruses (54, 55). Mucosal immunity, therefore, is important in diminishing infectious diseases by pathogens which colonize on or invade through a mucosal surface.

Humoral immunity is mediated by circulating antibodies, primarily IgG and IgM, in the blood. These antibodies facilitate phagocytosis and complement-mediated cytotoxicity, both of which lead to the death of the invading microorganism, antitoxic activity, and viral neutralization. Humoral immunity is, therefore, important in controlling those infectious diseases in which an organism possesses systemic phases of infection in the blood or in extracellular spaces within the body.

Cellular immunity consists of several types. One is termed a delayed-type hypersensitivity response, which causes T lymphocytes to stimulate macrophages to kill bacterial, protozoan, and mycotic intracellular pathogens. A second type, production of cytotoxic T lymphocytes, is directed at killing host cells infected with viruses. In the third type, natural killer cells are stimulated to kill virus-infected host cells.

Cellular immunity is therefore critically important in infections with bacterial and protozoan intracellular parasites and viruses.

The historical development and current status of vaccines against bacterial pathogens have been reviewed recently (26). Parenteral immunization with purified components of pathogens to induce protective immunity has given promising results in experimental animal model systems, but these vaccines tend to be expensive to produce, and few have been effectively reduced to use in immunizing humans or animals in medical and veterinary practice, respectively. Killed-bacteria (bacterin) vaccines have been used for quite some time (e.g., in typhoid fever, diphtheria, and cholera vaccines). Injection of bacterin vaccines induces humoral immunity but seldom gives long-lasting protection and therefore necessitates periodic booster immunizations. In addition, parenteral immunizations with some bacterins are associated with adverse side effects.

Live attenuated bacteria used for immunization do, however, induce long-lasting immunity. Also, live vaccines are inexpensive to prepare and easier to administer than are subunit and bacterin vaccines. One potential problem with live vaccines is that the gene which has been altered to attenuate the live vaccine strain can revert so that the agent regains full virulence and, thus, causes disease. In addition, live vaccines might persist in the environment with remote, yet possible, opportunities for gene transfer and recombination with other bacteria.

DISCOVERIES LEADING TO A STRATEGY FOR ORAL IMMUNIZATION

The idea to use avirulent salmonellae expressing colonization and/or virulence antigens specified by genes cloned from other pathogens as a means for oral immunization to elicit secretory, humoral, and cellular immunity against the pathogen supplying those genes was developed as a result of four lines of study.

The first discovery of importance was that enteric bacteria can be attenuated by mutation without impairing immunogenicity. Bacon et al. (3, 4) were the first to investigate the virulence of auxotrophic mutants of *Salmonella typhi* and noted that mutants with requirements for purines, *p*-aminobenzoic acid (*p*ABA), and aspartate had reduced virulence for mice. Germanier and Fürer first investigated use of *galE* mutants of *Salmonella typhimurium* for avirulence and immunogenicity in mice (27) and then proposed use of the *S. typhi galE* mutant Ty21a as a vaccine against typhoid fever in humans (28). Hoiseth and Stocker (34) used transposon mutagenesis with Tn*10* followed by selection for fusaric acid resistance which selects for deletional loss of Tn*10* and adjacent DNA sequences to yield mutations unable to revert. (Reversion was a problem that was apparent in the mutants isolated by Bacon et al. [4]). Hoiseth and Stocker initially isolated Δ*aroA* mutants impaired in the ability to synthesize the aromatic amino acid family of compounds, including *p*ABA, needed for folate biosynthesis, and dihydroxybenzoic acid, a precursor to enterochelin needed for iron transport. Recently they combined the Δ*aroA* mutation with a deletion mutation blocking adenine biosynthesis (Δ*purA*) (43). We have used Tn*10* insertions adjacent to the *asd* gene and subsequent selection for fusaric acid resistance to generate Δ*asd* mutations which impose a requirement for diaminopimelic acid to render *S. typhimurium* avirulent without impairing its ability to induce a generalized secretory immune response (15a). Many species of *Salmonella*, including *S. typhimurium* (29a, 30, 33, 38, 56), possess plasmids which contribute to virulence, and plasmid-cured derivatives have been investigated and proposed for use as live vaccines (53).

The second discovery was that orally fed *S. typhimurium* initially attaches to, invades, and proliferates in the gut-associated lymphoid tissue (GALT) in mice before infecting the liver and spleen (12). In other words, the *Salmo-nella*-host interaction has evolved so that the GALT serves as the portal entry of *Salmonella* species to reach deep tissues. Presumably, *Salmonella* species causing invasive disease in other host organisms also reach deep tissues by attaching to, invading, and persisting in the GALT, although data to substantiate this hypothesis are by and large absent. Table 1 presents data from an experiment in which mice were orally fed a mixture of differentially labeled drug-resistant bacteria and the fate of these bacteria was monitored as a function of time. *Streptococcus mutans*, which normally attaches to salivary glycoproteins on the tooth surface, passed through the gastrointestinal tract. *Escherichia coli*, which normally colonizes the colon, persisted for some time but also disappeared by day 4. *S. typhimurium*, on the other hand, attached to the small intestinal wall and attached to, invaded, and persisted in Peyer's patches. *S. typhimurium* also persisted in the contents of the small and large intestine. Unlike *Streptococcus mutans* and *E. coli*, *S. typhimurium* reached the spleen in high titers to result in typhoid fever and the death of the animal.

The third discovery was that antigen delivery to the GALT or Peyer's patches leads to a generalized secretory immune response at other mucosal sites such as the lamina propria of the pulmonary tract, urinary tract, and the gastrointestinal tract, and also secretions such as tears, saliva, milk, and colostrum (10, 13, 48). It is presumed that the mucosal immune system in a diversity of avian and mammalian species, although possibly differing in detail, is, in general, functionally analogous to the system as studied in mice and humans.

The final discovery was a composite of many discoveries from many laboratories, namely the identification in specific biochemical terms of colonization and virulence attributes of a large number of bacterial pathogens infectious to humans or animals. The cloning of the genes for these colonization and virulence antigens by recombinant DNA techniques affords the opportunity to construct avirulent derivatives of *Salmonella* species expressing these colonization and

TABLE 1
Bacterial titers in mice after oral feeding[a]

Bacterial species (inoculum [CFU]) and time after infection	CFU of bacteria in indicated location:				
	Peyer's patches	Small intestinal wall[b]	Small intestinal contents	Colon contents	Spleen
Streptococcus mutans (2×10^8)					
1 h	<10	<10	1×10^3	$>5 \times 10^4$	
5 h	<10	<10	<10	2×10^5	
26 h	<10	<10	<10	<10	
4 days	<10	<10	<10	<10	<10
Escherichia coli (2×10^8)					
1 h	8×10^1	3×10^3	2×10^5	$>1 \times 10^5$	
5 h	<10	<10	2×10^3	5×10^7	
26 h	<10	<10	<10	1×10^4	
4 days	<10	<10	<10	<10	<10
Salmonella typhimurium (1×10^8)					
1 h	7×10^1	4×10^2	2×10^5	$>1 \times 10^5$	
5 h	6×10^1	3×10^1	5×10^2	9×10^7	
26 h	6×10^2	<10	1×10^1	2×10^4	
4 days	5×10^4	5×10^3	1×10^5	2×10^4	6×10^5

[a]Mice were mixedly infected with *E. coli* (resistant to streptomycin and nalidixic acid), *S. typhimurium* (resistant to tetracycline and nalidixic acid), and *S. mutans* (resistant to streptomycin and spectinomycin). These antibiotics were used to monitor the recovery of each strain from mouse tissue with Penassay base agar (Difco Laboratories, Detroit, Mich.) (*E. coli* and *S. typhimurium*) and brain heart infusion agar (Difco) (*S. mutans*) used as basal media.
[b]Small intestinal wall other than Peyer's patches.

virulence antigens and to use the strains as bivalent oral vaccines. Several groups have made use of avirulent salmonellae to express colonization and virulence antigens specified by genes from other enteric pathogens by using classical (20) as well as recombinant DNA techniques (14, 15a, 45, 46, 68, 70) as means of gene transfer. We have used this approach to endow avirulent salmonellae with the ability to produce the *Streptococcus mutans* surface protein antigen A (SpaA) and glucosyltransferase A (GtfA) proteins and to elicit secretory and humoral antibodies against the streptococcal antigens as well as against *Salmonella* species (15a). Based on the initial studies, it is evident that bivalent avirulent *Salmonella* strains have the capacity to induce secretory, humoral, and cellular immune responses against the foreign antigen expressed by the avirulent *Salmonella* species. It should be emphasized that data pertaining to

induction of protective immunity against the pathogen supplying the colonization or virulence antigen are still not available.

STUDIES OF *S. TYPHIMURIUM* PATHOGENICITY

Although *S. typhimurium* LT2 has been one of the most studied organisms from a genetic point of view, knowledge of the genetic control over the ability of *S. typhimurium* to colonize and cause disease is fragmentary at best. We have, therefore, embarked on a series of studies to delineate the stages of the disease process and to identify genes involved and their means of genetic control. Although these studies have value in their own right, it should be evident that information pertaining to mechanisms of *Salmonella* pathogenesis could also augment knowledge as to how best to modify *Salmonella* species for use as the vector components for recombinant bivalent vaccine strains.

S. typhimurium strains have been known for some time to possess a large cryptic plasmid (2, 5, 18, 67). However, Jones et al. (38) demonstrated that this plasmid was not cryptic, but rather played an important role in the virulence of *S. typhimurium*. Although the exact role of the plasmid in virulence is not resolved (29a, 30, 33, 38, 56), the consensus is that the plasmid is involved with the invasion by *S. typhimurium* from the gut to the spleen and liver. Gulig and Curtiss (29a) developed an efficient method of curing the virulence plasmid by using transposon Tn*minitet* (71) to label the plasmid with a stable tetracycline resistance marker. Upon transposition from specialized vectors, the Tn*minitet* element cannot mediate its own transposition or deletion because Tn*minitet* does not encode transposase (71). Thus, Tn*minitet* insertions in the virulence plasmid are as stable as the plasmid itself. *S. typhimurium* with Tn*minitet*-labeled virulence plasmid was grown in novobiocin or at $43°C$ as curing regimens. Isolates that lost the virulence plasmid and Tn*minitet* were selected on fusaric acid-containing media (11, 44) by virtue of being tetracycline sensitive. Curing rates of 10^{-6} to 10^{-7} per cell per generation were observed, confirming the stability of the virulence plasmid. To ensure that the plasmid had not integrated into the chromosome (5, 38), cured derivatives were examined by Southern blot hybridization with a ^{32}P-labeled virulence plasmid.

Curing wild-type *S. typhimurium* SR-11 strain χ3306 yielded χ3337, which possessed a peroral (p.o.) 50% lethal dose (LD_{50}) more than 1,000-fold higher than that of χ3306 (Table 2). χ3337 was not completely avirulent by the p.o. route, however, because mice inoculated with 10^8 to 10^9 CFU became ill, and some deaths were observed. As an important control absent in many plasmid studies, reintroduction of the virulence plasmid into χ3337, yielding χ3338, restored wild-type virulence, thus confirming that the only genetic lesion of χ3337 was loss of the plasmid. In contrast to the differences observed in p.o. LD_{50}s, all three SR-11 strains had intraperitoneal (i.p.) LD_{50}s of less than 50 CFU. The mean day of death for plasmid-cured χ3337 (day 12.3) was significantly greater than that of χ3306 (day 7.3). Both wild-type and cured SR-11 cells colonized Peyer's patches to equal degrees for up to 1 week after p.o. inoculation with 10^9 CFU (Fig. 1). χ3337 persisted in Peyer's patches for as long as a month postinoculation, while mice infected with χ3306 died by day 8 postinoculation. The major difference in virulence between χ3306 and χ3337 was in invasiveness to spleens after p.o. infection (Fig. 2). As many as 100-fold more χ3306 than χ3337 cells were recovered from the spleens of mice 1 week after p.o. inoculation; however, χ3337 persisted in spleens for as long as 1 month postinoculation. The great differences in splenic infection indicate that cured χ3337 is less able to invade spleens, is killed more rapidly in spleens, grows more slowly in spleens, or a combination of these factors. These data are in agreement with

TABLE 2
Mouse LD_{50}s[a] for wild-type and plasmid-cured *S. typhimurium* strains

S. typhimurium strain	100-Kilobase plasmid	LD_{50}s (CFU) by infection method:	
		p.o.	i.p.
χ3306	+	3×10^5	<50
χ3337	−	$>10^8$	<50[b]
χ3338	+	10^5	<50

[a]Determined by the method of Reed and Muench (60) up to 30 days postinfection. +, Plasmid containing; −, plasmid cured.
[b]Mean day of death for χ3337 (12.3 days) was greater than that for χ3306 (7.3 days); $P < 0.001$ (Student's *t* test).

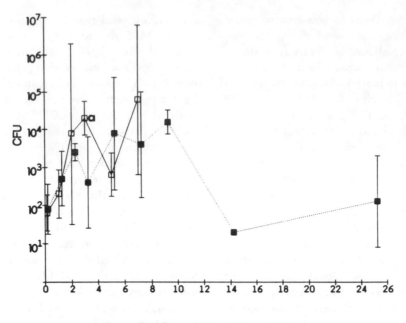

DAYS   POST-INOCULATION

FIGURE 1. Total CFU in Peyer's patches after p.o. inoculation of mice with 10^9 CFU of *S. typhimurium* SR-11 wild-type strain χ3306 (□) and virulence plasmid-cured χ3337 (■). Values are geometric means plus or minus standard deviations ($n = 2$ to 7 mice). *P* values in one-tailed Student's *t* test for CFU of χ3306 greater than χ3337; a in figure indicates $P < 0.0125$. Reproduced from reference 29a.

the results of Hackett et al. (30) and Pardon et al. (56). We also determined that the virulence plasmid was not involved in phagocytosis or killing by murine peritoneal macrophages or resistance to bactericidal activity of normal serum (complement). This latter result is in contrast to those of others (30, 31, 33).

Since plasmid-cured *S. typhimurium* strains retain normal tissue tropism for the GALT and are relatively avirulent, one can consider, as originally suggested by Nakamura et al. for *Salmonella enteritidis* (53), the possibility of using plasmid-cured derivatives as vaccine strains. On the other hand, the long-term persistence of the cured strains in spleens, the occasional deaths of mice after p.o. inoculation, and the high virulence by the i.p. route would suggest that other means for attenuation of *Salmonella* species are necessary to ensure a safe vaccine strain.

CONSTRUCTION AND TESTING OF AVIRULENT *SALMONELLA* STRAINS WITH IMPROVED ATTRIBUTES OF AVIRULENCE AND IMMUNOGENICITY

Although each of the previously cited means for rendering salmonellae avirulent by the presence of specific mutations without impairing immunogenicity has merit, all of these means have problems. *galE* mutants are difficult to grow so as to maintain immunogenicity since they are galactose sensitive (27, 28), but *galE* strains must be grown in the presence of galactose to produce normal lipopolysaccharide essential for immunogenicity (27, 29). However, growth in the presence of galactose selectively leads to galactose-resistant mutants that are irreversibly rough and no longer immunogenic (27). Δ*aroA* mutants abolish the syn-

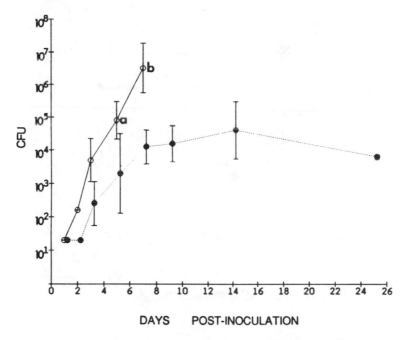

FIGURE 2. Total CFU in spleens after p.o. inoculation of mice with 10^9 CFU of *S. typhimurium* SR-11 wild-type χ3306 (○) and virulence plasmid-cured χ3337 (●). Values are geometric means plus or minus standard deviations ($n = 2$ to 7 mice). *P* values in one-tailed Student's *t* test for CFU of χ3306 greater than χ3337: a, <0.0125; b, <0.0005. Reproduced from reference 29a.

thesis of both enterochelin and folic acid. However, the conclusions of Yancey et al. (74) regarding the necessity of enterochelin for *S. typhimurium* virulence have been disputed by the results of Benjamin et al. (9). The latter demonstrated that mutations which interfere with the ability of *S. typhimurium* to chelate and transport iron are without significant effect on virulence. Therefore, the avirulence of ΔaroA mutants is most likely due to the inability to synthesize *p*ABA and subsequently folic acid. Since Bacon et al. (4) observed that administering *p*ABA in the diet of mice infected with mutants unable to synthesize *p*ABA led to wild-type levels of virulence, one must be concerned with phenotypic reversal of avirulence in vaccine strains due to dietary consumption of metabolites whose synthesis is blocked in the avirulent mutants. Although not having some of these other difficulties, the Δasd mutants rapidly die after oral inoculation and invasion of

the GALT. Thus, they are effective only at eliciting mucosal immunity and are partially and totally ineffective at inducing humoral and cellular immunity, respectively (15a).

Therefore, we began to investigate the use of transposon-induced mutations for which the impairment leading to avirulence could not be compensated by either diet or the animal host. To accomplish this, we screened a Tn10 mutant library of *S. typhimurium* prepared as depicted in Fig. 3 for mutants that were avirulent yet immunogenic. We also evaluated existing Tn10 insertion mutants with gene defects that we deemed likely to lead to avirulence and in which the metabolite whose synthesis is blocked could not be supplied by either diet or host; in addition, we hoped that the mutants would be immunogenic. Following introduction of a large number of Tn10-induced mutations into the mouse-virulent *S. typhimurium* SR-11 strain χ3306, each mutant

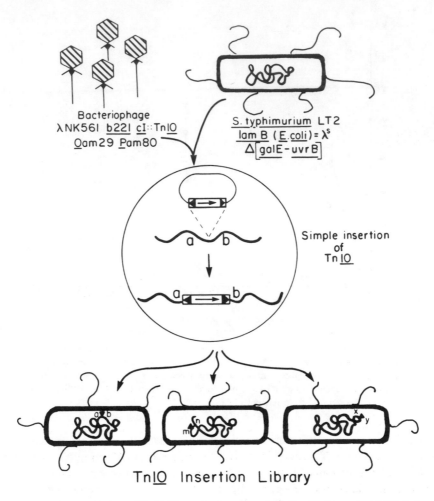

Bacteriophage
λNK561 b221 cI::Tn10
Oam29 Pam80

S. typhimurium LT2
lam B (E.coli) = λ^s
Δ[galE - uvrB]

Simple insertion
of
Tn 10

Tn10 Insertion Library

FIGURE 3. Construction of Tn*10* library in *S. typhimurium*. The Tn*10* vector λNK561 is used to infect a restriction-deficient, modification-proficient, bacteriophage λ-sensitive derivative of *S. typhimurium* (*hsdL6* Δ[*gal-uvrB*]-*1005 flaA66 rpsL120 xyl-404 lamB*+ Δ[*zja*::Tn*10*] [from *E. coli*] *hsdSA29*). Since phage λ is unable to replicate in *S. typhimurium* (6, 7), all tetracycline-resistant isolates must have Tn*10* transposed from the λ genome to a site within the *S. typhimurium* genome.

was evaluated. One mouse was challenged orally with 10^9 mutant cells and i.p. with 10^5 mutant cells. If these mice survived 30 days, they were challenged with either 10^9 or 10^5 virulent wild-type *S. typhimurium* cells orally or i.p., respectively. If these mice survived, larger experiments were conducted to quantitate (i) titers of mutant bacteria in intestinal contents, Peyer's patches, and spleens as a function of time after p.o. inoculation; (ii) LD$_{50}$ doses; (iii) level and duration of protection; and (iv) IgA

and IgG titers in saliva and serum, respectively.

Cyclic 3′,5′-AMP (cAMP) and the cAMP receptor protein (CRP) are necessary for the transcription of many genes and operons concerned with the transport and breakdown of nutrients (1). Systems used for transporting energy and carbon sources are generally under positive control by cAMP as are several amino acid permeases (1). In addition, the cAMP concentration in cells also influences lysogenization by temperate phages (35, 59), synthesis of pili and fimbriae (62), synthesis of flagella (42, 57, 75), and synthesis of at least one outer membrane protein (52). Although cAMP is present in mammalian cells, the concentrations of 0.1 to 1.0 µM present in gastrointestinal tissues and fluids and other cells (32, 64) which *S. typhimurium* can invade and multiply within are well below the concentration range of 0.1 (42) to 1.0 mM (1) necessary to allow *cya* mutants lacking adenylate cyclase to exhibit a wild-type phenotype in vitro. Furthermore, the inclusion of a *crp* mutation to eliminate CRP should abolish any benefit that could accrue from uptake of cAMP in vivo by *cya* mutants. We therefore constructed *S. typhimurium* SR-11 strains with *cya*::Tn*10* and *crp*::Tn*10* mutations (originally obtained from P. W. Postma [58]) eliminating the ability to synthesize adenylate cyclase (ATP pyrophosphate-lyase [cyclizing]; EC 4.6.1.1) and CRP, respectively. We initially observed that these mutants were avirulent but able to induce a high level of protective immunity (15b).

Figure 4 depicts the construction of the SR-11 strain with the *cya*::Tn*10* mutation and the derivation of the Δ*cya* mutation after selection for fusaric acid resistance. After the Δ*cya* defect was introduced, the *crp*::Tn*10* mutation was added and then deleted via a fusaric acid resistance selection regimen.

Table 3 presents data to demonstrate that the Δ*cya* Δ*crp* virulence plasmid-containing strain χ4064 is completely avirulent even when the inoculating dose represents 10,000 times the LD$_{50}$ of wild-type SR-11 cells and when given on 3 successive days.

Table 4 presents additional data demonstrating that strains with only the Δ*cya* mutation, whether or not they contain the virulence plasmid, are as avirulent as are the Δ*cya* Δ*crp* double mutants. Additional data from different experiments are presented by Curtiss and Kelly (15b). These studies indicated that 4-week-old mice were also unaffected by oral doses of 10^9 cells of various plasmid-containing and plasmid-free Δ*cya* and Δ*cya* Δ*crp* mutant strains.

Figures 5 and 6 present data on the fate of orally fed χ3456, a tetracycline-resistant derivative of the mouse-virulent wild-type SR-11 strain, and of χ4064, the Δ*cya* Δ*crp* avirulent mutant. It is evident that both strains attach to, colonize, and persist in the Peyer's patches to an equal extent (Fig. 5), but that the Δ*cya* Δ*crp* strain χ4064 is impaired in its ability to reach or to survive in spleens compared with the mouse-virulent strain χ3456 (Fig. 6). Thus, the Δ*cya* Δ*crp* mutations do not impair the initial tissue tropism but diminish the capacity of strains to invade deep tissues and cause disease. In these regards, the mutations cause a phenotype similar to that associated with plasmid curing. Independent of the virulence plasmid, Δ*cya* and Δ*cya* Δ*crp* mutants grow more slowly than do their wild-type parents (1, 15b, 17, 39), and this attribute undoubtedly contributes to their avirulence.

Table 5 presents data which demonstrate that mice immunized with 1×10^7, 1×10^8, or 1×10^9 cells of the Δ*cya* Δ*crp* virulence plasmid-containing strain χ4064 acquired immunity to challenge with either 2×10^8 or 2×10^9 wild-type *S. typhimurium* SR-11 χ3306 cells.

Preliminary data to assess the duration of protective immunity by using a number of different avirulent *S. typhimurium* immunizing strains are presented in Table 6. In this case, the challenge dose of wild-type SR-11 cells was only 100 times the LD$_{50}$ for unimmunized animals. Nevertheless, all of the animals immunized with Δ*cya* Δ*crp* double mutants survived when challenged either 30 or 60 days after immunization. In other experiments reported by Curtiss and Kelly (15b), it is demonstrated that 4-week-old mice immunized once with 10^9 avirulent *S. typhimurium* cells acquired immunity to challenge with the equivalent of 10^4 LD$_{50}$s of wild-type virulent SR-11 cells.

We also have investigated the stability of Δ*cya*, Δ*crp*, and Δ*cya* Δ*crp* mutants. Δ*cya* mutants are able to revert or mutate presumably to give rise to *crp** mutations (25, 63) which permit transcription of genes and operons requiring activation by the CRP in the absence

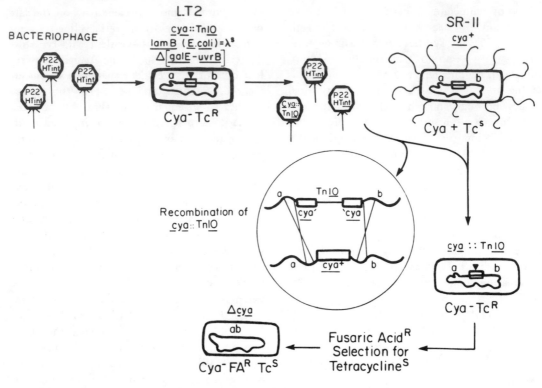

FIGURE 4. P22HT *int*-mediated transduction of *cya*::Tn*10* from an *S. typhimurium* LT2 strain to the mouse-virulent *S. typhimurium* SR-11 strain followed by selection for fusaric acid resistance to obtain deletion mutants lacking Tn*10* and adjacent DNA sequences.

of cAMP and also *csm* suppressor mutations that are closely linked to the *crp* gene (50) and can also obviate the need for cAMP in *cya* mutants. Even though these revertants or mutants were isolated, those tested for avirulence remained avirulent. All revertants or mutants obtainable from Δ*cya* Δ*crp* mutants were able to grow only on the carbon source used to select the revertant or mutant. These revertants also retained the avirulence properties of their parents. In

TABLE 3
Mortality of 8-week-old BALB/c mice 30 days after p.o. inoculation of avirulent *S. typhimurium* SR-11 Δ*cya* Δ*crp* χ4064 containing the virulence plasmid[a]

Immunizing dose (CFU)	Immunization schedule		Survival ratio (live/total mice) at 30 days postinoculation
	No. of doses	Time (days) between doses	
10^7	1		12/12
10^8	1		12/12
10^9	1		12/12
10^7	3	1	12/12
10^8	3	1	12/12
10^9	3	1	12/12

[a]After a 4-h food and water fast, animals were inoculated p.o. with the indicated strains and doses. Food and water were returned 30 min after inoculation.

TABLE 4
Mortality of BALB/c mice 30 days after p.o. inoculation with avirulent *S. typhimurium* SR-11 Δ*cya*
and Δ*cya* Δ*crp* strains[a]

Strain	Relevant genotype	Virulence plasmid	Inoculating dose (CFU)	Survival ratio (live/total mice) at 30 days postinoculation
χ4032	Δ*cya*	+	1×10^9	20/20
χ4060	Δ*cya*	−	9×10^8	20/20
χ4062	Δ*cya* Δ*crp*	−	7×10^8	20/20
λ4064	Δ*cya* Δ*crp*	+	1×10^9	20/20

[a]After a 4-h food and water fast, animals were inoculated p.o. with the indicated strains and doses. Food and water were returned 30 min after inoculation.

spite of these results, which suggest that suppressor-type mutations can occur but cannot completely obviate the need for wild-type *cya* or wild-type *crp* gene, we consider it wise to include both Δ*cya* and Δ*crp* mutations in any avirulent *Salmonella* strains to be used as vaccine candidates.

We have now begun to use these Δ*cya* Δ*crp* avirulent *S. typhimurium* mutants as the vector components for recombinant bivalent vaccines. A number of plasmid cloning vectors have been introduced into χ4062 and χ4064 and found to be more stable than the same cloning vectors in other avirulent *S. typhimurium* strains. Furthermore, χ4064 expresses the *Streptococcus sob-*

rinus SpaA antigenic determinant as well as or better than do *E. coli* K-12 strains or other avirulent *S. typhimurium* strains. Studies to evaluate immunogenicity of these strains to elicit antibodies against the *Streptococcus sobrinus* SpaA protein are in progress.

VIRULENCE GENES OF *BORDETELLA AVIUM*

Bordetella avium is the etiological agent of coryza or rhinotracheitis in avian species (41, 66). Although DNA-rRNA hybridization studies, nutritional analyses, and serological

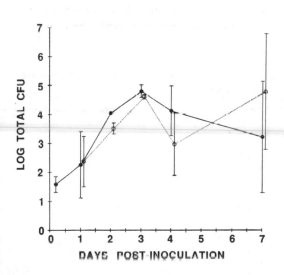

FIGURE 5. Recovery of *S. typhimurium* Δ*cya* Δ*crp* χ4064 (●) and wild-type χ3456 (○) from Peyer's patches at specified times after oral inoculation with 7.4×10^8 CFU of χ4064 and 4.0×10^8 CFU of χ3456. Vertical bars, Standard deviations. Reproduced from reference 15b.

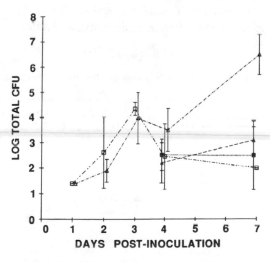

FIGURE 6. Recovery of *S. typhimurium* Δ*cya* Δ*crp* χ4064 (■, ▲) and wild-type χ3456 (□, △) from mesenteric lymph nodes (■, □) and spleen (▲, △) at specified times after p.o. inoculation with 7.4×10^8 CFU of χ4064 and 4.0×10^8 CFU of χ3456. Vertical bars, Standard deviations. Reproduced from reference 15b.

TABLE 5

Effectiveness of immunization with avirulent *S. typhimurium* SR-11 Δ*cya* Δ*crp* virulence plasmid-containing χ4064 and subsequent challenge with wild-type virulent *S. typhimurium* SR-11 χ3306[a]

Dose (CFU) of immunizing strain χ4064	Immunization schedule		Wild-type challenge dose (CFU)	Survival ratio (live/total mice) at 30 days postinoculation
	No. of doses	Time (days) between doses		
10^7	1		2×10^8	5/6
			2×10^9	6/6
	3	1	2×10^8	6/6
			2×10^9	6/6
10^8	1		2×10^8	6/6
			2×10^9	6/6
	3	1	2×10^8	5/6
			2×10^9	6/6
10^9	1		2×10^8	6/6
			2×10^9	6/6
	3	1	2×10^8	6/6
			2×10^9	6/6

[a]Thirty days after immunization with χ4064, each group of 8-week-old mice immunized with one or three consecutive daily doses of χ4064 was challenged with a p.o. dose of 2×10^8 and 2×10^9 CFU, respectively.

studies have indicated that *B. avium* is related to *Bordetella pertussis, Bordetella parapertussis,* and *Bordetella bronchiseptica, B. avium* does not produce a pertussislike toxin (16, 41; C. R. Gentry-Weeks, B. T. Cookson, and R. Curtiss III, Abstr. Annu. Meet. Am. Soc. Microbiol. 1987,

B82, p. 38) or adenylate cyclase toxin (Gentry-Weeks et al., Abstr. Annu. Meet. Am. Soc. Microbiol. 1987). Putative virulence factors of *B. avium* which are analogous to virulence factors of *B. pertussis* include a heat-labile dermonecrotic toxin which is lethal when injected

TABLE 6

Long-term protection of 8-week-old BALB/c mice immunized with avirulent *S. typhimurium* strains against challenge with wild-type virulent *S. typhimurium* SR-11 χ3306

Group[a] and immunizing strain	Relevant genotype	Virulence plasmid	Challenge dose (CFU)	Survival ratio (live/total mice) at 30 days postinoculation
I				
Control			6×10^7	0/5
χ4032	Δ*cya*	+	4×10^7	4/5
χ4060	Δ*cya*	−	6×10^7	4/5
χ4062	Δ*cya* Δ*crp*	−	6×10^7	5/5
χ4064	Δ*cya* Δ*crp*	+	6×10^7	5/5
II				
Control			2×10^7	1/5
χ4032	Δ*cya*	+	4×10^7	5/5
χ4060	Δ*cya*	−	2×10^7	5/5
χ4062	Δ*cya* Δ*crp*	−	2×10^7	5/5
χ4064	Δ*cya* Δ*crp*	+	2×10^7	5/5

[a]Groups I and II were challenged on days 30 and 60 postimmunization, respectively, after receiving ~10^9 CFU of the Δ*cya* or Δ*cya* Δ*crp* strains.

i.p. into poults (61; Gentry-Weeks et al., Abstr. Annu. Meet. Am. Soc. Microbiol. 1987) and a 1-kilodalton tracheal cytotoxin which destroys the ciliated tracheal epitheal cells, resulting in loss of clearance of oppotunistic pathogens (15). In addition, B. avium produces a heat-stable toxin, which is lethal when injected i.p. into mice (65), and a guinea pig hemagglutinin (37). The precise biochemical basis of colonization of B. avium in avian species is unknown. Presumably, outer membrane proteins which also function as hemagglutinins or fimbrial antigens might be involved in adherence and colonization of B. avium on the tracheal epithelium (36, 37). To elucidate the biochemical mechanism of adherence and to confirm the role of the putative virulence factors in disease, a λgt11 (76) library of B. avium DNA was constructed (Fig. 7). The library was screened immunologically with antisera against dermonecrotic toxin, provided by Richard Rimler, and antisera against B. avium outer membrane proteins, produced in this laboratory. Several bacteriophage plaques were identified which specify dermonecrotic toxin and outer membrane proteins. After λ plaques were identified which react with antibodies against the B. avium dermonecrotic toxin, lysogens were prepared to yield protein extracts that could be evaluated by Western blot analysis (Fig. 8). E. coli clones were identified that contained the dermonecrotic toxin antigenic determinants fused to the 116,000-molecular-weight LacZ fragment. In some cases, the toxin antigen was expressed in E. coli as a nonfusion protein. However, in either case, the protein was not toxic to mice when injected i.p. or to guinea pigs when injected intradermally. This could be due to lack of the entire structural gene, of an additional peptide encoded by another gene required for toxicity, or of modification or processing in E. coli.

The importance of these cloned genes in the virulence of B. avium will be determined by two different approaches. The first approach will involve inactivation of the cloned gene sequence by insertion of a transposon, and the inactivated gene sequence will be transferred

into a virulent B. avium strain. Recombination of the inactivated gene sequence with the intact gene will generate a mutant B. avium which lacks a functional protein. The mutant B. avium will be inoculated into turkey poults and investigated for the ability to colonize and cause disease. Infection of turkey poults with B. avium which contains a specific insertionally mutagenized gene and has reduced ability to cause disease will allow identification of those genes involved in colonization and disease. The second approach will involve the use of avirulent Salmonella mutants expressing B. avium genes which encode potential colonization or virulence attributes or both. Turkey and chicken poults will be immunized with these Salmonella strains and later challenged with B. avium to determine whether an immune response against a specified protein will preclude colonization or manifestation of a virulence attribute by virulent B. avium.

THE M PROTEIN OF *STREPTOCOCCUS EQUI*

Streptococcus equi causes strangles in the equidae. One of the virulence factors of this organism is the M protein, a surface molecule with antiphagocytic activity (8, 73). Contrary to observations regarding the M protein of other streptococci (19, 51), the *Streptococcus equi* M protein presents no size or antigenic variation (24a, 69). The M protein of *Streptococcus equi* possesses determinants which induce serum opsonic (21) and protective mucosal antibodies in the horse (22, 23). In addition, studies have implicated the M protein in the pathogenesis of purpura hemorrhagica, an immune-complex-mediated disease of the horse often seen as a sequela of strangles (24).

Galan and Timoney have cloned and expressed in E. coli the entire structural gene for the M protein of *Streptococcus equi* (24, 24a). The recombinant protein possesses the determinants that induce opsonic and mucosal antibodies as well as those determinants found in immune complexes of horses with purpura hemorrhagica. We have now expressed the *Strep-*

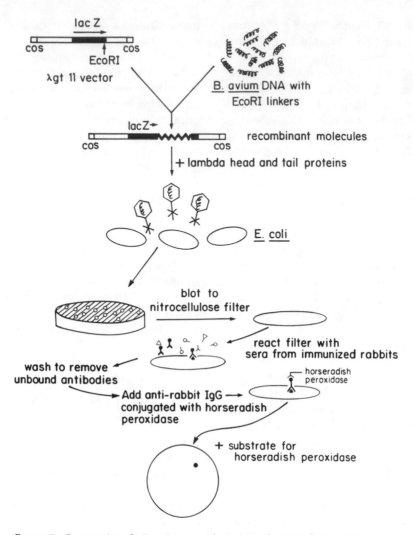

FIGURE 7. Construction of a *B. avium* gene library in the λgt11 (76) expression vector.

tococcus equi M protein gene in the avirulent *cya crp S. typhimurium* χ4062 and χ4064. As indicated by the Western blot analysis (Fig. 9), the *S. equi* M protein is expressed very efficiently by both *Salmonella* strains. Epitope mapping of the M protein gene is now in progress with the ultimate goal of dissecting the protective determinants from those involved in the development of purpura hemorrhagica. Success of these endeavors would result in the construction of a recombinant bivalent *Salmonella* vaccine strain which should induce protective mucosal and humoral immune responses against *Streptococcus equi* infections.

CONCLUSION

Avirulent *S. typhimurium* derivatives can be constructed with different mutations that define their period of survival and multiplication in the GALT and spleen and so regulate whether and to what level they induce secretory, humoral, and cellular immunity. The mutations responsible for these attributes can be transferred to other *Salmonella* species which have specificities for unique animal host species. Administration of live recombinant avirulent *S. typhimurium* strains expressing colonization and virulence protein antigens can induce

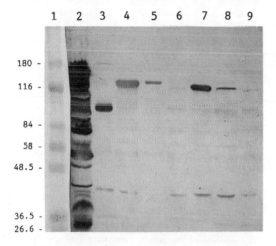

FIGURE 8. Western blot analysis of λgt11 clones specifying all or parts of the gene for *B. avium* dermonecrotic toxin. Lysates of *E. coli* lysogens were reacted with antisera against dermonecrotic toxin. Lanes: 1, molecular weight standards; 2, *B. avium* proteins; 3, 4, 5, 7, and 8, cross-reactive proteins from *E. coli* lysogens; 6 and 9, proteins from *E. coli* lysogens which lack cross-reactivity with antisera against dermonecrotic toxin. Further experiments have shown that lane 3 contains protein fused to β-galactosidase while lanes 4, 5, 7, and 8 contain nonfused proteins.

secretory, humoral, and cellular immune responses against the pathogen supplying the genes for the colonization or virulence antigens or both. Since many bacterial, viral, and fungal pathogens colonize or invade through a mucosal surface, effective secretory immunity would be an important first line of defense in reducing the spread of infectious diseases caused by these pathogens. Such recombinant bivalent live vaccines should also be inexpensive to produce and easy to administer.

In addition to the practical applications of the methods described, the system developed should be useful to study the secretory immune system in various animal species. More specifically, it should enable a better understanding of the basis for memory and of suppression (i.e., oral tolerances).

ACKNOWLEDGMENTS. Research was supported by Molecular Engineering Associates, Inc.; Public Health Service grant R01 DE06669 and fellowships F32 AI07168 to P.A.G. and F32 AI07628 to C.R.G.-W.; and U.S. Department of Agriculture grant GAM H86-CRSR-2-2854.

LITERATURE CITED

1. Alper, M. D., and B. N. Ames. 1978. Transport of antibiotics and metabolite analogs by systems under cyclic AMP control: positive selection of *Salmonella typhimurium cya* and *crp* mutants. *J. Bacteriol.* 133:149–157.

2. Anderson, E. S., and H. R. Smith. 1972. Fertility inhibition in strains of *Salmonella typhimurium*. *Mol. Gen. Genet.* 118:79–84.

3. Bacon, G. A., T. W. Burrows, and M. Yates. 1950. The effects of biochemical mutation on the virulence of *Bacterium typhosum*: the virulence of mutants. *Br. J. Exp. Pathol.* 31:714–724.

4. Bacon, G. A., T. W. Burrows, and M. Yates. 1951. The effects of biochemical mutation on the virulence of *Bacterium typhosum*: the loss of virulence of certain mutants. *Br. J. Exp. Pathol.* 32:85–96.

5. Bagdasarian, M., M. Hryniewicz, M. Zdzienicka, and M. Bagdasarian. 1975. Integrative suppression of a *dnaA* mutation in *Salmonella typhimurium*. *Mol. Gen. Genet.* 139:213–231.

6. Baron, L. S., E. Penido, I. R. Ryman, and S. Falkow. 1970. Behavior of coliphage lambda in hy-

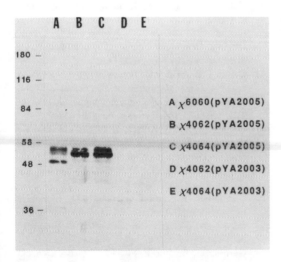

FIGURE 9. Western blot analysis of lysates from *E. coli* χ6060(pYA2005) (lane A) and *S. typhimurium* χ4062 (Δ*cya* Δ*crp*, virulence plasmid cured) and χ4064 (Δ*cya* Δ*crp*, virulence plasmid containing) carrying the plasmid pYA2005 (containing the M protein gene) (lanes B and C) or pYA2003 (plasmid vector) (lanes D and E). The blot was reacted with rabbit anti-*S. equi* M protein.

A χ6060(pYA2005)

B χ4062(pYA2005)

C χ4064(pYA2005)

D χ4062(pYA2003)

E χ4064(pYA2003)

brids between *Escherichia coli* and *Salmonella. J. Bacteriol.* 102:221–233.

7. Baron, L. S., I. R. Ryman, E. M. Johnson, and P. Gemski, Jr. 1972. Lytic replication of coliphage lambda in *Salmonella typhosa* hybrids. *J. Bacteriol.* 110:1022–1031.

8. Bazely, P. L. 1943. Studies with streptococci. V. Some relations between virulence of *S. equi* and immune response in the host. *Aust. Vet. J.* 19:62–85.

9. Benjamin, W. H., Jr., C. L. Turnbough, Jr., B. S. Posey, and D. E. Briles. 1985. The ability of *Salmonella typhimurium* to produce the siderophore enterobactin is not a virulence factor in mouse typhoid. *Infect. Immun.* 50:392–397.

10. Bienenstock, J., M. McDermott, D. Befus, and M. O'Neill. 1978. A common mucosal immunologic system involving the bronchus, breast, and bowel. *Adv. Exp. Med. Biol.* 107:53–59.

11. Bochner, B. R., H.-C. Huang, G. L. Schieven, and B. N. Ames. 1980. Positive selection for loss of tetracycline resistance. *J. Bacteriol.* 143:926–933.

12. Carter, P. B., and F. M. Collins. 1974. The route of enteric infection in normal mice. *J. Exp. Med.* 139:1189–1203.

13. Cebra, J. J., P. J. Gearhart, R. Kamat, S. M. Robertson, and J. Tseng. 1976. Origin and differentiation of lymphocytes involved in the secretory IgA response. *Cold Spring Harbor Symp. Quant. Biol.* 41:201–215.

14. Clements, J. D., F. L. Lyon, K. L. Lowe, A. L. Farrand, and S. El-Morshidy. 1986. Oral immunization of mice with attenuated *Salmonella enteritidis* containing a recombinant plasmid which encodes for production of the B subunit of heat-labile *Escherichia coli* enterotoxin. *Infect. Immun.* 53:685–692.

15. Cookson, B. T., and W. E. Goldman. 1987. Tracheal cytotoxin: a conserved virulence determinant of all *Bordetella* species. *J. Cell. Biochem.* 11B(Suppl.):124.

15a. Curtiss, R., III, R. Goldschmidt, S. M. Kelly, M. Lyons, S. Michalek, R. Pastian, and S. Stein. 1987. Recombinant avirulent *Salmonella* for oral immunization to induce mucosal immunity to bacterial pathogens, p. 261–271. *In* H. Kohler and P. T. LaVerde (ed.), *Vaccines: New Concepts and Developments.* Proceedings of the 10th International Convocation on Immunology. Longman Scientific and Technical, Harlow, Essex, Great Britain.

15b. Curtiss, R., III, and S. M. Kelly. 1987. *Salmonella typhimurium* deletion mutants lacking adenylate cyclase and cyclic AMP receptor protein are avirulent and immunogenic. *Infect. Immun.* 55:3035–3043.

16. DeLey, J., P. Segers, K. Kersters, W. Mannheim, and A. Lievens. 1986. Intra- and intergeneric similarities of the *Bordetella* ribosomal ribonu-

cleic acid cistrons: proposal for a new family *Alcaligenaceae. Int. J. Syst. Bacteriol.* 36:405–414.

17. Den Blaauwen, J. L., and P. W. Postma. 1985. Regulation of cyclic AMP synthesis by enzyme III^{Glc} of the phosphoenolpyruvate:sugar phosphotransferase system in *crp* strains of *Salmonella typhimurium. J. Bacteriol.* 164:477–478.

18. Dowman, J. E., and G. G. Meynell. 1970. Pleiotropic effects of derepressed bacterial sex factors on colicinogeny and the cell wall structure. *Mol. Gen. Genet.* 109:57–68.

19. Fischetti, V. A., K. F. Jones, and J. R. Scott. 1985. Size variation of the M protein in group A streptococci. *J. Exp. Med.* 160:1384–1401.

20. Formal, S. B., L. S. Baron, D. J. Kopecko, O. Washington, C. Powell, and C. A. Life. 1981. Construction of a potential bivalent vaccine strain: introduction of *Shigella sonnei* form I antigen genes into the *galE Salmonella typhi* Ty21a typhoid vaccine strain. *Infect. Immun.* 34:746–750.

21. Galán, J. E., and J. F. Timoney. 1985. Mucosal nasopharyngeal immune response of horses to protein antigens of *Streptococcus equi. Infect. Immun.* 47:623–628.

22. Galán, J. E., and J. F. Timoney. 1985. Immune complexes in purpura hemorrhagica of the horse contain IgA and M antigen of *Streptococcus equi. J. Immunol.* 135:3134–3137.

23. Galán, J. E., and J. F. Timoney. 1986. Passive transfer of mucosal antibody to *Streptococcus equi* in the foal. *Infect. Immun.* 54:202–206.

24. Galán, J. E., and J. F. Timoney. 1987. Molecular and genetic analysis of the M protein of *Streptococcus equi*, p. 181–184. *In* J. J. Ferretti and R. Curtiss III (ed.), *Streptococcal Genetics.* American Society for Microbiology, Washington, D.C.

24a. Galán, J. E., and J. F. Timoney. 1987. Molecular analysis of the M protein of *Streptococcus equi* and cloning and expression of the M protein gene in *Escherichia coli. Infect. Immun.* 55:3181–3187.

25. Garges, S., and S. Adhya. 1985. Sites of allosteric shift in the structure of the cyclic AMP receptor protein. *Cell* 41:745–751.

26. Germanier, R. (ed.). 1984. *Bacterial Vaccines.* Academic Press, Inc., New York.

27. Germanier, R., and E. Fürer. 1971. Immunity in experimental salmonellosis. II. Basis for the avirulence and protective capacity of *gal E* mutants of *Salmonella typhimurium. Infect. Immun.* 4:663–673.

28. Germanier, R., and E. Fürer. 1975. Isolation and characterization of Gal E mutant Ty21a of *Salmonella typhi*: a candidate strain for a live, oral typhoid vaccine. *J. Infect. Dis.* 131:553–558.

29. Gilman, R. H., R. B. Hornick, W. E. Woodward, H. L. DuPont, M. J. Snyder, M. M. Levine, and J. P. Libonati. 1977. Evaluation of a UDP-glucose-4-epimeraseless mutant of *Salmonella typhi*

as a live oral vaccine. *J. Infect. Dis.* 136:717–723.

29a. Gulig, P. A., and R. Curtiss III. 1987. Plasmid-associated virulence of *Salmonella typhimurium. Infect. Immun.* 55:2891–2901.

30. Hackett, J., I. K. Kotlarski, V. Mathan, K. Francki, and D. Rowley. 1986. The colonization of Peyer's patches by a strain of *S. typhimurium* cured of the cryptic plasmid. *J. Infect. Dis.* 153:1119–1125.

31. Hackett, J., P. Wyk, P. Reeves, and V. Mathan. 1987. Mediation of serum resistance in *Salmonella typhimurium* by an 11-kilodalton polypeptide encoded by the cryptic plasmid. *J. Infect. Dis.* 155:540–549.

32. Hahn, P., W. Cannon de Rodriguez, and J. P. Skala. 1986. Effect of age and diet on cyclic nucleotide concentrations in the intestinal mucosa of developing rats. *J. Nutr.* 116:887–891.

33. Helmuth, R., R. Stephen, C. Bunge, B. Hoog, A. Steinbeck, and E. Bulling. 1985. Epidemiology of virulence-associated plasmids and outer membrane protein patterns within seven common *Salmonella* serotypes. *Infect. Immun.* 48:175–182.

34. Hoiseth, S. K., and B. A. D. Stocker. 1981. Aromatic-dependent *Salmonella typhimurium* are nonvirulent and effective as live vaccines. *Nature* (London) 291:238–239.

35. Hong, J., G. R. Smith, and B. N. Ames. 1971. Adenosine 3':5'-cyclic monophosphate concentration in the bacterial host regulates the viral decision between lysogeny and lysis. *Proc. Natl. Acad. Sci. USA* 68:2258–2262.

36. Jackwood, M. W., and Y. M. Saif. 1987. Pili of *Bordetella avium:* expression, characterization, and role in in vitro adherence. *Avian Dis.* 31:277–286.

37. Jackwood, M. W., Y. M. Saif, P. D. Moorhead, and R. N. Dearth. 1985. Further characterization of the agent causing coryza in turkeys. *Avian Dis.* 29:690–705.

38. Jones, G. W., D. K. Rabert, D. M. Svinarich, and H. J. Whitfield. 1982. Association of adhesive, invasive, and virulence phenotypes of *Salmonella typhimurium* with autonomous 60-megadalton plasmids. *Infect. Immun.* 38:476–486.

39. Jovanovich, S. B. 1985. Regulation of a *cya-lac* fusion by cyclic AMP in *Salmonella typhimurium. J. Bacteriol.* 161:641–649.

40. Keren, D. F., G. H. Lowell, R. Rappvoli, and L. Nencioni. 1984. IgA-dependent cell-mediated activity against enteropathogenic bacteria: distribution, specificity, and characterization of the effector cells. *J. Immunol.* 133:988–992.

41. Kersters, K., K.-H. Hinz, A. Hertle, P. Segers, A. Lievens, O. Siegmann, and J. DeLey. 1984. *Bordetella avium* sp. nov. isolated from the respiratory tracts of turkeys and other birds. *Int. J. Syst. Bacteriol.* 34:56–70.

42. Komeda, Y., H. Suzuki, J. Ishidsu, and T. Iino.

1975. The role of cAMP in flagellation of *Salmonella typhimurium. Mol. Gen. Genet.* 142:289–298.

43. Levine, M. M., D. Herrington, J. G. Morris, G. Losonsky, J. Murphy, B. Tall, and B. Stocker. 1987. Safety, infectivity, immunogenicity and in vivo stability of two attenuated auxotrophic mutant strains of *Salmonella typhi,* 541Ty and 543Ty, used as oral vaccines in man. *J. Clin. Invest.* 79:888–902.

44. Maloy, S. R., and W. D. Nunn. 1981. Selection for loss of tetracycline resistance by *Escherichia coli. J. Bacteriol.* 145:1110–1112.

45. Maskell, D., F. Y. Liew, K. Sweeney, G. Dougan, and C. Hormaeche. 1986. Attenuated *Salmonella typhimurium* as live oral vaccines and carriers for delivering antigens to the secretory immune system, p. 213–217. *In* F. Brown, R. M. Chanock, and R. A. Lerner (ed.), *Vaccines 86.* Cold Spring Harbor Laboratory, Cold Spring Harbor, N.Y.

46. Maskell, D., K. J. Sweeney, D. O'Callaghan, C. E. Hormaeche, F. Y. Liew, and G. Dougan. 1987. *Salmonella typhimurium aroA* mutants as carriers of the *Escherichia coli* heat-labile enterotoxin B subunit to the murine secretory and systemic immune systems. *Microb. Pathogen.* 2:211–221.

47. Maurelli, A. T., B. Blackmon, and R. Curtiss III. 1984. Temperature-dependent expression of virulence genes in *Shigella* species. *Infect. Immun.* 43:397–401.

48. McCaughan, G., and A. Basten. 1983. Immune system of the gastrointestinal tract. *Int. Rev. Physiol.* 28:131–157.

49. McNabb, P. C., and T. B. Tomasi. 1981. Host defense mechanisms at mucosal surfaces. *Annu. Rev. Microbiol.* 35:477–496.

50. Melton, T., L. L. Snow, C. S. Freitag, and W. J. Dobrogosz. 1981. Isolation and characterization of cAMP suppressor mutants of *Escherichia coli* K-12. *Mol. Gen. Genet.* 182:480–489.

51. Moore, B. O., and J. T. Bryans. 1970. Type specific antigenicity of Group C streptococci from disease of the horse, p. 231–238. *In* J. T. Bryans and H. Gerber (ed.), *Proceedings of the Second International Conference on Equine Infectious Diseases,* Paris, 1969. S. Karger, Basel.

52. Movva, R. N., P. Green, K. Nakamura, and M. Inouye. 1981. Interaction of cAMP receptor protein with the *ompA* gene, a gene for a major outer membrane protein of *Escherichia coli. FEBS Lett.* 128:186–190.

53. Nakamura, M., S. Sato, T. Ohya, S. Suzuki, S. Ikeda, and T. Koeda. 1985. Plasmid-cured *Salmonella enteritidis* AL1192 as a candidate for a live vaccine. *Infect. Immun.* 50:586–587.

54. Ogra, P. L., and D. T. Karzon. 1969. Poliovirus antibody response in serum and nasal secretions following intranasal inoculation with inactivated poliovirus. *J. Immunol.* 102:15–23.

55. **Ogra, P. L., and D. T. Karzon.** 1969. Distribution of poliovirus antibody in serum, nasopharynx and alimentary tract following segmental immunization of lower alimentary tract with poliovirus. *J. Immunol.* **102**:1423–1430.

56. **Pardon, P., M. Y. Popoff, C. Coynault, J. Marly, and I. Miras.** 1986. Virulence-associated plasmids of *Salmonella* serotype typhimurium in experimental murine infection. *Ann. Microbiol.* (Paris) **137B**:47–60.

57. **Pastan, I., and S. Adhya.** 1976. Cyclic adenosine 5'-monophosphate in *Escherichia coli*. *Bacteriol. Rev.* **40**:527–551.

58. **Postma, P. W., H. G. Keizer, and P. Koolwijk.** 1986. Transport of trehalose in *Salmonella typhimurium*. *J. Bacteriol.* **168**:1107–1111.

59. **Rao, N. R., and C. V. S. Raj.** 1973. *Salmonella typhimurium* mutants affecting establishment of lysogeny. *Mol. Gen. Genet.* **125**:119–123.

60. **Reed, L. J., and H. Muench.** 1938. A simple method of estimating fifty percent endpoints. *Am. J. Hyg.* **27**:493–497.

61. **Rimler, R. B.** 1985. Turkey coryza: toxin production by *Bordetella avium*. *Avian Dis.* **29**:1043–1047.

62. **Saier, M. H., Jr., M. R. Schmidt, and M. Leibowitz.** 1978. Cyclic AMP-dependent synthesis of fimbriae in *Salmonella typhimurium*: effects of *cya* and *pts* mutations. *J. Bacteriol.* **134**:356–358.

63. **Scholte, B. J., and P. W. Postma.** 1980. Mutation in the *crp* gene of *Salmonella typhimurium* which interferes with inducer exclusion. *J. Bacteriol.* **141**:751–757.

64. **Schwartzel, E. H., Jr., S. Bachman, and R. A. Levine.** 1977. Cyclic nucleotide activity in gastrointestinal tissues and fluids. *Anal. Biochem.* **78**:395–405.

65. **Simmons, D. G., C. Dees, and L. P. Rose.** 1986. A heat-stable toxin isolated from the turkey coryza agent, *Bordetella avium*. *Avian Dis.* **30**:761–765.

66. **Simmons, D. G., J. G. Gray, L. P. Rose, R. C.** Dillman, and S. E. Miller. 1979. Isolation of an etiologic agent of acute respiratory disease (rhinotracheitis) of turkey poults. *Avian Dis.* **23**:194–203.

67. **Smith, H. R., G. O. Humphreys, N. D. F. Grindley, J. N. Grindley, and E. S. Anderson.** 1973. Molecular studies of an *fi*⁺ plasmid from strains of *S. typhimurium*. *Mol. Gen. Genet.* **143**:143–151.

68. **Stevenson, G., and P. A. Manning.** 1985. Galactose epimeraseless (*galE*) mutant G30 of *Salmonella typhimurium* is good potential live oral vaccine carrier for fimbrial antigens. *FEMS Microbiol. Lett.* **28**:317–321.

69. **Timoney, J. F., and T. Trachman.** 1985. Immunologically reactive proteins of *Streptococcus equi*. *Infect. Immun.* **48**:29–30.

70. **Tramont, E. C., R. Chung, S. Berman, D. Keren, C. Kapfer, and S. B. Formal.** 1984. Safety and antigenicity of typhoid-*Shigella sonnei* vaccine (strain 5076-1C). *J. Infect. Dis.* **149**:133–136.

71. **Way, J. C., D. Davis, D. E. Roberts, and N. Kleckner.** 1984. New Tn*10* derivatives for transposon mutagenesis and for construction of *lacZ* operon fusions by transposition. *Gene* **32**:369–379.

72. **Williams, R. C., and R. J. Gibbons.** 1972. Inhibition of bacterial adherence by secretory immunoglobulin A: a mechanism of antigen disposal. *Science* **177**:697–699.

73. **Woolcock, J. B.** 1974. Purification and antigenicity of an M-like protein of *Streptococcus equi*. *Infect. Immun.* **10**:116–122.

74. **Yancey, R. J., S. A. L. Breeding, and C. E. Lankford.** 1979. Enterochelin (enterobactin): virulence factor for *Salmonella typhimurium*. *Infect. Immun.* **24**:174–180.

75. **Yokota, R., and J. S. Gots.** 1970. Requirement of adenosine 3', 5'-cyclic phosphate for flagella formation in *Escherichia coli* and *Salmonella typhimurium*. *J. Bacteriol.* **103**:513–516.

76. **Young, R. A., and R. W. Davis.** 1983. Efficient isolation of genes by using antibody probes. *Proc. Natl. Acad. Sci. USA* **80**:1194–1198.

Chapter 20

Enhancement of Nonspecific Resistance to Bacterial Infection by Biologic Response Modifiers

JAMES A. ROTH

Department of Veterinary Microbiology and Preventive Medicine
Iowa State University
Ames, Iowa 50011

INTRODUCTION

Metchnikoff observed at the end of the 19th century that previous bacterial infection can increase the resistance of an animal to unrelated pathogenic bacteria (55). His observation could be compared to the more well-known observation that infection with one virus may interfere with infection by a second, unrelated virus. Indeed, it is now apparent that some of the same molecules mediate nonspecific interference with both bacterial and viral infection.

In recent years numerous compounds, referred to as biologic response modifiers (BRMs), have been shown to increase nonspecific host resistance to bacterial infection. The mechanism of action of these compounds is, in most cases, not well understood. It is clear that they do not act directly on the bacterial organism, but rather act to enhance the defense mechanisms of the host. The majority of research on BRMs has evaluated their efficacy in tumor, fungal, or viral infection models. This is especially true for the molecularly defined endogenous BRMs (i.e., interferons, interleukins, tumor necrosis factors [TNFs],

colony-stimulating factors [CSFs], and thymus hormones). In this report I focus on the role of BRMs in enhancing resistance to bacterial infection.

BRMs are agents that alter the normal host defense mechanism or immune response. Several BRMs that are potentially useful therapeutically have been purified and their molecular structures have been determined. This has allowed them to be prepared in high purity and in sufficient quantity to be evaluated in vitro and in vivo. Therefore, their individual properties can be assessed, free of contaminating substances. In general, BRMs can be divided into two categories: (i) those that are produced by the host normally and are products of the host genome (endogenous BRMs) and (ii) those that are not products of the mammalian genome (exogenous BRMs), but whose mechanisms of action include induction of endogenous BRMs and alteration of the biologic response of the individual. The efficacy of BRMs in enhancing resistance to bacterial infection has been evaluated by using a variety of animal models (usually mice). Some models involve the use of bacteria which are virulent in normal animals, while other models incorporate immunosuppression as a prerequisite for infection. For a BRM to be effective in the first type of model, it would presumably need to enhance the ability of the host to overcome the bacterial virulence factor(s). In the second type of model the BRM may have an effect by overcoming aspects of the immunosuppression. A brief description of some of the better-characterized BRMs which have been shown to nonspecifically enhance resistance to bacterial infection is included here.

TYPES OF BRM

Exogenous BRMs

Bacteria and Bacterial Derivatives

The bacteria and bacterial derivatives which have been used to enhance nonspecific resistance to bacterial infection are summarized in Table 1. With only one exception, all of the research cited in Table 1 was performed with mice (*Corynebacterium parvum* was evaluated for enhancing resistance to *Listeria monocytogenes* in rabbits [4]). A common finding was that the BRM had to be given before challenge (usually at least 24 h before) to induce improved resistance to disease.

The first bacterial organism to be extensively investigated as a BRM was the mycobacterium bacillus Calmette-Guérin (*Mycobacterium bovis* BCG). Living or killed BCG is capable of enhancing host resistance to a number of bacterial pathogens (Table 1). Subsequent efforts focused on purifying the active component(s) of BCG, beginning with the use of a methanol extraction residue of BCG and culminating with the identification of biologically active molecules associated with BCG. Trehalose-6,6'-dimycolate (cord factor) and muramyl dipeptide are two molecules found in BCG, each of which is capable of enhancing nonspecific resistance to bacterial infection (Table 1). A number of biologically active analogs of muramyl dipeptide have also been produced. Other bacterial cells apart from mycobacteria

have been shown to enhance nonspecific resistance to infection, including *C. parvum, Streptococcus pyogenes, Lactobacillus casei,* and *Corynebacterium granulosum* (Table 1).

Lipopolysaccharide extracted from gram-negative organisms (endotoxin) is capable of enhancing nonspecific resistance to bacterial infection if given between 6 and 48 h before challenge (65). When lipopolysaccharide is administered at the time of or after challenge, it induces a negative phase during which the host is more susceptible and can even be killed by a normally nonvirulent strain of bacteria (27, 52). Monophosphoryl lipid A is an immunostimulatory substance prepared by acid hydrolysis of bacterial endotoxin (71). This derivative of bacterial lipopolysaccharide has lost its toxicity and pyrogenicity but has retained a variety of effects on immune reactivity (70), including the enhancement of host resistance to bacterial infection (15).

Fauve and Hevin (29) reported that a phospholipid extract of either *L. monocytogenes* or *Salmonella typhimurium* was capable of enhancing nonspecific resistance to bacterial infection. This activity was apparently not due to endotoxin, since extracts of both gram-positive and gram-negative bacteria were equally active and the phospholipid extract did not have endotoxinlike toxic activities.

Pharmacologic Compounds

A number of BRMs which are not of bacterial or host origin have been found to enhance nonspecific resistance to bacterial infection (Table 2). Levamisole is a widely used anthelmintic which also has been shown to have immunopotentiating properties, which are apparently due to stimulation of lymphocyte, macrophage, and neutrophil function (35, 69). A single dose of levamisole given 24 h before *Staphylococcus aureus* challenge in a rat or 30 days before *Corynebacterium pseudotuberculosis* challenge in a mouse significantly enhanced resistance to challenge.

Lipoidal amines are relatively simple synthetic compounds that resemble natural mem-

TABLE 1

Bacteria and bacterial derivatives that have been shown to enhance nonspecific resistance to bacterial infection[a]

Bacterial organism or derivative used as BRM	Challenge organism (reference)
Mycobacteria	
Bacillus Calmette-Guérin	*S. enteritidis* (40); *S. aureus* (26, 91); *S. typhimurium* (9, 87); *L. monocytogenes* (9); *E. coli* (77); *K. pneumoniae* (65); *B. abortus* (95)
Methanol extraction residue	*Yersinia pestis* (101); *K. pneumoniae* (102); *S. typhimurium* (102); *S. aureus* (91, 102); *S. pneumoniae* (102); *Proteus mirabilis* (102); *P. aeruginosa* (102); *S. pyogenes* (102)
Cord factor	*K. pneumoniae* (64); *L. monocytogenes* (64); *S. typhi* (107); *S. typhimurium* (107)
Muramyl dipeptide (and analogs)	*K. pneumoniae* (2, 14, 16, 24, 63); *S. pneumoniae* (42); *P. aeruginosa* (32, 33, 54); *L. monocytogenes* (32); *S. enteritidis* (61)
C. parvum	*Bordetella pertussis* (1); *S. aureus* (1, 91); *B. abortus* (1, 36); *S. enteritidis* (21); *E. coli* (12); *L. monocytogenes* (4, 56, 57)
S. pyogenes (OK-432)	*M. intracellulare* (78); *P. aeruginosa* (78, 81, 82)
L. casei (LC 9018)	*M. intracellulare* (79); *S. marcescens* (80); *K. pneumoniae* (80); *P. aeruginosa* (81, 91); *L. monocytogenes* (83)
C. granulosum	*K. pneumoniae* (65)
Endotoxin	*K. pneumoniae* (27, 65); *S. aureus* (27); *M. tuberculosis* (27); *Francisella tularensis* (34); *S. pneumoniae* (34)
Monophosphoryl lipid A	*E. coli* (15); *S. epidermidis* (15)
Bacterial phospholipid extract	*L. monocytogenes* (29); *S. typhimurium* (29)

[a]All challenge experiments were done in mice, except for those described in reference 4, which were done in rabbits.

brane lipids in their amphipathic nature (i.e., they have both hydrophilic and hydrophobic regions) and solubility properties. This family of compounds has been used experimentally to increase resistance to tumors and infectious agents and has also proved to be effective as adjuvants for enhancing cellular and humoral immune responses to antigens (38). Two lipoidal amine compounds (CP 20,961 and CP 46,665) have been shown to be capable of enhancing nonspecific resistance to bacterial infection (Table 2). CP 20,961 [N,N-dioctadecyl-N',N'-bis(2-hydroxyethyl)propane diamine] is an interferon inducer which is also known as avridine (45). This compound was found to enhance resistance of mice to challenge with *L. monocytogenes* but did not protect against challenge with *S. typhimurium*. Avridine has been used experimentally in cattle.

Neutrophils taken from cattle treated with avridine had increased bactericidal activity against *Escherichia coli* (106) and increased functional activity (75). The increase in functional activity of neutrophils was more pronounced in immunosuppressed cattle (75). CP-46,665 is a lipoidal amine that does not elicit measurable interferon but is capable of activating macrophages and enhancing nonspecific resistance to bacterial infection (45) (Table 2).

Malic anhydride divinyl ether is a synthetic polyanionic copolymer that is capable of activating macrophages and of increasing the resistance of mice to infection with *L. monocytogenes* (57).

The mechanisms of action of both types of exogenous BRMs (bacterial and pharmacologic) in enhancing resistance to bacterial infection are not well understood. In some cases

TABLE 2

Pharmacologic compounds that have been shown to enhance nonspecific resistance to bacterial infection through their activity as BRMs

Pharmacologic compound	Challenge organism (reference)
Levamisole	S. aureus (30); C. pseudotuberculosis (43)
Lipoidal amines	
CP 46,665	P. aeruginosa (94); Bacteroides fragilis (98); E. coli (97)
CP 20,961	L. monocytogenes (57, 104)
Malic anhydride divinyl ether	L. monocytogenes (57)
Interferon inducers [poly-(I:C), statolon, pyran, tilorone]	F. tularensis (34); S. pneumoniae (34); K. pneumoniae (68)

information is available to indicate changes in host cell function under the influence of a BRM, but information is generally not available regarding alterations in molecular aspects of the interaction of the bacterial pathogen with altered host defense mechanisms (perhaps mimicking a cell-mediated immune response). It is assumed that most of the activity of the exogenous BRMs is due to the induction of endogenous BRMs which have direct and indirect effects on immune cell physiology, including enhancement of macrophage and neutrophil bactericidal activity.

Endogenous BRMs

In recent years several cytokines which modulate host defense mechanisms have been isolated and characterized. These molecules have been investigated extensively in vitro and in vivo for effects on immune cell functions and the immune response. Most have also been extensively investigated for their influence on neoplastic and viral diseases of mice. Much less emphasis has been placed on evaluating their ability to enhance nonspecific resistance to bac-

terial infection. The biologic activities of those endogenous BRMs which suggest that they may be effective in enhancing resistance to bacterial infection are briefly reviewed here, and examples are cited (when I have been able to find them) of experimental evidence demonstrating enhancement of nonspecific resistance to bacterial infection.

IL-1

Interleukin-1 (IL-1) is a cytokine produced mainly by mononuclear phagocytes. It has been known as endogenous (or leukocytic) pyrogen because it induces fever (25). IL-1 has been shown to activate a variety of phagocyte functions (49, 50) and to attract phagocytes to inflammatory sites (84). Recombinant human IL-1a has been shown to increase the survival rate of mice challenged with *Pseudomonas aeruginosa* or *Klebsiella pneumoniae* (62).

IL-2

Interleukin-2 (IL-2) is a glycoprotein secreted by T lymphocytes after antigen and IL-1 stimulation. IL-2 is required for the proliferation of activated T cells, natural killer (NK) cells, and other cytotoxic effector cells (103). Administration of IL-2 has been shown to enhance survival of mice infected with *Trypanosoma cruzi* or *Toxoplasma gondii* (20, 90), but there are few reports of the prophylactic efficacy of IL-2 in bacterial infection. Chong (19) demonstrated that when administered prophylactically, IL-2 protected approximately 80 to 90% of mice from lethal challenge with *E. coli* or *P. aeruginosa*. The effect was dose dependent and was fully inducible as early as 1 h and up to 18 h after a single administration of IL-2. When IL-2 and challenge bacteria were given by the same route (either intravenously or intraperitoneally) protection was observed, but when IL-2 and challenge bacteria were given by different routes there was little effect (19). The author (19) suggested that the IL-2 effect may have been due to macrophage activation. Although IL-2 has not been shown to activate macrophages directly, it is capable of inducing mouse and human lymphocytes in culture to produce gamma interferon (37, 46, 99), which has been shown to be a potent inducer of macrophage (60, 86) and neutrophil (67, 88, 93) activation.

Interferons

There are three general types of interferon: alpha, beta, and gamma. Alpha interferons are produced by leukocytes in response to a variety of inducers, such as viruses, bacterial products, polynucleotides, and tumor cells. At least 15 subtypes of human alpha interferon have been described. Even though alpha interferons are secreted by T and B lymphocytes (and other leukocytes), they are not considered to be lymphokines because their production is not induced by contact with the antigen-specific receptor and is not limited to clones of cells that specifically recognize the antigen. Beta interferon is produced by fibroblasts or epithelial cells in response to the same types of inducers (viruses, bacterial products, and polynucleotides) as alpha interferons. Gamma interferon is produced by T lymphocytes in response to specific antigenic stimulation or the presence of IL-2 (39).

All three types of interferon control the replication of certain viruses by inhibiting the production of viral protein in infected cells. The interferons can also modify a variety of biologic activities and therefore have important regulatory functions. Gamma interferon is an especially active BRM. It is at least one of the lymphokines capable of neutrophil and macrophage activation and migration inhibition activity. Gamma interferon also enhances the activity of NK cells (39).

Purified mouse fibroblast interferon (alpha and beta) was shown to reduce the lethality of intragastrically administered S. typhimurium in infant mice. The protective effect of the interferon was prevented by neutralizing it with anti-interferon globulin. The fibroblast interferon was shown to reduce the invasiveness of S. typhimurium for intestinal epithelial cells both in vitro and in vivo, thus inhibiting the estab-

lishment of intracellular infection (10). Human leukocytic interferon inhibited the invasion of HEp-2 tissue culture cells by Salmonella and Shigella spp. (11). This appears to be an example of a BRM specifically overcoming an important virulence attribute of a bacterial pathogen (invasiveness for intestinal epithelial cells).

Bovine alpha-1 interferon (recombinant) has been evaluated for its ability to prevent Pasteurella haemolytica pneumonia in a viral immunosuppression challenge model (3). Cattle infected with infectious bovine rhinotracheitis virus followed 4 days later by an aerosol of Pasteurella haemolytica typically develop a severe Pasteurella pneumonia. When recombinant bovine alpha-1 interferon was administered 24 to 72 h before the infectious bovine rhinotracheitis virus challenge, there was a significant increase in the ability of the animals to withstand the Pasteurella haemolytica challenge. The reduction in viral bacterial synergy did not appear to be due to a direct effect of the interferon on virus replication, since there was no significant difference in the amount of virus shedding from the upper respiratory tract between the treated and control groups. Since differences in neutrophil function were observed between the two groups, it was suggested that the protection from Pasteurella haemolytica pneumonia may have been due to an immunomodulatory effect rather than a direct antiviral effect (3). Recombinant bovine alpha and gamma interferons have been shown to have in vitro and in vivo immunomodulatory effects on bovine lymphocyte and neutrophil function (7, 93).

Gamma interferon has been shown to be a potent macrophage-activation (60, 86) and neutrophil-activating (67, 88, 93) factor. Human gamma interferon in vitro inhibited the intracellular multiplication of Legionella pneumophila (6) and Chlamydia psittaci (76). Treatment of mice with sera containing gamma interferon significantly increased the survival of mice subsequently challenged with S. typhimurium (44). It was suggested that the enhanced survival was due to more-efficient killing of bacteria by phagocytic cells. Since this experimentation was not done with purified gamma interferon, it is difficult to be sure that the biologic activity was due to gamma interferon. In vitro treatment with recombinant human gamma interferon enhanced the antimicrobial activity of dexamethasone-treated human macrophages against *L. monocytogenes* and *S. typhimurium* (85). In vivo treatment of mice with recombinant murine gamma interferon provided protection against infection with *L. monocytogenes* (47).

TNFs

Tumor necrosis factor alpha (TNF-alpha) (also known as cachectin) is a soluble protein secreted by macrophages after treatment with endotoxin or certain other stimulants (31). TNF-beta is a lymphokine (also referred to as lymphotoxin) which has about 30% homology with the functionally similar TNF-alpha (66). Both TNF-alpha and TNF-beta have been shown to be potent stimulators of neutrophil activity, especially phagocytosis, oxidative metabolism, and cytotoxicity (48, 67, 88, 89). TNF-alpha can be detected in serum samples from animals that have been sequentially treated with certain intracellular pathogens (*M. bovis, C. parvum*) and endotoxin (31). These properties of the TNFs suggest that they may be capable of enhancing resistance to bacterial infection.

CSF

Colony-stimulating factor (CSF) refers to a group of glycoproteins that stimulate monocyte-macrophage and granulocyte production by the bone marrow. Many cell types, including macrophages, fibroblasts, and endothelial cells, have been shown to produce CSF without an apparent stimulus. Lymphocytes stimulated with mitogens also produce various CSFs (105). Trudgett et al. (96) investigated changes in CSF levels in serum in response to *Salmonella* infection in mice. Since a large and sustained elevation in CSF was noted during infection, they postulated that CSF may have a direct role in host defenses. They published data suggesting

that macrophages incubated with unpurified CSF had greater bactericidal activity against *Salmonella* spp. than controls did. More recently, purified natural granulocyte-macrophage CSF and recombinant granulocyte-macrophage CSF have been shown to be neutrophil-activating factors (100). They apparently have not been evaluated for their ability to enhance nonspecific resistance to bacterial infection.

Tuftsin

Tuftsin is a tetrapeptide (N^2-[1-(N^2-L-threonyl-L-lysyl)-L-prolyl]-L-arginine) that is an integral part of the heavy chain of immunoglobulin G (in humans at least) (59). Tuftsin is liberated from the immunoglobulin G molecule through the sequential action of two enzymes, one located in the spleen and the other located on the membrane of phagocytes. Individuals who have undergone splenectomy are deficient in tuftsin and have an increased susceptibility to bacterial infection. Tuftsin activates many aspects of both neutrophil and macrophage function and has been shown to augment the bactericidal activity of murine macrophages toward *E. coli, Staphylococcus aureus, S. typhimurium,* and *L. monocytogenes.* Tuftsin also enhanced clearance of *Staphylococcus aureus, L. monocytogenes, E. coli,* and *Serratia marcescens* from the blood of infected mice and increased the survival rate of mice infected with *Streptococcus pneumoniae.*

Thymic Hormones

It is now well established that the thymus functions as an endocrine gland and produces a number of peptides or proteins that have important effects on the immune system, primarily through influencing T-cell maturation. Studies of thymus hormones initially involved the use of partially purified extracts of thymus glands (e.g., thymosin fraction 5). Later, individual peptides were isolated and characterized (thymosin alpha-1, thymosin beta-4, thymulin, thymopoietin, and thymic humoral factor) (17). Thymus hormones have been shown to have some efficacy in reducing the incidence of bacterial infection. Thymostimulin reduced the rate of postoperative infections from 28.6 to 4.8% in anergic patients (28). Thymopentin, a pentapeptide which contains the active site of the thymopoietin molecule, improved survival in an animal burn wound sepsis model (94) and in a peritonitis model (98). Subsequently, thymopentin was shown to improve both neutrophil and macrophage ability to kill *P. aeruginosa* in burned guinea pigs (97). Thymosin alpha-1 has been shown to increase resistance of mice to systemic *Candida albicans* infection by enhancing the candidacidal activity of neutrophils (8). This increase in neutrophil function may be indirect and may be due to the ability of thymosin alpha-1 to stimulate the production of interferon and IL-2 (17).

Interactions of Exogenous and Endogenous BRMs

The evidence cited above indicates that several endogenous cytokines act as BRMs and are capable of enhancing host resistance to bacterial infection when injected into animals. Many of these cytokines would be released during an immune response to infection and are important components of cell-mediated immunity. When multiple cytokines are released during a cell-mediated immune response, they may act synergistically to enhance resistance to bacterial infection. In a similar manner, the exogenous BRMs may cause the release of several cytokines which may act synergistically. The injection of a purified cytokine may also induce the secretion of other cytokines. Further research is needed to characterize the synergistic or antagonistic effects of multiple cytokines in resistance to bacterial infection.

SELECTION OF A BRM FOR A SPECIFIC BACTERIAL INFECTION

The selection of a BRM for use in prevention or therapy of a specific bacterial infection requires an understanding of the pathogenesis of the disease process and of the mechanism of action of the BRM. Tables 1 and 2 cite examples in which BRMS were found to reduce the severity of bacterial disease when they were used prophylactically (i.e., prior to the bacterial challenge in most cases). The purpose of these tables is to demonstrate that BRMs can enhance resistance to bacterial infection. There are also reports in the literature (not cited here) which show that some of these BRMs were not effective in reducing disease symptoms in a particular bacterial challenge model. Since the cellular and molecular basis for the pathogenesis of infection in the various challenge models is often not well characterized, it is difficult to reach conclusions about why the BRM was ineffective. It is, of course, not valid to conclude that a BRM which was ineffective in a particular bacterial challenge model has no potential for enhancing resistance to bacterial infection under different circumstances.

For opportunistic or secondary bacterial infections, the critical element in the pathogenesis of the infection may be the dysfunction of one or more aspects of normal host defense. In these situations, reversal of the immunosuppression by a BRM may prevent or alleviate the clinical disease. Therefore, in selecting a BRM, it would be helpful to understand the cellular and molecular basis of the immunosuppression and of the mechanism of action of the BRM. Many of the examples of BRMs that enhance resistance to bacterial infection (Table 1) involved immunosuppression in the bacterial challenge model (e.g., burns, surgery, and viral infection). In other types of bacterial infection, especially with facultative intracellular pathogens, the critical element in the pathogenesis of the infection may be the action of specific bacterial virulence factors on host defense mechanisms. If the actions of the virulence factors or the nature of the immunosuppression were understood at the cellular and molecular level, it may be possible to select a BRM which could specifically antagonize them and be prophylactically or therapeutically useful. Recent research on *Brucella abortus* is summarized below to illustrate an approach to defining a bacterial virulence factor and then testing a BRM to specifically overcome that virulence factor.

B. abortus (the causative agent of brucellosis in cattle and undulant fever in humans) is a facultative intracellular parasite capable of surviving within nonactivated macrophages and neutrophils (58, 92). A cell-mediated immune response (but not a humoral immune response) can provide protection against clinical disease. The use of exogenous BRMs (BCG and *C. parvum*) has been shown to nonspecifically enhance resistance to *B. abortus* infection (1, 36, 95). These observations suggest that a more thorough understanding of the cellular and molecular basis for *B. abortus* virulence and the mechanism of action of BRMs may lead to a place for BRMs in management of *B. abortus* infections. It may also help in research on vaccine development by defining the important aspects of a cell-mediated immune response which must be induced by vaccination (i.e., the endogenous BRMs that are most beneficial for protection).

Both smooth and rough strains of *B. abortus* have been shown to be readily ingested by human and bovine neutrophils but are resistant to killing, with the smooth strain being more resistant than the rough strain (51, 73, 74). Robertson and co-workers (51, 73, 74) also observed that either viable or killed *B. abortus* organisms inhibited neutrophil degranulation and release of lysosomal enzymes. It was shown by using granule extracts that the myeloperoxidase-H_2O_2-halide system was effective in killing *B. abortus* if the system was allowed to function normally (74). Thus, inhibition of degranulation would appear to be an important factor in the intracellular survival of *B. abortus*.

We have demonstrated that GMP and adenine are associated with the surface of *B. abortus* and are easily released into the suspending medium (13, 14). These two components are capable of inhibiting neutrophil primary granule degranulation and therefore the activity of the myeloperoxidase-H_2O_2-halide antibacterial system of the neutrophil (5). *Haemophilus somnus* (another bacterial pathogen which can survive after being phagocytosed by bovine neutrophils) (23) also inhibits the myeloperoxidase-H_2O_2-halide system by releasing the purines

guanine and adenine from its surface (18, 41). The inhibition of phagocyte degranulation may be a general property of purine ribonucleotides, ribonucleosides, and bases. Riches et al. (72) indicated that adenosine, AMP, ADP, ATP, and related structural analogs of adenosine were inhibitory to lysosomal secretion by mouse macrophages. Guanosine was one of the structural analogs that was found to be inhibitory.

It is not clear how the adenine, guanine, or GMP is released from the bacterium. *H. somnus* was found to release both purine and pyrimidine ribonucleotides, ribonucleosides, and bases into phosphate-buffered saline solution at 37°C (18). Deoxyribonucleotides, deoxyribonucleosides, and thymidine were not found. Corbel and Brewer (22) have shown that supernatant fluids from continuous cultures of *B. abortus* contain up to 100 mg of soluble RNA per liter. These observations suggest that perhaps both of these organisms produce RNA that is loosely associated with their surface and is therefore easily released and hydrolyzed.

The observations that adenine, guanine, or GMP was released by viable facultative intracellular pathogens and that these molecules inhibited the myeloperoxidase-H_2O_2-halide antibacterial activity of the neutrophil (apparently through inhibition of primary granule degranulation) were both unexpected. It may seem less surprising if one considers that a bacterium destroyed within the phagolysosome would be expected to be degraded by lysosomal hydrolytic enzymes, which would liberate nucleotides, nucleosides, and bases from intracellular RNA. These substances may then serve as a signal to stop degranulation into the phagolysosome containing degraded bacteria, thus conserving the remaining lysosomes. A bacterium which has evolved to release purines into its surroundings may be able to inhibit phagosome-lysosome fusion and enhance its intracellular survival by being perceived by the phagocyte as already degraded. It would appear to be advantageous for a bacterium to use purines or purine nucleotides as virulence factors, because under normal conditions the host immune system could not be induced to produce humoral or cell-mediated immunity to these compounds because of their small molecular size.

If GMP and adenine are important virulence factors for *B. abortus*, then a BRM which overcomes the inhibition of primary granule degranulation induced by GMP and adenine should enhance neutrophil-mediated killing of *B. abortus*. We have evaluated recombinant bovine gamma interferon in vitro for its influence on the function of normal neutrophils and neutrophils exposed in vitro to GMP and adenine or *B. abortus*. Lymphokine (containing gamma interferon) and recombinant bovine gamma interferon were each shown to influence a number of activities of normal bovine neutrophils in vitro (53, 93), including the iodination response of neutrophils stimulated with suboptimal concentrations of opsonized zymosan (P. C. Canning and J. A. Roth, submitted for publication). When neutrophils were preincubated with recombinant bovine gamma interferon in vitro, the suppression of iodination induced by GMP, adenine, or *B. abortus* was partially prevented. These neutrophils also showed a small but significant increase in brucellacidal activity in vitro. Treatment with gamma interferon in vitro also enhanced the ability of the neutrophils to produce superoxide anion (Canning and Roth, submitted).

Treatment of adult cattle with 0.5 mg of recombinant bovine gamma interferon per animal enhanced the in vitro brucellacidal activity of peripheral blood neutrophils (Canning and Roth, submitted). However, the enhancement of bacterial killing was small, and a significant proportion of the *Brucella* organisms survived after a 90-min incubation with the activated neutrophils. The enhanced bactericidal activity of the neutrophils correlated with the enhancement of iodination by gamma interferon-treated cattle neutrophils which were incubated in the presence of *B. abortus* or adenine and GMP. There is thus an association between the ability of gamma interferon to enhance neutrophil function in the face of the potential bacterial virulence factors (adenine and GMP) and the ability of gamma interferon to

enhance neutrophil brucellacidal activity. Similar results were observed after in vitro treatment of the neutrophils with gamma interferon and after in vivo treatment of the animal. This implies that the gamma interferon is acting directly on the neutrophils in vivo.

The enhanced brucellacidal activity of neutrophils after gamma interferon treatment may be due to the prevention of degranulation inhibition, to the enhanced superoxide anion generation, or to a combination of both effects plus perhaps other unmeasured neutrophil functions. Gamma interferon would be expected to be released during a cell-mediated immune response and may be partially responsible for the relative degree of protection associated with cell-mediated immunity.

This research has focused on only one cell of the host defense system, one potential virulence factor of *B. abortus* (there are undoubtedly more), and one cytokine. It is useful to study the interactions of individual components such as this, but it must be kept in mind that the interaction between the host and *B. abortus* is quite complex and involves many more factors than the ones we examined. Understanding the individual components may eventually allow a better understanding of the entire host-pathogen interaction and lead to effective prophylactic or therapeutic intervention for the benefit of the host.

LITERATURE CITED

1. Adlam, C., E. S. Broughton, and M. T. Scott. 1972. Enhanced resistance of mice to infection with bacteria following pretreatment with *Corynebacterium parvum*. *Nature* (London) *New Biol.* 235:219–220.

2. Ausobsky, J. R., M. Scuitto, L. S. Trachtenberg, and H. C. Polk, Jr. 1984. The role of muramyl dipeptide in the therapy of established experimental bacterial infection. *Br. J. Exp. Pathol.* 65:1–9.

3. Babiuk, L. A., H. Bielfeldt-Ohmann, G. Gifford, C. W. Carniecki, V. T. Scialli, and E. B. Hamilton. 1985. Effect of bovine alpha interferon on bovine herpesvirus type 1-induced respiratory disease. *J. Gen. Virol.* 66:2383–2394.

4. Baughn, R. E., D. M. Musher, and J. M. Knox. 1977. Effect of sensitization with *Propionibacterium*

acnes on the growth of *Listeria monocytogenes* and *Treponema pallidum* in rabbits. *J. Immunol.* 118:109–113.

5. Bertram, T. A., P. C. Canning, and J. A. Roth. 1986. Preferential inhibition of primary granule release from bovine neutrophils by an extract from *Brucella abortus*. *Infect. Immun.* 52:285–292.

6. Bhardway, N., T. W. Nash, and M. A. Horwitz. 1982. Interferon-gamma-activated human monocytes inhibit the intracellular multiplication of *Legionella pneumophila*. *J. Immunol.* 137:2662–2669.

7. Bielfeldt-Ohmann, H., and L. A. Babiuk. 1986. Alteration of some leukocyte functions following *in vivo* and *in vitro* exposure to recombinant bovine alpha- and gamma-interferon. *J. Interferon Res.* 6:123–136.

8. Bistoni, F., M. Baccarini, E. Blasi, C. Riccardi, P. Marconi, and E. Garaci. 1985. Modulation of polymorphonucleate-mediated cytotoxicity against *Candida albicans* by thymosin alpha1. *Thymus* 7:69–84.

9. Blanden, R. V., M. J. Lefford, and G. B. Mackaness. 1969. The host response to *Calmette-Guerin bacillus* infection in mice. *J. Exp. Med.* 129:1079–1101.

10. Bukholm, G., B. P. Berdal, C. Haug, and M. Degré. 1984. Mouse fibroblast interferon modifies *Salmonella typhimurium* infection in infant mice. *Infect. Immun.* 45:62–66.

11. Bukholm, G., and M. Degré. 1983. Effect of human leukocyte interferon on invasiveness of *Salmonella* species in HEp-2 cell cultures. *Infect. Immun.* 42:1198–1202.

12. Calhoun, K., L. Trachtenberg, K. Hart, and H. C. Polk. 1980. *Corynebacterium parvum*: immunomodulation in local bacterial infections. *Surgery* 87:52–58.

13. Canning, P. C., J. A. Roth, and B. L. Deyoe. 1986. Release of 5'-guanosine monophosphate and adenine by *Brucella abortus* and their role in the intracellular survival of the bacteria. *J. Infect. Dis.* 154:464–470.

14. Canning, P. C., J. A. Roth, L. B. Tabatabai, and B. L. Deyoe. 1985. Isolation of components of *Brucella abortus* responsible for inhibition of function in bovine neutrophils. *J. Infect. Dis.* 152:913–921.

15. Chase, J. J., W. Kubey, M. H. Dulek, C. J. Holmes, M. G. Salit, F. C. Pearson III, and E. Ribi. 1986. Effect of monophosphoryl lipid A on host resistance to bacterial infection. *Infect. Immun.* 53:711–712.

16. Chedid, L., M. Parant, F. Parant, P. Lefrancier, J. Choay, and E. Lederer. 1977. Enhancement of nonspecific immunity to *Klebsiella pneumoniae* infection by a synthetic immunoadjuvant (N-acetylmuramyl-L-alanyl-D-isoglutamine) and several analogs.

Proc. Natl. Acad. Sci. USA 74:2089–2093.

17. Chen, J., and A. L. Goldstein. 1985. Thymosins and other thymic hormones, p. 121–140. *In* P. F. Torrence (ed.), *Biological Response Modifiers. New Approaches to Disease Intervention.* Academic Press, Inc., Orlando, Fla.

18. Chiang, Y. W., M. L. Kaeberle, and J. A. Roth. 1986. Identification of the suppressive components in *Haemophilus somnus* fractions which inhibit bovine polymorphonuclear leukocyte function. *Infect. Immun.* 52:792–797.

19. Chong, K.-T. 1987. Prophylactic administration of interleukin-2 protects mice from lethal challenge with gram-negative bacteria. *Infect. Immun.* 55:668–673.

20. Choromanski, L., and R. Kuhn. 1985. Interleukin-2 enhances specific and nonspecific immune responses in experimental Chagas' disease. *Infect. Immun.* 50:354–357.

21. Collins, F. M., and M. T. Scott. 1974. Effect of *Corynebacterium parvum* treatment on the growth of *Salmonella enteritidis* in mice. *Infect. Immun.* 9:863–869.

22. Corbel, M. J., and R. A. Brewer. 1980. Isolation and properties of an RNA fraction present in *Brucella* culture supernatants. *J. Hyg.* 84:223–236.

23. Czuprynski, C. J., and H. L. Hamilton. 1985. Bovine neutrophils ingest but do not kill *Haemophilus somnus* in vitro. *Infect. Immun.* 50:431–436.

24. Dietrich, F. M., W. Sackman, O. Zak, and P. Dukor. 1980. Synthetic muramyl dipeptide immunostimulants: protective effects and increased efficacy of antibiotics in experimental bacterial and fungal infections in mice, p. 1730–1732. *In* J. D. Nelson and C. Grassi (ed.), *Current Chemotherapy and Infectious Disease: Proceedings of the 11th International Congress of Chemotherapy and the 19th Interscience Conference on Antimicrobial Agents and Chemotherapy,* vol. 2. American Society for Microbiology, Washington, D.C.

25. Dinarello, C. A., and S. M. Wolff. 1982. Molecular basis of fever in humans. *Am. J. Med.* 72:799–819.

26. Dubos, R. J., and R. W. Schaedler. 1957. Effects of cellular constituents of mycobacteria on the resistance of mice to heterologous infections. *J. Exp. Med.* 106:703–717.

27. Dubos, R. J., and R. W. Schaedler. 1956. Reversible changes in the susceptibility of mice to bacterial infections. *J. Exp. Med.* 104:53–65.

28. Farina, E. C., M. Garino, and G. Balbo. 1986. Thymostimulin prophylaxis of postoperative infections in anergic patients. *Can. J. Surg.* 29:445–446.

29. Fauve, R. M., and B. Hevin. 1974. Immunostimulation with bacterial phospholipid extracts. *Proc. Natl. Acad. Sci. USA* 71:573–577.

30. Fischer, G. W., J. K. Podgore, J. W. Bass, J.

L. Kelley, and G. Y. Kobayashi. 1975. Enhanced host defense mechanisms with levamisole in suckling rats. *J. Infect. Dis.* 132:578–581.

31. Flick, D. A., and G. E. Gifford. 1985. Tumor necrosis factor, p. 171–218. *In* P. F. Torrence (ed.), *Biological Response Modifiers. New Approaches to Disease Intervention.* Academic Press, Inc., Orlando, Fla.

32. Fraser-Smith, E. B., and T. R. Matthews. 1981. Protective effect of muramyl dipeptide analogs against infections of *Pseudomonas aeruginosa* or *Candida albicans* in mice. *Infect. Immun.* 34:676–683.

33. Fraser-Smith, E. B., R. V. Waters, and T. R. Matthews. 1982. Correlation between in vivo anti-*Pseudomonas* and anti-*Candida* activities and clearance of carbon by the reticuloendothelial system for various muramyl dipeptide analogs, using normal and immunosuppressed mice. *Infect. Immun.* 35:105–110.

34. Giron, D. J., J. P. Schmidt, R. J. Ball, and F. F. Pindak. 1972. Effect of interferon inducers and interferon on bacterial infections. *Antimicrob. Agents Chemother.* 1:80–81.

35. Hadden, J. W., A. England, and J. R. Sadlik. 1979. The comparative effects of isoprinosine, levamisole, muramyl dipeptide, and SM 1213 on lymphocyte and macrophage proliferation and activation in vitro. *Int. J. Immunopharmacol.* 1:17–27.

36. Halpern, B., A. Fray, Y. Crepin, O. Platica, A. M. Lorinet, A. Rabourdin, L. Sparros, and R. Isaac. 1973. *Corynebacterium parvum*, a potent immunostimulant in experimental infections and in malignancies, p. 217–236. *In* G. E. W. Wolstenholm and J. Wright (ed.), *Immunopotentiation.* CIBA Foundation symposium 18. Associated Scientific Publishers, London.

37. Handra, K., R. Suzuki, H. Matsui, Y. Shimizu, and K. Kumagai. 1983. Natural killer (NK) cells as a responder to interleukin 2 (IL 2). II. IL 2-induced interferon gamma production. *J. Immunol.* 130:988–992.

38. Hoffman, W. H. 1984. Lipoidal amines, p. 121–132. *In* R. L. Fenichel and M. A. Chirigos (ed.), *Immune Modulation Agents and Their Mechanisms.* Marcel Dekker, Inc., New York.

39. Hooks, J. J., and B. Detrick. 1985. Immunoregulatory functions of interferon, p. 57–75. *In* P. F. Torrence (ed.), *Biological Response Modifiers. New Approaches to Disease Intervention.* Academic Press, Inc., Orlando, Fla.

40. Howard, J. G., G. Biozzi, B. N. Halpern, C. Stiffel, and D. Mouton. 1959. The effect of *Mycobacterium tuberculosis* (BCG) infection on the resistance of mice to bacterial endotoxin and *Salmonella enteritidis* infection. *Br. J. Exp. Pathol.* 40:281–290.

41. Hubbard, R. D., M. L. Kaeberle, J. A. Roth, and Y. W. Chiang. 1986. *Haemophilus somnus*-induced interference with bovine neutrophil func-

tions. *Vet. Microbiol.* 12:77–85.

42. Humphres, R. C., P. R. Henika, R. W. Ferraresi, and J. L. Krahenbuhl. 1980. Effects of treatment with muramyl dipeptide and certain of its analogs on resistance to *Listeria monocytogenes* in mice. *Infect. Immun.* 30:462–466.

43. Irwin, M. R., and H. D. Knight. 1975. Enhanced resistance to *Corynebacterium pseudotuberculosis* infections associated with reduced serum immunoglobulin levels in levamisole-treated mice. *Infect. Immun.* 12:1098–1103.

44. Izadkhah, Z., A. D. Mandel, and G. Sonnenfeld. 1980. Effect of treatment of mice with sera containing gamma interferon on the course of infection with *Salmonella typhimurium* strain LT-2. *J. Interferon Res.* 1:137–145.

45. Jensen, K. E. 1986. Synthetic adjuvants: avridine and other interferon inducers, p. 79–89. *In* R. M. Nervig (ed.), *Advances in Carriers and Adjuvants for Veterinary Biologics.* Iowa State University Press, Ames.

46. Kawase, I., C. G. Brooks, K. Kuribayashi, S. Olabuenaga, W. Newman, S. Gillis, and C. S. Henney. 1982. Interleukin 2 induces gamma-interferon production: participation of macrophages and NK-like cells. *J. Immunol.* 131:288–292.

47. Kiderlen, A. F., S. H. E. Kaufmann, and M.-L. Lohmann-Matthes. 1984. Protection of mice against the intracellular bacterium *Listeria monocytogenes* by recombinant immune interferon. *Eur. J. Immunol.* 14:964–967.

48. Klebanoff, S. J., M. A. Vadas, J. M. Harlan, L. H. Sparks, J. R. Gamble, J. M. Agosti, and A. M. Waltersdorph. 1986. Stimulation of neutrophils by tumor necrosis factor. *J. Immunol.* 136:4220–4225.

49. Klempner, M. S., and C. A. Dinarello. 1979. Stimulation of neutrophil oxygen dependent metabolism by human leukocytic pyrogen. *J. Clin. Invest.* 64:996–1002.

50. Klempner, M. S., C. A. Dinarello, and J. I. Gallin. 1978. Human leukocytic pyrogen induces release of specific granule contents from human neutrophils. *J. Clin. Invest.* 61:1330–1336.

51. Kreutzer, D. L., L. A. Dreyfus, and D. C. Robertson. 1979. Interactions of polymorphonuclear leukocytes with smooth and rough strains of *Brucella abortus*. *Infect. Immun.* 23:737–742.

52. Landy, M. 1956. Increase in resistance following administration of bacterial lipopolysaccharides. *Ann. N.Y. Acad. Sci.* 66:292–303.

53. Lukacs, K., J. A. Roth, and M. L. Kaeberle. 1985. Activation of neutrophils by antigen-induced lymphokine with emphasis on antibody-independent cytotoxicity. *J. Leukocyte Biol.* 38:557–572.

54. Matthews, T. R., and E. B. Fraser-Smith. 1980. Protective effect of muramyl dipeptide and analogs

against *Pseudomonas aeruginosa* and *Candida albicans* infections of mice, p. 1734–1735. *In* J. D. Nelson and C. Grassi (ed.), *Current Chemotherapy and Infectious Disease: Proceedings of the 11th International Congress of Chemotherapy and the 19th Interscience Conference on Antimicrobial Agents and Chemotherapy,* vol. 2. American Society for Micriobiology, Washington, D.C.

55. Metchnikoff, E. 1907. *Immunity in Infective Diseases,* p. 300–324. Cambridge University Press, Cambridge. (Translation by F. G. Binnie.)

56. Morahan, P. S., P. H. Coleman, S. S. Morse, and A. Volkman. 1982. Resistance to infections in mice with defects in the activities of mononuclear phagocytes and natural killer cells: effects of immunomodulators in beige mice and ^{89}Sr-treated mice. *Infect. Immun.* 37:1079–1085.

57. Morahan, P. S., W. L. Dempsey, A. Volkman, and J. Connor. 1986. Antimicrobial activity of various immunomodulators: independence from normal levels of circulating monocytes and natural killer cells. *Infect. Immun.* 51:87–93.

58. Moulder, J. W. 1974. Intracellular parasitism: life in an extreme environment. *J. Infect. Dis.* 130:300–306.

59. Najjar, V. A. 1985. Tuftsin (thr-lys-pro-arg): a natural activator of phagocytic cells with antibacterial and antineoplastic activity, p. 141–169. *In* P. F. Torrence (ed.), *Biological Response Modifiers. New Approaches to Disease Intervention.* Academic Press, Inc., Orlando, Fla.

60. Nathan, C. F., H. W. Murray, M. E. Wiebe, and B. Y. Rubin. 1983. Identification of interferon-gamma as the lymphokine that activates human macrophage oxidative metabolism and antimicrobial activity. *J. Exp. Med.* 158:670–689.

61. Onozuka, K., T. Saito-Taki, and M. Nakano. 1984. Augmentation of protective and antibacterial activity induced by muramyl dipeptides in CBA/N defective mice with X-linked immunodeficiency for *Salmonella enteritidis* infection. *Infect. Immun.* 45:424–427.

62. Ozaki, Y., T. Ohashi, A. Minami, and S.-I. Nakamura. 1987. Enhanced resistance of mice to bacterial infection induced by recombinant human interleukin-1a. *Infect. Immun.* 55:1436–1440.

63. Parant, M., F. Parant, and L. Chedid. 1978. Enhancement of the neonate's nonspecific immunity to *Klebsiella* infection by muramyl dipeptide, a synthetic immunoadjuvant. *Proc. Natl. Acad. Sci. USA* 75:3395–3399.

64. Parant, M., F. Parant, L. Chedid, J. C. Drapier, J. F. Petit, J. Wietzerbin, and E. Lederer. 1977. Enhancement of nonspecific immunity to bacterial infection by cord factor (6,6'-trehalose dimycolate). *J. Infect. Dis.* 135:771–777.

65. Parant, M., F. Parant, L. Chedid, and L. Minor.

1975. Immunostimulants bacteriens et protection de la souris enfectée par *Klebsiella pneumoniae* resistante aux antibiotiques par mutation ou par transfert de plasmides. *Ann. Immunol.* (Paris) 126C:319–326.

66. Pennica, D., G. E. Nedwin, J. S. Hayflick, P. H. Seeburg, R. Derynck, M. A. Palladino, W. J. Kohr, B. B. Aggarwal, and D. V. Goeddel. 1984. Human tumor necrosis factor: precursor structure, expression and homology to lymphotoxin. *Nature* (London) 312:724–729.

67. Perussia, B., M. Kobayashi, M. E. Rossi, I. Anegon, and G. Trinchieri. 1987. Immune interferon enhances functional properties of human granulocytes: role of Fc receptors and effect of lymphotoxin, tumor necrosis factor, and granulocyte-macrophage colony-stimulating factor. *J. Immunol.* 138:765–774.

68. Pindak, F. F. 1970. Protection of mice against bacterial infection by interferon inducers. *Infect. Immun.* 1:271–273.

69. Repine, J. E., and S. D. Douglas. 1977. Effect of levamisole on morphology, bactericidal activity, and metabolism of human neutrophils in vitro. *Proc. Soc. Exp. Biol. Med.* 156:527–530.

70. Ribi, E. 1986. Structure-function relationship of bacterial adjuvants, p. 35–49. *In* R. M. Nervig (ed.), *Advances in Carriers and Adjuvants for Veterinary Biologics.* Iowa State University Press, Ames.

71. Ribi, E. 1984. Beneficial modification of the endotoxin molecule. *J. Biol. Response Modif.* 3:1–9.

72. Riches, D. W. H., J. L. Watkins, P. M. Henson, and D. R. Stanworth. 1985. Regulation of macrophage lysosomal secretion by adenosine, adenosine phosphate esters, and related structural analogues of adenosine. *J. Leukocyte Biol.* 37:545–557.

73. Riley, L. K., and D. C. Robertson. 1984. Ingestion and intracellular survival of *Brucella abortus* in human and bovine polymorphonuclear leukocytes. *Infect. Immun.* 46:224–230.

74. Riley, L. K., and D. C. Robertson. 1984. Brucellacidal activity of human and bovine polymorphonuclear leukocyte granule extracts against smooth and rough strains of *Brucella abortus. Infect. Immun.* 46:231–236.

75. Roth, J. A., and M. L. Kaeberle. 1985. Enhancement of lymphocyte blastogenesis and neutrophil function by avridine in normal and dexamethasone-treated cattle. *Am. J. Vet. Res.* 46:53–57.

76. Rothermel, C. D., B. Y. Rubin, and H. W. Murray. 1983. Gamma interferon is the factor in lymphokine that activates human macrophages to inhibit intracellular *Chlamydia psittaci* replication. *J. Immunol.* 131:2542–2544.

77. Rouben, D. P., K. Fagelman, M. T. McCoy, and H. C. Polk, Jr. 1977. Enhancement of non-specific host defenses against local bacterial challenge. *Surg. Forum* 28:44–45.

78. Saito, H., K. Nagashima, and H. Tomioka. 1983. Effects of bacterial immunopotentiators, LC 9018 and OK-432, on the resistance against *Mycobacterium intracellulare* infection in mice. *Hiroshima J. Med. Sci.* 32:145–148.

79. Saito, H., T. Watanabe, and Y. Horikawa. 1982. Protective effects of a *Lactobacillus casei* preparation, LC 9018, on the experimental *Pseudomonas aeruginosa* infection in mice. *Med. Biol.* 104:283–287.

80. Saito, H., T. Watanabe, Y. Horikawa, and O. Tado. 1980. Enhanced resistance to *Serratia marcescens, Klebsiella pneumoniae* and *Candida albicans* infections in mice pretreated with *Lactobacillus casei*. *Med. Biol.* 101:29–32.

81. Saito, H., T. Watanabe, T. Kitagawa, and K. Asano. 1985. Protective effects of bacterial immunostimulants, OK-432 and LC 9018, on *Pseudomonas aeruginosa* infection in tumor-bearing mice. *Hiroshima J. Med. Sci.* 34:459–462.

82. Saito, H., T. Watanabe, H. Tomioka, K. Sato, and T. Kitagawa. 1983. Enhanced resistance to *Pseudomonas aeruginosa* infection in mice pretreated with OK-432. *Hiroshima J. Med. Sci.* 32:235–239.

83. Sato, H. 1984. Enhancement of host resistance against *Listeria* infection by *Lactobacillus casei*: role of macrophages. *Infect. Immun.* 44:445–451.

84. Saunder, D. N., N. L. Mounessa, S. I. Katz, C. A. Dinarello, and J. I. Gallin. 1984. Chemotactic cytokines: the role of leukocytic pyrogen and epidermal cell thymocyte-activating factor in neutrophil chemotaxis. *J. Immunol.* 132:828–832.

85. Schaffner, A. 1985. Therapeutic concentrations of glucocorticoids suppress the antimicrobial activity of human macrophages without impairing their responsiveness to gamma interferon. *J. Clin. Invest.* 76:1755–1764.

86. Schreiber, R. D., and A. Celada. 1985. Molecular characterization of interferon gamma as a macrophage activating factor, p. 87–118. *In* E. Pick (ed.), *Lymphokines*, vol. 11. Academic Press, Inc., New York.

87. Senterfitt, V. C., and J. W. Shands, Jr. 1970. Salmonellosis in mice infected with *Mycobacterium bovis* BCG. *Infect. Immun.* 1:583–586.

88. Shalaby, M. R., B. B. Aggarwal, E. Rinderknecht, L. P. Svedersky, B. S. Finkle, and M. A. Palladino, Jr. 1985. Activation of human polymorphonuclear neutrophil functions by interferon-gamma and tumor necrosis factors. *J. Immunol.* 135:2069–2073.

89. Shalaby, M. R., M. A. Palladino, Jr., S. E. Hirabayashi, T. E. Eessalu, G. D. Lewis, H. M. Shepard, and B. B. Aggarwal. 1987. Receptor binding and activation of polymorphonuclear neutrophils by tumor necrosis factor-alpha. *J. Leukocyte Biol.* 41:196–204.

90. Sharma, S. D., J. M. Hofflin, and J. S. Remington. 1985. In vivo recombinant interleukin 2 administration enhances survival against a lethal challenge with *Toxoplasma gondii*. *J. Immunol.* 135:4160–4163.

91. Sher, N. A., S. D. Chaparas, L. E. Greenburg, and S. Bernard. 1975. Effects of BCG, *Corynebacterium parvum*, and methanol-extraction residue in the reduction of mortality from *Staphylococcus aureus* and *Candida albicans* infections in immunosuppressed mice. *Infect. Immun.* 12:1325–1330.

92. Smith, H. 1977. Microbial surfaces in relation to pathogenicity. *Bacteriol. Rev.* 41:475–500.

93. Steinbeck, M. J., J. A. Roth, and M. L. Kaeberle. 1986. Activation of bovine neutrophils by recombinant interferon-gamma. *Cell. Immunol.* 98:137–144.

94. Stinnett, J. D., L. D. Loose, P. Miskell, C. L. Tenney, S. J. Gonce, and J. W. Alexander. 1983. Synthetic immunomodulators for the prevention of fatal infections in a burned guinea pig model. *Ann. Surg.* 198:53–57.

95. Sulitzeanu, D., A. Bekierkunst, L. Groto, and J. Loebel. 1962. Studies on the mechanism of nonspecific resistance to *Brucella* induced in mice by vaccination with BCG. *Immunology* 5:116–128.

96. Trudgett, A., T. A. McNeill, and M. Killen. 1973. Granulocyte-macrophage precursor cell and colony-stimulating factor responses of mice infected with *Salmonella typhimurium*. *Infect. Immun.* 8:450–455.

97. Waymack, J. P., S. Gonce, P. Miskell, and J. W. Alexander. 1985. Mechanisms of action of two new immunomodulators. *Arch. Surg.* 120:43–48.

98. Waymack, J. P., P. Miskell, S. J. Gonce, and J. W. Alexander. 1984. Immunomodulators in the treatment of peritonitis in burned-malnourished animals. *Surgery* 96:308–314.

99. Weigent, D. A., G. J. Stanton, and H. M. Johnson. 1983. Interleukin-2 enhances natural killer cell activity through induction of gamma interferon. *Infect. Immun.* 41:992–997.

100. Weisbart, R. H., D. W. Golde, S. C. Clark, G. G. Wong, and J. C. Gasson. 1985. Human granulocyte-macrophage colony-stimulating factor is a neutrophil activator. *Nature* (London) 314:361–363.

101. Weiss, D. W. 1960. Enhanced resistance of mice to infection with *Pasteurella pestis* following vaccination with fractions of phenol-killed tubercle bacilli. *Nature* (London) 186:1060–1061.

102. Weiss, D. W., R. S. Bonhag, and J. A. Parks. 1964. Studies on the heterologous immunogenicity of a methanol-insoluble fraction of attenuated tubercle bacilli (BCG). *J. Exp. Med.* 119:53–70.

103. Welte, K., and R. Mertesmann. 1985. Human interleukin 2: biochemistry, physiology, and possible pathogenetic role in immunodeficiency syn-

dromes. *Cancer Invest.* 31:35–49.

104. **Wing, E. J., and S. Boehmer.** 1984. Dissociative effects of a novel immunomodulating agent (CP-20,961) on host defenses of mice. *J. Immunopharmacol.* 6:339–358.

105. **Wing, E. J., and R. K. Shadduck.** 1985. Colony-stimulating factor, p. 219–243. *In* P. F. Torrence (ed.), *Biological Response Modifiers. New Approaches to Disease Intervention.* Academic Press, Inc., Orlando, Fla.

106. **Woodward, L. F., R. L. Jasman, D. O. Farrington, and K. E. Jensen.** 1983. Enhanced antibody-dependent bactericidal activity of neutrophils from calves treated with a lipid amine immunopotentiator. *Am. J. Vet. Res.* 44:389–394.

107. **Yarkoni, E., and A. Bekierkunst.** 1976. Nonspecific resistance against infection with *Salmonella typhi* and *Salmonella typhimurium* induced in mice by cord factor (trehalose-6,6'-dimycolate) and its analogs. *Infect. Immun.* 14:1125–1129.

Chapter 21

Approaches to Identify and Neutralize Virulence Determinants of *Fusobacterium* and *Bacteroides* spp.

DAVID L. EMERY

Commonwealth Scientific and Industrial Research Organisation, Division of Animal Health
Animal Health Research Laboratory
Parkville 3052, Victoria
Australia

INTRODUCTION

Owing to their ubiquity in soil and in proximity to the various mucosal surfaces of humans and domestic animals, the obligate anaerobic bacteria are generally opportunistic pathogens whose invasion is facilitated by devitalization of host tissue and disruption of the integrity of epithelial surfaces. Three principal genera are important for domestic animals: *Clostridium, Bacteroides,* and *Fusobacterium.* Those of lesser importance at present include members of the families *Veillionaceae, Propionobacteriaceae,* and *Actinobacillaceae* and the genus *Leptotricha* (family *Bacterioidaceae*). The ability of the pathogenic anaerobes to survive in the environment as spores (*Clostridium* spp.) or proliferate in the gut with guaranteed transmission from dam to offspring ensures that eradication of pathogens is not possible and that each generation of animals is equally at risk from infection. Since the mortalities arising from clostridial intoxications have prompted the development and release of a variety of effective clostridial vaccines, I intend to discuss the

progress toward developing equally efficient control measures against disease caused by *Bacteroides* and *Fusobacterium* spp. Organisms of importance to veterinary medicine are emphasized, but additional studies of human pathogens are also mentioned.

A principle feature of tissue infections is that a mixed microflora is often isolated, such that identification of anaerobic bacteria as causal agents is often complicated by the presense of aerobes and microbial synergism. Retrospectively, causation can be deduced by vaccination against infection, whereas in other instances it serves only to highlight the mixed flora of the lesion. For example, ovine and bovine footrot can be prevented and cured by the administration of vaccines containing pilated *Bacteroides nodosus* (15, 23), whereas vaccination of mice with capsular material from *Bacteroides fragilis* only serves to eliminate this organism from the mixed flora of experimental abdominal abscesses induced by autochthonous intestinal bacteria (62). Direct evidence for pathogenicity and causation of disease is obtained by the reproduction of clinical syndrome following inoculation of pure cultures of the organism. Thus, footrot can be induced experimentally by the application of pure cultures of *B. nodosus* to the macerated feet of sheep, and lesions typical of clinical foot or liver abscess can be elicited with pure cultures of *Fusobacterium necrophorum* containing more than 10^8 bacteria (14, 23, 43, 53, 56). The pathogenesis of foot infections in ruminants is unclear, and the above studies do not preclude interactions between *B. nodosus* and *F. necrophorum* and other organisms including *Corynebacterium pyogenes* (54, 80), *Bacteroides melaninogenicus* (7, 63), or microaerophilic cocci (86). However, they suggest that *B. nodosus* and *F. necrophorum* are responsible for either the ultimate development of the infection or the maintenance of the lesion. Thus, *B. nodosus* is considered the causal agent of ovine footrot and interdigital dermatitis of ruminants (15, 23, 27), and toxigenic biovars of *F. necrophorum* cause necrobacillosis (43, 47, 66, 82). Necrobacillosis describes a spectrum of clinical entities including foot and liver abscesses of ruminants, calf diphtheria, necrotic enteritis of pigs, epithelial ulcers, and dental and soft-tissue cellulites in a variety of species (66). Although conditions such as liver abscess occur throughout the year, foot and epithelial infections have a seasonal occurrence during periods of high rainfall and humidity, lush pasture growth, and muddy conditions; the spring and autumn of temperate climates. Generally, older animals are more at risk in the field (B. L. Clark, *in* J. R. Egerton, W. K. Yong, and G. G. Rifkin, ed., *Footrot and Other Bacterial Diseases of the Feet of Ruminants*, in press).

PRELIMINARY CONSIDERATIONS FOR STRATEGIC INTERVENTION IN ANAEROBIC INFECTION

Epidemiology

Footrot is an insidious, contagious infection with close to 100% morbidity in climatic conditions favorable for transmission. In contrast to many *Fusobacterium* and *Bacteroides* strains, *B. nodosus* is not found among the in-

testinal microflora and appears to weather climatic extremes in sequestered infective and necrotic foci in the feet of carrier sheep (94). Thus, control of infection and carrier animals could eradicate the disease. The seasonal recurrence of footrot during periods of high rainfall indicates that immune responses of limited protective value and duration emanate from natural infections (38). For organisms such as *Clostridium* spp., other *Bacteroides* spp. (e.g., *B. fragilis* and *B. gingivalis*), and *F. necrophorum,* which are present in either the gut or the soil, devitalization of tissue as a result of trauma, gut stasis, or concurrent infections (e.g., interdigital dermatitis) predispose wound contamination or overgrowth of the anaerobes (12, 38, 60, 98). Immunity to these infections could only ameliorate the severity of clinical lesions rather than eradicate the causal organisms, but apart from animals surviving clostridial infections, immunity appears short lived or subliminal. However, increases in titers of antifusobacterial immunoglobulin in serum can be detected during the periods of transmission whether or not animals develop clinical infections (D. L. Emery, *in* J. R. Egerton, W. K. Yong, and G. G. Rifkin, ed., *Footrot and Other Bacterial Infections of the Feet of Ruminants,* in press). A consideration of the predisposing causes of this category of infections may enable preventative management procedures to be instigated.

Pathology and Pathogenesis

A detailed analysis of the histopathology of disease during the establishment of infection provides useful insights concerning the location and progress of the lesion and the types of host cells involved at various stages. This, in turn, gives some indication of the type of immunity which should be elicited by specific vaccination and may identify possible virulence determinants of the causal agent by their effects on host cells and tissue. Detailed descriptions of the histopathology of ovine footrot, foot abscess, and liver abscess are available (29, 48, 80, 101; D. J. Stewart, *in* J. R. Egerton, W.

K. Yong, and G. G. Rifkin, ed., *Footrot and Other Bacterial Diseases of the Feet of Ruminants,* in press), and only a brief description relevant to bacterial pathogenesis and the development of immunity is reiterated in this paper.

The severity of ovine footrot is the net result of three factors: the temperature and humidity of the relevant season, which determines morbidity or transmissibility of the infection, the virulence of the strain of *B. nodosus,* and the innate resistance of the host. Three syndromes are recognized, ranging in severity from benign footrot (also known as interdigital dermatitis or foot scald), usually associated with *F. necrophorum* or benign strains of *B. nodosus* (e.g., cattle strains in sheep [15]), to intermediate and severe footrot, which involve underrunning lesions and severe lameness (29). Regardless of the final lesion, ovine footrot commences as an interdigital dermatitis that develops on macerated skin and extends into the epidermal matrix of the hoof, progressively underrunning the horn of the heel and hoof (29). The infection with *B. nodosus* is restricted to the relatively avascular area between the stratum spinosum and stratum granulosum, distal to the germinal epithelium (54). In this area, the lesion is not accompanied by infiltrates of inflammatory cells (29). Progressive erosion of the support for the keratinized layers of the hoof results in physical separation of the hoof with accompanying inflammation, pain, and lameness. Part of this effect is also due to the presence of *F. necrophorum,* which is found consistently in the deeper tissues of the hoof epithelium, where tissue damage occurs (54) and inflammation is pronounced (29). Two other gram-negative bacteria, in intimate proximity, are noted in close association with *F. necrophorum* (54). From this observation, and the enhancement of growth of *F. necrophorum* by cultures of *B. nodosus,* footrot is considered an example of pathogenic synergism (80). It is envisaged that the erosive lesions caused by *B. nodosus* weaken the ability of hoof to resist normal wear and tear and expose it to separation and destructive infections caused in part by *F. necrophorum.*

In foot abscess, which usually proceeds from interdigital dermatitis or traumatic, penetrating wounds to the foot, coagulative necrosis of the skin and connective tissue occurs, with the resultant production of a purulent cellulitis containing abundant *F. necrophorum* and a few leukocytes (48), but surrounded by an area of intense hyperemia. By comparison, experimental inoculation of *F. necrophorum* into the portal circulation results in the rapid formation of microabscesses and foci of bacterial emboli (74). Neutrophils appear to be lysed rapidly, and the lesion develops over several days to present as a necrotic center with a transitional zone of inflammation containing progressively larger proportions of macrophages than polymorphonuclear leukocytes (PMN) and an outer organized layer of reticular fibers and fibroblasts (74, 80).

Examination of the epidemiology and pathogenesis of infections caused by *B. nodosus* and *F. necrophorum* indicates that in ovine footrot the insidious nature of the lesion emanates in part from the relative sequestration of the infective focus from the immune and inflammatory system of the host. This conjecture is consistent with the failure of a natural infection to elicit a durable immunity (38), the progress of infection despite the ability of ovine PMN and macrophages to phagocytose *B. nodosus* efficiently (37), and the curative effects of systemic immunization (23), which boost the titers of specific antibody induced by a concurrent infection.

Infections caused by *F. necrophorum* are noncontagious and acute prior to sequestration of the lesion, requiring a primed and fast-acting immunity to prevent the initial multiplication of the organism. Although acquired immunity to *F. necrophorum* is debatable (see below), it is known that in closed herds of ruminants the incidence of foot abscess decreases with time. Whether this is due to management procedures or the development of immunity to the incumbent strains of *F. necrophorum* has not been analyzed. This effect may also explain the high incidence of liver abscess in feedlots where large introductions of stock occur regularly.

Virulence Determinants of Anaerobic Bacteria

Bacterial virulence is a relative term and has been defined as the ability to cause death or disease in the host or the capacity to surmount available host defenses (88). To this end, a virulence determinant is considered to be a bacterial attribute or metabolite which provides the organism with a selective advantage to establish infection or to ensure its own reproduction. Virulence factors may act either singly or in combination at the various arbitrary stages of infection, namely adherence, local proliferation, tissue invasion, and systemic dissemination. For synergistic infections, virulence factors may also encompass products which are of mutual benefit to the microflora in clinical lesions. Since virulence determinants are considered essential for bacteria to initiate infections, they are obvious candidates for protective vaccines, and their study is pertinent to both prophylaxis and pathogenesis.

A list of proposed virulence determinants for *B. nodosus* and *F. necrophorum* is given in Table 1. It is apparent that the range of virulence determinants is similar to that exhibited by other aerobic and anaerobic bacteria. The virulence determinants have been identified by their capacity to duplicate pathogenetic effects in vitro (i.e., adherence to cells, destruction of cells, or proteolysis) and in vivo (i.e., induction of cellulitis) or to induce protective immunity when purified material is used as an immunogen. For *B. nodosus*, the virulence determinants currently investigated include pili (or fimbriae), outer membrane proteins (OMP), lipopolysaccharide (endotoxin, LPS), and proteases. Virulence determinants of *F. necrophorum* include capsules, OMP, LPS, and a cytolytic exotoxin. There is little evidence that *F. necrophorum* produces proteases, although it elaborates lipase (B. L. Clark, J. A. Vaughan, and D. L. Emery, *in* J. R. Egerton, W. K. Yong, and G. G. Rifkin, ed., *Footrot and Other Bacterial Diseases of the Feet of Ruminants,* in press). In addition, several virulence-associated phenomena including hemagglutination (47), platelet aggregation (49), and fimbriae (83) are also characteristic of virulent strains of *F. necrophorum* (see below).

Response of the Host

When vaccination of animals presents the most economical means of controlling or eradicating an infectious disease, the rational formulation of an efficient vaccine requires a balanced knowledge of the interaction between microbial pathogenicity and host immunity. This is rarely achieved, especially in synergic

TABLE 1
Virulence determinants of *B. nodosus* and *F. necrophorum*

Organism and virulence determinant	Pathogenetic effect	Biochemistry	MW	References
B. nodosus				
Pili	Adherence (?)	Protein polymers	15,000–19,000	32, 44, 68, 69
OMP	Unknown	Five glycoproteins	Various	34
LPS	Low toxicity	Enterobacterial	>100,000	34, 89
Proteases	Digest hoof matrix	Proteins (ca. five isoenzymes)	40,000	45, 83
F. necrophorum				
Capsules (?)	Prevent phagocytosis	Polysaccharide (?)	High	Unpublished
OMP	Serum resistance (?)	Ca. eight glycoproteins	Various	This paper
LPS	Cell toxicity	Enterobacterial	High	8, 100
Pili (?)	Unknown	Protein polymer	High (polymer)	84
Hemagglutinin	Adherence	Protein	19,000	59, 61, 73
Cytolysin	Destroys phagocytes	Protein	High (>300,000) Low (<10,000)	18, 35, 46, 58, 81

infections, such that the development of current bacterial vaccines has generally involved empirical refinement of whole-cell antigens through the protection generated by successive immunizations and challenges. This approach has enabled protective immune responses to be defined retrospectively.

Nonspecific Host Responses

Phagocytic cells, including mononuclear phogocytes, PMN, and serum opsonins (complement components, natural antibody, and β-lysins), are the major nonspecific effector mechanisms against gram-negative anaerobes in ruminants. Phagocytosis of B. nodosus is rapidly effected by ovine and bovine PMN and adherent monocytes, and the rate of uptake is enhanced by anti-pilus immunoglobulin G2 or immunoglobulin G1 and immunoglobulin M, respectively (37; D. Emery and J. Rothel, unpublished data). Three other features of the response in vitro indicate that professional phagocytes does not constitute a major mechanism of resistance in natural infections. First, virulent and benign strains of B. nodosus are phagocytosed with equal facility, and the rate of uptake is not affected by a concurrent infection (37). Second, the rate of phagocytosis of B. nodosus is similar when PMN derived from breeds of sheep which differ in susceptibility to footrot are used (37). Although phagocytic cells may contribute to resolution of the infection, the underrunning lesions of the hoof do not attract inflammatory cells prior to physical breakdown of the epithelium (54); this event also provides the major stimulus to the host immune system during natural infections (38).

Both AB and B biovars of F. necrophorum are also phagocytosed by bovine PMN, but the rate of uptake, as determined by chemiluminescence, is depressed in a dose-dependent fashion by culture supernatants from toxigenic biovars (Emery and Rothel, unpublished data). These results are consistent with the rapid pathogenic effects on PMN of the leucocidin produced by AB biovars (35) and the destruction of PMN in abscesses initiated by F. necrophorum (82).

Although serum from ruminants exhibits bactericidal activity against gram-negative aerobes such as Escherichia coli (71), activity against anaerobes has been difficult to demonstrate. In ovine footrot, benign strains of B. nodosus and some virulent strains which have been propagated in vitro are killed by ovine serum (24, 33). In contrast, the growth of virulent bacteria of recent isolation from lesions has not been impeded by up to 40% (vol/vol) newborn ovine serum or serum from infected or immunized sheep (33). Although these results may reflect technical inadequacies in the assay, the weak bactericidal activity of ovine serum against B. nodosus may reflect both the biological impotence of B. nodosus LPS (89) and the relatively weak cross-protection engendered by immunization with cell wall preparations from B. nodosus (41, 92). By comparison, the growth of AB biovars of F. necrophorum has not been impeded in vitro by up to 40% (vol/vol) bovine serum from any source (D. Emery, unpublished data).

Innate Resistance

The detailed examination of resistance to particular infectious diseases is a plausible method to identify markers for genetic selection or to discover protective mechanisms and the microbial antigens which induce them. Under climatic conditions conducive to moderate transmission of footrot, strong-wooled breeds of sheep are more resistant to footrot than are fine-wooled Merinos (26, 38, 85). Severe challenges with virulent organisms abrogate the phenomenon (38). Resistance manifests as a failure of the infection to progress past initial interdigital lesions (benign footrot [38]). Several experimental results suggest that the character of the interdigital epithelium is of central importance to the resistant phenotype. First, scarification of interdigital skin prior to experimental infection abolished resistance (38, 75). In addition, the rates of phagocytosis, serum bactericidal activity, and kinetics of antibody formation after infection were similar in resistant and susceptible sheep (33, 38). In terms of genetic markers, the heritability of resistance among progeny of resistant sires averaged 0.30 (84), and an association between the resistant phenotype and the ovine class I antigen SY6 of the major histocompatibility complex has been noted (P. Outteridge and D. Stewart, unpublished data). One practical aspect of vaccinating resistant sheep is that an interaction between innate and acquired immunity reduces the amount of antigen required to elicit comparable levels of protection against footrot in resistant animals compared with susceptible sheep (95).

Calves from three inbred sire lines at the Commonwealth Scientific and Industrial Research Organisation differ in their susceptibility to experimental and natural infections with *F. necrophorum* (B. Clark and J. Dufty, unpublished data). Calves from resistant sires are also high responders, showing faster elaboration of higher titers of agglutinating and anticellular antibodies against *F. necrophorum* and increased neutralizing titers against the leucocidin (J. Dufty and D. Emery, unpublished data). Although the high response was associated with possession of major histocompatibility complex class I antigen MB6 (W9), MB10 was associated with depressed antibody titers and poor lymphocyte transformation (J. Dufty, unpublished data). Whether the association between antibody responses and decreased incidence of infection reflected a true causal relationship or resulted from an increased incidence of infection in young suckling calves is currently under study.

Acquired Immunity

In contrast to the sequelae of clostridial infections in which a minority of animals survive and are resistant to subsequent reinfection, there are few deaths but scant durable immunity elicited by infections with other anaerobic gram-negative bacteria. For foot infections, seasonal recurrence of infection is predictable in stock exposed previously, and for liver abscess, new lesions appear to establish readily despite preexisting pathology. Natural infections certainly boost antibody titers against most antigens of *B. nodosus* and *F. necrophorum*, but the effect is generally suboptimal and transient (Emery, in press). For example, titers of agglutinating antibodies to the pili from the infecting strain of *B. nodosus* rarely exceed 2,000 during natural infections (38), which is well below the level of 3,000 deemed predictive of protective immunity (99). The heartening feature of footrot is that empirical immunization of sheep with whole-cell cultures of *B. nodosus* converts a subliminal immunity into systemic protection (23) and has allowed the progressive definition of the protective immune response and the relevant antigens of *B. nodosus* (90). Apart from the proliferative responses of T lymphocytes from immunized sheep to antigens of *B. nodosus* in lymphocyte transformation assays in vitro, there is no evidence that typical cytotoxic or delayed-type hypersensitivity activity is involved in immunity against footrot (Emery, in press). That protection is antibody mediated is evidenced by the ability to transfer immunity passively to naive recipients by using immunoglobulin G from immune donors (25). In addition, antipilus immunity can be abrogated by chemical modification of the antigen so that its ability to elicit antibody detected in agglutination assay, but not enzyme-linked immunosorbent assay (ELISA), is lost (39). Effective prolongation of immunity requires the use of adjuvants to potentiate antibody responses, and susceptibility returns as the serum titer declines (77). The specificity of protective antibodies is discussed below.

Whether immunity to *F. necrophorum* can be acquired is still subject to debate, since apart from findings that the incidence of foot abscess in closed flocks or herds decreases with time, most commercial or experimental vaccines either have not been evaluated or unreliably induce protection of less than 70% (Emery, in press). This arises in part from the lack of a suitable model to examine the pathogenesis of infection, since although it has been easy to induce abscesses by inoculation with *F. necrophorum* (in large numbers) (2, 8, 15, 43), application of pure cultures of AB biovars of *F. necrophorum* to devitalized skin or by intradermal inoculation has produced foot abscess only sporadically (15; B. Clark, unpublished data). In addition, the delineation of any protective response against *F. necrophorum* is complicated (see below).

Although no evidence for cellular immunity has been advanced for *F. necrophorum,* inoculation with complete Freund adjuvant can enhance resistance to a challenge infection nonspecifically (17, 42). This effect occurs when the routes of immunization and challenge are similar (i.e., intraperitoneal) and was manifested in mice as a five- to eightfold increase in the 50% lethal dose (42); the effect was not observed when foot abscess was produced experimentally in sheep (see Table 6).

VIRULENCE DETERMINANTS

Virulence Determinants of *B. nodosus* and *F. necrophorum*

B. nodosus

Pili (or fimbriae). Pili are filamentous appendages emanating from the polar ends of *B. nodosus* and are helical protein polymers of pilin monomers with subunit molecular weights (MWs) ranging from 15,000 to 19,000 (44). In cultures of *B. nodosus,* pili are responsible for twitching motility, which in turn is a property related to virulence but is not the sole criterion for virulence (22, 97). Although attempts to establish models of pilus activity in vitro have not been successful to date, it is considered, by analogy with other bacterial models, that pili are involved in the adherence of *B. nodosus* to epithelial cells in the hoof. Inoculation of purified pili into sheep induces synthesis of agglutinating antibodies, which in turn are used to serogroup strains of *B. nodosus* (16, 90). Thus far, 8 to 10 major serogroups have been determined, and current commercial vaccines contain organisms representative of each (77). A number of serogroups have also been subtyped on the basis of partial agglutination reactions; whether these represent additional

serogroups is still unresolved (C. M. Thorley, quoted in reference 96, p. 171). Amino acid sequencing of pili has identified a monomer containing 151 residues; the N-terminal 24 amino acids are predominantly hydrophobic and are almost identical to those in pili from *Neisseria gonorrhoeae, Moraxella nonliquefaciens,* and *Pseudomonas aeruginosa* (68). Further sequences of pili have been deduced from gene sequences (30). The capacity of pilin to elicit agglutinating antibodies is dependent on an intrachain disulfide bond (39), and counterimmunoelectrophoresis, immunogold labeling, and analysis of pilus structure with monoclonal antibodies (MAbs) have shown that two to four antigenic epitopes are present on the molecule (20, 40; D. Young, unpublished data).

OMP. Owing to the regular coprecipitation of pili with an OMP of MW 78,000 to 80,000 (a doublet in some strains [34]), it is thought that this protein anchors the pili to the cell wall of *B. nodosus* as does the basal protein of *E. coli.* In addition to this protein, five other OMPs (including pili) are consistently extracted from the cell wall of *B. nodosus* (34), and have MWs of 50,000, 38,000, 34,500, and 26,500. Most of these proteins have similar antigenicity in the majority of strains examined, and their relative mobility and patterns of antigenicity do not reflect patterns of cross-protection in vivo (33, 41, 97). In benign strains, OMP and LPS may be targets for the bactericidal activity of ovine serum, since this is diminished following incubation of serum with whole bacteria (33).

LPS-endotoxin. Examination of the LPS of gram-negative anaerobes has revealed two types. *Fusobacterium, Veillonella,* and *Leptotrichia* spp. possess typical enterobacterial LPS in which the core sugars and heptose are linked via 2-keto-3-deoxyoctulosonate to lipid A (55). The biological potency of LPS from *B. nodosus* is low, and it is the only *Bacteroides* species possessing enterobacterial-type LPS (34, 89). In all other *Bacteroides* spp. examined, the LPS does not contain 2-keto-3-deoxyoctulosonate or heptose (55). Owing to its low potency, *B. nodosus* LPS does not account for the differences in virulence among clinical isolates.

Proteases. In contrast to pili, OMP, and LPS, the proteolytic activity of culture supernatants from *B. nodosus* can readily distinguish benign strains of the organism from those of intermediate and high virulence (21, 27), although no single laboratory test can discriminate between the last two types (97). Physically, the proteases from virulent strains are more thermostable and possess greater and more rapid proteolytic and elastolytic activity than those from benign strains (91, 97). Functionally, *B. nodosus* elaborates serine proteases which have activity similar to that of chymotrypsin, requiring divalent calcium ions for activity (65), and which are inhibited by α_2-macroglobulin from ovine serum (70). Biochemically, the protease isoenzymes have MW 40,000, and on zymograms after electrophoretic separation the patterns of activity of the four or five isoenzymes are characteristic for benign and virulent strains (45, 64). Antigenically, the proteases from *B. nodosus* appear similar in that antisera from vaccinated sheep can neutralize proteolytic activity in vitro (70) and precipitate proteases in agarose gels (93). Mixtures of protease isoenzymes from a virulent strain of *B. nodosus* are prophylactic in vivo (93). The functional significance of the protease is not known, but it may be required to harvest nutrients.

F. necrophorum

Strains of *F. necrophorum* isolated from clinical lesions or from normal tissue have been assigned to biovars on the basis of cultural characteristics (47). Two biovars, A and B, and an intermediate type, AB (resembling more closely the A biovars in character), have been identified (47). A and AB biovars are more frequently isolated from lesions, are virulent for ruminants and mice (35, 47, 81, 82), produce exotoxin, and are hemolytic for a range of erythrocytes (35, 47). In contrast, B biovars predominate in the environment and among the gut microflora (47, 60, 82). They are avirulent for ruminants (14, 35), nonhemolytic, and nontoxigenic (35). Therefore, immunity must

be induced against A and AB biovars, but identification of unique molecules on these strains is complicated by cross-reactions with antigens on commensal B biovars. However, the obvious differences in virulence between A and B biovars imply that properties restricted to the A or AB biovar could be virulence determinants. These features include capsules, LPS, OMP, and exotoxins.

Capsules. In an examination of 12 strains of AB and B biovars of *F. necrophorum,* only the former, grown on solid or in liquid medium, elaborated mucoid capsules as identified with Maneval stain (S. Vicino, D. Emery, and J. Vaughan, unpublished data). The degree of encapsulation diminished with prolonged cultivation in vitro, but the structure, chemical composition, and antigenicity of this material remain to be examined.

OMP. Around six or seven major groups of proteins are extracted from cells of *F. necrophorum* by use of potassium thiocyanate (72), but are shared between A and B biovars. The function of OMP in resistance to inhibition of growth by the presence of up to 40% (vol/vol) fresh ovine antisera is currently unknown.

LPS. Fusobacteria possess a typical enterobacterial-type LPS which activates both the alternate complement pathway (10) and Hagemann factor (11). The content of 2-keto-3-deoxyoctulosonate in fusobacterial LPS is low (0.8%), and the 50% lethal dose was 0.002 μg (16.8 mg/kg) (100). Limited studies on the LPS from *F. necrophorum* indicated that A and B biovars possess LPSs of equivalent biological potency (8), although Inoue et al. (56) suggested that LPS from an A biovar was more toxic than that from a B biovar. Antigenically, the LPSs from A and B biovars appear similar when reacted with polyclonal antisera in immunoblots (Emery, unpublished data).

Pili (fimbriae). Although we have not observed fimbriae among 12 strains of *F. necrophorum* at the Commonwealth Scientific and Industrial Research Organisation, Shinjo and Kiyoyama (83) examined the pathogenicity of fimbriate hemagglutinating (HA$^+$) and HA$^-$ mutants of the same A biovar and found that the HA⁻ mutant was less pathogenic. Although changes in the antigenicity of the fimbriae with the mutation could not be excluded, the results imply that fimbriae are not responsible for hemagglutination or virulence and are consistent with correlations between hemagglutination and virulence (47). The ultrastructure of fimbriae from *F. necrophorum* appears similar to that of fimbriae from other bacteria (83), but the MW of any monomer has not been determined.

Hemagglutinin. The morphology of the hemagglutinin from *F. necrophorum* resembles that of LPS, and its chemical properties are analogous to those of pili (73). It is apparently associated with the cell wall, is heat labile, and has a subunit MW of 19,000 (73). More research on this product is required before its pathogenetic activity can be assessed, although the purified material adhered to Vero cells and bovine hepatocytes and could be inhibited by antihemagglutinin sera (59, 61).

Other cellular virulence-associated determinants have been reported for *F. necrophorum*. Platelet aggregation appears to be related to the virulence of the organism (49), probably as a result of the capacity of fusobacterial cell walls to activate complement (10). However, AB biovars did not aggregate platelets (49), so that the role of this phenomenon in clinical infections is still speculative.

Exotoxins. Certain strains of *F. necrophorum* produce a cytolysin which is destructive for leukocytes, erythrocytes, and a variety of cultivated cells including macrophages, kidney cells, and fibroblasts (19, 35, 46, 47, 50, 58, 79). The supernatants initiate degenerative changes and production of cellulitis in the skin of rabbits (9, 79). The exotoxin(s) has been termed hemolysin, cytotoxin, or leucocidin, but correlations between the titers of each activity (35) and between respective neutralization titers in serum from immunized animals suggest that all effects could be mediated by a common molecule (43). The activity of the hemolysin is comparable to that of phospholipase A and lysophospholipase (2). Correlations between the pathogenicity of strains of *F. necrophorum* and

levels of leucocidin implicate this product as a virulence determinant (8, 14, 19, 43).

The location and biochemical properties of the leucocidin are less clear. Cytotoxic activity has been found in cytoplasmic extracts of *F. necrophorum* (50), but the majority of activity appears extracelullarly and not in the cell wall (43). Two main forms of the molecule have been reported: a large, heat-labile moiety of MW ca. 300,000, which is produced by AB biovars, with maximum titers produced after 18 h of logarithmic growth in vitro (18, 35), and a smaller species (MW < 500), which is heat stable and is produced by all biovars during a 7-day period in vitro (46, 81). Partial purification of the larger moiety by gel filtration resulted in identification of MW 13,000, 14,000, and 103,000 components in immunoblots from toxigenic strains, whereas nontoxigenic B biovars possessed only an MW 13,500 fragment (36). The MWs of the smaller components of the exotoxin were similar to the estimates of 5,000 to 10,000 reported by Kanoe et al. (58). Whether the larger exotoxin can form aggregates with LPS in culture supernatants (36) or is degraded during extended culture periods to smaller active components is not known. The capacity of antisera to neutralize the leucocidin from several strains of *F. necrophorum* suggested that the molecule could be variable antigenically (36).

STRATEGIC MITIGATION OF INFECTIONS CAUSED BY ANAEROBIC BACTERIA

Factors Influencing the Choice of Strategy

The strategy selected to minimize the impact of infectious disease is ultimately dependent on the net profitability of each strategy to the producer. This cost-benefit analysis is influenced externally only by direct government regulations and is exemplified in Australia by efforts to eradicate ovine footrot by the imposition of quarantine orders on affected properties. In contrast, the presence of *F. nec-*

rophorum among the autochthonous microflora necessitates control of infections, rather than eradication. The remaining variable concerns prevention of infection or curing a current outbreak. The choices confronting producers are usually fourfold: changes in management practices, genetic selection of resistant stock, chemotherapy, and vaccination. Since descriptions of management changes are outside the scope of this review and since no satisfactory markers are available to select stock for resistance to anaerobic bacterial infections (nor is it warranted to select stock on this basis alone), the following discussion focuses on chemotherapy and vaccination as exemplified by infections caused by *B. nodosus* and *F. necrophorum*.

Chemotherapy

For curing ruminant footrot, two chemotherapeutic approaches are possible: foot bathing and systemic treatment with antibiotics (penicillin and streptomycin) (28; for a review, see reference 96). The recent rekindling of interest in formulations of zinc sulfate for topical application has prompted attempts to eradicate footrot from infected flocks. However, treatment with zinc sulfate also requires thorough inspection of treated flocks 14 to 21 days after the final treatment and rigorous culling (4). The cure rate with foot bathing and inspection (ca. 80%) was not improved by paring of feet prior to foot bathing with or without additional antibiotic treatment or a single dose of a commercial vaccine (67). Other workers reported that foot bathing did not have any advantage over thorough foot paring (76) and that the optimal procedures for foot bathing may vary with the season and the nature of the outbreak. The administration of a single intramuscular dose of penicillin-streptomycin is at least as effective as foot paring and application of topical agents (22). Vaccination, although curative, takes at least 3 to 4 weeks to diminish the infection, owing to the period taken to generate effective levels of specific antibody.

For treatment of infections caused by *F. necrophorum,* antibiotics are the method of choice.

Generally, for foot infections, the lesion rapidly resolves with chemotherapy, provided that (i) dependent drainage of the purulent contents is achieved and (ii) the joint and joint capsule are not involved (reviewed by Clark [in press]). It is speculative whether antibiotic feed additives reduce the incidence of liver abscesses in feedlot cattle. In human medicine, in which cost is less accountable, infections caused by *Fusobacterium* and *Bacteroides* species (*B. fragilis, B. gingivalis,* and *B. melaninogenicus*) are routinely treated with antibiotics, and prophylaxis by vaccination is not being contemplated. Alternative preventative measures against foot and liver abscess include the provision of Formalin footbaths (48) or the administration of ethylenediamine dihydroiodide in the feed (6).

Vaccination

Three major considerations dictate the widespread acceptance of vaccination when economic benefits can be sustained. First, when mortalities following infection with obligate anaerobes are high, as in the clostridial intoxications, routine vaccination of young and pregnant stock is regularly practiced. Second, since most pathogenic anaerobes are present in the environment or as commensal organisms, control of the disease, rather than eradication, necessitates the continued use of the vaccine. Third, when eradication is possible (e.g., for ovine footrot), different combinations of conventional treatments and vaccination from those used simply to control morbidity and mortality may be adopted.

Vaccination against ovine footrot. Vaccines have been used and are currently used to protect sheep effectively against infection with *B. nodosus* and to reduce the numbers of infected sheep for control of an outbreak of the disease. Since the cure rate of the vaccine in infected sheep decreases as the climatic conditions become more favorable for transmission, eradication of the disease also involves regular and stringent inspection and culling (77).

The first type of vaccines used are pilusbased vaccines. Serotype-specific immunity is elicited in sheep inoculated with as little as 5 μg of purified pilus protein incorporated into oil-based adjuvants (93). Since serotyping of *B. nodosus* based on pilus agglutination reactions can be used to predict protection, the current commercial vaccines contain piliated strains of *B. nodosus* representing 8 to 10 serogroups (77). Adequate quantities of pili are necessary on *B. nodosus* to elicit protection, since depiliated organisms are poorly protective (94). However, the fastidiousness, slow growth, and variable pilus production of *B. nodosus* in vitro, together with the granulomata produced at the site of inoculation of whole-cell vaccines incorporated into oil adjuvants, have prompted investigators to perform research to develop purified pilus vaccines produced from recombinant DNA technology or synthetic peptides. Consequently, the pilus gene from *B. nodosus* was isolated and expressed in *E. coli* downstream of a heat shock promoter in the plasmid pBR322 (30, 31). However, the product was expressed as the pilin monomer, copurified with the cytoplasmic membrane of *E. coli,* and was of limited protective value in vivo (31, 40). Because of the sequence homology between the hydrophobic N-terminal regions of pili from *B. nodosus* and *P. aeruginosa* (32, 68, 69), the gene was recloned in the latter organism. The product was polymeric, filamentous, and effective as a vaccine (95). Additionally, the recombinant material was as effective as native pili in reducing the percentage of severe footrot in an infected flock to less than 5% over 50 days after two doses of vaccine 1 month apart; an incidence of around 40% severe footrot was observed after the same period in unvaccinated sheep (95). Field trials with recombinant pili from the eight major serogroups will commence shortly.

The possibility of reducing the number of serotypes needed for producing comprehensive protection by using pilus-based vaccines has been addressed by attempting to define the location and nature of pilus epitopes. MAbs and clones of ovine helper T lymphocytes are being used to define epitopes recognized by B and T lymphocytes, respectively, so that a synthetic peptide could be constructed incorporating both epitopes (since this construction will have to be recognized during a challenge infection). The current collection of MAbs have identified at least four epitopes on pili (Table 2), including the agglutinating epitope (Young, unpublished data), probably corresponding to those detected by using polyclonal antisera (20, 40). Of interest is that although the agglutinating epitope is conformational (nonlinear) and serotypically restricted, at least three other linear epitopes have been identified, two of which are also serotypically restricted (Table 2). Given the correlations between protection and titers of agglutinating antibody, we presently have no idea of the titers of antibody against, and immonogenicity of, linear epitopes either serotypically restricted or shared between serogroups. Several assays, including competitive and direct ELISAs and immonoblots, have located a determinant detected by an MAb which is shared by serogroups A, B, C, E, F, and G but is not common to serogroups D and H (D. Young and D. Emery, submitted for publication) (Table 2). The same pattern of reactivity is exhibited by ovine antisera raised against the hydrophobic N-terminal region of pili (Table 3; Emery, unpublished data). It is also the pattern of reactivity of leukocytes harvested from immunized sheep and incubated with pili from several serogroups in vitro (J. Rothel and D. Emery, unpublished data) (Table 3). These findings are consistent with the relatively high sequence homology (around 70%) among pili from serogroups A, B, C, and E, (68, 69; N. McKern, personal communication). Since the cross-reactive MAb was raised against serogroup F, this would suggest that pili from serogroup F and perhaps serogroup G would also be contained in this group (Young, unpublished data). In contrast, pili from serogroup H show little sequence homology with those from the above serogroups (32), and (from the data in Tables 2 and 3) pili from serogroup D are also in another category. Although the N-terminal region of the molecule probably contains these cross-reactive T- and B-cell epitopes, other T-cell epitopes have been defined

TABLE 2

Reactivity of anti-pilus MAbs with pili from different serogroups of B. nodosus[a]

No. of MAbs (immunogens)	Serogroup restriction (no. of agglutinating pili)	Serogroups recognized	Nature of epitope	No. of epitopes detected[b]
13 (A, F, H)	Yes (4)	Subtype of immunogen only	Discontinuous	1
			Linear (9 nonagglutinating MAbs)	2
5 (F)	No (0)	A, B, C, E, F, G	Linear (5)	1

[a]MAbs were produced against pili from B. nodosus serogroups A (strain 198), F (strain 336), and H (strain 265) and were screened in ELISAs with pili from different serogroups. The capacity of MAbs to recognize linear or discontinuous epitopes was determined by assaying on dissociated, reduced, and alkylated pili.

[b]The number of epitopes on pili from each serogroup recognized by the MAbs was determined in competitive ELISAs with pilus fragments or ovine antisera, or in additivity ELISAs where the optical density at 450 nm was augmented >25% when two MAbs were reacted with pili compared with result with each MAb bound separately (D. Young, D. Emery, and D. J. Stewart, manuscript in preparation).

in the mid- and C-terminal region of the molecule by using synthetic peptides and T-cell clones raised against serogroup A pili from B. nodosus. In these results, two of six clones reacted with peptides 3 and 7, which overlap in sequence with the C terminus of pilin (Table 4). One clone reacted with peptide 2, in the central region of the molecule. Although these regions are not B-cell epitopes in terms of their inability to react with a panel of MAbs, their protective capacity is not known. A more-detailed definition of these epitopes is being attempted. Since the agglutinating epitope is conformational, the production of a synthetic peptide to mimic its structure is complicated.

Indeed, whether it is possible to produce a synthetic peptide vaccine against ovine footrot to reduce either the cost of the inoculum or the number of pilus serogroups needed to promote a comprehensive protection requires further research. The current technology allows this problem to be addressed.

The second type of vaccines used are whole-cell vaccines. A limited degree of cross-protective immunity against strains of B. nodosus from heterologous serogroups is induced by immunization of sheep with depilated B. nodosus or extracts of OMP (92; Table 5). Contamination of pilus preparations with small amounts of OMP meant that cross-protection was also in-

TABLE 3

Comparative reactivity of MAbs, polyclonal ovine antisera, and ovine peripheral blood leukocytes against pili from different serogroups of B. nodosus

Reagent (serogroup of immunogen)[a]	Antibody titers and cpm in lymphocyte transformations with pili from serogroups:								
	None	A	B	C	D	E	F	G	H
Bulk PBL (A)	1,500	8,400	5,500	4,526	1,650	2,980	2,680	1,590	1,490
Bulk PBL (H)	3,675	9,680	3,010	8,750	46,870	3,780	9,460	2,780	52,680
Antipilus serum (A)	120	185,000	71,200	15,200	20,300	25,800	47,900	36,240	48,875
Antipilin serum (A)	160	105,000	28,800	29,800	8,500	24,500	15,680	17,500	5,500
Anti-N-terminal serum (a)	130	2,500	2,200	4,100	600	1,700	1,000	1,700	340
Cross-reactive MAb (F)	<100	25,000	25,600	22,800	<100	20,000	16,400	17,100	<100

[a]For peripheral blood leukocytes, results are mean responses from duplicate cultures in three experiments with 10 sheep, for which the leukocytes were incubated with pili (1 μg/ml) for 4 days. Antibody titers are the reciprocal of that dilution of ovine serum with an optical density at 450 nm of 0.3 in ELISAs. Antipilus serum was raised against native pili, antipilin serum was produced after immunization with dissociated-reduced pili (39), and immunization with the N-terminal fragment (ca. 30% of the pilin monomer [39]) resulted in specific antiserum. The cross-reactive MAb was produced by D. Young (submitted). PBL, Peripheral blood leukocytes.

TABLE 4

Comparative reactivity of ovine peripheral blood leukocytes and T-lymphocyte clones against pili and pilus-based peptides from B. nodosus serogroup A[a]

Responder cells	cpm of cells incubated with following antigen:								
	None	Pili	Pep-1	Pep-2	Pep-3	Pep-4	Pep-5	Pep-7	ConA/IL-2
Sheep 1 PBL	440	9,260	2,520	2,350	1,730	827	355	1,780	15,600
Sheep 7 PBL	8,887	32,404	11,243	7,461	21,816	10,743	20,270	33,280	176,800
Clone 1	466	1,625	535	860	840	710	320	846	3,980
Clone 2	643	3,190	1,220	1,076	2,280	1,163	1,230	2,345	11,790
Clone 3	560	2,472	580	372	1,972	976	582	2,463	10,492
Clone 4	340	780	390	520	610	430	256	343	1,006
Clone 5	256	1,496	343	180	340	502	198	390	870
Clone 6	490	2,997	580	2,116	488	598	722	508	10,226

[a] T-lymphocyte clones were cultivated from sheep 1, cloned at limiting dilutions, and expanded with recombinant human interleukin-2 (10 U/ml weekly). At mid-week, cells were harvested and subcultivated with autologous antigen-presenting cells, which were peripheral blood leukocytes incubated with pili (1 μg/ml) or peptides (25 μg/ml) for 2 h prior to being inactivated with 5,000 rads of γ-irradiation or 20 μg of mitomycin C per ml for 30 min. cpm are expressed for duplicate cultures after 4 day of incubation (Emery and Rothel, manuscript in preparation). Responses to third-party antigens (tetanus toxoid, keyhole limpet hemocyanin, and ovalbumin) were less than 150% of cpm without antigen in column 2. PBL, Peripheral blood leukocytes; ConA, concanavalin A; IL-2, interleukin 2.

duced when more potent adjuvants were used in inocula (93). However, cross-protection was usually operative against B. nodosus strains of intermediate or reduced virulence or under climatic conditions less favorable for transmission (i.e., less than 50% of feet affected in a flock) (42). Thus, cross-protection is of little practical value, but may serve to support pilus-based protection when strains from serogroups other than those in the commercial vaccines cause infection. The immunological mechanism for cross-protection is not known, but since it is independent of antipilus ELISA or agglutination titers and of anti-LPS activity, it may be bactericidal in nature (41). The structural integrity of the OMP is required for induction of cross-protective immunity, since the reactivity of sera raised against five individual OMPs

TABLE 5

Cross-protection against B. nodosus using whole-cell vaccines and purified proteases[a]

Vaccine	% of feet with underrunning lesions (severe footrot) after challenge with:		
	Strain A (virulent)	Strain C (intermediate)	Strain E (intermediate)
Whole cells (+ pili) (strain A)	2.1[b]	22.5[b]	5.6
OMP (strain A)	34.7	35.0	11.2
Pili (strain A)	0.0[b]	40.0	18.1
Purified protease (V2) (strain A)	21.0[b]		
Purified proteases (V2, V3, V5) (strain A)	6.3[b]	15.0[b]	2.8[b]
Whole cells (+ pili) (strain C)	32.4	2.0	
Whole cells (+ pili) (strain C)			0.0[b]
Controls	83.3	57.5	20.8

[a] Sheep were inoculated twice with antigen incorporated 1:2 in incomplete Freund adjuvant prior to being challenged on pasture (strain A) or in pens (strains C and E). The results are mean cumulative percentages of feet with >3c lesions over 8 to 15 weeks after challenge. Table is compiled from data in references 41 and 93.
[b] Significant protection, P < 0.05.

did not match the spectrum of cross-protection observed in vivo (41).

In cattle, autogenous, pilated, whole-cell vaccines containing organisms of *B. nodosus* from serogroups B and G significantly reduced the incidence of interdigital dermatitis for up to 1 year (15).

The third type of vaccines used are protease-based vaccines. Recently, cross-protective immunity against strains of both intermediate and high virulence has been elicited in sheep inoculated with extracellular proteases produced by a virulent A strain (93) (Table 5). A positive correlation was observed between the degree of protective immunity and the anti-protease ELISA titers in ovine serum assayed against a combination of purified virulent protease isoenzymes (93). In addition, a combination of protease isoenzymes (V2, V3, and V5) induced a more effective immunity than did V2 alone (93). Although the antigenicity of most protease isoenzymes appears identical, immunoprecipitation and immunoblotting techniques have shown that the virulent isoenzyme V_2 possesses a different or additional determinant from the others (97). A provisional patent covering the development of a protease-based vaccine has been filed (Commonwealth Scientific and Industrial Research Organisation, U.S. patent PG8700-84, December, 1984), and the protease gene has been cloned into *E. coli* and expressed by the surrogate organism. The protective capacity of antiprotease immunoglobulin presumably neutralize the activity of the molecule by inhibiting its binding to its substrate or receptor (70).

Vaccination against F. necrophorum.   Given that vaccination would attempt to control, rather than eradicate, infections with *F. necrophorum,* preparations which elicit protection are dependent upon the species studied. In mice, the incidence of deaths or lesions after a challenge infection with *F. necrophorum* has been reduced by previous sublethal infections (17), repeated inoculations of fixed or heat-killed cells (1, 3, 43), LPS (52), cytoplasmic toxoid (53), ribosomal fractions (5), or culture supernatants containing leucocidin (42). Cytoplasmic tox-

oids without adjuvants have been used successfully to reduce the prevalence of liver abscess in sheep and cattle (51, 53), and culture supernatants emulsified in incomplete Freund adjuvant gave cattle significant protection against an experimental challenge infection (14). Subsequent studies have given less reproducible results, and the efficacy of our current vaccines is less than 50% (Table 6) (43; B. Clark, unpublished data). In addition, inactivated material from *F. necrophorum* inoculated as a single dose into mice and rabbits has been relatively unsuccessful in inducing immunity (9, 13, 17, 79, 87).

There are several reasons why vaccination against *F. necrophorum* appears stalemated and empirical at present. (i) The pathogenesis of infections is not known. Although inoculation of pure cultures can reproduce the clinical lesion, the synergistic contribution of other bacteria such as *B. melaninogenicus* (7, 63), *C. pyogenes* (78), or microaerophilic cocci (86) is not known. (ii) There is no definitive serotyping system for *F. necrophorum* (which is indicative of protective immunity, if any) (47). Serological cross-reactions between virulent organisms and gut commensals render interpretations difficult (47). In addition, all adult animals possess substantial antibody titers against *F. necrophorum* (47), and since adult animals are most at risk, these antibodies could be deemed not protective. This conundrum could be resolved only by analysis of epitopes on bacterial antigens and antigen-specific isotypes of antibody to see whether differences exist between naive and resistant livestock and between virulent and nonpathogenic biovars of *F. necrophorum.* (iii) The mechanism of immunity to *F. necrophorum* has not been determined, although a concept of activated macrophages (1) is supported by the nonspecific resistance and increased 50% lethal dose observed after inoculation of mice with Freund complete adjuvant (17, 42). However, that effect is not observed in sheep inoculated with oil-based adjuvants (Table 6), and this raises the next point. (iv) A definitive experimental challenge model has not been es-

TABLE 6

Protective capacity of antigens from *F. necrophorum* against experimental foot abscess in sheep[a]

Vaccine	Aggregate lesion score	% Protection
10^{10} heat-killed cells	44	54.2[b]
LPS (from 10^{10} cells)	59	38.5
Concentrated culture supernatant (10^{10} cells)	63	32.3
Semipurified leucocidin (10^{10} cells)	65	32.3
Adjuvant alone	90	6.4
Unvaccinated controls	96	0.0

[a]Groups of 20 sheep were inoculated twice with antigens emulsified 1:2 in incomplete Freund adjuvant prior to the inoculation subcutaneously in the interdigital skin with 1.4×10^8 toxigenic *F. necrophorum* cells from the vaccine strain. Aggregate lesion scores are the sum of the lesions among sheep from each group and incorporate both the degree and the duration of the experimental infection (maximum score of 6 for each foot and 480 for each group [43]). Results are compiled from two experiments (43 and my unpublished data).
[b]Significant protection ($P < 0.05$).

tablished, to the extent that inoculation of *F. necrophorum* directly into feet, peritoneal cavity, or blood may override any protective effects operating during natural infections. Evaluation of putative vaccines in extensive laborious field trials is urgently required to determine definitely whether immunity is attainable. For foot abscess, with a maximum incidence of around 4 to 25% depending on the season, extremely large groups of animals are needed. (v) Immunity may be elicited more effectively in the peritoneal cavity than in the feet, as suggested by the contrasting results obtained from using semipurified leucocidin in mice and sheep (43). The inoculation of *F. necrophorum* subcutaneously into the interdigital skin may allow the growth of the organism to outpace immune effector mechanisms in comparison with the arrest of *F. necrophorum* in liver and lymph nodes in the abdomen. Thus, immunity may be more effective when both immunization and challenge are given intraperitoneally, since similar preparations appear more effective in preventing liver abscess in ruminants (50, 53) than for use in immunizing against foot abscess (14, 43). It should be appreciated that the mode of challenge may also contribute to these differences in experimental results (see above).

CONCLUDING REMARKS

Infections caused by *B. nodosus* and *F. necrophorum* highlight the contrasting approaches to the strategic control of anaerobic bacterial infections which do not present with the high mortalities of clostridial intoxications. On one hand, *B. nodosus* is not found in the normal gastrointestinal microflora, survives poorly in the environment, and is amenable to eradication. The disease it produces is insidious and contagious and produces little durable immunity. The choices confronting producers regarding control are dependent upon whether they are containing an outbreak or preventing an infection. For the former, labor-intensive foot inspection, foot paring, and foot bathing with or without chemotherapy is required, whereas specific vaccination is effective for prophylaxis. An analysis of the virulence determinants of *B. nodosus* and the pathology and pathogenesis of the infection has enabled progressive refinement of footrot vaccines, providing a definitive role for vaccines in the control and eradication of the disease. This is due principally to the establishment of a serogrouping system which is directly relevant to protective immunity.

The situation for *F. necrophorum* is stark by contrast. Control measures must limit the impact of the infection rather than eradicate the organism or the disease. The infection itself is rapid in onset and noncontagious and causes low morbidity and mortality. Little is known of the pathogenesis of infection, and experimental models to study the microbial interactions early in the infection and to evaluate vaccines have been difficult to establish. Owing to the failure of putative virulence determinants of *F. necrophorum* to induce immunity consistently, a serological analysis of strains of the organism which is relevant to protection has not been forthcoming, and only empirical analyses of bacterial antigens or extracts have been conducted. These constraints to the progress of research with *F. necrophorum* emphasize the importance of knowledge of microbial pathogenesis, virulence determinants, host immunity, and their interactions in addressing vaccination against anaerobic bacteria. At present, infections caused by *F. necrophorum* are contained by antibiotics, but technical advances to address some of the above problems may widen the choice of control measures that are available in the future.

ACKNOWLEDGMENTS. I am extremely grateful for constructive discussion with and access to unpublished data of Neil McKern, John Dufty, and Dianne Young and for the excellent technical assistance of James Rothel. I also appreciate beneficial collaborative research with David Stewart and Bruce Clark at the Commonwealth Scientific and Industrial Research Organisation.

LITERATURE CITED

1. Abe, P. M., J. W. Holland, and L. R. Stauffer. 1978. Immunization of mice against *Fusobacterium necrophorum* infection by parenteral or oral administration of vaccine. *Am. J. Vet. Res.* 39:115–118.
2. Abe, P. M., C. J. Kendall, L. R. Stauffer, and J. W. Holland. 1979. Hemolytic activity of *Fusobacterium necrophorum* culture supernatants due to presence of phospholipase A and lysophospholipase. *Am. J. Vet. Res.* 40:92–96.
3. Abe, P. M., E. S. Lennard, and J. W. Holland. 1976. *Fusobacterium necrophorum* infection in mice as a model for the study of liver abscess formation and induction of immunity. *Infect. Immun.* 13:1473–1478.
4. Atkins, J. W. 1986. The use of zinc sulphate formulation for the eradication of footrot during a period favouring spread of the disease, p. 43–46. *In* D. J. Stewart, J. E. Petersen, N. M. McKern, and D. L. Emery (ed.), *Footrot in Ruminants.* Commonwealth Scientific and Industrial Research Organisation Division of Animal Health and Australian Wool Corporation, Glebe, New South Wales, Australia.
5. Berg, J. N. 1982. Toxicity associated with *Fusobacterium necrophorum* vaccines, p. 267–269. *In* J. Espinasse (ed.), *Fourth International Symposium on Disorders of the Ruminant Digit.* Société Française de Buratrie, Alfort, Paris, France.
6. Berg, J. N., L. N. Brown, P. G. Ennis, and L. H. Self. 1976. Experimentally induced footrot in feedlot cattle fed rations containing organic iodide (ethylenediamine dihydriodide) and urea. *Am. J. Vet. Res.* 37:509–512.
7. Berg, J. N., and R. W. Loan. 1975. *Fusobacterium necrophorum* and *Bacteroides melaninogenicus* as etiological agents of footrot in cattle. *Am. J. Vet. Res.* 36:1115–1120.
8. Berg, J. N., and C. M. Scanlan. 1982. Studies of *Fusobacterium necrophorum* from bovine hepatic abscesses: biotypes, quantitation, virulence, and antibiotic susceptibility. *Am. J. Vet. Res.* 43:1580–1586.
9. Beveridge, W. I. B. 1934. A study of twelve strains of *Bacillus necrophorus,* with observations on the oxygen intolerance of the organism. *J. Pathol. Bacteriol.* 38:467–491.
10. Bjornson, A. B. 1984. Role of complement in host resistance against members of the *Bacteroidaceae. Rev. Infect. Dis.* 6(Suppl. 1):S34–S39.
11. Bjornson, H. S. 1984. Enzymes associated with the survival and virulence of gram-negative anaerobes. *Rev. Infect. Dis.* 6(Suppl. 1):S21–S24.
12. Border, M., B. D. Firehammer, D. S. Shoop, and L. L. Myers. 1985. Isolation of *Bacteroides fragilis* from the feces of diarrheic calves and lambs. *J. Clin. Microbiol.* 21:472–473.
13. Cameron, C. M., and W. J. P. Fuls. 1977. Failure to induce in rabbits effective immunity to a mixed infection of *Fusobacterium necrophorum* and *Corynebacterium pyogenes* with a combined bacterin. *Onderstepoort J. Vet. Res.* 44:253–256.
14. Clark, B. L., and D. L. Emery, D. J. Stewart, J. H. Dufty, and D. A. Anderson. 1986. Studies into immunisation of cattle against interdigital necrobacillosis. *Aust. Vet. J.* 63:107–110.
15. Clark, B. L., D. J. Stewart, D. L. Emery, J. H. Dufty, and R. G. Jarrett. 1986. Immunisation of cattle against interdigital dermatitis (footrot) with an autogenous *Bacteroides nodosus* vaccine. *Aust. Vet. J.* 63:61.
16. Claxton, P. D., L. A. Ribeiro, and J. R. Egerton. 1983. Classification of *Bacteroides nodosus* by agglutination tests. *Aust. Vet. J.* 60:331–334.
17. Conlon, P. J., K. P. Hepper, and G. W. Teresa. 1977. Evaluation of experimentally induced *Fusobacterium necrophorum* infections in mice. *Infect. Immun.* 15:510–517.
18. Coyle-Dennis, J. E., and L. H. Lauerman. 1978. Biological and biochemical characteristics of *Fusobacterium necrophorum* leukocidin. *Am. J. Vet. Res.* 39:1790–1793.

19. Coyle-Dennis, J. E., and L. H. Lauerman. 1979. Correlations between leukocidin production and virulence of two isolates of *Fusobacterium necrophorum*. *Am. J. Vet. Res.* 40:274–276.

20. Day, S. E. J., C. M. Thorley, and J. E. Beesley. 1986. Serotyping of *Bacteroides nodosus:* proposal for 9 further serotypes (J-R) and study of the antigenic complexity of *B. nodosus* pili, p. 147–159. *In* D. J. Stewart, J. E. Peterson, N. M. McKern and D. L. Emery (ed.), *Footrot in Ruminants*. Commonwealth Scientific and Industrial Research Organisation Division of Animal Health and Australian Wool Corporation, Glebe, New South Wales, Australia.

21. Depiazzi, L. J., and R. B. Richards. 1979. A degrading protease test to distinguish benign and virulent ovine isolates of *Bacteroides nodosus*. *Aust. Vet. J.* 55:25–28.

22. Depiazzi, L. J., and R. B. Richards. 1985. Motility in relation to virulence of *Bacteroides nodosus*. *Vet. Microbiol.* 10:107–116.

23. Egerton, J. R., and D. H. Burrell. 1970. Prophylactic and therapeutic vaccination against ovine footrot. *Aust. Vet. J.* 46:517–522.

24. Egerton, J. R., and G. C. Merritt. 1970. The occurrence of bactericidal antibodies against *Fusiformis nodosus* in sheep serum. *J. Comp. Pathol.* 80:369–376.

25. Egerton, J. R., and G. C. Merritt. 1973. Serology of footrot: antibodies against *Fusiformis nodosus* in normal, infected, vaccinated and passively immunised sheep. *Aust. Vet. J.* 49:139–145.

26. Egerton, J. R., and I. R. Morgan. 1972. Treatment and preventation of footrot in sheep with *Fusiformis nodosus* vaccine. *Vet. Rec.* 91:453–456.

27. Egerton, J. R., and I. M. Parsonson. 1969. Benign footrot—a specific interdigital dermatitis of sheep associated with infection by less proteolytic strains of *Fusiformis nodosus*. *Aust. Vet. J.* 45:345–349.

28. Egerton, J. R., I. M. Parsonson, and N. P. H. Graham. 1968. Parenteral chemotherapy of ovine footrot. *Aust. Vet. J.* 44:275–283.

29. Egerton, J. R., D. S. Roberts, and I. M. Parsonson. 1969. The aetiology and pathogenesis of ovine footrot. A histological study of the bacterial invasion. *J. Comp. Pathol.* 79:207–215.

30. Elleman, T. C., P. A. Hoyne, D. L. Emery, D. J. Stewart, and B. L. Clark. 1984. Isolation of the gene encoding pilin of *Bacteroides nodosus* (strain 198), the causal organism of ovine footrot. *FEBS Lett.* 173:103–107.

31. Elleman, T. C., P. A. Hoyne, D. L. Emery, D. J. Stewart, and B. L. Clark. 1986. Expression of the pilin gene from *Bacteroides nodosus* in *Escherichia coli*. *Infect. Immun.* 51:187–192.

32. Elleman, T. C., P. A. Hoyne, N. M. McKern, and D. J. Stewart. 1986. Nucleotide sequence of

the gene encoding the two-subunit pilin of *Bacteroides nodosus* 265. *J. Bacteriol.* 167:243–250.

33. Emery, D. L. 1984. Reactivity of sera from sheep immunised with individual outer membrane proteins of *Bacteroides nodosus* against heterologous bacterial strains. *Vet. Microbiol.* 9:453–466.

34. Emery, D. L., B. L. Clark, D. J. Stewart, I. J. O'Donnell, and D. R. Hewish. 1984. Analysis of the outer membrane proteins of *Bacteroides nodosus*, the causal organism of ovine footrot. *Vet. Microbiol.* 9:155–168.

35. Emery, D. L., J. H. Dufty, and B. L. Clark. 1984. Biochemical and functional properties of a leucocidin produced by several strains of *Fusobacterium necrophorum*. *Aust. Vet. J.* 61:382–387.

36. Emery, D. L., R. D. Edwards, and J. S. Rothel. 1986. Studies on the purification of the leucocidin of *Fusobacterium necrophorum* and its neutralization by specific antisera. *Vet. Microbiol.* 11:357–372.

37. Emery, D. L., and D. J. Stewart. 1984. Phagocytosis of *Bacteroides nodosus* by ovine peripheral blood leucocytes. *Vet. Microbiol.* 9:169–179.

38. Emery, D. L., D. J. Stewart, and B. L. Clark. 1984. The comparative susceptibility of five breeds of sheep to footrot. *Aust. Vet. J.* 61:85–88.

39. Emery, D. L., D. J. Stewart, and B. L. Clark. 1984. The structural integrity of pili from *Bacteroides nodosus* is required to elicit protective immunity against footrot in sheep. *Aust. Vet. J.* 61:237–238.

40. Emery, D. L., D. J. Stewart, B. L. Clark, and T. C. Elleman. 1986. Protective parts of pili from *Bacteroides nodosus*, p. 207–210. *In* D. J. Stewart, J. E. Peterson, N. M. McKern, and D. L. Emery (ed.), *Footrot in Ruminants*. Commonwealth Scientific and Industrial Research Organisation Division of Animal Health and Australian Wool Corporation, Glebe, New South Wales, Australia.

41. Emery, D. L., D. J. Stewart, B. L. Clark, T. C. Elleman, and N. McKern. 1985. Identification of protective antigens of *Bacteroides nodosus* by the immune response against footrot in sheep. *Annu. Proc. Sheep Vet. Soc.* 9:23–25.

42. Emery, D. L., and J. A. Vaughan. 1986. Generation of immunity against *Fusobacterium necrophorum* in mice inoculated with extracts containing leucocidin. *Vet. Microbiol.* 12:255–268.

43. Emery, D. L., J. A. Vaughan, B. L. Clark, and D. J. Stewart. 1986. Virulence determinants of *Fusobacterium necrophorum* and their prophylactic potential in animals, p. 267–274. *In* D. J. Stewart, J. E. Petersen, N. M. McKern, and D. L. Emery (ed.), *Footrot in Ruminants*. Commonwealth Scientific and Industrial Research Organisation Division of Animal Health and Australian Wool Corporation, Glebe, New South Wales, Australia.

44. Every, D. 1979. Purification of pili from *Bacteroides nodosus* and an examination of their chemical, phys-

ical and serological properties. *J. Gen. Microbiol.* 115:309–316.

45. **Every, D.** 1982. Proteinase isoenzyme patterns of *Bacteroides nodosus*: distinction between ovine virulent isolates, ovine benign isolates and bovine isolates. *J. Gen. Microbiol.* 128:809–812.

46. **Fales, W. H., J. F. Warner, and G. W. Teresa.** 1977. Effects of *Fusobacterium necrophorum* leukotoxin on rabbit peritoneal macrophages *in vitro*. *Am. J. Vet. Res.* 38:491–495.

47. **Fievez, L.** 1963. *Comparative Study of Strains of Sphaerophorus necrophorus Isolated from Man and Animals.* European Academic Press, Brussels. (In French.)

48. **Flint, J. C., and R. Jensen.** 1951. Pathology of necrobacillosis of the bovine foot. *Am. J. Vet. Res.* 12:5–12.

49. **Forrester, L. J., B. J. Campbell, N. J. Berg, and J. T. Barrett.** 1985. Aggregation of platelets by *Fusobacterium necrophorum*. *J. Clin. Microbiol.* 22:245–249.

50. **Garcia, M. M., D. C. Alexander, and K. A. McKay.** 1975. Biological characterization of *Fusobacterium necrophorum* cell fractions in preparation for toxin and immunization studies. *Infect. Immun.* 11:609–616.

51. **Garcia, M. M., W. J. Dorward, D. C. Alexander, S. E. Magwood, and K. A. McKay.** 1974. Results of a preliminary trial with *Sphaerophorus necrophorus* toxoids to control liver abscesses in feedlot cattle. *Can. J. Comp. Med.* 38:222–226.

52. **Garcia, M. M., K. M. Charlton, and K. A. McKay.** 1975. Characterization of endotoxin from *Fusobacterium necrophorum*. *Infect. Immun.* 11:371–379.

53. **Gargia, M. M., and K. A. McKay.** 1978. Intraperitoneal immunization against necrobacillosis in experimental animals. *Can. J. Comp. Med.* 42:121–127.

54. **Hine, P. M.** 1984. Ovine footrot: histopathology of a synergic disease, p. 85–98. *In* M. J. Hill (ed.), *Models of Aerobic Infection. Proceedings of the Third Anaerobe Discussion Group Symposium.* Martinus Nijhoff, The Hague, The Netherlands.

55. **Hofstad, T.** 1974. The distribution of heptose and 2-keto-deoxy-octonate in *Bacteroidaceae*. *J. Gen. Microbiol.* 85:314–320.

56. **Inoue, T., M. Kanoe, N. Goto, K. Matsumura, and K. Nakano.** 1975. Chemical and biological properties of lipopolysaccharides from *Fusobacterium necrophorum* biovar A and biovar B strains. *Jpn. J. Vet. Sci.* 47:639–645.

57. **Jensen, R., J. C. Flint, and L. A. Griner.** 1954. Experimental hepatic necrobacillosis in beef cattle. *Am. J. Vet. Res.* 15:5–14.

58. **Kanoe, M., T. Ishii, K. Mizutani, and H. Blobel.** 1986. Partial characterisation of leukocidin from *Fusobacterium necrophorum*. *Zentralbl. Bakteriol. Mikrobiol. Hyg. Ser. A* 261:170–176.

59. **Kanoe, M., and K. Iwaka.** 1986. Adherence of *Fusobacterium necrophorum* to bovine hepatic cells. *FEMS Microbiol. Lett.* 35:245–248.

60. **Kanoe, M., Y. Izuchi, and M. Toda.** 1978. Isolation of *Fusobacterium necrophorum* from bovine ruminal lesions. *Jpn. J. Vet. Sci.* 40:275–281.

61. **Kanoe, M., S. Nagai, and M. Toda.** 1985. Adherence of *Fusobacterium necrophorum* to Vero cells. *Zentralbl. Bakteriol. Mikrobiol. Hyg. Ser. A* 260:100–107.

62. **Kasper, D. L.** 1986. Bacterial capsule—old dogmas and new tricks. *J. Infect. Dis.* 153:407–415.

63. **Kaufman, E. J., P. A. Mashimo, E. Hausmann, C. T. Hanks, and S. A. Ellison.** 1972. Fusobacterial infection: enhancement by cell free extracts of *Bacteroides melaninogenicus* possessing collagenolytic activity. *Arch. Oral Biol.* 17:577–580.

64. **Kortt, A. A., J. E. Burns, and D. J. Stewart.** 1983. Detection of the extracellular proteases of *Bacteroides nodosus* in polyacrylamide gels: rapid method of distinguishing virulent and benign ovine isolates. *Res. Vet. Sci.* 35:171–174.

65. **Kortt, A. A., I. J. O'Donnell, D. J. Stewart, and B. L. Clark.** 1982. Activities and partial purification of extracellular proteases of *Bacteroides nodosus* from virulent and benign footrot. *Aust. J. Biol. Sci.* 35:481–489.

66. **Langworth, B. F.** 1977. *Fusobacterium necrophorum:* its characteristics and role as an animal pathogen. *Bacteriol. Rev.* 41:373–390.

67. **Malecki, J. C., and L. Coffey.** 1986. Effectiveness of treatment programs based on footbathing with zinc sulphate formulation for virulent *Bacteroides nodosus* infections in sheep, p. 51–55. *In* D. J. Stewart, J. E. Petersen, N. M. McKern, and D. L. Emery (ed.), *Footrot in Ruminants.* Commonwealth Scientific and Industrial Research Organisation Division of Animal Health and Australian Wool Corporation, Glebe, New South Wales, Australia.

68. **McKearn, N. M. I. J. O'Donnell, A. S. Inglis, D. J. Stewart, and B. L. Clark.** 1983. Amino acid sequence of pilin from *Bacteroides nodosus* (strain 198), the causative organism of ovine footrot. *FEBS Lett.* 164:149–153.

69. **McKern, N. M., I. J. O'Donnell, D. J. Stewart, and B. L. Clark.** 1985. Primary structure of pilin protein from *Bacteroides nodosus* (strain 216): comparison with the corresponding protein from strain 198. *J. Gen. Microbiol.* 131:1–6.

70. **Merritt, G. C., and J. R. Egerton.** 1978. IgG_1 and IgG_2 immunoglobulins to *Bacteroides (Fusiformis) nodosus* protease in infected and immunized sheep. *Infect. Immun.* 22:1–4.

71. **Mittall, K. R., and D. G. Ingram.** 1975. Bactericidal and opsonic activities of normal sheep serum against gram-negative bacteria. *Am. J. Vet. Res.* 36:1189–1193.

72. Mukker, T. K. S. 1979. Immunogenicity of a chaotropically extracted protective antigen(s) of *Pasteurella multocida* type A (bovine origin) against experimental pasteurellosis in mice. *J. Gen. Microbiol.* 113:37–43.

73. Nagai, S., M. Kanoe, and M. Toda. 1984. Purification and partial characterization of *Fusobacterium necrophorum* haemagglutinin. *Zentralbl. Bacteriol. Mikrobiol. Hyg. Ser. A* 258:232–241.

74. Nakajima, Y., H. Ueda, Y. Yagi, K. Nakamura, Y. Motoi, and S. Takeuchi. 1986. Hepatic lesions in cattle caused by experimental infection of *Fusobacterium necrophorum. Jpn. J. Vet. Sci.* 48:509–515.

75. Parker, C. F., R. F. Cross, and K. L. Hamilton. 1985. Genetic resistance to footrot in sheep. *Annu. Proc. Sheep Vet. Soc.* 9:16–19.

76. Plant, J. W., and P. D. Claxton. 1986. Efficacy of paring, footbathing and vaccination in the treatment of footrot, p. 57–62. *In* D. J. Stewart, J. E. Peterson, N. M. McKern, and D. L. Emery (ed.), *Footrot in Ruminants.* Commonwealth Scientific and Industrial Research Organisation Division of Animal Health and Australian Wool Corporation, Glebe, New South Wales, Australia.

77. Reed, G. A. 1986. The role of footrot vaccines in Australia, p. 173–176. *In* D. J. Stewart, J. E. Peterson, N. M. McKern, and D. L. Emery (ed.), *Footrot in Ruminants.* Commonwealth Scientific and Industrial Research Organisation Division of Animal Health and Australian Wool Corporation, Glebe, New South Wales, Australia.

78. Roberts, D. S. 1967. The pathogenic synergy of *Fusiformis necrophorus* and *Corynebacterium pyogenes.* 1. Influence of a leucocidal exotoxin of *F. necrophorus. Br. J. Exp. Pathol.* 48:665–673.

79. Roberts, D. S. 1970. Toxic, allergenic and immunogenic factors of *Fusiformis necrophorus. J. Comp. Pathol.* 80:247 257.

80. Roberts, D. S., and J. R. Egerton. 1969. The aetiology and pathogensis of ovine footrot. *J. Comp. Pathol.* 79:217–227.

81. Scanlan, C. M., J. N. Berg, and F. F. Campbell. 1986. Biochemical characterization of the leukotoxins of three bovine strains of *Fusobacterium necrophorum. Am. J. Vet. Res.* 47:1422–1425.

82. Scanlan, C. M., and T. L. Hathcock. 1983. Bovine rumenitis— liver abscess complex: a bacteriological review. *Cornell Vet.* 73:288–297.

83. Shinjo, T., and H. Kiyoyama. 1986. Pathogenicity of a non-haemagglutinating mutant strain of *Fusobacterium necrophorum* biovar A in mice. *Jpn. J. Vet. Sci.* 48:523–527.

84. Skerman, T. M. 1986. Genetic variation and inheritance of susceptibility to footrot in sheep, p. 73–75. *In* D. J. Stewart, J. E. Petersen, N. M. McKern, and D. L. Emery (ed.), *Footrot in Ruminants.* Commonwealth Scientific and Industrial Research Organisation Division of Animal Health and Australian Wool Corporation, Glebe, New South Wales, Australia.

85. Skerman, T. M., S. K. Erasmuson, and D. Every. 1981. Differentiation of *Bacteroides nodosus* biotypes and colony variants in relation to their virulence and immunoprotective properties in sheep. *Infect. Immun.* 32:788–795.

86. Slee, K. J. 1985. A microaerophilic coccus in pyogenic infections of ruminants. *Aust. Vet. J.* 62:57–59.

87. Smith, G. R., J. C. Oliphant, and R. Parsons. 1984. The pathogenic properties of *Fusobacterium* and *Bacteroides* species from wallabies and other sources. *J. Hyg.* 92:165–175.

88. Sparling, P. F. 1983. Bacterial virulence and pathogenesis: an overview. *Rev. Infect. Dis.* 5(Suppl. 4):S637–S646.

89. Stewart, D. J. 1977. Biochemical and biological studies on lipopolysaccharide of *Bacteroides nodosus. Res. Vet. Sci.* 23:319–325.

90. Stewart, D. J. 1978. The role of various antigenic fractions of *Bacteroides nodosus* in eliciting protection against footrot in vaccinated sheep. *Res. Vet. Sci.* 24:14–19.

91. Stewart, D. J. 1979. The role of elastase in the differentiation of *Bacteroides nodosus* infections in sheep and cattle. *Res. Vet. Sci.* 27:99–105.

92. Stewart, D. J., B. L. Clark, D. L. Emery, J. E. Peterson, and K. J. Fahey. 1983. A *Bacteroides nodosus* immunogen, distinct from the pilus, which induces cross-protective immunity in sheep vaccinated against footrot. *Aust. Vet. J.* 60:83–85.

93. Stewart, D. J., B. L. Clark, D. L. Emery, J. E. Peterson, and A. A. Kortt. 1986. The phenomenon of cross protection against footrot induced by vaccination of sheep with *Bacteroides nodosus* vaccine, p. 185–192. *In* D. J. Stewart, J. E. Peterson, N. M. McKern and D. L. Emery (ed.), *Footrot in Ruminants.* Commonwealth Scientific and Industrial Research Organisation Division of Animal Health and Australian Wool Corporation, Glebe, New South Wales, Australia.

94. Stewart, D. J., B. L. Clark, J. E. Petersen, D. A. Griffiths, and E. F. Smith. 1982. Importance of pilus-associated antigen in *Bacteroides nodosus* vaccines. *Res. Vet. Sci.* 32:140–147.

95. Stewart, D. J., and T. C. Elleman. 1987. A *Bacteroides nodosus* pili vaccine produced by recombinant DNA for the prevention and treatment of foot-rot in sheep. *Aust. Vet. J.* 64:79–81.

96. Stewart, D. J., J. E. Peterson, N. M. McKern, and D. L. Emery (ed.). 1986. *Footrot in Ruminants.* Commonwealth Scientific and Industrial Research Organisation Division of Animal Health and Australian Wool Corporation, Glebe, New South Wales, Australia.

97. Stewart, D. J., J. E. Peterson, J. A. Vaughan, B. L. Clark, D. L. Emery, J. B. Caldwell, and A. A. Kortt. 1986. Clinical and laboratory diagnosis of benign, intermediate and virulent strains of *Bacteroides nodosus*, p. 81–91. *In* D. J. Stewart, J. E. Peterson, N. M. McKern, and D. L. Emery (ed.), *Footrot in Ruminants*. Commonwealth Scientific and Industrial Research Organisation Division of Animal Health and Australian Wool Corporation, Glebe, New South Wales, Australia.

98. Sweeney, C. R., T. J. Divers, and C. E. Benson. 1985. Anaerobic bacteria in 21 horses with pleuropneumonia. *J. Am. Vet. Med. Assoc.* 187:721–724.

99. Thorley, C. M., and J. R. Egerton. 1981. Comparison of alum-absorbed and non-alum absorbed oil emulsion vaccines containing either pilate or nonpilated *Bacteroides nodosus* cells in inducing and maintaining resistance of sheep to experimental footrot. *Res. Vet. Sci.* 30:32–37.

100. Warner, J. F., W. H. Fales, R. C. Sutherland, and G. W. Teresa. 1975. Endotoxin from *Fusobacterium necrophorum* of bovine hepatic abscess origin. *Am. J. Vet. Res.* 36:1015–1019.

101. West, D. M. 1983. Observations on an outbreak of foot abscess in sheep. *N.Z. Vet. J.* 31:71–74.

Section VI: Past, Present, and Future Studies

Chapter 22

The State and Future of Studies
on Bacterial Pathogenicity

H. SMITH

Department of Microbiology
University of Birmingham
Birmingham B15 2TT
United Kingdom

INTRODUCTION

The present state of studies of bacterial pathogenicity may be described under the following headings: (i) establish a method for comparing the virulence of strains in either the natural host or a relevant animal model; (ii) obtain strains of high and low virulence; (iii) compare strains of differing virulence in biological tests related to pathogenicity; (iv) identify the determinant that causes the chosen biological property; (v) prove relevance of the biological property and its determinant to infection in vivo; and (vi) relate the chemical structure of the virulence determinant to the mechanisms of its biological action. Also, a section on the impact of genetic manipulation on proof of causation and of relevance in vivo is included.

One challenge for the future is to take more and more virulence determinants up this progressive research ladder. The other is to attend to neglected areas, such as the determinants of countering commensal protection of mucous surfaces; the factors which turn some mucosal commensals into pathogens; the relation of bacterial nutrition and metabolism to growth in vivo; latent and carrier states; the determi-

nants of immunopathological damage; the bases for host and tissue specificities; and the microbial interactions of mixed infections.

My brief was to summarize the symposium contributions, to describe the state of knowledge on bacterial pathogenicity, and to point out unanswered questions for future research. I shall combine the first two parts by using the papers in this volume as some examples in a description of the present state of studies on bacterial pathogenicity. Then I shall go on to discuss the challenge for the future.

STEPS IN STUDYING BACTERIAL PATHOGENICITY

Recognizing that pathogenicity is a multifactorial property (39, 68, 70, 73) requiring for any bacterial species the action in vivo of a number of determinants, the goal of our studies is to recognize each determinant of pathogenicity, to identify it, and to relate its chemical structure to biological action. The logical steps to achieve this goal for each determinant are summarized above. All these steps have been achieved only for a few bacterial toxins. The difficulties involved in each step and the extent of fulfilment are discussed below, and a section on genetic manipulation is included because of its special contribution to proof of causation and of relevance in vivo. To illustrate the principles, I use examples from the five cardinal requirements of pathogenicity: infection of mucous surfaces; entry to the host tissues through these surfaces; multiplication in the environment in vivo; interference with host defense mechanisms; and damage to the host. All these aspects are covered in this volume, although in various degrees of detail.

Establish a Method for Comparing the Virulence of Strains in either the Natural Host or a Relevant Animal Model

The procedure for comparing virulence of strains is simple. By inoculating animals with graded doses of the different strains, the numbers of each strain which produce a standard disease effect are obtained. Statistical methods for providing quantitative assessments of virulence are also well established. The snags are often the inability to use the natural host and the questionable validity of the animal model, not only in relation to species differences in disease syndromes but also in relation to unnatural routes of inoculation. It is not surprising that the major advances in knowledge of bacterial and viral diarrheas have come first from studies of veterinary diseases in which both the host and route of infection can be natural. Isaacson (Chapter 2 of this volume) refers to this point in studies of adherence by *Escherichia coli*. Even with veterinary diseases, however, financial considerations sometimes dictate the use of animal models, which is mostly mandatory for human disease; however, comparison of strain virulence for some less-dangerous human pathogens, e.g., enterobacterial vaccine strains, has been done with volunteers. No animal model can substitute entirely for the natural disease. Some models, such as infection of guinea pigs by using aerosols containing *Legionella pneumophila,* oral infection of primates with shigellae, and gut infection of young rab-

bits or mice with *Vibrio cholerae,* are clearly better than injecting mice with these or other bacteria. However, the latter procedure sometimes continues because of convenience, habit, and sometimes unexplained parallelism with field results. The current situation on acquired immune deficiency syndrome research epitomizes the persistent and often unavoidable constraint put on studies of pathogenicity by lack of relevant models.

Obtain Strains of High and Low Virulence

Comparisons between strains of high and low virulence are more discerning than experiments with single strains for probing the multifactorial nature of pathogenicity. Early on, strains of differing virulence were obtained by surveying naturally occurring strains, by lowering the virulence of fresh isolates through passage in vitro, by raising the virulence of laboratory strains through animal passage, and by induced mutation using colony form or nutritional deficiencies to select the mutants (4, 16). Sometimes colony form was correlated with differences in virulence, e.g., smooth and rough forms of enterobacteria and pneumococci. The presence or absence of particular virulence attributes in available strains was largely a matter of chance; e.g., the avirulent Sterne strain of *Bacillus anthracis* lacked a capsule but produced the toxin, whereas the avirulent HM strain had a capsule but did not form toxin (62).

In the late 1960s, plasmid-mediated transfer of virulence attributes was demonstrated by Smith and Linggood (74) for mucosal adherence and toxin production in *E. coli* infections of piglets. The successful use of plasmids for preparing strains of various degrees of virulence was then compounded by recombinant DNA technology and sophisticated methods of mutation. Now, virulent strains can be produced from avirulent strains at will and vice versa, and often the changes can be related to the presence or absence of specific virulence attributes. The full impact of modern genetic manipulation on the production of differing strains is described by Curtiss et al. (Chapter 19 of this volume) and in a later section of this paper.

Compare Strains of Differing Virulence in Biological Tests Related to Pathogenicity

The aim is to demonstrate for a virulent strain a pertinent biological action which is absent or much reduced in an avirulent strain, thus providing a basis for subsequent identification of the determinant concerned. The biological tests should be related to mucosal infection, mucosal invasion, growth in vivo, interference in host defense, or host damage. More importantly, they must be relevant to the pattern of infection caused in vivo by the pathogen under consideration. The first requirement is discussed here, and the second is discussed below.

Up to the 1950s, only resistance to serum killing, interference with phagocytosis, and toxicity in animals had received much attention (16). Now, many biological tests span all facets of pathogenicity with various degrees of validity. Many of them owe much to the development of tissue and organ culture techniques in virology. Tests bearing on mucosal adherence of bacteria involve, with decreasing validity, the use of whole animals, organ cultures of mucosal pieces, fresh suspensions of primary epithelial cells scraped or otherwise removed from mucosal surfaces, and tissue culture cells. Little attention is given to adherence to glycocalices which can overlay mucosal cells, except in histological examination of sections from whole-animal infection, for which the glycocalyx can be stabilized by treatment with antibody (25, 51; Chapters 1, 2, and 3 of this volume). Investigations aimed at explaining the invasion of mucous surfaces have, for convenience, concentrated on the entry into epithelial cell lines or HeLa cells in tissue culture, with penetration of guinea pig conjunctivae (the Sereny test) and the mucosal cells of organ cultures or intestinal loops as more valid tests (24, 53, 80; Chapter 4 of this volume).

Factors affecting growth in vivo can be in-dicated by studying growth rates and yields of virulent and avirulent strains in body fluids, in tissue extracts, and in culture media with and without nutrients (e.g., iron and erythritol) which may limit or stimulate growth in vivo (56, 64). Turning to inhibition of host defense, all the following aspects have been probed by numerous biological tests: inhibition of humoral bactericidins (20, 42, 70; Chapter 6 of this volume); interference with chemotaxis, opsonization, ingestion, and intracellular killing in phagocytosis experiments (20, 42, 70; Chapters 9, 10, and 11 of this volume); prevention of complement activation or action (20, 42, 68, 70; Chapter 7 of this volume); and suppression of or interference with the immune response (20, 42, 70; Chapter 6 of this volume). Toxins are still detected by tissue damage in skin tests, fluid loss from the gut, and lethality, but there is increasing use of tissue culture cells to monitor specific effects (70, 79; Chapters 14 and 15 of this volume). As regards immunopathological damage, it is possible to detect immediate- and delayed-type hypersensitivity, cytotoxic reactions, and Arthus-type reactions by a variety of immunological tests (28, 43).

In summary, there is no difficulty in finding biological tests related to pathogenicity; the question is whether they are relevant to the specific infection in vivo (see below).

Identify the Determinant that Causes the Chosen Biological Property

The classical chemical approach to identification of the virulence determinant is discussed here; genetic manipulation is considered below.

The bacterial toxins have been relatively easy to handle, since most of them are excreted and act extracellularly. Once toxic activity has been demonstrated in culture filtrates by an appropriate biological test, purification can follow by using the biological activity for assaying fractions until the toxin is shown to be pure by the usual biochemical criteria. Proof of causation is provided throughout the process by the biological assay, and it can be reinforced by neutralization of the toxic activity with specific antisera. This was done for the classical toxins (diphtheria, tetanus, and botulinum toxins) before sophisticated biochemical methods for separating large molecules were available (84). These biochemical methods have revolutionized toxinology in the past 20 years, so that purification, identification, and proof of causation are commonplace for toxins, as contributors to this book have made clear (Chapters 13, 14, 15, and 16 of this volume).

If the putative virulence determinant is a surface component, identification is more difficult and proof of causation is even more so. The first step in identification is to demonstrate an association between a surface component and biological activity by examining more- and less-active strains for differences in capsulation, pilation, outer membrane proteins, lipopolysaccharide (LPS) components, lipids, teichoic acids, peptidoglycan composition, or any other cell wall constituents. A combination of morphological and chemical methods can be used with sodium dodecyl sulfate-polyacrylamide gel electrophoresis as a powerful tool. Removal or destruction of selected components by chemicals (e.g., periodate) or enzymes (e.g., neuraminidase, hyaluronidase, and proteases) can also be related to biological activity. Such experiments were used early in studies of pathogenicity to associate capsular and surface components of various pathogens with resistance to phagocytosis, e.g., the capsular polysaccharides of pneumococci, the hyaluronic acid capsule and M protein of *Streptococcus pyogenes,* the VI antigen of *Salmonella typhi,* and envelope fraction I of *Yersinia pestis* (16, 92). They are now perhaps the most prevalent experiments in the subject, associating many bacterial components with various mucosal interactions and with resistance to all aspects of host defense (17, 43, 65; Chapters 4 and 5 of this volume). One point should be stressed at this juncture: demonstration of association is not proof of causation (for discussion of this point, see references 67 and 76). Sometimes this is forgotten.

The surface component that has been associated with biological activity must now be removed from the bacteria, purified, and examined chemically. Removal from the bacterial surface does not present much difficulty, because simple washing or use of detergents and other agents is quite effective. Some difficulty can be encountered in liberating individual components from outer membrane or cell wall complexes, but methods are available (32). Once the components have been liberated, biochemical purification is fairly easy with the versatility of the present methods for separating large molecules.

Proving that an isolated putative determinant causes the particular biological effect when it is present in situ on the bacterial surface is not easy (67). Often the biological activity, e.g., inhibition of phagocytosis, may be demonstrated by conducting the appropriate test with an otherwise inactive avirulent strain in a medium containing the putative determinant. Sometimes such tests are used as biological assays for the putative determinant during its removal from the surface and subsequent purification. In these tests, however, the putative determinant may act extracellularly and not at the bacterial surface, e.g., neutralization of opsonins by pneumococcal polysaccharides (49). Ideally, if genetic manipulation (see below) is excluded, the purified determinant should be either attached to the surface of an avirulent strain that lacks it or reattached to the surface of the virulent strain from which it had been removed, thereby conferring the particular biological activity. Hence, the bacteria must be pretreated with the putative determinant and the subsequent procedure must be conducted after removing free determinant and washing. Any biological activity demonstrated will then be due to the surface-attached determinant. Such attachment can be checked by gold labeling and electron microscopy or fluorescent-antibody testing. Unfortunately, this goal is not usually achieved, because reattachment to the surface does not occur in the pretreatment. For example, a surface antigen of virulent *Brucella abortus* strongly associated with resistance to intracellular killing by bovine phagocytes was not able to confer such resistance on an attenuated susceptible strain (26), and noninvasive shigellae could not be rendered invasive by treatment with proteins b and c, which are coded for by the *Shigella* invasion plasmid and may be the determinants concerned (Chapter 4 of this volume; T. L. Hale, personal communication). Occasional successes have occurred when the test bacteria were closely related to the source of the putative determinant. A complete LPS (i.e., with a full polysaccharide side chain), extracted from a serum-resistant *E. coli* strain, attached to the surface and conferred serum resistance onto otherwise sensitive, LPS-deficient organisms harvested from early exponential growth; and LPS from three different virulent enterobacteria did not confer resistance (1). More recently, a 20-kilodalton (kDa) lipoprotein, strongly associated with the resistance to human phagocyte-mediated intracellular killing of an in vivo selected strain of *Neisseria gonorrhoeae,* conferred resistance on a closely related susceptible strain, in contrast to purified pili, which had not been associated with such resistance (44).

The main method of strengthening the evidence for causation is to neutralize the biological activity of intact virulent organisms by specific antibody raised against the purified putative determinant. This method was used early in studies of pathogenicity to show that many capsular materials were determinants of bacterial resistance to phagocytosis (16, 49, 92). It is now used for all aspects of pathogenicity, e.g., in indicating lipoteichoic acid and pili, respectively, as the determinants of streptococcal and *E. coli* K99 adhesion to mucous surfaces (3; Chapter 2 of this volume) and a 20-kDa lipoprotein as a determinant of gonococcal resistance to intracellular killing (44). Antibody specificity is crucial. Monoclonal antibodies could be a boon in this respect, but although they have been used extensively in identifying bacterial surface components, their use in proving causation of biological effect is still limited (77). Examples are as follows: a reduction of resistance of K1 strains of *E. coli* to ingestion

by phagocytes by treatment with monoclonal antibodies against the LPS (34); and blockage of attachment of *Mycoplasma pneumoniae* to chicken erythrocytes by monoclonal antibodies against mycoplasmal proteins, not those against lipids (40). Sometimes monoclonal antibodies may fail to neutralize the biological activity because they are directed against the wrong epitopes.

Loss of a bacterial surface component may contribute to virulence, bringing specific difficulties to the proof of causation. Gonococci grown in vivo are resistant to killing by fresh human serum, but this resistance is lost phenotypically on subculture in vitro. It is restored by incubating a host-derived, small molecular factor present in genital secretions, serum, and extracts of erythrocytes, and its restoration is associated with loss of high-M_r components of the LPS which, in serum-susceptible gonococci, may be the targets for bactericidal immunoglobulin M in fresh human serum (45, 81). Evidence for causation would be provided by showing that the LPS components present in susceptible gonococci but not resistant gonococci neutralize the bactericidal activity of fresh human serum and that LPS components of resistant organisms lack neutralizing activity.

Prove Relevance of the Biological Property and Its Determinant to Infection In Vivo

Four aspects of proving the relevance of the biological property to infection in vivo are discussed below. In all of them we should be aware of the difference between relevance to infection in vivo in an animal model and that in the natural host. Proof of both is possible for veterinary diseases, but for human diseases we often only get as far as the first. Results from animal models are indications, not solid evidence, of relevance to infection in humans unless they are supported by direct observations. These observations are limited to the use of body fluids and cells for tests in vitro, to occasional volunteer studies, and to active or passive protective measures based on knowledge derived from animal models.

Base biological tests on in vivo observations. Before the quest for the determinant begins, the scene on relevance should be set by properly choosing the biological test which is to form the basis of the search. It should be related to an aspect of the disease process which has been either directly observed or unequivocally described in the literature. Light and electron microscopy of early interactions of pathogens with mucous surfaces, including an overlying glyocalyx if it is present, should indicate which biological tests for adherence and penetration might be valid and which might not (25). Comparison of the rate of increase in population in vivo with that in laboratory media might indicate whether bacterial nutrients are scarce or abundant. Localized growth in particular tissues might reflect the distribution of preferred nutrients. Turning to methods of interference with host defenses, relevant tests can be indicated by histological observations of the early stages of infection in subcutaneous tissue, in the peritoneal cavity, on mucous surfaces, or in tissue chambers. Are large numbers of virulent bacteria seen extracellularly compared with avirulent strains, indicating resistance to both humoral bactericidins and ingestion by phagocytes; are virulent strains seen intact within phagocytes, suggesting resistance to intracellular killing; are phagocytes scarce in the lesions, indicating subversion of the inflammatory response; or are phagocytes damaged, indicating possible cytotoxins? As regards tests for toxins, subcutaneous infections may show edema, hemorrhage, or lysis of a particular tissue (e.g., muscle, collagen), indicating what to look for in subsequent injections of culture filtrates. Also, what are the main clinical and pathological effects of infection (e.g., diarrhea, hemorrhage, and neurological disturbances) to be reproduced in tests for toxins?

No one would argue against the logic of making such preliminary observations to prompt the use of relevant biological tests. Sometimes, however, a biological test is chosen for ease of routine operation either without the prelimi-

nary checks or with little reference to them. Lethality for mice after intraperitoneal, intravenous, or intracerebal injections of bacteria which cause enteric or respiratory infections is a good example. The discovery of the cholera toxin by use of rabbit intestinal loops and oral inoculation after much irrelevant injection of bacterial extracts into mice is the warning here. Resistance to complement-mediated serum killing is another frequently used test which may or may not be relevant to the particular infection in vivo. Tests of adherence to, penetration of, and toxicity to various types of tissue culture cells are finding increasing use. Such tests often have the advantages of being quantitative and repeatable, which adds to their attraction. However, their connection with the in vivo situation may be tenuous, e.g., an adherence test with tissue culture cells for a pathogen which sticks to the glycocalyx in vivo. Alternatively, they may reflect only part of the overall infection pattern; e.g., penetration of HeLa cells by shigellae is sufficient to detect the effects of the 120- to 140-kilobase invasion plasmid, but penetration of intact mucosae in rabbit intestinal loops or whole animals requires the expression of chromosomal elements (Chapter 4 of this volume). If such tests are used to speed progress, periodic testing should be done in more complex but relevant systems, e.g., rabbit intestinal loops for enterotoxins (Chapter 15 of this volume).

Show that the putative determinant is present in vivo. Extracellular toxins or their antibodies can be detected in tissue samples and blood by serological methods. Bacterial components can be demonstrated either by fluorescent reactions of monospecific (preferably monoclonal) antibodies with bacteria in tissue sections or by biochemical (e.g., sodium dodecyl sulfate-polyacrylamide gel electrophoresis) and antigenic (Western blotting [immunoblotting]) analysis of bacteria isolated from infected animals (8, 63). In vivo production of surface components can also be demonstrated by detecting their corresponding antibodies, such as those against the invasion proteins of shigellae (Chapter 4 of this volume) and the iron-regulated proteins of *E. coli* (Chapter 8 of this volume).

Demonstrate biological activity in vivo. Direct demonstration of the biological relevance of extracellular toxins is relatively easy. Very early, the toxic effects of injected diphtheria, tetanus, and botulinum toxins were seen to be identical with those of the disease (84) and this has now been demonstrated for many other toxins (79), not the least the various enterotoxins (Chapter 15 of this volume). In many cases, direct demonstration of relevant toxic activity has been backed by passive and active immunoprotection of animals and humans against infections such as tetanus, diphtheria, botulism, various enteric infections, and those caused by *Pasteurella haemolytica* (79; Chapters 13, 14, and 15 of this volume).

Direct demonstration of the biological effects of surface virulence determinants in vivo is well-nigh impossible. Most of these determinants are involved in complex interactions with mucous surfaces and/or host defenses which occur concurrently with other surface interactions between the bacteria and the host. The once much-used aggressin test (promotion by the putative determinant of lethal infection with an otherwise sublethal dose of organisms), shown, for example, by pneumococcal polysaccharides (92), merely testifies to an overall interference with host defense, not inhibition of a particular aspect. Promotion of early infection could be monitored histologically in a local site, but the precise role of the determinant in the complex interactions with the inflammatory responses would not be identified. Evidence for relevance has to come indirectly, namely by passively protecting an animal against infection with the specific antibody to the determinant which neutralizes its particular biological effect. Monoclonal antibodies have an obvious role. Neonatal infection of calves with *E. coli* was prevented by monoclonal antibodies against the K99 adherence antigen (Chapter 18 of this volume). Similarly, monoclonal antibodies against meningococcal capsular material (an inhibitor of serum lysis and of phagocytosis [68]) protected mice against infection (5). Also,

monoclonal antibodies against the capsular polysaccharide of *Haemophilus influenzae*, an inhibitor of complement activation and ingestion by phagocytes, protected infant rats against a lethal infection (30). Also, monoclonal antibodies against LPS protected against several gram negative infections (Chapter 18 of this volume). As mentioned above, more than one aspect of virulence may be neutralized by antibody if the bacterial component concerned is the determinant of several properties. Lack of protection does not necessarily mean that the determinant is irrelevant to infection, because some virulence determinants are either not antigenic or poorly so, e.g., the capsular poly-D-glutamic acid of *B. anthracis* (69).

Search in vivo for unknown virulence attributes. During infection, the growth conditions for bacterial pathogens are complex, constantly changing, and different from those in laboratory cultures. Hence, some virulence determinants may be expressed only under the conditions in vivo and, owing to phenotypic change and the selection of types, bacteria grown in vitro may be deficient in such determinants (8, 62, 63). This premise is merely a promulgation of the cardinal principle of biology, namely that behavior is determined by genes and environment. The importance of this principle in studies of pathogenicity is at last being recognized. When experiments with organisms grown in vitro fail to provide answers to important aspects of pathogenicity, direct examinations of organisms grown in vivo might give clues to further advance. This philosophy was behind the discovery of the anthrax toxin, which solved one of the enigmas of pathogenicity: the cause of death in anthrax. The toxin was found in the blood of guinea pigs dying of the disease (71) and was later produced in vitro (72). Also, the observations of De and Chatterji (12) that *V. cholerae* caused fluid to accumulate in ligated rabbit intestinal loops heralded the recognition of the cholera toxin (22).

Recently, interest in organisms in vivo has increased, the trend being hastened by modern techniques such as sodium dodecyl sulfate-polyacrylamide gel electrophoresis and Western blotting, which allow meaningful examination of unfractionated surface components in the relatively small numbers of bacteria that can be obtained from in vivo sources (8). Examples are as follows. Wild-type *E. coli* and K-12 strains containing the ColV plasmid differed in serum sensitivity and envelope protein profiles when grown in vivo and in vitro (23). *Bacteroides fragilis* had more capsule and more phagocytosis resistance and survived better in chambers implanted intraperitoneally into rabbits when grown in vivo compared with cultures grown in the laboratory (61). In rabbit tissue cages, group B streptococci produced more virulence-determining capsular polysaccharide than in vitro (85). Staphylococci grown in dialysis bags in the peritoneal cavities of sheep were more resistant to phagocytosis and more virulent than those grown in vitro, and they had an extra antigen and a different amino acid composition (87). *Pseudomonas aeruginosa* obtained directly from a cystic fibrosis patient contained three outer membrane proteins not shown by organisms grown in vitro unless grown, as in vivo, under iron-restricted conditions (7). Similarly, urine-derived enterobacteria (*E. coli, Proteus mirabilis,* and *Klebsiella pneumoniae*) showed two or more outer membrane proteins not found in vitro unless grown under iron-restricted conditions (36, 58). Similar results were obtained for *E. coli* and *V. cholerae* obtained directly from infected animals (Chapter 8 of this volume). Gonococci from patients and those grown in subcutaneous chambers in guinea pigs were more resistant to killing by human serum and by human phagocytes than organisms grown in vitro (45). The resistance in vivo to serum killing was phenotypically determined, was lost on subculture in vitro, was restored by incubation with a host product present in urogenital secretions and probably derived from erythrocytes, and was possibly due to the lack of target LPS antigens for bactericidal immunoglobulin M (45, 81). The resistance to intracellular killing by human phagocytes was a selective effect of the in vivo conditions and was determined by a 20-kDa outer membrane lipoprotein (44, 45).

This increasing interest in direct examination of organisms grown in vivo has been accompanied by the realization that chemostat culture might mimic the growth conditions that occur in vivo. In some cases, these conditions appear to be limiting, because bacterial multiplication is slow early in infection (8, 65). The resistance of some gram-positive bacteria to lysozyme and of *P. aeruginosa* to killing by phagocytes was increased by Mg^{2+} limitation, and the toxicity of *E. coli* cell walls was increased by glycerol limitation (18, 21, 46). Production of pili by *E. coli* and the serum resistance of *E. coli, N. gonorrhoeae,* and *Pseudomonas* species are affected by nutrient limitation (9). Bacteria from chemostat culture could be used as a source of virulence determinants, provided that the cultural conditions do reflect, as distinct from might reflect, the environment in vivo. For iron limitation, we can be sure: iron is limited in vivo; iron limitation in chemostat culture induces siderophore formation and new outer membrane proteins; the same outer membrane proteins are present in organisms grown in vivo; and antibodies to the proteins are found in patients (2, 7, 8, 58; Chapter 8 of this volume). The role of each protein either in iron uptake or any other aspect of pathogenicity is not yet fully clarified. This work on iron limitation indicates the potential of first learning more about the nutrients which restrict or promote growth in vivo and then studying their influence on bacterial components and virulence attributes in chemostat culture.

Impact of Genetic Manipulation on Proof of Causation and of Relevance In Vivo

The essence of the genetic approach is either to remove a virulence-related biological property from a positive strain or to confer it on a deficient strain by deletion or transfer of a single gene whose product—the virulence determinant—is known or can be identified (76, 77, 88; Chapter 19 of this volume). Genetic manipulation, particularly induced mutation, has been used in studies of pathogenicity since the

1950s, but the versatility and precision of the method has been increased enormously in the past 10 to 15 years, first by the use of plasmid-encoded determinants and then by recombinant DNA technology. The method has a particular advantage over chemical extraction (see above) for proving causation and relevance for virulence determinants on bacterial surfaces, because they are either formed or not formed on the intact organisms depending on the presence or absence of the gene. The difficulty of reattachment of an isolated determinant is not encountered, and the need for neutralization by antibody is obviated. In the main, genetic manipulation has been used for proving causation and relevance in vivo of putative virulence determinants indicated by other studies, rather than for discovering new determinants, although there are notable exceptions, e.g., the invasion determinants of the shigellae (Chapter 4 of this volume). Below are summarized different aspects of genetic manipulation, their difficulties, and their successes. Details should be sought elsewhere (19, 59, 76, 77, 88; Chapter 19 of this volume).

Use of mutants. Mutants lacking the putative virulence determinant are compared with the wild type in the appropriate biological test and in virulence tests in vivo.

Chemical mutagenesis, e.g., with *N*-methyl-*N'*-nitro-*N*-nitroguanidine, often produces multiple mutations. The mutations should therefore be reintroduced into a nonmutagenized isogenic recipient strain to remove unwanted silent mutations as much as possible before the biological and biochemical changes are studied in relation to the problem in hand. Sometimes this is not possible (77), and even when it is, the mutants must be subjected to critical biochemical and genetic analyses to ensure the absence of more than one mutation. Failure to carry out such analysis complicated attempts to identify the determinants of serum and phagocytosis resistance in *Salmonella typhimurium* (76, 77). Nevertheless, classical mutation has been used to prove causation and relevance in vivo for many putative virulence determinants such as the coagulase of staphy-

lococci and the exotoxin A of *P. aeruginosa* (76, 77). Curtiss et al. (Chapter 19 of this volume) describe other examples for the salmonellae.

Recently, transposon-induced mutagenesis has added a new dimension to studies of pathogenicity. Insertion of transposons (e.g., Tn5 or Tn7) into the DNA of either bacterial chromosomes or plasmids deletes the activity of genes. The transposons are labeled by coding for antibiotic resistance. Hence, although the transposon insertions are at random, the particular gene deleted can be identified by genetic mapping or DNA hybridization techniques or both (89; Chapter 19 of this volume). Thus, specific mutations can be identified and the mutants can be examined biologically and biochemically for the absence of both virulence properties and putative determinants. Sometimes difficulties are encountered in introducing transposons into relevant strains of the pathogen (88). Nevertheless, the technique is finding increasing application and success in studies of pathogenicity. Examples are the demonstration of causation and relevance in vivo for exoenzyme S of *P. aeruginosa* (41) and the hemolysin of *Listeria monocytogenes* (27). Others are the distinguishing of the multiple virulence attributes of *Bordetella pertussis* (88–90) and *Yersinia* species (47, 48). Still another is the attenuation of *Salmonella* species for possible oral vaccination by deletion of genes coding for specific virulence factors (Chapter 19 of this volume).

Even more recently, site-directed mutagenesis (52) has been used to obtain nontoxigenic mutants of *V. cholerae* for vaccines (33). The gene of interest in a known gene sequence of a cloned DNA fragment (see below) from the bacterium under examination is either mutagenized by transposon insertion (52) or replaced by another gene by using restriction enzymes and ligases (33). Then, by recombination between the host organism for this cloning and the wild type pathogen under examination, the gene sequences of the latter containing the gene of interest are replaced by the mutant sequences from which this gene has been removed. The method is complex but very specific. It could be useful in studies of pathogenicity in which the putative virulence gene has been located.

Use of plasmid-encoded determinants. Plasmid transfer between positive and negative strains, together with analysis of the plasmid gene products, was a major factor in proving that adherence antigens, the heat-labile and heat-stable enterotoxins, and the hemolysin were virulence determinants of *E. coli,* active in vivo (15, 19, 74, 77). It has also contributed substantially to knowledge of mucosal invasion by shigellae (24, 53; Chapter 4 of this volume), and there are many other examples (Chapters 2, 8, and 14 of this volume). Nevertheless, like mutagenesis, plasmid transfer must be analyzed critically both genetically and biochemically to provide solid evidence of causation and relevance. Plasmids contain a few to several hundred kilobases and thus can code for many polypeptides. The multiple products and biological properties encoded by plasmids are exemplified by the enterotoxin, the colonization antigen, and the RG5 and ColV plasmids of *E. coli.* The latter, for example, codes for colicin V production, serum resistance, and ion-sequestering mechanisms (19, 55). Hence, as for chromosomal DNA (see below), the DNA of complex plasmids must be critically examined and cloned to identify the single gene responsible for the chosen product and biological activity. This has been accomplished in some cases. The K88 adherence antigen gene was cloned into a recombinant plasmid from the relatively small but still complex K88 plasmid. When the recipient *E. coli* strain was inoculated orally into piglets, it colonized the bowels with the bacteria close to the epithelial surface and evoked K88 antibody (15). Similarly, the structural genes have been identified for the K99 adherence antigen (Chapter 2 of this volume) and a hemolysin (Chapter 14 of this volume) of *E. coli,* both on complex plasmids. On the other hand, dissection of the large, 140-MDa plasmid, associated with the ability of shigellae to invade epithelial cells (53), to identify the product(s) responsible for invasive ability has proved difficult because of the large

number of other genes present and their products (29, 38, 54, 86). At last, however, it appears that proteins b (57 kDa) and c (43 kDa), products of the 22-MDa fragment of the large plasmid, may be the determinants of cell invasion (Chapter 4 of this volume). These examples illustrate the range of difficulty in analyzing plasmids and their products to prove causation and relevance.

Use of gene cloning. The method for use of gene cloning is summarized here; details are given elsewhere (88; Chapter 19 of this volume). There are many cloning strategies, mostly invoking *E. coli.* For example, in cosmid cloning (10) the total DNA of the chosen pathogen is split into fragments by ultrasonic waves or restriction endonucleases or both and the fragments are packaged into plasmids containing the *cos* gene of lambda bacteriophage within the phage heads. The phage is then used to transduce the *E. coli* so that it contains the DNA fragments as part of a recombinant plasmid. A genetic library of the total DNA is thus constructed within several hundred *E. coli* colonies. The colony with the required DNA segment is identified by culturing the colonies and examining their products either biologically (e.g., toxic activity) or, more usually, chemically (e.g., in sodium dodecyl sulfate-polyacrylamide gel electrophoresis). Next, the DNA piece in the plasmid is reduced to the smallest DNA unit (optimally a single gene) encoding the putative determinant by paring down with restriction endonucleases and sequential subcloning via the vector. Provided that expression of the cloned gene can be enhanced, the resultant *E. coli* K-12 can be used to demonstrate directly the biological activity of the putative determinant and also to produce it. This aspect has been particularly helpful in producing relevant surface components of bacteria that cannot be grown in vitro, such as *Mycobacterium leprae* and *Treponema pallidum,* by cloning DNA from organisms obtained from animals (83). More importantly, the cloned gene can then be reintroduced into deficient strains of the original pathogen, thereby conferring the biological property and virulence in vivo. Also, since its position and properties are known, the gene can be deleted specifically by transposon-induced or site-directed mutagenesis (see above) from either *E. coli* K-12 or the pathogen with consequent loss of biological effect and virulence in vivo.

The success of this method depends on accurate transcription and translation and adequate expression of the vector-cloned DNA insert within the host cell and on effective transfer of the cloned gene from the host cell to the appropriate pathogen. Problems were not evident when *E. coli* K-12 was the host cell and the putative virulence determinants of pathogenic *E. coli* were being studied. Indeed, gene cloning first showed its strength by adding weight to the evidence that the adherence antigens, the heat-labile and heat-stable enterotoxins, and the hemolysins of *E. coli* are virulence determinants relevant in vivo (15, 19, 59, 91; Chapter 2 of this volume). However, problems have been encountered with pathogens other than *E. coli,* for example, for the multiple virulence factors of *B. pertussis* and *Yersinia* species, for which transposon-induced mutagenesis has provided the way forward (48, 88, 89). Nevertheless, in many cases the difficulties have been overcome, with consequent benefit to studies on causation and relevance. The cloned gene for the toxin causing toxic shock was introduced into a negative staphylococcal strain, which then formed the toxin in vitro and produced toxic shock effects in rabbits when the staphylococci were grown in an intravaginal chamber; also, specific deletion of the gene removed the ability to produce such effects (13). Also, a gonococcal strain from which the cloned gene from the immunoglobulin A1 protease of gonococci had been specifically deleted colonized fallopian tube epithelium just as well as the protease positive strain did, thus indicating that the protease may not be a significant factor in mucosal colonization (11, 35). Further examples for *Streptococcus equi, Bordetella avium,* and *Haemophilus somnus* are given elsewhere (Chapters 18 and 19 of this volume). For some gram-positive pathogens, e.g., *B. anthracis,* preliminary cloning in *Bacillus subtilis*

may have advantages (31). Gene cloning has proved difficult for capsular carbohydrates and LPSs (77), but progress is being made, for example, with the capsular polysaccharide of K1 *E. coli* (60, 82).

Special problems of gene manipulation. Close linkage of genes may make it difficult to identify the altered gene in mutation studies (77). Also, a virulence property may depend on complex interaction of the multiple products of a gene cluster as for the five genes specifying the aerobactin iron-uptake system (9). Pleiotropy may occur, i.e., when the gene product under examination may not be the virulence determinant, but a mediator of either the formation or the action of the real determinant. Finally, tests in vitro may show that a particular strain has the necessary gene for encoding a putative virulence determinant, but this gene may not be expressed in the environment in vivo.

Relate the Chemical Structure of the Virulence Determinant to the Mechanism of Its Biological Action

Only for the bacterial toxins has the chemical structure of the determinant been related to its mechanism of action to any significant extent. A few bacterial toxins have been investigated at the highest level of molecular biology, entailing intricate protein and enzyme chemistry and membrane interactions. I shall not repeat here, even in summary, the exceptional and erudite work on the classical bacterial toxins which still continues at the level of sequencing, of X-ray analysis of crystals, and of mapping of epitopes by monoclonal antibodies to provide the complete primary and three-dimensional structures of the molecules and pinpoint the sites that determine toxic activity. The work is very well known and is described in detail elsewhere (79; Chapter 13 of this volume). Also, during the past 20 years, these studies on diphtheria, cholera, *E. coli,* tetanus, and botulinum toxins have provided templates for similar work on other toxins (79), including enterotoxins (Chapter 15 of this volume), membrane-damaging toxins (Chapter 16 of this volume), and Shiga and pasteurella toxins (Chapter 14 of this volume).

Studies on structure and function of virulence determinants other than toxins have yet to appear in quantity and at the high level of those on toxins. The structures of some adherence antigens and their variations have been obtained by sequencing and other methods, e.g., the structures of the pili of gonococci (57, 75) and *E. coli* (Chapters 1 and 2 of this volume). Also, the general nature of some host receptors is known, e.g., the mannosides and globotetraosylceramide, respectively, for mannose-susceptible and -resistant pili for *E. coli* (68), and the low-molecular-weight carbohydrate receptor for the adhesion antigen of 987P *E. coli* (Chapter 2 of this volume). Some attention has been given to the molecular interactions of some adhesins with relevant host cells, e.g., the pili of gonococci (57), and to the influence of hydrophobicity and charge on such interactions (Chapter 1 of this volume). Nevertheless, structure and function studies on adhesin-receptor interaction at the detailed chemical level comparable to studies on toxins have not yet been done.

Studies of the determinants of mucosal invasion are not yet at a point at which structure and function can be investigated. As regards multiplication in vivo, the influence of iron-limiting conditions on the growth of *E. coli* has been studied molecularly (Chapter 8 of this volume), but this is the only example.

The chemistry of some determinants of interference with host defense mechanisms is beginning to emerge, especially for LPS and capsular polysaccharides (50). We have considerable knowledge of the mechanisms of certain host defense systems such as the insertion of the C3b-9 bactericidal component of complement into bacterial cell membranes (Chapter 7 of this volume) and the modes of intracellular killing by phagocytes (Chapter 9 of this volume). Also, we have some ideas on how bacterial components can overcome these defense mechanisms (Chapters 5, 6, 7, and 9 of this volume). Furthermore, work with mutants has coupled the

resistance of *E. coli* to phagocytosis with colitose residues in the LPS side chain and that of *S. typhimurium* to phagocytosis with abesquosyl-mannosyl-rhamnosyl-galactose sequences in its LPS (65). Finally, physicochemical investigations of bacterium-phagocyte reactions have begun (78). These are steps in the right direction. We still, however, await deeper studies of the relation of the chemical structure of, say, a capsular polysaccharide with its ability to inhibit the biochemical mechanisms of complement killing or ingestion and destruction by phagocytes.

THE CHALLENGE FOR THE FUTURE

The challenge for the future is twofold. First, more and more virulence attributes related to the five requirements of pathogenicity must be taken up the research ladder, namely, from observation of a relevant biological property through identification of the putative determinant and proof of causation and relevance in vivo to structure and function investigations by the methods outlined in the previous sections. A topic ripe for detailed chemical studies of structure and function is bacterial adherence to mucous membranes, now that the receptors for known adherence antigens are being recognized. At present, invasion of epithelial cells by shigellae, gonococci, and other mucosal invaders is entering the determinant stage, which, with proof of causation and relevance in vivo, should take some time to complete before structure and function studies can begin. The well-defined determinants of interference with host defense are long overdue for studies of structure and function, especially since, as stated above, the chemical composition and action of complement are becoming clearer as are the membrane components, the ingestion processes, and the intracellular killing mechanisms of phagocytes. This also applies to the immunological processes that are sometimes perturbed by bacterial products and components (20, 42). Toxinology is so well established and popular that many more toxins will be taken through to studies of structure and function at the highest levels of molecular biology.

Second, attention must be given to important areas of pathogenicity that are either neglected or inadequately studied. Examples are as follows.

Despite the well-proven, powerful, and to some extent explained protective effect of the prolific normal flora of the lower bowel, the upper respiratory tract, and the female lower urogenital tract (66; Chapters 3 and 18 of this volume), some pathogenic species, e.g., the shigellae, streptococci, and *E. coli,* can, in small numbers, infect these mucous membranes. How do they overcome the protective effect of the commensals? This crucial early stage of mucosal infection is a mystery and should be investigated at the biological and determinant levels as soon as possible. Studies by R. Freter (Chapter 3 of this volume) provide a basis. Research in this area is warranted by the worldwide distress caused by enteritis, respiratory infections, and urogenital infections.

The old problem, commensal-pathogen conversion, should be investigated by all modern techniques in relation to meningococcal outbreaks, nosocomial staphylococcal infections, and mucosal and systemic candidiasis. What microbial and host factors determine the transformation from commensal to pathogenic manifestations? Does the transformation occur in a single individual or is transfer to another host necessary? The major problem is the absence of relevant animal models.

The articles reported in this volume underline the neglect of the influence of bacterial nutrition and metabolism on pathogenicity, i.e., the study of bacterial growth in vivo. Only one paper deals with this topic (Chapter 8 of this volume), compared with massive treatment of the other facets of pathogenicity. This is not the fault of the symposium organizers; there simply is not enough research in this area. Rate of growth is one of the most important factors in pathogenicity, especially in the early stages of infection. If it is fast, the host defenses are less able to cope with the invasion than if it is slow. What nutrients determine the growth rate of particular pathogens in vivo at different stages of infection? How do they affect metabolism? The lack of research in this area is surprising, because for a long time the successful studies on the influence of iron shortage on pathogenicity (Chapter 8 of this volume) have been well recognized, and they show the way forward. Other nutrients which limit bacterial growth in vivo should be recognized, leading to similar molecular investigations on their action. The nutrients that become available in late stages of infection, which may determine the rapid bacterial growth, should also be identified. If their molecular influence on bacterial growth is studied, means other than the use of antibiotics to arrest the overwhelming infection may be indicated. Also, again taking the work on iron and pathogenicity as an example, the influence of either nutrient deficiency or addition (for nutrients that appear later in infection) on production of potential virulence determinants in chemostat culture could be related to the composition of organisms grown in vivo (8). The possibility that preferred nutrients localized in certain tissues may determine tissue specificity should be borne in mind. This possibility was raised by the identification of erythritol as the cause of localization of brucellae in fetal tissues of cattle, sheep, and pigs: tissue extracts were fractionated for a stimulant of *Brucella* growth in vitro followed by promotion of infection in vivo by the isolated erythritol (64). This and similar work on the influence of urea on certain kidney infections (64) opened a channel for studies of pathogenicity that has never been exploited. Again, if nutrients determining tissue localization were identified, their influence on the production of virulence determinants could be studied in chemostat culture. Specific, nutritionally deficient mutants could be used in all aspects of the above investigations. To sum up, one of the most pressing needs for further knowledge of pathogenicity is for experts in microbial metabolism to follow the molecular biologists into the field.

Perturbation of host defense mechanisms by bacteria is receiving adequate attention at the determinant level in all areas except one: the carrier state. Any attention to this problem, i.e., long-term survival of bacteria in vivo despite the presence of immunospecific defenses, has been largely observational and speculative. For example, in a recent article (20) my colleagues and I suggested that immunosuppression, poor antigenicity of virulence determinants, antigenic shift, antibody proteases, and intracellular habitat either in nonprofessional phagocytes such as epithelial cells or in impaired macrophages might be important in bacterial persistence of some carrier states. However, there is neither proof that they are the main factors concerned nor identification of the determinants if they are involved. Carrier and latent states in human and veterinary medicine are perhaps the most serious of current epidemiological problems, since they provide foci for future infection. They should be investigated fully at the determinant level.

Toxins are receiving overwhelming attention. In contrast, the determinants of immunopathological damage are largely neglected. Some studies have taken place, particularly the relation to heart and kidney damage of streptococcal cell wall antigens including the M protein (93). Nevertheless, despite their clinical importance, many cytotoxic, Arthus-type, delayed-type hypersensitivity, and autoimmune reactions found in bacterial infections have not been investigated at the determinant level (43, 93).

Tissue and host specificity of bacterial infections, phenomena of fundamental importance, are not sufficiently studied. Explanations require investigation of variations of the host, not the bacteria. As regards mucosal colonization, the presence in or absence from certain tissues or hosts of the receptors required for adherence antigens (Chapter 2 of this volume) or the presence or absence of enzymes that can destroy adherence or invasion determinants of bacteria (Chapter 4 of this volume) may be a factor. The influence of preferred nutrients in some tissues or hosts has been discussed above.

The presence or absence of nonspecific host defense mechanisms and aspects of the immune response has been given some attention in studies with inbred strains of mice (14, 37), but this attention could be increased.

Finally, mixed infections of viruses and bacteria, of different bacteria, and of bacteria with fungi or protozoa are important clinical problems. These infections have received spasmodic attention over many years and, when investigated at a fundamental level, considerable success has been achieved. Examples are heel abscess in sheep, periodontal disease, and abdominal abscess. In all these cases, knowledge at the determinant level has been obtained from investigations involving the use of either the natural host or animal models (6, 66). These successes should encourage further work. Viral-bacterial interactions are gaining more attention (66), which, it is hoped, will be extended to reactions between other microorganisms.

CONCLUSION

Our subject has made great progress and is in good heart. There is much to do in the future. What more could we wish?

LITERATURE CITED

1. Allen, R. J., and G. K. Scott. 1981. Comparison of the effects of different lipopolysaccharides on the serum bactericidal reactions of two strains of *Escherichia coli*. *Infect. Immun.* 31:831–832.
2. Anwar, H., M. R. W. Brown, A. Day, and P. H. Weller. 1984. Outer membrane antigens of mucoid *Pseudomonas aeruginosa* isolated directly from the sputum of a cystic fibrosis patient. *FEMS Microbiol. Lett.* 24:235–239.
3. Beachey, E. H. 1981. Bacterial adherence: adhesin-receptor interaction mediates the attachment of bacteria to mucosal surfaces. *J. Infect. Dis.* 143:325–345.
4. Braun, W. 1953. *Bacterial Genetics*. The W. B. Saunders Co., Philadelphia.
5. Brodeur, B. R., Y. Larose, P. Tsang, J. Hamel, F. Ashton, and A. Ryan. 1985. Protection against infection with *Neisseria meningitidis* group B serotype 2b by passive immunization with serotype-specific monoclonal antibody. *Infect. Immun.* 50:510–516.
6. Brook, I. 1986. Encapsulated anaerobic bacteria in

synergistic infections. *Microbiol. Rev.* 50:452–457.

7. Brown, M. R. W., H. Anwar, and P. A. Lambert. 1984. Evidence that mucoid Pseudomonas aeruginosa in cystic fibrosis lung grows under iron-restricted conditions. *FEMS Microbiol. Lett.* 21:113–117.

8. Brown, M. R. W., and P. Williams. 1985. The influence of environment on envelope properties affecting survival of bacteria in infection. *Annu. Rev. Microbiol.* 39:527–556.

9. Carbonetti, N. H., and P. H. Williams. 1984. A cluster of five genes specifying the aerobactin iron uptake system of plasmid ColV-K30. *Infect. Immun.* 46:7–12.

10. Collins, J. 1979. *Escherichia coli* plasmids packageable *in vitro* in λ bacteriophage particles. *Methods Enzymol.* 68:309–326.

11. Cooper, M. D., Z. A. McGhee, M. H. Mulks, J. M. Koomey, and T. L. Hindman. 1984. Attachment to and invasion of human fallopian tube mucosa by an IgA1-protease deficient mutant of *Neisseria gonorrhoea* and its wild-type parent. *J. Infect. Dis.* 150:737–744.

12. De, S. N., and D. N. Chatterji. 1953. An experimental study of the mechanism of action of *Vibrio cholerae* on the intestinal mucous membrane. *J. Pathol. Bacteriol.* 66:559–562.

13. de Azavendo, J. C. S., T. J. Foster, P. J. Hartigan, J. P. Arbuthnott, M. O'Reilly, B. N. Kreiswirth, and R. P. Novick. 1985. Expression of the cloned toxic shock syndrome toxin 1 gene (*tst*) in vivo with a rabbit uterine model. *Infect. Immun.* 50:304–309.

14. Dissel, J. T., P. C. J. Leijh, and R. van Furth. 1985. Differences in initial role of intracellular killing of *Salmonella typhimurium* by resistant peritoneal macrophages from various mouse strains. *J. Immunol.* 134:3404–3410.

15. Dougan, G., R. Sellwood, D. Maskill, K. Sweeney, F. Y. Liew, J. Beesley, and C. Hormaeche. 1986. In vivo properties of a cloned K88 adherence antigen determinant. *Infect. Immun.* 52:344–347.

16. Dubos, R. J., and J. C. Hirsch. 1965. *Bacterial and Mycotic Infections of Man*, 4th ed. J. B. Lippincott Co., Philadelphia.

17. Easmon, C. S. F., J. Jeljaszewiez, M. R. W. Brown, and P. A. Lambert. 1983. The role of the envelope in survival of bacteria in infection. *Medical Microbiology*, vol. 3. Academic Press, Inc. (London), Ltd., London.

18. Ellwood, D. C., and D. W. Tempest. 1972. Effects of environment on bacterial wall content and composition. *Adv. Microb. Physiol.* 7:83–117.

19. Elwell, L. P., and P. L. Shipley. 1980. Plasmid-mediated factors associated with virulence of bacteria to animals. *Annu. Rev. Microbiol.* 34:465–496.

20. Falconi, G., M. Campa, H. Smith, and G. M. Scott. 1984. *Bacterial and Viral Inhibition and Modulation of Host Defenses*. Academic Press, Inc. (London), Ltd., London.

21. Finch, J. E., and M. R. W. Brown. 1978. Effect of growth environment on *Pseudomonas aeruginosa* killing by rabbit polymorphonuclear leucocytes and cationic proteins. *Infect. Immun.* 20:340–346.

22. Finkelstein, R. A., and J. J. La Spalluto. 1970. Production, purification and assay of cholera toxin. *J. Infect. Dis.* 121(Suppl.):63–73.

23. Finn, T. M., J. P. Arbuthnott, and G. Dougan. 1982. Properties of *Escherichia coli* grown *in vivo* using a chamber implant system. *J. Gen. Microbiol.* 128:3083–3091.

24. Formal, S. B., T. L. Hale, and E. C. Boedeker. 1983. Interactions of enteric pathogens and the intestinal mucosa. *Philos. Trans. R. Soc. London Ser. B* 303:65–73.

25. Freter, R., and G. W. Jones. 1983. Models for studying the role of bacterial attachment in virulence and pathogenesis. *Rev. Infect. Dis.* 5:S647–S658.

26. Frost, A. J., H. Smith, K. Witt, and J. Keppie. 1972. The chemical basis of the virulence of *Brucella abortus*. X. A surface virulence factor which facilitates intracellular growth of *Brucella abortus* in bovine phagocytes. *Br. J. Exp. Pathol.* 53:587–596.

27. Gaillard, J. L., P. Berche, and P. J. Sansonetti. 1986. Transposon mutagenesis as a tool to study the role of hemolysin in the virulence of *Listeria monocytogenes*. *Infect. Immun.* 52:50–55.

28. Gell, P. G. H., and R. R. A. Coombs. 1968. *Clinical Aspects of Immunology*. Blackwell Scientific Publications, Ltd., Oxford.

29. Hale, T. L., E. V. Oaks, and S. B. Formal. 1985. Identification and antigenic characterization of virulence-associated plasmid-coded proteins of *Shigella* spp. and enteroinvasive *Escherichia coli*. *Infect. Immun.* 50:620–629.

30. Hunter, K. W., Jr., V. G. Hemming, G. W. Fischer, S. R. Wilson, R. J. Hartzmann, and J. N. Woody. 1982. Antibacterial activity of human monoclonal antibody to *Haemophilus influenzae* type B capsular polysaccharide. *Lancet* ii:798–799.

31. Ivins, B. E., and S. L. Welkos. 1986. Cloning and expression of the *Bacillus anthracis* protective gene in *Bacillus subtilis*. *Infect. Immun.* 54:537–542.

32. Johnston, K. H. 1978. Antigenic profile of an outer membrane complex of *Neisseria gonorrhoeae* responsible for serotypic specificity, p. 121–129. *In* G. F. Brooks, E. C. Gotschlich, K. K. Holmes, W. D. Sawyer, and F. E. Young (ed.), *Immunobiology of Neisseria gonorrhoeae*. American Society for Microbiology, Washington, D.C.

33. Kaper, J. B., H. Lockman, M. M. Baldini, and M. M. Levine. 1984. Recombinant nontoxigenic *Vibrio cholerae* strains as attenuated cholera vaccine candidates. *Nature* (London) 308:655–658.

34. Kaufmann, B. M., A. S. Cross, S. L. Futrovsky, H. F. Sidberry, and J. C. Sadoff. 1986. Monoclonal antibodies reactive with K-1 encapsulated *Escherichia coli* lipopolysaccharide are opsonic and protect mice against lethal challenge. *Infect. Immun.* 52:617–619.

35. Koomey, J. M., R. E. Gill, and S. Falkow. 1982. Genetic and biochemical analysis of gonococcal IgA1 protease; cloning in *Escherichia coli* and construction of mutants of gonococci that fail to produce activity. *Proc. Natl. Acad. Sci. USA* 79:7881–7885.

36. Lam, C., F. Turnowksy, E. Schwarzinger, and W. Neruda. 1984. Bacteria recovered without subculture from infected human urines expressed iron regulated outer membrane proteins. *FEMS Microbiol. Lett.* 24:255–259.

37. Lissner, C. R., R. N. Swanson, and A. D. O'Brien. 1983. Genetic control of the innate resistance of mice to *Salmonella typhimurium* expression of the *ity* gene in peritoneal and splenic macrophages isolated in vitro. *J. Immunol.* 131:3006–3013.

38. Maurelli, A. T., B. Baudry, D. d'Hauteville, T. L. Hale, and P. J. Sansonetti. 1985. Cloning of plasmid DNA sequences involved in invasion of HeLa cells by *Shigella flexneri*. *Infect. Immun.* 49:164–171.

39. Mims, C. A. 1982. *The Pathogenesis of Infectious Disease*. Academic Press, Inc. (London), Ltd., London.

40. Morrison-Plummer, J., D. K. Leith, and J. B. Baseman. 1986. Biological effects of anti-lipid and anti-protein monoclonal antibodies on *Mycoplasma pneumoniae*. *Infect. Immun.* 53:398–403.

41. Nicas, T. I., and B. H. Iglewski. 1984. Isolation and characterization of transposon-induced mutants of *Pseudomonas aeruginosa* deficient in production of exoenzyme S. *Infect. Immun.* 45:470–474.

42. O'Grady, F., and H. Smith. 1981. *Microbial Perturbation of Host Defences*. Academic Press, Inc. (London), Ltd., London.

43. Parish, W. E. 1972. Host damage resulting from hypersensitivity to bacteria. *Symp. Soc. Gen. Microbiol.* 22:157–192.

44. Parsons, N. J., A. A. Kwaasi, P. V. Patel, C. A. Nairn, and H. Smith. 1986. A determinant of resistance of *Neisseria gonorrhoeae* to killing by human phagocytes; an outer membrane lipoprotein of about 20 kDa with a high content of glutamic acid. *J. Gen. Microbiol.* 132:3277–3287.

45. Parsons, N. J., P. V. Patel, P. M. V. Martin, M. Goldner, and H. Smith. 1985. Gonococci in vitro and in vivo: studies of the host and bacterial determinants of gonococcal resistance to killing by human serum and by phagocytes, p. 487–494. *In* G. K. Schoolnik, G. F. Brooks, S. Falkow, C. E. Frasch, J. S. Knapp, J. A. McCutchan, and S. A. Morse (ed.), *The Pathogenic Nesseriae*. American Society for Microbiology, Washington, D.C.

46. Pearson, A. D., and D. C. Ellwood. 1974. Growth environment and bacterial toxicity. *J. Med. Microbiol.* 7:391–393.

47. Portnay, D. A., H. F. Blark, D. T. Kingsbury, and S. Falkow. 1983. Genetic analysis of essential plasmid determinants of pathogenicity in *Yersinia pestis*. *J. Infect. Dis.* 148:297–304.

48. Portnay, D. A., and R. J. Martinez. 1985. Role of a plasmid in the pathogenicity of *Yersinia* species. *Curr. Top. Microbiol. Immunol.* 118:29–51.

49. Quie, P. G., G. S. Giebink, and P. K. Peterson. 1981. Bacterial mechanisms for inhibition of ingestion of phagocytic cells, p. 121–142. *In* F. O'Grady and H. Smith (ed.), *Microbial Perturbation of Host Defences*. Academic Press Inc. (London), Ltd., London.

50. Robbins, J. B., R. Schneerson, W. B. Egan, W. Vann, and D. T. Liu. 1980. Virulence properties of bacterial capsular polysaccharides—unanswered questions, p. 115–132. *In* H. Smith, J. J. Skehel, and M. J. Turner (ed.), *The Molecular Basis of Microbial Pathogenicity*. Verlag Chemie, Weinheim, Federal Republic of Germany.

51. Rozee, K. R., D. Cooper, K. Lam, and J. W. Costerton. 1982. Microbial flora of the mouse ileum mucous layer and epithelial surface. *Appl. Environ. Microbiol.* 43:1451–1463.

52. Ruvkun, G. B., and F. M. Ausubel. 1981. A general method for site-directed mutagenesis. *Nature* (London) 289:85–88.

53. Sansonetti, P. J., D. J. Kopecko, and S. B. Formal. 1982. Involvement of a plasmid in the invasive ability of *Shigella flexneri*. *Infect. Immun.* 35:852–860.

54. Sasakawa, C., S. Makino, K. Kamata, and M. Yoshikawa. 1986. Isolation, characterization, and mapping of Tn5 insertions into the 140-megadalton invasion plasmid defective in the mouse Sereny test in *Shigella flexneri* 2a. *Infect. Immun.* 54:32–36.

55. Saunders, J. R. 1981. Plasmids and bacterial pathogens. *Nature* (London) 290:362.

56. Schade, A. L., and L. Caroline. 1946. An iron binding component in human blood plasma. *Science* 104:340–341.

57. Schoolnik, G. K., R. Fernandez, J. Y. Tai, J. B. Rothbard, and E. C. Gotschlich. 1984. Gonococcal pili: primary structure and receptor binding domain. *J. Exp. Med.* 159:1351–1370.

58. Shand, G. H., H. Anwar, J. Kadurugamuna, M. R. W. Brown, S. H. Silverman, and J. Melling. 1985. In vivo evidence that bacteria in urinary tract infection grow under iron-restricted conditions. *Infect. Immun.* 48:35–39.

59. Shipley, P. L., W. S. Dallas, G. Dougan, and S. Falkow. 1979. Expression of plasmid genes in pathogenic bacteria, p. 176–180. *In* D. Schlessinger (ed.), *Microbiology—1979*. American Society for Microbiology, Washington, D.C.

60. Silver, R. P., C. W. Finn, W. F. Vann, W. Aar-

onson, R. Schneerson, P. J. Kretschmer, and C. F. Garon. 1981. Molecular cloning of the KI capsular polysaccharide genes of *E. coli*. *Nature* (London) 289:696–698.

61. Simon, G. L., M. S. Klempner, D. L. Kasper, and S. L. Gorbach. 1982. Alteration in opsonophagocytic killing by neutrophils of *Bacteriodes fragilis* associated with animal and laboratory passage: effect of capsular polysaccharide. *J. Infect. Dis.* 145:72–77.

62. Smith, H. 1958. The use of bacteria grown *in vivo* for studies on the basis of their pathogenicity. *Annu. Rev. Microbiol.* 12:77–102.

63. Smith, H. 1964. Microbial behaviour in natural and artificial environments. *Symp. Soc. Gen. Microbiol.* 14:1–29.

64. Smith, H. 1968. Biochemical challenge of microbial pathogenicity. *Bacteriol. Rev.* 32:164–184.

65. Smith, H. 1977. Microbial surfaces in relation to pathogenicity. *Bacteriol. Rev.* 41:475–500.

66. Smith, H. 1982. The role of microbial interactions in infectious disease. *Philos. Trans. R. Soc. London Ser. B* 297:551–561.

67. Smith, H. 1983. The elusive determinants of bacterial interference with non-specific host defences. *Philos. Trans. R. Soc. London Ser. B* 303:99–113.

68. Smith, H. 1984. The biochemical challenge of microbial pathogenicity. *J. Appl. Bacteriol.* 57:395–404.

69. Smith, H. 1984. Bacterial subversion rather than suppression of immune defences, p. 171–190. *In* G. Falconi, M. Campa, H. Smith, and G. M. Scott (ed.), *Bacterial and Viral Inhibition and Modulation of Host Defences*. Academic Press, Inc. (London), Ltd., London.

70. Smith, H., J. P. Arbuthnott, and C. A. Mims. 1983. *The Determinants of Bacterial and Viral Pathogenicity*. The Royal Society, London.

71. Smith, H., and J. Keppie. 1954. Observations on experimental anthrax: demonstration of a specific lethal factor produced *in vivo* by *Bacillus anthracis*. *Nature* (London) 173:869–870.

72. Smith, H., and H. B. Stoner. 1967. Anthrax toxic complex. *Fed. Proc.* 26:1554–1557.

73. Smith, H., and J. H. Pearce. 1972. *Microbial Pathogenicity in Man and Animals*. Cambridge University Press, Cambridge.

74. Smith, H. W., and M. A. Linggood. 1971. Observations on the pathogenic properties of the K88, HLY and ENT plasmids of *Escherichia coli* with particular reference to porcine diarrhoea. *J. Med. Microbiol.* 4:467–485.

75. So, M., E. Billyard, C. Deal, E. Getzoff, P. Hagblom, T. F. Meyer, E. Segal, and T. Tainer. 1985. Gonococcal pilus: genetics and structure. *Curr. Top. Microbiol. Immunol.* 118:13–28.

76. Sparling, P. F. 1979. Use of microbial genetics in the study of pathogenicity: differentiation between correlation and causation, p. 249–253. *In* D. Schles-

singer (ed.), *Microbiology—1979*. American Society for Microbiology, Washington, D.C.

77. Sparling, P. F. 1983. Applications of genetics to studies of bacterial virulence. *Philos. Trans. R. Soc. London Ser. B* 303:199–207.

78. Stendahl, O. 1983. The physiocochemical basis of surface interaction between bacteria and phagocytic cells, p. 137–153. *In* C. S. F. Easmon, J. Jeljaszewicz, M. R. W. Brown, and P. A. Lambert (ed.), *The Role of the Envelope in the Survival of Bacteria in Infection*. Academic Press, Inc. (London), Ltd., London.

79. Stephen, J., and R. A. Pietrowski. 1986. *Bacterial Toxins*, 2nd ed. Thomas Nelson and Sons, Ltd., Walton-on-Thames, England.

80. Stephens, D. S., L. H. Hoffman, and Z. A. McGee. 1983. Interaction of *Neisseria meningitidis* with human nasopharyngeal mucosa: attachment and entry into columnar epithelial cells. *J. Infect. Dis.* 148:369–377.

81. Tan, E. L., P. V. Patel, N. J. Parsons, P. M. V. Martin, and H. Smith. 1986. Lipopolysaccharide alteration is associated with induced resistance of *Neisseria gonorrhoeae* to killing by human serum. *J. Gen. Microbiol.* 132:1407–1413.

82. Timmis, K. N., G. J. Boulnois, D. Bitter-Suermann, and F. C. Cabello. 1985. Surface components of *Escherichia coli* that mediate resistance to the bactericidal activities of serum and phagocytes. *Curr. Top. Microbiol. Immun.* 118:197–218.

83. van Embden, J. D., H. J. van der Donk, R. V. van Eijk, H. G. van der Heide, J. A. de Jong, M. F. van Olderen, A. D. Osterhaus, and L. M. Schouls. 1983. Molecular cloning and expression of *Treponema pallidum* DNA in *Escherichia coli* K-12. *Infect. Immun.* 42:187–196.

84. van Heyningen, W. E. 1955. The role of toxins in pathology. *Symp. Soc. Gen. Microbiol.* 5:16–39.

85. Wagner, M., S. E. Holm, and B. Wagner. 1982. Growth of group B streptococci and development of surface antigens in tissue cages implanted into rabbits. *Zentralbl. Bakteriol. Hyg. Abt. 1 Orig. Reihe A* 252:287–298.

86. Watanabe, H., and A. Nakamura. 1986. Identification of *Shigella sonnei* form I plasmid genes necessary for cell invasion and their conservation among *Shigella* species and enteroinvasive *Escherichia coli*. *Infect. Immun.* 53:352–358.

87. Watson, D. W. 1983. Models to study antigenic and virulence properties of *Staphylococcus aureus* grown under *in vivo* conditions, p. 85–90. *In* G. Keusch and T. Wadstrom (ed.), *Experimental Bacterial and Parasitic Infections*. Elsevier Biomedical Press, Amsterdam.

88. Weiss, A. A., and S. Falkow. 1983. The use of molecular techniques to study microbial determinants of pathogenicity. *Philos. Trans. R. Soc. London Ser. B* 303:219–225.

89. Weiss, A. A., and E. L. Hewlett. 1986. Virulence

factors of *Bordetella pertussis*. *Annu. Rev. Microbiol.* 40:661–686.

90. Weiss, A. A., E. L. Hewlett, G. A. Myers, and S. Falkow. 1984. Pertussis toxin and extracytoplasmic adenylate cyclase as virulence factors of *Bordetella pertussis. J. Infect. Dis.* 150:219–222.

91. Welch, R. A., E. P. Dellinger, B. Minshew, and S. Falkow. 1981. Haemolysin contributes to virulence of extra-intestinal *E. coli* infections. *Nature* (London) 294:665–667.

92. Wilson, G. S., and A. A. Miles. 1946. *Topley and Wilson's Principles of Bacteriology and Immunity,* 3rd ed. Edward Arnold Ltd., London.

93. Zabriskie, J. B. 1983. Immunopathological mechanisms in bacterial host interactions. *Philos. Trans. R. Soc. London Ser. B* 303:177–187.

INDEX